Handbook of Statistical Methods for Case-Control Studies

Chapman & Hall/CRC
Handbooks of Modern Statistical Methods

Series Editor
Garrett Fitzmaurice, *Department of Biostatistics, Harvard School of Public Health, Boston, MA, U.S.A.*

The objective of the series is to provide high-quality volumes covering the state-of-the-art in the theory and applications of statistical methodology. The books in the series are thoroughly edited and present comprehensive, coherent, and unified summaries of specific methodological topics from statistics. The chapters are written by the leading researchers in the field, and present a good balance of theory and application through a synthesis of the key methodological developments and examples and case studies using real data.

Longitudinal Data Analysis
Edited by Garrett Fitzmaurice, Marie Davidian, Geert Verbeke, and Geert Molenberghs

Handbook of Spatial Statistics
Edited by Alan E. Gelfand, Peter J. Diggle, Montserrat Fuentes, and Peter Guttorp

Handbook of Markov Chain Monte Carlo
Edited by Steve Brooks, Andrew Gelman, Galin L. Jones, and Xiao-Li Meng

Handbook of Survival Analysis
Edited by John P. Klein, Hans C. van Houwelingen, Joseph G. Ibrahim, and Thomas H. Scheike

Handbook of Mixed Membership Models and Their Applications
Edited by Edoardo M. Airoldi, David M. Blei, Elena A. Erosheva, and Stephen E. Fienberg

Handbook of Missing Data Methodology
Edited by Geert Molenberghs, Garrett Fitzmaurice, Michael G. Kenward, Anastasios Tsiatis, and Geert Verbeke

Handbook of Design and Analysis of Experiments
Edited by Angela Dean, Max Morris, John Stufken, and Derek Bingham

Handbook of Cluster Analysis
Edited by Christian Hennig, Marina Meila, Fionn Murtagh, and Roberto Rocci

Handbook of Discrete-Valued Time Series
Edited by Richard A. Davis, Scott H. Holan, Robert Lund, and Nalini Ravishanker

Handbook of Big Data
Edited by Peter Bühlmann, Petros Drineas, Michael Kane, and Mark van der Laan

Handbook of Spatial Epidemiology
Edited by Andrew B. Lawson, Sudipto Banerjee, Robert P. Haining, and María Dolores Ugarte

Handbook of Neuroimaging Data Analysis
Edited by Hernando Ombao, Martin Lindquist, Wesley Thompson, and John Aston

Handbook of Statistical Methods and Analyses in Sports
Edited by Jim Albert, Mark E. Glickman, Tim B. Swartz, Ruud H. Koning

Handbook of Methods for Designing, Monitoring, and Analyzing Dose-Finding Trials
Edited by John O'Quigley, Alexia Iasonos, Björn Bornkamp

Handbook of Quantile Regression
Edited by Roger Koenker, Victor Chernozhukov, Xuming He, and Limin Peng

Handbook of Environmental and Ecological Statistics
Edited by Alan E. Gelfand, Montserrat Fuentes, Jennifer A. Hoeting, Richard L. Smith

For more information about this series, please visit: https://www.crcpress.com/go/handbooks

Handbook of Statistical Methods for Case-Control Studies

Ørnulf Borgan
Norman E. Breslow
Nilanjan Chatterjee
Mitchell H. Gail
Alastair Scott
Christopher J. Wild

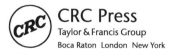

CRC Press
Taylor & Francis Group
Boca Raton London New York

CRC Press is an imprint of the
Taylor & Francis Group, an **informa** business

A CHAPMAN & HALL BOOK

CRC Press
Taylor & Francis Group
6000 Broken Sound Parkway NW, Suite 300
Boca Raton, FL 33487-2742

First issued in paperback 2020

© 2018 by Taylor & Francis Group, LLC
CRC Press is an imprint of Taylor & Francis Group, an Informa business

No claim to original U.S. Government works

Version Date: 20180518

ISBN 13: 978-0-367-57137-5 (pbk)
ISBN 13: 978-1-4987-6858-0 (hbk)

Visit the Taylor & Francis Web site at
http://www.taylorandfrancis.com

and the CRC Press Web site at
http://www.crcpress.com

Contents

Preface

This book grew out of the vision of the late Norman Breslow, the unrivaled giant of case-control studies. Norman instigated the book, helped select the editors, topics, and authors and wrote two chapters before dying during its production. His early work and classic books,[a][b] in 1980 and 1987 with Nick Day, codified methods for case-control studies through careful attention to methodologic detail, cogent examples, and the introduction of modeling approaches, including logistic regression for matched and unmatched designs. These books set the standard as teaching texts and authoritative references on the design and analysis of case-control (and cohort) studies for decades and are still among the most widely used and cited texts on epidemiologic methods.[c]

Nonetheless, there has been a profusion of research clarifying and extending the range of theory and applications of the case-control design in the past 38 years. Norman Breslow contributed importantly to that research. He recognized the need for a new Handbook that could bring readers up to date on theoretical developments while meeting the needs of the practicing epidemiologist by illustrating new methods with practical examples. Even a Handbook of manageable length cannot address all the important work in this period, but Norman Breslow and the other editors have attempted to cover key areas in a way that will allow the reader to understand the major developments and have references to a broader literature.

The book consists of 28 chapters that we have divided into five parts covering distinct areas, but with some overlap. Part I reviews the evolution and history of the case-control design (Chapter 1) and gives a brief synopsis of design options and approaches to analysis (Chapter 2).

Part II describes basic concepts and approaches to analysis in greater detail (Chapter 3) and includes chapters on special designs including matched case-control designs (Chapter 4), designs with multiple case and control types (Chapter 5), and the self-controlled case-crossover design (Chapter 7). These chapters provide numerous examples and stress special strengths, weakness, and approaches to analysis for these designs. Chapter 6 on causal inference for case-control studies defines causal parameters and intervention effects and relates classical analytic procedures and threats to validity to causal graphs and methods. Chapters on analytic methods describe: how to analyze studies with small samples (Chapter 8); sample size calculations for unconditional multivariate logistic models and for studies with other special features, such as many potential exposures or measurement error (Chapter 9); and designs and analytic approaches for handling covariate measurement error (Chapter 10).

The case-control methods discussed in Part II do not assume knowledge of the sampling fractions from a well-defined cohort. In Part III, it is assumed that the case-control study is sub-sampled from a cohort with a well-defined sampling plan or otherwise supplemented

[a]Breslow, N. E. and Day, N. E. (1980). *Statistical Methods in Cancer Research. Volume I - The Analysis of Case-Control Studies.* International Agency for Research on Cancer, Lyon.

[b]Breslow, N. E. and Day, N. E. (1987). *Statistical Methods in Cancer Research, Volume II: The Design and Analysis of Cohort Studies.* International Agency for Research on Cancer, Lyon.

[c]Day, N. E. and Gail, M. H. (2007). Norman Breslow, an architect of modern biostatistics. *Lifetime Data Analysis*, **13**, 435-438.

by whole-cohort information. Chapter 11 describes the added flexibility in risk modeling that is possible for cohort data, and how such models can be estimated from case-control data when sampling fractions are known. Chapter 12 treats the case-control study as the second phase of a two-phase sample from a cohort and presents both likelihood-based and survey-based analytical approaches. Chapter 13 concentrates on survey methods for the two-phase design and shows how survey calibration that uses information from all cohort members increases the efficiency of the case-control analysis. Chapter 14 shows how unbiased estimates of exposure effects on a secondary outcome can be obtained from case-control data for a different primary outcome, provided the primary case-control data are a second-phase sample from a known cohort (see also Chapter 28). These ideas extend to sampling of individuals with longitudinal measurements when the sampling depends in a well-defined manner on the longitudinal outcomes (Chapter 15).

Part IV concerns case-control studies that take place within a well-defined cohort, where the cases are assumed to occur according to a Cox regression model or another hazards regression model for time-to-event data. The two main types of case-control studies for time-to-event data are the nested case-control design and the case-cohort design. Chapter 16 gives an overview of these designs and reviews methods for inference under the Cox proportional hazards model. Chapter 16 also serves as an introduction to the later chapters in Part IV. Chapter 17 considers case-cohort studies, and describes a sample survey approach to analysis of case-cohort data under both the Cox model and an additive hazards model. In particular, it is described how one may use survey calibration on covariates measured on the entire cohort to improve efficiency. Inference for Cox regression for nested case-control data is discussed in Chapter 18. It is shown how a counting process approach provides a framework that allows for a unified treatment of various sampling designs for the controls, including random and counter-matched sampling. Chapter 19 shows how nested case-control data may be considered as case-cohort data with a nonstandard sampling scheme for the sub-cohort. Thereby one may overcome some of the limitations of nested case-controls studies; in particular it becomes possible to reuse the controls for the study of secondary end-points. Chapter 20 treats members of the cohort who are not sampled in phase two of a nested case-control study or case-cohort study as having missing data on the phase-two variables. One can then impute the full cohort data and use multiple imputation for inference with improved efficiency. Chapter 21 describes maximum likelihood estimation, using all available cohort data, for nested case-control and case-cohort samples under semiparametric transformation models that include the Cox model as a special case. The self-controlled case series method is considered in Chapter 22. The method uses only cases to evaluate the association between occurrences of the event of interest and time-varying exposures. The method is related to the case-crossover method discussed in Chapter 7.

Part V describes the use of case-control methods in genetic epidemiology. Chapter 23 provides general overview and principles of case-control studies for conducting modern genome-wide association studies. Chapter 24 describes tests for a gene-environment interaction based on the prospective likelihood for case-control data. The case-only approach has more power but requires that the gene and environmental factors be independent in the source population. A full logistic analysis is also possible from the retrospective likelihood under the independence assumption, but empirical Bayes shrinkage is recommended to guard against violations of the independence assumption. In a genome-wide association study (GWAS), there are hundreds of thousands of genetic variants (single nucleotide polymorphisms or SNPs) to examine (Chapter 25). To avoid loss of power to detect SNP-environment interactions from Bonferroni correction for multiplicity, one can pre-screen the SNPs and then apply the Bonferroni correction only to those SNPs that pass the prescreen, provided the screening statistic is independent of the interaction test statistic (Chapter 25). Family-based case-control designs, such as the case-parents design or the case-sibling design, are robust to confounding from population stratification that can affect population-based case-control studies, but family-based designs have power limitations, and only certain parameters of interest are estimable (Chapter 26). Chapter 27 describes the challenges of using mixed linear models to estimate associations and to develop risk predictors from genome-wide association (case-control) data. Once SNP data have been collected from a GWAS for a particular disease phenotype, it is desirable to determine whether the SNPs are associated with some other phenotype. Methods for such secondary analyses are described in Chapter 28 (see also Chapter 14).

Norman Breslow contributed to and inspired research in many of the areas above. Unfortunately, he died before this project could be completed, as did his friend and co-Editor, Alastair Scott, who was a leader in introducing survey sampling and profile likelihood methods into case-control analysis. It has been an honor for the remaining editors to complete this project, which stands as a reminder of Norman Breslow's vision and contributions to biostatistics and epidemiology.

The editors would like to thank the authors who have used their expertise and valuable time to write all the insightful chapters for the handbook. Without their efforts this book would never have existed. In addition, we thank John Kimmel of CRC Press, who has been our helpful contact with the publisher.

For many of the chapters, the authors have provided data sets, R code, and other supplementary material. This material can be found on a special website for the handbook, which is accessible via the CRC Press website: `https://www.crcpress.com/9781498768580`.

Ørnulf Borgan
Nilanjan Chatterjee
Mitchell H. Gail
Chris J. Wild

About the Editors

Ørnulf Borgan is a Professor in Statistics at the University of Oslo in Norway, and he has a M.Sc. and PhD in statistics from the same university. His main research interest has been statistical methods for survival and event history data, including nested case-control and case-cohort designs. He is co-author on two books on the use of counting processes and martingales in survival and event history analysis, and he has been editor of the Scandinavian Journal of Statistics. Borgan is a Fellow of the American Statistical Association and member of the Norwegian Academy of Science and Letters.

Norman E. Breslow was, at the time of his death, Professor Emeritus in the Department of Biostatistics, University of Washington, Seattle and Member of the Fred Hutchinson Cancer Research Center. He earned his PhD in Statistics from Stanford University. He was a founding member and longtime statistical collaborator for the National Wilms Tumor Study. He made seminal theoretical contributions to survival analysis and epidemiological methods, and his two books on cohort and case-control studies with Nick Day became touchstones for teaching and authoritative guidance for decades. In addition to receiving many awards for scholarship, including the Mortimer Spiegelman Award and R.A. Fisher Award, he was a member of the Institute of Medicine of the National Academy of Sciences and President of the International Biometric Society. Norman Breslow was admired by many friends, colleagues, and trainees, including 13 doctoral students who together would constitute a world class biostatistics department.

Nilanjan Chatterjee is a Bloomberg Distinguished Professor at the Johns Hopkins University with joint appointments in the Departments of Biostatistics and Oncology. During 2008-15, he was the Chief of the Biostatistics Branch of the Division of Cancer Epidemiology and Genetics at the National Cancer Institute. He conducted his PhD dissertation research on two-phase designs during 1996-1999 under the supervision of Dr. Norman Breslow and Dr. Jon Wellner at the University of Washington, Seattle. He leads a broad research program in developing and applying statistical methods for modern large scale biomedical studies, including large scale genetic association studies in case-control settings. He is a Fellow of the American Statistical Association, an elected member of the American Epidemiologic Society, and has received numerous awards, including the notable Committee of the Presidents of Statistical Society (COPSS) award for outstanding contribution by a statistician under the age of 41.

Mitchell H. Gail is a Senior Investigator at the Biostatistics Branch of the Division of Cancer Epidemiology and Genetics, National Cancer Institute (NCI). He earned an M.D. from Harvard Medical School and a PhD in statistics from George Washington University. His work at NCI has included studies on the motility of cells in tissue culture, clinical trials of lung cancer treatments and preventive interventions for gastric cancer, assessment of cancer biomarkers, AIDS epidemiology, and models to project the risk of breast cancer. Dr. Gail's current research interests include statistical methods for the design and analysis of epidemiologic studies and models to predict the absolute risk of disease. He is also working on methods of calibration and seasonal adjustment for multi-center molecular-epidemiologic studies and analytic methods for microbiome studies. Dr. Gail is a Fellow and former President of the American Statistical Association and a member of the National Academy of Medicine of the U.S. National Academy of Sciences.

Alastair Scott was, at the time of his death, Emeritus Professor of Statistics at the University of Auckland in New Zealand where he had a 45-year career. After a M.Sc. from Auckland he earned a PhD in statistics from the University of Chicago. He was one of the major contributors to the field of survey sampling. He worked also in biostatistics, primarily on methods for fitting models to response-selective data (e.g., case-control studies) bringing in his sampling expertise. He was a former President of the New Zealand Statistical Association and a Fellow of the American Statistical Association, the Institute of Mathematical Statistics, and the Royal Society of New Zealand.

Chris J. Wild is a Professor of Statistics at the University of Auckland in New Zealand. After a M.Sc. from Auckland he earned a PhD in statistics from the University of Waterloo in Canada in 1979. His research interests have included nonlinear regression in which he has an often-cited book with G.A.F. Seber and on methods for fitting models to response-selective data (e.g., case-control studies) and data with structured missing data. He is a Fellow of the American Statistical Association and a Fellow of the Royal Society of New Zealand and a former President of the International Association for Statistical Education.

List of Contributors

Editors

Ørnulf Borgan
Department of Mathematics
University of Oslo
Oslo, Norway

Norman E. Breslow
Department of Biostatistics
University of Washington
Seattle, Washington

Nilanjan Chatterjee
Department of Biostatistics
Johns Hopkins University
Baltimore, Maryland

Mitchell H. Gail
Division of Cancer Epidemiology and
   Genetics
National Cancer Institute
Rockville, Maryland

Alastair Scott
Department of Statistics
University of Auckland
Auckland, New Zealand

Chris J. Wild
Department of Statistics
University of Auckland
Auckland, New Zealand

Authors

Gustavo Amorim
Department of Statistics
University of Auckland
Auckland, New Zealand

William E. Barlow
Department of Biostatistics
University of Washington
Seattle, Washington

Raymond J. Carroll
Department of Statistics, Texas A&M
   University, College Station, Texas
and School of Mathematical and
   Physical Sciences, University of
   Technology, Sydney, Australia

John B. Cologne
Department of Statistics
Radiation Effects Research Foundation
Hiroshima, Japan

James Y. Dai
Division of Public Health Sciences
Fred Hutchinson Cancer Research Center
Seattle, Washington

Joseph A. "Chris" Delaney
Department of Epidemiology
University of Washington
Seattle, Washington

Guoqing Diao
Department of Statistics
George Mason University
Fairfax, Virginia

Vanessa Didelez
Leibniz Institute for Prevention Research
    and Epidemiology - BIPS,
and Faculty of Mathematics/Computer
    Science, University of Bremen
Bremen, Germany

Robin J. Evans
Department of Statistics
University of Oxford
Oxford, United Kingdom

Paddy Farrington
School of Mathematics and Statistics
The Open University
Milton Keynes, United Kingdom

David Golan
Faculty of IE&M
Technion - Israel Institute of Technology
Haifa, Israel

Jinko Graham
Department of Statistics and Actuarial
    Science
Simon Fraser University
Burnaby, Canada

Summer S. Han
Quantitative Sciences Unit
Stanford University School of Medicine
Stanford, California

Sebastien Haneuse
Department of Biostatistics, Harvard
    T.H. Chan School of Public Health
Harvard University
Boston, Massachusetts

Patrick J. Heagerty
Department of Biostatistics
University of Washington
Seattle, Washington

Li Hsu
Division of Public Health Sciences
Fred Hutchinson Cancer Research Center
Seattle, Washington

Jie Kate Hue
Department of Biostatistics
University of Washington
Seattle, Washington

Ruth H. Keogh
Department of Medical Statistics
London School of Hygiene and Tropical
    Medicine
London, United Kingdom

Charles Kooperberg
Division of Public Health Sciences
Fred Hutchinson Cancer Research Center
Seattle, Washington

Dan-Yu Lin
Department of Biostatistics
University of North Carolina
Chapel Hill, North Carolina

Thomas Lumley
Department of Statistics
University of Auckland
Auckland, New Zealand

Barbara McKnight
Department of Biostatistics
University of Washington
Seattle, Washington

Brad McNeney
Department of Statistics and Actuarial
    Science
Simon Fraser University
Burnaby, Canada

Robert Platt
Department of Epidemiology,
    Biostatistics, and Occupational Health
McGill University
Montreal, Canada

Paul J. Rathouz
Department of Biostatistics & Medical
 Informatics
University of Wisconsin School of
 Medicine & Public Health
Madison, Wisconsin

Saharon Rosset
Department of Statistics
Tel Aviv University
Tel Aviv, Israel

Sven Ove Samuelsen
Department of Mathematics
University of Oslo
Oslo, Norway

Jonathan S. Schildcrout
Department of Biostatistics
Vanderbilt University Medical Center
Nashville, Tennessee

Min Shi
Biostatistics and Computational Biology
 Branch
National Institute of Environmental
 Health Sciences
Durham, North Carolina

Nathalie Støer
Oslo University Hospital
Oslo, Norway

Samy Suissa
Department of Epidemiology and
 Biostatistics, McGill University
and Centre for Clinical Epidemiology,
 Jewish General Hospital
Montreal, Canada

Duncan C. Thomas
Department of Preventive Medicine
University of Southern California
Los Angeles, California

David M. Umbach
Biostatistics and Computational Biology
 Branch
National Institute of Environmental
 Health Sciences
Durham, North Carolina

Clarice R. Weinberg
Biostatistics and Computational Biology
 Branch
National Institute of Environmental
 Health Sciences
Durham, North Carolina

Noel S. Weiss
Department of Epidemiology
University of Washington
Seattle, Washington

Heather Whitaker
School of Mathematics and Statistics
The Open University
Milton Keynes, United Kingdom

Leila R. Zelnick
Department of Medicine
University of Washington
Seattle, Washington

Donglin Zeng
Department of Biostatistics
University of North Carolina
Chapel Hill, North Carolina

Part I

Introduction

1

Origins of the Case-Control Study

Norman E. Breslow and Noel Weiss

University of Washington

1.1 Statistics in medicine

The origins of epidemiology and demography are often traced to Graunt's (1662) production of vital statistics through his observations on the London Bills of Mortality and to Halley's (1693) construction of a life table for the city of Breslau. The following century witnessed rapid developments in probability theory and mathematical statistics through the work of Legendre, Laplace, Bayes, Gauss, and many others. Medicine, however, as practiced well into the nineteenth century, remained largely in the dark ages, with heavy reliance on questionable theories and appeal to authority. There was little or no attempt to develop treatment plans, or to counsel preventive measures, on the basis of scientific data analysis.

1.1.1   The *méthode numérique* of PCA Louis

Armitage (1983) traces the origin of clinical statistics to the renaissance in French medicine that was inspired by the revolution of 1789-99. He cites in particular the work of Philippe Pinel, who advocated empiricism to evaluate the efficacy of treatments, and of Pierre Charles Alexandre Louis. PCA Louis is perhaps best known for the *méthode numérique* he developed to study the efficacy of bloodletting, which was widely used at the time to treat a host of "inflammatory" diseases (Louis, 1835). His numerical method involved the careful collection, tabulation and analysis of statistical data, a refinement of the approach advocated earlier by Pinel. Louis recorded the duration of episodes of pneumonia according to the number of days elapsed until first bleeding since onset of disease, separately for those who lived and died, and compared the average durations for those bled between 1-4 and 5-9 days. He concluded that bloodletting had a much smaller therapeutic effect than commonly believed.

1.1.2   Louis' impact on scientific medicine

Louis had enormous impact on the subsequent development of scientific medicine. His Paris lectures were widely attended, including by many British and American physicians. The Americans returned home with his latest publications, each of which was published in Boston in translation, followed by lengthy review articles in the American Journal of Medical Sciences. His British students included William Farr and William Guy, two of the most influential figures in the development of medical statistics during the 19th century. Farr spent most of his life working in the General Register Office (GRO), where he greatly influenced the development of public health statistics (Farr, 1885). Demonstrating his enthusiasm for the new methods he had learned from Louis, Guy (1839, p. 35) wrote

> "Already has the application of the numerical method to the varying conditions and social relations of mankind given birth to a science of vast extent and of unequalled interest — the science of Statistics."

A professor of forensic medicine and Dean of the Faculty of Medicine at King's College London (1846-1858), Guy was also very active in the Royal Statistical Society, serving as its president (1873-1875). The Society still presents in his memory the prestigious Guy medals in bronze, silver and gold.

1.2   The earliest case-control studies

1.2.1   Louis' contributions to case-control reasoning

PCA Louis was just as enthusiastic about the potential of his numerical method to unravel the causes of disease as he was about its utility in the evaluation of treatments. Paneth *et al.* (2002) open their paper on the origins of the case-control study with the quotation:

> "Judging from the manner in which the subject is usually handled, the study of the etiology of diseases is generally undertaken with great levity, even by men of high acquirement. Some slight general knowledge, supported by a little more or a little less common sense, is quite sufficient to fit its possessor for the discovery of the causes of disease, in other words, to qualify him for the most complicated problem within the whole range of pathology" (Louis, 1844).

TABLE 1.1
Disease diagnosis by category of
occupation for 1,659 outpatients at King's
College Hospital (Guy, 1843, p. 203).

Exertion required	Diagnosis		
by occupation	TB	Other	Odds
Little	125	385	0.325
Varied	41	136	0.301
More	142	630	0.225
Great	33	167	0.198
Totals	341	1,318	0.259

In his book on tuberculosis, from which the quote is taken, Louis himself demonstrated the type of reasoning that underlies the case-control approach. He took issue with the claim of a hereditary influence on tuberculosis by one of his colleagues, who had noted that 36 of 99 tubercular patients had parents who had died of the disease. Louis recognized that this probability of "exposure" among the case series was insufficient on its own to conclude that offspring of tubercular patients were more likely than others to develop the disease. He speculated that, if the same proportion of deaths were due to tuberculosis in the hospital from which the cases were drawn, then "hereditary influence would be shown not to exist at all." A greater proportion exposed among the case series than among a control series was needed to suggest the "influence" of exposure.

1.2.2   Guy's study of occupational exertion and tuberculosis

The first case-control study, published just a few years after his stay in Paris with Louis, is in fact often attributed to William Guy (1843). Using data on male outpatients from King's College Hospital who worked at indoor occupations, Guy constructed a table that is summarized here in Table 1.1. This showed numbers of patients cross-classified according to the level of exertion required by their occupation and according to disease diagnosis. He also calculated the odds of tuberculosis, i.e., the ratio of the number with tuberculosis (cases) to the number with other diagnoses (controls), for each exertion level. Noting that the odds of tuberculosis decreased with the exertion level, he concluded that "strong exercise is favorable to health," or at least to the absence of tuberculosis. Had he taken the final step in a modern treatment of these data, dividing each of the odds by that for a baseline category (e.g., little exertion), he could have quantified the association between increasing exercise and the relative risk of disease.

1.2.3   Snow, Whitehead, and the London cholera epidemic

A classic story in the annals of epidemiology is that of John Snow's 1854 investigation of the outbreak of cholera in the Soho district of London, his construction of a map showing the location of cases in relation to the Broad Street pump, leading to the removal of the pump handle, and his subsequent studies of the companies that supplied water to households with and without cholera. Snow's work was assisted and his results were eventually confirmed by William Farr (1885), though Farr himself did not immediately accept Snow's hypothesis that cholera resulted from contaminated water. The crucial contributions to this investigation made by the young curate of the parish that included Broad Street, the Reverend Henry Whitehead, are less well known (Whitehead, 1855; Chave, 1958). Initially skeptical of Snow's claims, Whitehead attempted to interview every family living on Broad Street at the time

TABLE 1.2
Exposure to Broad Street
pump water for cholera cases
and controls.

	Case	Control
Exposed	80	57
Unexposed	20	279

OR = 19.6, $p < 0.001$

of the outbreak. Excluding uncertain responses, he ascertained that among 58 individuals who died of cholera, 45 had drunk water from the pump just prior to the outbreak. This was also true of 35 of 42 cholera survivors but only 57 of 336 unaffected residents. He summarized his findings by noting the great difference in the ratio 80:20 of drinkers versus nondrinkers of well water among the affected cases and the ratio 57:279 among those not affected by the disease. Today his data would be summarized as shown in Table 1.2, where, of course, the addition of the odds ratio (OR) and p-value is a modern embellishment of little consequence here to the causal argument. Some epidemiologists regard Whitehead's as the first case-control study (Paneth *et al.*, 2002).

1.3   Towards the modern case-control study

Further applications of the case-control approach, including one on marital status, fertility and breast cancer published in 1862, one on smoking and lip cancer in 1920 and another on diet and pellagra in 1920, were reviewed by Paneth *et al.* (2002), who concluded that they had done little to attract others to implement the newly developing methodology.

1.3.1   Janet Elizabeth Lane-Claypon

Janet Elizabeth Lane-Claypon, a brilliant English physician who earned both an MD and a PhD in physiology, is credited with a number of "firsts" in epidemiology and biostatistics. Her 1912 report on the value of cow's milk versus breast milk as food for infants may have been the first retrospective cohort study and also the first to investigate the potential effects of a confounder, social class (Winkelstein, 2004). It was among the earliest studies to employ Student's t-test, most likely at the suggestion of the well-known statistician Major Greenwood. Lane-Claypon employed the test to investigate the anomalous difference between mean weights of infants during their first eight days for the breast versus cow's milk fed groups compared with the differences found thereafter. She concluded that the apparent advantage of cow's milk during the first eight days, based on only 10 and 24 measurements, respectively, was likely due to sampling error. The clear advantage of breast milk in terms of weight gain during later periods, however, was not.

1.3.2 Lane-Claypon's study of breast cancer

In 1923 Neville Chamberlain, then the British Minister of Health, appointed a Committee on Cancer "to consider available information with regard to the causation, prevalence and treatment of cancer." Having decided to first study cancer of the breast, the Committee hired Lane-Claypon to review the relevant literature. It then commissioned her to "investigate a sufficient and suitable series of cases of cancer of the breast in regard to specified antecedent conditions, and at the same time a parallel and equally representative series of control cases, i.e., women whose conditions of life were broadly comparable to the cancer series but who had no sign of cancer" (Lane-Claypon, 1926).

In order to enroll a sufficient number of cases and controls, eventually 508 and 509, respectively, Lane-Claypon enlisted the participation of other physicians she knew, mostly women. Eventually subjects were drawn from 8 hospitals in London and 3 in Glasgow. In view of the excessive time required to collect a large number of incident cases, all women who had been treated previously for breast cancer and who lived within about 20 miles of each hospital were invited to return to the hospital for a medical evaluation and to complete a questionnaire. No further attempt at contact was made for those who failed to respond to the letter of invitation. "The patients here under consideration represent, therefore, only an unknown proportion of those who were still alive, while those who were dead do not enter the investigation at all" (Lane-Claypon, 1926). Roughly 80% of controls were surgical or medical in-patients who were free of cancer. They were selected so that most were between 45 and 70 years of age; the rest of the controls were outpatients of similar age.

Lane-Claypon developed a detailed, structured questionnaire that she reproduced in her report. She was quite aware of the potential for recall bias, noting that cases with breast cancer might be psychologically disposed to over-emphasize antecedent "troubles" with their breasts, whereas controls might well have forgotten them.

1.3.3 Reproductive factors and the risk of breast cancer

The first step in the data analysis was to ascertain whether or not the data on cases and controls were "suitable for comparison." Lane-Claypon concluded that they were based on similarity in age, nationality (mostly English and Scotch), marital status and social status. There were somewhat more single women among cases and married women among controls, however, and she remarked that "in view of the known prevalence of cancer of the breast among single women this difference was perhaps to be anticipated." Lane-Claypon then investigated the influence of various features of reproductive life on breast cancer risk. She was the first to demonstrate that age at marriage of (married and widowed) cases was significantly higher than for controls. Taking age at marriage as a surrogate for age at first birth, this was the first demonstration of the well-known fact that early pregnancy lowers breast cancer risk.

Lane-Claypon then proceeded to establish, again for the first time, the strong relationship between fertility and risk. Indeed, a total of 1,521 pregnancies were reported by control women versus only 1,023 by cases. She was not content with this simple comparison, however, since it failed to account for the potential confounding effects of age at and duration of marriage. The statistician, Major Greenwood, constructed a multiple regression equation to predict the number of children expected among married case women as a function of marital age and duration, and similarly for control women. When the equation for the case series was applied to the controls, 3.89 children per women were predicted whereas an average of 5.34 were observed. Conversely, applying the control equation to the cases, an average of 4.72 children were expected, whereas the observed number was 3.48. Both differences were highly significant.

Among other "antecedent" factors that Lane-Claypon investigated was age at menarche. She observed that 20.0% of control women reported menarche before 13 years versus 13.3% for the breast cancer cases. The percentages for onset of menarche over 15 years were 25.7% and 22.4%, respectively. Apparently unaware of the development of the chi-squared test in the early 1900's by Pearson and Fisher, she remarked, "It is not possible, at present to say whether there is any significance in these variations." Using odds ratios and confidence intervals in a re-analysis of her data, Press and Pharoah (2010) showed the observed differences would indeed be regarded as significant by current standards. They also showed that mothers who breast-fed their babies for a year or more had half the risk of breast cancer compared to those who either did not breast-feed or for whom the duration of lactation was 3 months or less. Lane-Claypon herself observed that "It was somewhat surprising to find the large numbers of children who were fed for over a year, especially in the control series," but in her summary conclusions calls attention only to the excess of case mothers who either failed to suckle or suckled for a "very long period."

Lane-Claypon is deservedly credited with having performed the first "modern" case-control study. She started with well-conceived questions and developed the means to answer them, in particular, via a multi-center study using a structured questionnaire in the hands of trained interviewers. She was aware of problems of recall bias and confounding and was meticulous in her approach to data analysis and interpretation. Her pathbreaking work stimulated a successful attempt to replicate her study in the United States (Wainwright, 1931). Her results have stood the test of time, and account for a good portion of what is known today about breast cancer risk factors.

1.4   Doll and Hill's study of smoking and lung cancer

Further development of case-control studies took place during the later 1920's, 1930's and 1940's. Lilienfeld and Lilienfeld (1979) called attention to early use of the methodology by sociologists and to a 1947 study of the relationship between sex hygiene and penile cancer. Morabia (2010) reviewed four German studies of smoking and lung cancer published in 1938 and 1943. He noted that all the studies prior to 1950, including that of Lane-Claypon, were strictly focused on a comparison of antecedent exposures in cases and controls, with no attempt to interpret the results in terms of disease risk. Since the latter was of primary scientific interest, the potential of case-control methodology was at the time widely underappreciated. Four case-control studies of cigarette smoking and lung cancer were published in 1950 that galvanized the attention of the medical community and ultimately led to the famous Surgeon General's Report on Smoking and Health in 1964. The study by Doll and Hill (1950) was the most influential of the four. It opened a new era in which the case-control approach gained wide acceptance as a valid method for elucidating the causes of disease.

1.4.1   Background and conduct of the study

In 1947 Austin Bradford Hill, revered as the father of the randomized clinical trial, was director of the Medical Research Council (MRC) statistical research unit and Professor of Medical Statistics and Epidemiology at the London School of Hygiene and Tropical Medicine. The MRC had just been asked by the Ministry of Health to find an explanation for the huge increase in lung cancer deaths between the two world wars. When Hill was approached about undertaking a large-scale etiologic study, he invited a young physician, whom he knew to be statistically competent and interested in cancer, to direct the study. Thus began the long collaboration between Richard Doll and AB Hill.

Twenty London hospitals were asked to participate by notifying the MRC unit of all patients admitted with carcinoma of the lung, stomach or large bowel. One of four full-time workers interviewed each patient using a "set questionary" that included a detailed smoking history. The interviewer was instructed to query in the same manner, in the same hospital and at about the same time, a control patient of the same gender and 5-year category of age who did not have cancer. In their 1950 report, Doll and Hill first presented the data in much the same fashion as for earlier case-control studies. They noted the similarity in age and gender between lung cancer cases and their respective controls, a result of the matching, a minor difference in social class and a substantial difference in place of residence, due to the cases having been drawn from further afield than the controls. The difference in place of residence disappeared when cases and controls were restricted to district hospitals without special treatment facilities. They then showed the differences between lung cancer cases and matched controls as regards duration and intensity of smoking, age started and stopped smoking and an estimate of the total amount of tobacco ever consumed.

1.4.2   Estimation of absolute and relative risks

A final table in the discussion of Doll and Hill's 1950 report presented a type of analysis of case-control data never seen before. Restricting attention to cases from Greater London, where they had some idea regarding the demographics of the underlying population, they applied the frequency distribution of daily cigarette consumption among controls of a given age to the estimated population of the same age to arrive at an estimated population denominator for the number of cases in each age by smoking category. Lacking detailed information on the fraction of the Greater London population covered by the 20 hospitals, they were justifiably cautious in their interpretation, asserting that the ratios of cases to denominators in each cell of the table "are not measures of the actual risks of developing carcinoma of the lung, but are put forward very tentatively as proportional to these risks." Averaging results for the top three age categories, they concluded "If the risk among non-smokers is taken as unity ... the relative risks become 6, 19, 26, 49 and 65" for smoking categories of an average of 3, 10, 20, 35 and 60 cigarettes per day compared to nonsmokers.

Doll and Hill continued to collect cases and controls and to expand their roster of hospitals, publishing the final results of their investigation two years later (Doll and Hill, 1952). With the addition of crucial information not used earlier, namely the age-specific numbers of deaths from lung cancer and population denominators in Greater London for the year 1950, they were able to estimate absolute death rates by smoking category from their case-control data. Table 1.3, reconstructed from Table XII in their 1952 report, shows the case-control data upon which this calculation was based. The male population of Greater London aged 45-64 in 1950 was 937,000, among whom 1,474 lung cancer deaths were reported. By applying the proportion of cases in each smoking category in their study to this population number, they could estimate the number of lung cancer deaths by amount smoked. This involved the assumption that the smoking patterns among lung cancer cases were similar to those among persons who died of the disease, which seemed reasonable in view of the very high mortality. Thus, for example, they estimated that $(197/539) \times 1,474 = 538.7$ deaths occurred among those smoking 5-14 cigarettes per day. Similarly, applying the control proportions to the population, they estimated that $(397/932) \times 937,000 = 399,130$ men aged 45-64 in the population smoked 5-14 cigarettes per day. Dividing the estimated numbers of cases by the estimated population, they calculated that $538.7/399.1 = 1.35$ deaths per 1,000 population occurred due to lung cancer.

Thus Doll and Hill's first publication demonstrated that, if one could assume the controls

TABLE 1.3
Number of lung cancer cases and controls in Greater London
among males aged 45-64 years, by average amount smoked
in the preceding 10 years, with estimated death rates of lung
cancer per 1,000 persons per year.

| | Average daily number of cigarettes | | | | | | |
	0	1-4	5-14	15-24	25-49	50+	Total
Controls	38	87	397	279	119	12	932
Cases	2	19	197	171	129	21	539
Rates	0.14	0.59	1.35	1.67	2.95	4.96[1]	1.57

[1]Corrected from 4.74 shown by Doll and Hill

were representative of the population at risk vis-à-vis exposure, case-control data were
sufficient to estimate relative risks. The second demonstrated that absolute risks were also
estimable provided one knew the overall population risk or, equivalently, the proportion
of that population sampled as controls. These results were obtained using Hill's inimitable
numerical style without recourse to mathematical formalism. The formulas came later in
the work of Cornfield (1951) on relative risk and Neutra and Drolette (1978) on absolute
risk.

1.4.3   Addressing criticisms of the case-control method

The statistical advances were by no means the only innovations, however. Through careful
analysis of the available data, Doll and Hill provided evidence to counter some of the major
criticisms of the case-control method. They argued for lack of selection bias among controls
by demonstrating that their smoking habits were similar to those of patients with gastric or
large bowel cancer. They countered possible claims of interviewer or recall bias likewise, by
demonstrating that the smoking habits of patients initially thought to have lung cancer, but
who were found on pathology examination after the interview not to have it, were similar
to those of controls. They excluded the possibility that place of residence might confound
the observed associations by a sub-analysis restricted to district hospitals, which yielded
the same overall results.

The Doll and Hill study set the standard for case-control research for years thereafter.
Beginning in the mid 1950's the number of case-control studies published in the medical
literature increased dramatically (Cole, 1979).

1.5   The distinctive contributions of case-control studies

Case-control studies sometimes can be relatively inexpensive and quick to conduct. In many
instances, such studies are the first in a sequence of increasingly rigorous efforts to investigate
an association between a risk factor and a disease. There are circumstances in which the
results of cohort studies are given more credence, due to their relative lack of recall and
control selection bias. The conclusions in the 1964 Surgeon General's Report on Smoking
and Health, for example, were based primarily on a review of data from seven large cohort
studies, rather than from the case-control studies that preceded them. Nonetheless, certain
questions are addressed most appropriately using case-control studies. Furthermore, the
results of well-done case-control studies can serve as the basis for public health or clinical

decisions well before the results of cohort studies, not to mention randomized trials, might become available. This concluding section identifies several scenarios where the case-control method has a distinct role to play in studies of the causation or prevention of disease.

1.5.1 Elucidation of the etiologies of uncommon diseases

In 1971, Herbst *et al.* (1971) compiled a series of eight cases of clear cell adenocarcinoma of the vagina in adolescents and young women diagnosed in the Boston area during 1966-1969. Up until that time, this condition had been viewed as being extraordinarily rare. Interviews with the mothers of these cases revealed that all but one had taken the synthetic hormone, diethylstilbestrol, during the pregnancy that resulted in the birth of their daughter. None of the mothers of 32 control subjects, matched for sex and hospital and date of birth, claimed to have taken diethylstilbestrol during pregnancy. A case-control study in New York conducted soon thereafter obtained a similar result (Greenwald *et al.*, 1971). At that time there was no clear understanding of the biological mechanism underlying the association, but nonetheless it was widely viewed as causal, and the US Food and Drug Administration specified pregnancy as a contraindication to the use of diethylstilbestrol.

1.5.2 Assessment of exposure-disease relations in which there is a short induction period

In response to mini-epidemics of an otherwise-rare condition, Reye's syndrome (a potentially life-threatening pediatric condition defined by the presence of liver injury and encephalopathy that can develop soon after an episode of flu or chicken pox), case-control studies were conducted to examine a broad range of potentially causative exposures. These studies (Halpin *et al.*, 1982) observed a very large difference between the proportions of cases and of controls who had been given aspirin during the antecedent illness. Later investigations, which employed a more rigorous case definition, obtained a greater degree of comparability of exposure ascertainment between cases and controls and had a more sensitive means of ascertainment of aspirin use, obtained very similar results (Hurwitz *et al.*, 1987; Forsyth *et al.*, 1989). Largely because of the results of these studies, the American Academy of Pediatrics proscribed the use of aspirin in children suspected of having flu or chicken pox.

Similarly, based primarily on the results of a number of case-control studies that observed, compared to controls, a far higher proportion of infants who succumbed to sudden infant death syndrome to have been put to sleep in the prone position, the American Academy of Pediatrics recommended that, as a general rule, infants should be put to sleep only on their back or side (Kattwinkel *et al.*, 1992).

1.5.3 Examination of potential exposure-disease associations when a disease outcome is not identifiable from routinely available sources

The presence of arteriosclerosis in the abdominal aorta, femoral arteries and/or popliteal arteries can lead to exertional leg pain termed intermittent claudication, akin to angina pectoris that is caused by arteriosclerosis in the coronary artery. A substantial fraction of patients with intermittent claudication receive only outpatient care, and so a cohort study in which hospital discharge diagnoses are scanned to enumerate potential cases would fail to identify many persons with this condition. The problem can be dealt with by case-control studies that enumerate cases from outpatient medical records. These studies, e.g., that by Weiss (1972), have established a relation between cigarette smoking and intermittent claudication that is the same strength as that between cigarette smoking and lung cancer.

1.5.4   Overcoming noncomparability of exposed and nonexposed subjects in cohort studies

Virtually all screening tests for cancer are introduced for general use on the basis of studies that document the sensitivity and specificity of the screening modality, together with the expectation that treatment of an early-diagnosed cancer case will, on average, lead to a better outcome than would later diagnosis, and thus later treatment. Formal evaluations of the efficacy of screening by means of randomized trials generally are not conducted until the screening modality has been in use for some time, and often are not conducted at all. Using a cohort study to evaluate screening efficacy in reducing cancer mortality can be problematic. Persons who undergo screening are, by definition, free of symptoms and signs of the cancer being screened for. Assuring that unscreened persons are similarly free of symptoms and signs of the cancer, however, requires a greater depth and frequency of exposure ascertainment than most cohort studies — even those that include direct contact with cohort members — are able to employ. If high-quality medical records are available in which to ascertain the presence of cancer screening, persons who died of the cancer in question can be compared to age-matched controls. The matched control is a person from the same underlying population who is at risk for the disease in question, born at the same time as the case and alive at the time of the case death. The comparison is made of the history of receipt of screening during that period of time prior to the case's diagnosis or first symptoms, or the corresponding period of calendar time for the matched control, in which it might be anticipated that a relatively more-treatable form of the disease, or of a disease precursor, would have been present.

The case-control approach was used to gauge the impact of screening sigmoidoscopy on mortality from colorectal cancer among members of a large prepaid medical care plan in which this form of early disease detection had been employed for a number of years (Selby *et al.*, 1992). Among persons who had been members of the plan for a minimum of one year, medical records revealed that 24.2% of controls had been screened, in contrast to only 8.8% of persons with fatal distal cancer, i.e., cancer that arose in the lower 20 centimeters of the colon and rectum, and so potentially was within the reach of the sigmoidoscope (adjusted odds ratio = 0.4). Arguing in support of a protective influence of screening was the observation that the proportion of cases of fatal colorectal cancer whose malignancy originated *above* the reach of a sigmoidoscope in whom screening had taken place was identical to that of controls. Ultimately, randomized trials of the efficacy of screening sigmoidoscopy were conducted, but the results of these trials did not become available until 20 years after the publication of the findings of the above case-control study. During those two decades the use of screening sigmoidoscopy (and then colonoscopy) became substantially more common in many parts of the world, no doubt in large part because of the strong association seen in this study and in case-control studies that followed.

Bibliography

Armitage, P. (1983). Trials and errors: The emergence of clinical statistics. *Journal of the Royal Statistical Society (Series A)*, **146**, 321–334.

Chave, S. P. W. (1958). Henry Whitehead and cholera in Broad street. *Medical History*, **2**, 92–108.

Cole, P. (1979). The evolving case-control study. *Journal of Chronic Disease*, **32**, 15–27.

Cornfield, J. (1951). A method of estimating comparative rates from clinical data. Applications to cancer of the lung, breast, and cervix. *Journal of the National Cancer Institute*, **11**, 1269–1275.

Doll, R. and Hill, A. B. (1950). Smoking and carcinoma of the lung. Preliminary report. *British Medical Journal*, **2**, 739–748.

Doll, R. and Hill, A. B. (1952). A study of the aetiology of carcinoma of the lung. *British Medical Journal*, **2**, 1271–1286.

Farr, W. H. (1885). *Vital Statistics: A Memorial Volume of Selections from the Reports and Writings of William Farr*. The Sanitary Institute of Great Britain, London.

Forsyth, B. W., Horwitz, R. I., Acampora, D., Shapiro, E. D., Viscoli, C. M., Feinstein, A. R., Henner, R., Holabird, N. B., Jones, B. A., Karabelas, A. D. E., Kramer, M. S., Miclette, M., and Wells, J. A. (1989). New epidemiologic evidence confirming that bias does not explain the aspirin Reye's syndrome association. *Journal of the American Medical Association*, **261**, 2517–2524.

Graunt, J. (1662). *Natural and Political Observations Mentioned in a Following Index, and Made upon the Bills of Mortality*. Roycroft, London.

Greenwald, P., Barlow, J. J., Nasca, P. C., and Burnett, W. S. (1971). Vaginal cancer after maternal treatment with synthetic estrogens. *New England Journal of Medicine*, **285**, 390–393.

Guy, W. A. (1839). On the value of the numerical method as applied to science, but especially to physiology and medicine. *Journal of the Statistical Society of London*, **2**, 25–47.

Guy, W. A. (1843). Contributions to a knowledge of the influence of employment on health. *Journal of the Statistical Society of London*, **6**, 197–211.

Halley, E. (1693). An estimate of the degrees of mortality of mankind, drawn from the curious tables of births and funerals in the city of Breslaw; with an attempt to ascertain the price of annuities upon lives. *Philosophical Transactions of the Royal Society of London*, **17**, 596–610.

Halpin, T. J., Holtzhauer, F. J., Campbell, R. J., Hall, L. J., Correavillasenor, A., Lanese, R., Rice, J., and Hurwitz, E. S. (1982). Reye's syndrome and medication use. *Journal of the American Medical Association*, **248**, 687–691.

Herbst, A. L., Ulfelder, H., and Poskanzer, D. C. (1971). Adenocarcinoma of vagina – association of maternal stilbestrol therapy with tumor appearance in young women. *New England Journal of Medicine*, **284**, 878–881.

Hurwitz, E. S., Barrett, M. J., Bregman, D., Gunn, W. J., Pinsky, P., Schonberger, L. B., Drage, J. S., Kaslow, R. A., Burlington, D. B., Quinnan, G. V., Lamontagne, J. R., Fairweather, W. R., Dayton, D., and Dowdle, W. R. (1987). Public Health Service study of Reye's syndrome and medications. Report of the main study. *Journal of the American Medical Association*, **257**, 1905–1911.

Kattwinkel, J., Brooks, J., and Myerberg, D. (1992). Positioning and SIDS. *Pediatrics*, **89**, 1120–1126.

Lane-Claypon, J. E. (1926). A further report on cancer of the breast, with special reference to its associated antecedent conditions. Reports on Public Health and Medical Subjects, pages 1–189. His Majesty's Stationery Office, London.

Lilienfeld, A. M. and Lilienfeld, D. E. (1979). A century of case-control studies: Progress? *Journal of Chronic Disease*, **32**, 5–13.

Louis, P. C. A. (1835). *Recherches sur les Effets de la Saignée*. Baillière, Paris.

Louis, P. C. A. (1844). *Researches on Phthisis, Anatomical, Pathological and Therapeutical*. The Sydenham Society, London.

Morabia, A. (2010). Janet Lane-Claypon – interphase epitome. *Epidemiology*, **21**, 573–576.

Neutra, R. R. and Drolette, M. E. (1978). Estimating exposure-specific disease rates from case-control studies using Bayes theorem. *American Journal of Epidemiology*, **108**, 214–222.

Paneth, N., Susser, E., and Susser, M. (2002). Origins and early development of the case-control study: Part 1, Early evolution. *Sozial- und Präventivmedizin*, **47**, 282–288.

Press, D. J. and Pharoah, P. (2010). Risk factors for breast cancer. A reanalysis of two case-control studies from 1926 and 1931. *Epidemiology*, **21**, 566–572.

Selby, J. V., Friedman, G. D., Quesenberry, C. P., and Weiss, N. S. (1992). A case-control study of screening sigmoidoscopy and mortality from colorectal-cancer. *New England Journal of Medicine*, **326**, 653–657.

Wainwright, J. (1931). A comparison of conditions associated with breast cancer in Great Britain and America. *American Journal of Cancer*, **15**, 2610–2645.

Weiss, N. S. (1972). Cigarette-smoking and arteriosclerosis obliterans: An epidemiologic approach. *American Journal of Epidemiology*, **95**, 17–25.

Whitehead, H. (1855). *Report on the Cholera Outbreak in the Parish of St. James, Westminster, during the Autumn of 1854*. Churchill, London.

Winkelstein, W. (2004). Vignettes of the history of epidemiology: Three firsts by Janet Elizabeth Lane-Claypon. *American Journal of Epidemiology*, **160**, 97–101.

2

Design Issues in Case-Control Studies

Duncan C. Thomas

University of Southern California

2.1 Rationale for case-control studies

The two principal analytical study designs used in traditional risk-factor epidemiology are *cohort* and *case-control* designs. In cohort studies, individuals are sampled and their exposure status is determined initially; subsequent disease status is the outcome variable. In case-control studies, cases and noncases are sampled, and the "outcomes" being compared are the covariates (including exposure). If the underlying cohort (or source population from which the cases arise) can be identified, the case-control study can be regarded as a special sampling design for efficiently learning about the risk factor associations in the cohort (Wacholder *et al.*, 1992a,b,c). Indeed, case-control studies are of great public health interest and utility because the odds ratio that can be estimated from a case-control study approximates the relative risk comparing exposed to unexposed in a cohort study (Cornfield, 1951). Cohort and case-control designs are distinguished primarily by the direction of inference: cohort studies reason forwards in time from an exposure to disease, while case-control studies reason the other direction from disease back to possible causes. It is this direction of inference – not the temporal sequence of data collection – that is conceptually important. Either type of study can be conducted "retrospectively" (using records from the past) or "prospectively" (collecting new observations as they occur in the future). Although some authors have used the terms prospective and retrospective to refer to cohort and case-control designs, respectively, it is better to be explicit about the time periods over which the data were collected, whether for a cohort study or case-control study.

The great advantage of the case-control design is that it does not require enormous sample sizes or a long period of follow-up – only enough to accrue a sufficient number of cases and a comparable number of controls. Thus the case-control design is ideal for studying rare diseases. With this design, more resources can be devoted to data quality, e.g., verifying the diagnosis of cases and unaffected status of controls and obtaining much more detailed information on exposure than is typically possible in a cohort study.

The case-control design begins with the ascertainment of a representative sample of cases of the disease of interest from a defined population (typically a geographic region and a time period), along with a suitably defined unaffected "control" group. (Note the potential confusion over use of the word "control" in the two designs: as unexposed in a cohort study but as a noncase in a case-control study; to avoid this confusion, the term "referent group" may be preferable for the unexposed comparison in either design.) Both the cases and controls are then assessed to determine their prior exposures over the period thought to be etiologically relevant, e.g., excluding the years immediately prior to diagnosis, which are unlikely to be causally related for diseases with long latency and when pre-diagnostic symptoms might have altered the case's exposure behavior. The case-control design may be more susceptible to various study biases described below, notably differences in the representativeness of cases and controls relative to their source populations and in the quality of the exposure information from each group. To minimize the effect of confounding (Section 2.2.5), controls are generally individually- or group-matched (Section 2.2.3) to cases on factors like age, gender, race, and other known risk factors that are not of primary interest but could also be related to exposure and thus distort the exposure-disease relationship of primary interest.

2.2   Basic design considerations

The basic design principle is that cases should be representative of all cases in the population and controls should be representative of the source population of cases (Wacholder *et al.*, 1992a). This is most easily accomplished in situations where there is a population-based disease registry and where there is some means of sampling from the total population. For some diseases like cancer, population-based registries may exist, like the National Cancer Institute's Surveillance, Epidemiology and End Results (SEER) registries that cover specific regions in the United States. But in the United States, there is no population registry, so sampling from a SEER coverage area requires other methods. For example, the CARE study (Marchbanks *et al.*, 2002) used cases from SEER and random-digit dialing (Section 2.2.2) to select controls from the same SEER region. Alternatively, a complete sampling frame for the population may exist for selecting controls, but there might be no population-based registry for the disease of interest. In this situation, cases are often recruited from hospitals, and for comparability, hospital-based controls are also used.

2.2.1 Population-based ascertainment of cases

A rigorous definition of the case series is an essential starting point. Ideally this is population-based, for example all cases identified by a registry covering some population defined by space and time, or for mortality, all deaths in a similarly defined population. But many diseases are not routinely recorded in any population-based registry, so one must resort to hospital- or clinic-based series or a special survey of the population. In such cases, it may be more difficult to identify the source population from which the identified cases arose, as hospitals typically do not have well-defined catchment areas from which all cases would come and different cases from the same area may go to different hospitals. Since the goal of etiologic research is studying the causes of disease incidence, cases should comprise representative series of newly diagnosed individuals, not prevalent cases at a particular point in time as would be identified by a cross-sectional survey; the latter would tend to over-represent long-duration cases, yielding associations either with incidence or disease duration (e.g., with case-fatality rates).

2.2.2 Sources of controls

Having defined the case series, there may be various ways of sampling from the population that gave rise to these cases. The ideal would be a random sample of the population, possibly stratified by such factors as age and gender to match the corresponding frequency distribution of cases, but this would require a sampling frame listing all the people eligible to be selected. While some countries (Australia and the Scandinavian countries, for example) maintain such population registers, many others, including the United States, do not. Even when registries are available, confidentiality policies may preclude access for research purposes. Some alternatives that have been widely used include:

- *Neighborhood controls:* The investigator makes a census of the neighborhood surrounding each case and selects an eligible control at random from that list. For example, a field worker may start at some pre-determined location near the case's residence (say the corresponding location one block away to preserve the anonymity of the case) and walk the neighborhood in a spiral pattern to obtain a list of potential control residences. At each door, the walker either asks for the identity of individuals who might be eligible as controls or leaves a request to call the investigator with this information if no one answers; the walk continues until some predetermined number of residences has been surveyed. Once complete, the first eligible person who agrees to participate is used as the control.

- *Random digit dialing controls:* Starting with the first few digits of a case's phone number, the remaining digits are selected at random and dialed. If a suitable control is available and willing to participate, he or she is included in the list of available controls to be sampled, or the first available control is selected.

- *Friend controls:* Each case is asked to list the names and contact information for a number of friends and one of these is selected at random.

- *Spouse controls:* For diseases of adulthood, the spouse of the case is selected.

- *Sibling controls:* A sibling who has attained the age of the case, still free of the disease under study, is selected as the control.

- *Birth registry controls:* For diseases of childhood, the child born immediately preceding or following the case may be used.

- *Hospital controls:* For hospital-based case series, individuals attending the same hospital for some condition(s) thought to be unrelated to the risk factors under study may be used as a control.

None of these is ideal (Wacholder *et al.*, 1992b). The three general principles for evaluating potential sources of controls are representativeness of the study base population, freedom from confounding, and comparability of data quality. Wacholder *et al.* (1992b) also discuss the relative efficiency of different control sources and whether it is advisable for cases and controls to have equal opportunity for exposure (Poole, 1986).

Neighborhood controls are likely to best represent the source population of cases (Robins and Pike, 1990), but obtaining them is laborious, and it may be impractical to survey some dangerous neighborhoods. Furthermore, for geographically determined exposures like air pollution, cases and controls would tend to have similar exposures, leading to "overmatching" and loss of efficiency. Random digit dialing controls are also labor intensive, typically requiring on average about 40 calls to identify each control and may be subject to various selection biases related to phone availability. Random digit dialing is becoming more and more difficult with the increasing prevalence of answering machines, caller id, and cell phones (Link and Kresnow, 2006; Kempf and Remington, 2007). Spouse controls are typically of the opposite gender and unsuitable for studying exposures that are sex-related. Many cases may also not have an eligible spouse or sibling control. Friend controls can be subject to various biases relating to differences between cases in their number of friends, the representativeness of their exposures, willingness of cases to name friends, and the risk of overmatching (Flanders and Austin, 1986; Siemiatycki, 1989; Robins and Pike, 1990; Thompson, 1990; Wacholder *et al.*, 1992b; Kaplan *et al.*, 1998; Ma *et al.*, 2004). These are more likely to pose a problem for environmental risk factors, particularly those related to social behaviors like smoking, than for genetic factors, however (Shaw *et al.*, 1991). Hospital controls are afflicted by some other condition that led them to the hospital. It can be difficult to choose conditions that are truly unrelated to the risk factors under study if particular diseases are to be used as controls or conversely which conditions to exclude if all others are to be used as controls. In addition, hospital controls suffer from another problem known as Berkson's bias (Westreich, 2012): individuals with multiple diseases are likely to be overrepresented because they have more opportunities to be sampled because they enter the hospital more frequently.

2.2.3   Matching and stratified sampling

Inherent in many of the control selection strategies described above is the idea of individual matching. Beyond providing a convenient way of selecting controls, it also serves the important function of ensuring the comparability of case and control series on factors that are not of particular interest but may be important risk factors for the disease. Matching can be done either individually or by strata. For the former, the control that most closely matches the case on the set of factors under study is selected (typically this may entail prioritizing the various factors, e.g., gender, followed by age within 5 years, followed by race, followed by education, etc.). For stratum (or frequency) matching, cases are divided into mutually exclusive strata and controls are selected at random from among eligible noncases in each stratum at a fixed ratio to the number of cases.

Individual matching is generally done by defining a sequence of criteria to be matched upon, beginning by requiring an exact match (for discrete variables, or for continuous variables a match within either strata or within some tolerance (Austin *et al.*, 1989)) on the most important criteria, and then seeking the closest available match on less critical factors, relaxing the closeness of matching as needed to find an acceptable control. Once selected as a control for one case, that individual is usually not eligible to be paired with another more closely matching case, so that the resulting set of pairs could be less than optimal overall. Such rules can be difficult to implement when several risk factors are to be matched for simultaneously. An attractive alternative is the use of optimal matching designs (Rosenbaum, 1989), typically involving minimization over all possible case-control pairs of some measure of multivariate distance on the set of matching factors. This minimization can be accomplished without having to enumerate all possible pairings using an efficient network algorithm. Cologne and Shibata (1995) compared two such approaches, one based on the propensity-score (the probability of being a case given the matching factors, as estimated from the entire pool of cases and potential controls (Rosenbaum and Rubin, 1985)) and a variance-weighted Euclidean distance between case-control pairs (Smith *et al.*, 1977). In a nested case-control study of liver cancer within the atomic bomb survivor cohort, where hepatitis B infection was considered as a potentially strong confounder or modifier, they concluded that the weighted-distance method produced better overall closeness across matched sets because the propensity score tended to be poorly estimated.

An advantage of individual matching is that cases and controls can be assigned comparable "reference dates" for evaluation of time-dependent exposure variables, such as one year before diagnosis of the case or the corresponding interval before interview, age, or calendar date for the matched control. Unless cases' and controls' reference dates are similar, the comparison of variables like cumulative exposure can be biased by lack of comparability of their times over which exposure is accumulated or their "opportunity for exposure." This is more difficult to accomplish for unmatched or frequency-matched case-control studies, for which it would be necessary to assign reference dates for controls corresponding to the distribution of reference dates for all cases in the same stratum; this would be difficult to accomplish until after all the cases have been enrolled.

2.2.4 Exposure assessment

The second major challenge in case-control study design is exposure assessment, particularly ensuring comparability of the quality of information from cases and controls. "Recall bias" is a particularly difficult challenge if exposure information is to be obtained by interview or questionnaire: cases may be more inclined to over-report exposures they think could have caused their disease or to deny exposure about which there is some stigma. Cases with advanced disease may be too ill to respond accurately to questions or it may be necessary to obtain exposure information from a proxy (e.g., next of kin) if the case is dead or too sick to respond (Nelson *et al.*, 1990; Wacholder *et al.*, 1992b). For this reason, Gordis (1982) suggested selecting dead controls for dead cases, so that exposure information would be obtained by proxy for both, but this violates the principle of controls' representativeness of the base population (McLaughlin *et al.*, 1985), even if it does tend to promote comparability of data quality.

Exposure measurement error has been widely discussed in the statistical and epidemiological literature (Carroll *et al.*, 2006) as summarized in Chapter 10 of this book. In case-control studies, if the exposure measurement error mechanism affects cases and controls similarly ("nondifferential" measurement error), odds ratios will tend to be attenuated toward 1. If the measurement error is differential, as from recall bias, odds ratio estimates can be seriously biased in either direction. In the "classical error" model, in which the measurement errors are uncorrelated with the true value of the exposure, the general effect is to dilute a true association (biasing its magnitude towards the null and reducing power). In the "Berkson error" model, measurement errors are independent of the assigned values. This arises commonly in experiments where target exposures are specified but individuals may differ in their actual exposures; in a case-control design, this error model may arise when a group mean is assigned to each individual in the group, such as the average exposure by job title. In this case there may be no bias towards the null, but the variance of the exposure-response slope estimate will be inflated. A variety of statistical methods are available to correct for these effects if the distribution of measurement errors is known, although the loss of power cannot generally be recovered by purely statistical methods (Thomas *et al.*, 1993). The usual bias towards the null in the classical error model may not apply in multivariate exposure models, however, as errors in measurement of a causal exposure can "spill over" into noncausal exposures, producing spurious associations (Armstrong *et al.*, 1989; Zeger *et al.*, 2000). Study designs that include multiple measurements or reference sub-studies with "gold standard" measurement tools may be helpful to estimate error distributions and correct for them (Greenland, 1988; Spiegelman and Gray, 1991). Such studies could take the form of external "validation" studies comparing the exposure assessment methods used in the case-control study with gold standard or repeated measurements, but may be more informative (particularly if one wishes to assess differential measurement errors between cases and controls) if conducted on subsets of the same case-control study subjects, perhaps using one of the hybrid designs discussed in Section 2.4 below.

2.2.5   Dealing with bias

"Bias" refers to any aspect of study design or analysis that would tend to make the result of a study differ on average from the true value. Epidemiologists usually rely on observational data and do not have the opportunity to test hypotheses by controlled experiments that rely on randomization to ensure comparability of the groups being compared (Greenland, 1990). Hence, the associations between risk factors and disease found in epidemiologic studies are subject to various biases and do not necessarily indicate causation. Dozens of specific biases have been described (Sackett, 1979), but epidemiologists generally classify them into three main types: confounding, selection, and information bias.

Confounding refers to underlying relationships of exposure and disease to other variables that can induce spurious relationships between them, mask a true relationship, or distort its magnitude. Unlike selection and information biases that relate to study design and analysis problems, confounding refers to fundamental relationships amongst variables in the source population. For example, the rates of most diseases increase with age and, of course, cumulative exposure must also increase with age; this alone would tend to make disease risk appear to be positively associated with cumulative exposure to almost anything, even if that exposure had nothing to do with disease. Epidemiologists address this problem by a variety of study design or analysis techniques, including matching cases and controls on potential confounding variables, restricting the study to only a single value of a potential confounder (e.g., only to males or to Caucasians), or by stratification or statistical adjustment in the analysis. While these techniques can eliminate confounding by known risk factors, it is never possible to know all the potential confounders, so the possibility of residual confounding will always remain in any observational study. Only a randomized experimental study can guarantee freedom from confounding, and then only in expectation.

To be a confounder, a factor must be related to exposure and be an independent risk factor for disease, i.e., not simply associated with disease indirectly through exposure. Controlling for a factor that is not independently related to disease is called "overmatching" or "overadjustment" (Day *et al.*, 1980). Although it would not bias the exposure-disease association, it would inflate its variance and reduce power by unnecessarily restricting the variability in exposure. This concept is related to the question of whether cases and controls should be required to be comparable in terms of "opportunity for exposure" (Poole, 1986; Wacholder *et al.*, 1992a).

Selection bias refers to any aspect of the study design that may tend to make the sample of study subjects unrepresentative of their source population. For example, in a case-control study, it may not be possible to include all cases within the defined geographic area or time period because some of them may have died, moved away, could not be located, or refused to participate; if exposure is related to case-fatality, for example, this will distort the true relationship with disease incidence. Likewise, controls should represent the source population that gave rise to the cases, but this is often difficult to accomplish if there is no population registry. Selection bias is difficult to assess quantitatively without data on the subjects who did not participate, hence it can be helpful to try to obtain at least limited demographic information on as many of them as possible. The potential for selection bias needs to be considered in hospital-based case-control studies. For example, cases with severe disease may be over-represented in a teaching hospital, and the patients with control diseases may not be representative of the source population with respect to the risk factor under study.

Information bias refers to any aspect of the collection of data on the subjects included in a study that will tend to distort the true values of the variables being collected. In Section 2.2.4 we mentioned recall bias and other forms of exposure measurement error that induce information bias. Mismeasurement of covariates used to control for confounding can also result in bias from incomplete control for confounding (Greenland, 1980; Greenland and Robins, 1985).

2.3 Overview of analysis approaches

Chapter 3 and subsequent chapters of this book will develop the various approaches to the analysis of case-control data in some detail, so here I simply outline the key concepts.

2.3.1 Basic unmatched and matched analyses of categorical data

Cohort studies provide direct estimators of the risk of disease in each exposure subgroup and hence their ratio estimates a quantity known as the relative risk. More precisely, the parameter of interest could be either the probability of disease incidence (risk) over a fixed time period like a pregnancy or a 5-year clinical trial, or the age-specific incidence rates over an extended time period. The age-standardized ratio of rates – the incidence rate ratio or hazard ratio – is then a weighted average of the ratio of age-specific incidence rates. In contrast, the proportions of cases out of all exposed and unexposed subjects in a case-control study are not directly interpretable owing to the different sampling fractions of cases and controls; their ratio does not estimate a meaningful population parameter.

More than 60 years ago, Cornfield (1951) showed that case-control data could be used to approximate the cohort relative risk by using instead the odds ratio, under the assumption that the disease was rare and that cases and controls were sampled without reference to their exposure status. This happens because the ratio of case and control sampling fractions cancels out in the calculation of the population odds ratio, which in turn approximates the population relative risk. This so-called "rare disease assumption" has been repeated in most of the classic epidemiologic textbooks, although there are circumstances where it is not really needed to estimate parameters of real interest. For example, in a matched case-control study where controls are sampled from the population at risk at the age at which each case occurs, the odds ratio is an exact estimator of the hazard ratio (Miettinen, 1976; Greenland and Thomas, 1982; Sheehe, 1962; Prentice and Breslow, 1978). Although matched case-control studies do not allow the main effects of the matching factors to be estimated, one can still study variation in exposure-disease odds ratio across levels of the matching variables (Section 2.3.3).

Most epidemiologic papers present key results in terms of categorical exposure variables. For unmatched case-control studies, this is easily done by means of a simple $2 \times K$ contingency table of counts, where $K \geq 2$ is the number of categories of the exposure variable. Effect estimates are then provided in the form of odds ratios, $OR_k = (n_{1k}n_{00})/(n_{0k}n_{10})$ with estimated variance of $\log(OR) = 1/n_{1k} + 1/n_{00} + 1/n_{0k} + 1/n_{10}$, where the first subscript indexes case-control status and the second indexes the exposure categories. In the 1:1 matched design with a binary exposure, the McNemar odds ratio is given by m_{10}/m_{01} with estimated variance of $\log(OR) = 1/m_{10} + 1/m_{01}$, where m_{10} is the number of pairs in which the case, but not the control, is exposed and m_{01} is the number of pairs with the control exposed but not the case. Closed form expressions for multiple controls or multi-level exposure categories are not available for matched studies, so maximum likelihood methods (Section 2.3.2) must be used instead. For unmatched, but stratified, case-control studies, the Mantel-Haenszel estimator of the odds ratio

$$OR_k = \frac{\sum_s n_{1ks}n_{00s}/n_{++s}}{\sum_s n_{10s}n_{0ks}/n_{++s}}$$

can be used, where s indexes the confounder strata, but its variance is more complex (Robins *et al.*, 1986). Again, maximum likelihood methods are more widely used.

2.3.2 Logistic regression

The logistic model for disease is given by

$$\text{logit}\,\{P(D = 1|\boldsymbol{x})\} = \alpha + \boldsymbol{x}^{\mathrm{T}}\boldsymbol{\beta},$$

where D denotes disease status ($D = 1$ for case, $D = 0$ for a control), $\boldsymbol{x}$ denotes a vector or risk factors, $\boldsymbol{\beta}$ a corresponding vector of regression coefficients (the log of their corresponding odds ratios), and $\text{logit}(p) = \log[p/(1 - p)]$. This can be written equivalently as

$$P(D = 1|\boldsymbol{x}) = \text{expit}(\alpha + \boldsymbol{x}^{\mathrm{T}}\boldsymbol{\beta}),$$

where $\text{expit}(x) = e^x/(1 + e^x)$. The model can be fitted to either cohort or case-control data by maximizing the likelihood

$$L(\alpha, \boldsymbol{\beta}) = \prod_{i=1}^{n} P(D_i \,|\, \boldsymbol{x}_i, \alpha, \boldsymbol{\beta}) = \prod_{i=1}^{n} \frac{e^{D_i(\alpha+\boldsymbol{x}_i^{\mathrm{T}}\boldsymbol{\beta})}}{1 + e^{\alpha+\boldsymbol{x}_i^{\mathrm{T}}\boldsymbol{\beta}}}.$$

The only difference between the two settings is that in a cohort study the intercept term α estimates the logit of the "baseline risk" (the risk to an individual with $\boldsymbol{x} = 0$), but in a case-control study it is offset by the log of the ratio of case to control sampling fractions and is usually of no particular interest. For individually matched case-control studies, the conditional likelihood is used instead:

$$L(\boldsymbol{\beta}) = \prod_{i=1}^{n} P(D_{i0} \,|\, \sum_j D_{ij} = 1, \{\boldsymbol{x}_{ij}\}, \boldsymbol{\beta}) = \prod_{i=1}^{n} \frac{e^{\boldsymbol{x}_{i0}^{\mathrm{T}}\boldsymbol{\beta}}}{\sum_{j=0}^{J} e^{\boldsymbol{x}_{ij}^{\mathrm{T}}\boldsymbol{\beta}}},$$

where the second subscript j indexes the members of matched set i, with $j = 0$ denoting the case and $j = 1, \ldots, J$ the matched controls. Note that no intercept term is needed in the conditional likelihood, as it cancels out even if each matched set were to have a different baseline risk. Maximum likelihood estimates of β can be found by an iterative search algorithm like the Newton-Raphson method. Significance tests and confidence intervals are based on standard theory for maximum likelihood (Cox and Hinkley, 1974), e.g., likelihood-ratio, score, and Wald tests for significance, inverse information for variance estimation.

2.3.3 Main effects, confounding, interactions

Logistic regression provides a flexible framework for modeling complex determinants of disease risk in either case-control or cohort studies. Multiple exposure variables can be included in the x vector and the corresponding components of β have the interpretation of the log relative risks adjusted for the other variables in the model. This applies as well to confounders, which can also be included in the x vector. For continuous exposure variables, β estimates the change in the log odds ratio per unit change of the covariate (the slope of its dose-response relationship on a logit scale). For very strong risk factors, one might want to add quadratic or other terms to the model to allow for nonlinearities on a log scale. Interactions ("effect modification" in epidemiologic parlance) can be tested by including products of main effect variables, with the corresponding regression coefficient having the interpretation of the log of the ratio of relative risks for one variable across the levels of the other. For example for the binary variables x_1 and x_2, the logit is $\alpha + \beta_1 x_1 + \beta_2 x_2 + \beta_{12} x_1 x_2$, and the interaction is

$$\beta_{12} = \log\left(\frac{OR(D, x_1 \mid x_2 = 1)}{OR(D, x_1 \mid x_2 = 0)}\right) = \log\left(\frac{OR(D, x_2 \mid x_1 = 1)}{OR(D, x_2 \mid x_1 = 0)}\right).$$

Interaction can be similarly defined for continuous variables, so that the interaction regression coefficient estimates the change in the slope of the logit dose-response curve of one variable per unit change of the other (or vice versa).

The logistic model is widely used because of its flexibility, attractive statistical properties, and readily available software. There is nothing biological about the form of the model, however. While many risk factors show monotonic gradients that can be at least roughly approximated by a logistic curve and multiple risk factors or confounders may tend to show roughly multiplicative joint effects on disease risk (or additivity on the logit scale), there is no guarantee that this is true. It therefore behooves the analyst to carefully assess the fit of the model, adding additional terms or transforming variables as needed, as in any other statistical analysis. Chapter 11 describes a number of nonstandard relative risk (or relative odds) functions that can be fit to case-control data. In some circumstances, more flexible models such as a generalized additive model (Hastie and Tibshirani, 1990) or splines (de Boor, 1978) might be used to model the relative risks. For models with latent variables, the probit model (Albert and Chib, 1993) may be more attractive, as it allows a closed-form expression for the marginal risk, which is not possible for the logistic model.

The dependence of disease risk on past exposures can be quite complex, with exposures at different ages or times prior to disease having different effects. Dose rate and duration of exposure can also modify the dose-response relationship. Such effects have been studied in detail for tobacco smoking (Lubin *et al.*, 2007), although there are many other examples in the radiation and occupational epidemiology literatures. See Thomas (1988) and Thomas (2009, chapter 6) for extensive discussions of approaches to modeling exposure-time-response relationships.

2.4   Designs for sub-sampling a well-defined cohort

In a cohort study, the base population from which cases arise is explicit. One of the major expenses of a cohort study is assembling the exposure information on the entire cohort. This may not be necessary if only a small portion of the cohort will develop the disease. For example, in an occupational study, obtaining exposure information on a large cohort can be very expensive. To minimize these costs, an efficient compromise can be to obtain this information only on the cases and a random sample of the rest of the cohort. There are two principal variants of this idea, the case-cohort and nested case-control designs, as well as numerous variations of these that are discussed in greater detail in Parts III and IV.

2.4.1   Case-cohort design

The basic idea of case-base sampling was first introduced by Mantel (1973), who proposed that controls (the "subcohort") be sampled at random from the entire cohort at the time of enrollment, irrespective of whether or not they later became cases; the analysis then compares the cases as a group to the controls. Thus, some cases will appear in the subcohort, and some outside it, but all cases are used. The original case-base design (Kupper *et al.*, 1975; Miettinen, 1982, 1985; Flanders *et al.*, 1990; Langholz and Goldstein, 2001) uses standard methods for estimating risk ratios (rather than rate ratios), with an adjustment to the variance to allow for the overlap between subjects appearing both as cases and as controls. This basic idea was later refined by Prentice (1986) in the case-cohort design to allow for censoring by estimating rate ratios using the Cox regression model. Key requirements are that baseline data and specimens need to be stored (but not analyzed) on all cohort members, and outcome data, such as time to disease and duration of follow-up, is needed for all members of the cohort. The main advantage of case-base sampling (with either analysis) is that the same control group can be used for comparison with different disease outcomes. Another potential advantage is that baseline data on the subcohort can be processed early in the study while the cases are accumulating (for example, occupational exposure records before baseline can be summarized and serum biomarkers of exposure could be measured for controls without waiting to see who will become cases). However, to control for temporal variation in laboratory assays, it may be preferable to analyze the cases and subcohort specimens at the same time, although it may still be necessary to allow for differences in the length of time specimens have been stored. The main disadvantages of case-base sampling are that a more complex analysis is required, and this design can be less efficient than a nested case-control design for studies of long duration with many small strata (Langholz and Thomas, 1990).

2.4.2   Nested case-control design

In the nested case-control design (Liddell *et al.*, 1977), controls are individually matched to each case by random sampling from the set of subjects who were at risk at the time that the case was diagnosed; the data are then analyzed as a matched case-control study. In this scheme, it is possible for a subject to be sampled as a control for more than one case, and for a case to serve as a control for an earlier case. This leads to unbiased estimation of the relative risk parameter. Excluding cases from eligibility to serve as controls for other cases (Hogue *et al.*, 1983) leads to a bias away from the null (Greenland *et al.*, 1986).

2.4.3   Two-phase designs

Sometimes data on crude measurements of exposure (e.g., smoker yes/no) or confounders are available on all the cases and controls ("phase 1 sample"), but it is expensive to get refined measurements. The two-phase case-control design (White, 1982) collects refined data on exposure, confounders, or modifiers in a subset ("phase 2") of the cases and controls chosen to take advantage of the crude measurements and have good power to detect main effects or interactions with the refined exposure (Breslow and Chatterjee, 1999). These designs entail independent subsampling within categories defined both by disease status and by categories of the crude exposure/covariate variables from phase 1, an approach that at face value would seem to violate the basic design principle that cases and controls be sampled independently of their exposure status. Data from both phases are combined in the analysis, with appropriate allowance for the biased sampling in phase 2. The optimal design entails over-representing the rarer cells, typically the exposed cases. Although most applications have focused on its use for improving exposure characterization for main effects or for better control of confounding, the two-phase design can also be highly efficient for studying interactions. For example, Li *et al.* (2000) used a two-phase design nested within the Atherosclerosis Risk in Communities (ARIC) study to estimate the interaction between GSTM1/GSTT1 and cigarette smoking on the risk of coronary heart disease. Their sampling scheme was not fully efficient for addressing this particular question because it stratified only on intima media thickness, not smoking, subsampled only the controls, and did not exploit the information from the original cohort in the analysis. Re-analyses of other data from the ARIC study (Breslow *et al.*, 2009) demonstrated the considerable improvement in efficiency that can be obtained by using the full cohort (crude) information. These designs are discussed further in Chapter 17 of this book.

2.4.4   Counter-matching

Counter-matching (Langholz and Goldstein, 1996) is essentially a matched variant of the two-phase design. Here one or more controls are selected for each case by systematically mismatching them to cases on the exposure surrogate variable available from phase I, such that each matched set contains the same number of exposed individuals. For example, a study of second (contralateral) breast cancers in relation to radiotherapy and DNA damage repair genes (Bernstein *et al.*, 2004) counter-matched each case to two controls with unilateral breast cancer, such that each matched set contained two subjects who had been treated by radiotherapy. Radiation doses to each quadrant of the contralateral breast were then estimated and DNA was obtained for genotyping candidate DNA repair genes and for a genome-wide association study. Considerable gains in power can be obtained compared to conventional nested case-control designs, both for main effects and for interactions. For gene-environment interactions, Andrieu *et al.* (2001) showed that a design that counter-matches on surrogates of both exposure and genotype was more powerful than conventional nested case-control studies or designs counter-matched on just one of these factors using the same number of controls per case.

2.4.5   Case-only, case-crossover, case-specular designs

Other nontraditional designs include the case-only design for gene-environment interactions (Section 2.5.3 and Chapter 24 in this book), the case-crossover design for studying short-term effects of time-varying exposures (Maclure, 1991), and the case-specular design for spatially varying exposures (Zaffanella *et al.*, 1998). These designs typically do not entail enrolling unaffected subjects as actual controls but use some aspect of the cases' own histories as controls. Thus, the case-only design relies on an assumption that genes and environments are independently distributed in the source population, while the case-crossover design compares the exposure of the case at the etiologically-relevant time to the same subject's exposure at some other time, and the case-specular design compares the exposure at the case's location to that at some other comparable location. The latter design has been used, for example, to compare radiation doses at the exact location of a tumor to the dose at other locations in the same organ (Cardis *et al.*, 2007; Langholz *et al.*, 2009), or the magnetic field strength at subject's homes to that at comparable locations that may not correspond to actual people's homes (Zaffanella *et al.*, 1998).

2.5 Case-control studies of genetics

Although each area of application has its own challenges, the field of genetics has spawned quite a number of unique developments. In this section, I briefly review some of these design and analysis issues to introduce the reader to the more detailed material in Part V of this book. I begin with a discussion of some family-based designs aimed at avoiding the problem of confounding by population substructure that can arise in traditional case-control designs with unrelated cases and controls. These issues are the same whether one is studying a single candidate gene or the entire genome. I then briefly introduce some approaches to genome-wide studies, including the problems of analyzing ultra high-dimensional data. I conclude with a discussion of gene-environment interactions and mediation of genetic and environmental factors through biomarkers of internal biological processes.

2.5.1 Family-based designs

The problem of population stratification refers to variation in genotype distributions across subpopulations with different ancestral origins. If these subpopulations also have differing disease risks for reasons apart from the genotypes, confounding of the association of disease with genotypes can result. These subpopulations may not be readily identifiable by self-report. Some studies have asked about race and/or ethnic origins of subjects' parents and grandparents, but not only is this information often inaccurate, it can also be particularly challenging for multi-racial subjects. Failure to account for population stratification can lead to both uncontrolled confounding and over-dispersion of test statistics, so that conventional significance tests will have size above the nominal significance level. For genome-wide association studies, a variety of statistical adjustment procedures have been developed under the general heading of "genomic control" (Section 2.5.2). Family-based designs completely avoid the problem by making comparisons within each family, as the offspring all have identical ancestral origins. There are two main variants of this design, one using unaffected relatives as controls and one relying on gene transmissions from parents to offspring.

The simplest of these designs is a case-sibling study, in which unaffected siblings of a case are treated as matched controls using a standard matched analysis. If only a single case and a single control per family are included, no special analysis issues arise, but if multiple cases or multiple controls are selected from the same family, the possible permutations of disease status against genotypes are not equally likely under the null hypothesis that the gene is not itself causal but is linked to a causal gene (Curtis, 1997), requiring the use of a robust variance estimator (Siegmund *et al.*, 2000). Unaffected cousins or other relatives could also be used as controls, but because they could have somewhat different ancestries, the control of population stratification is less complete than when using siblings. The main argument against using family members as controls is that they are more likely to have the same genotype as the case than are unrelated individuals. This "overmatching" results in loss of power, compared to using unrelated controls, although family-based designs can be more powerful for testing gene-environment interactions (Witte *et al.*, 1999).

The case-parent-triad basic design use genotype information from both parents and an affected child (case). This design can be thought of as a matched case-control study that compares the genotype of the case to those of hypothetical siblings that inherited the other possible genotypes from the parents. Thus the controls are "pseudo-sibs," rather than real siblings. For an additive genetic effect (a log relative risk that is a linear function of the number of variant alleles), the "transmission disequilibrium test" (Spielman *et al.*, 1993) is simply a McNemar test of the number of alleles transmitted from heterozygous parents to affected offspring compared with those not transmitted; for dominant or recessive models or for gene-environment interactions, conditional logistic regression can be used. The case-parent-triad design is generally more powerful than the case-sibling design per case, but requires three people to be genotyped per case, and enrolling complete triads can be difficult in practice.

2.5.2   Genome-wide association studies

Against a background of disappointing results from candidate gene studies, Risch and Merikangas (1996) suggested that it might soon be technically possible to test associations with the entire genome, relying on the phenomenon of linkage disequilibrium so that one need only genotype a subset of markers that are strongly correlated with the remaining common variants. The first such "genome-wide association studies" (GWAS) were published less than a decade later, using high-density genotyping arrays of single nucleotide polymorphisms (SNPs) selected based on the International Haplotype Mapping (HapMap) project. Since then, technological advances have dramatically increased the coverage of genotyping panels (now typically in the millions of variants) and lowered their costs, allowing thousands of studies to be done that have reported associations of thousands of SNPs with hundreds of diseases (Welter *et al.*, 2014). The vast majority of these associations would not have been contemplated as a priori hypotheses; indeed, most have not been with variants that alter the protein coding sequence of genes, but rather are located in regulatory regions of the genome, often previously thought of as "junk DNA." In the aggregate, however, they still account for only a small fraction of the presumed heritability of most chronic diseases estimated from family or twin studies (Gusev *et al.*, 2013). Furthermore, by the design of the genotyping platforms, such GWASs are limited to common variants (typically defined as those with minor allele frequencies $> 5\%$). Next generation sequencing platforms offer the prospect of truly genome-wide scans of all genetic variants, common or rare (Casey *et al.*, 2013), but with a total of about 3.3 billion base pairs in the human genome, of which at least 50 million vary across individuals, the problems of multiple comparisons and sparse data are daunting.

Two issues worth addressing are efficient study design for GWASs and analytical approaches to deal with the problem of population stratification. The traditional case-control design using unrelated controls has been the most widely used, as it is relatively easy to enroll the vast numbers of subjects needed to attain the level of genome-wide significance ($p < 5 \times 10^{-8}$ to allow for about a million effectively independent tests). For greater power, various groups have combined their data into large consortia, often involving tens of thousands of cases and controls, using meta-analysis of single-SNP summary statistics. For greater power in the face of multiple comparisons, two-stage or multi-stage designs have been widely used (Thomas *et al.*, 2009). Originally proposed by Satagopan and Elston (2003), a first sample is used for scanning associations with a large number of variables (e.g., millions of SNPs) and then a subset of the most promising of these are tested in a second, independent sample. This greatly reduces the multiple-testing penalty, thereby improving power. Statistical significance is determined in a joint analysis of the combined samples, with appropriate allowance for the staged testing. (Note that these two-stage designs are fundamentally different from the two-phase designs described earlier (Section 2.4.3), where the second phase is a stratified subsample of the first phase subjects rather than an independent sample.)

High-density genotyping panels also provide a way of addressing the problem of population stratification mentioned above by using a large number of markers to infer each individual's ancestral origins. The first approach proposed simply used the distribution of association test statistics to estimate an empirical null distribution allowing for over-dispersion (Devlin *et al.*, 2001), but more recently, methods using Bayesian clustering (Pritchard *et al.*, 2000), principal components (Price *et al.*, 2006), or mixed models (Yu *et al.*, 2005) have become more popular methods to control for population stratification. In admixed populations like African-Americans or Hispanics, the use of targeted panels of ancestry informative markers (Tian *et al.*, 2008) may be more efficient, but for most purposes, a subset of the same panel of GWAS markers (usually winnowed out to eliminate those in high correlation with each other) can be quite effective for use in these methods.

2.5.3   Gene-environment interactions

A portion of complex disease risk is probably due to the interaction of inherited genetic and environmental factors (G × E) (Manolio *et al.*, 2009; Thomas, 2010). To date, few such interactions have been found in population-based studies, however. Even for studying a priori hypotheses about specific exposures and specific genes, large sample sizes and accurate measurements of exposures, genes, and diseases are essential.

An attractive design specific to G × E studies is the case-only design that relies on an assumption of gene-environment independence in the source population in lieu of controls (Piegorsch *et al.*, 1994). Thus, the odds ratio for association between genotype and exposure in cases estimates the multiplicative interaction odds ratio from a case-control design, but with greater precision as the assumption that the population OR = 1 replaces the estimation of that association from controls. Of course, the validity of the approach depends critically on that independence assumption, and one cannot simply test that assumption in controls first to decide whether to use the case-only or case-control estimator of the interaction, as these two steps would not be independent (Albert *et al.*, 2001). However, empirical Bayes compromises between case-only and case-control estimators have been developed that offer the power advantage of the former and the robustness of the latter (Li and Conti, 2009; Mukherjee *et al.*, 2012). Alternatively, the full case-control data set can be analyzed under the assumption of G-E independence for greater power (Chatterjee and Carroll, 2005). Two-step methods (Hsu *et al.*, 2012; Gauderman *et al.*, 2013) also rely on exploiting G-E association or G-D marginal association in a first step for conducting genome-wide interaction studies (GWIS) with environmental factors one at a time.

2.5.4   Mediation by biomarkers

The previous sections have focused exclusively on germline variation, but this is just one of numerous high-dimensional "omics" technologies that are emerging: epigenomics, transcriptomics, metabolomics, proteomics, to name just a few. These have the potential to shed light on fundamental biological processes mediating the effects of genes and the environment on disease risks. Statistical methods here are in their infancy, with most of the work so far being focused on the relationship of these "omics" either to disease risk or treatment outcomes or to the factors influencing them, like environmental exposures. Nevertheless, there is a growing interest in using techniques like causal mediation analysis (Imai *et al.*, 2010; Pearl, 2014) to study the whole process. For example, in the genetics realm, Huang (2015) and Huang *et al.* (2015) have used this approach to model the pathway from germline variation through epigenetics to gene expression and ultimately to disease, while in the environmental realm Bind *et al.* (2016) have used it to model a pathway from air pollution exposure through methylation to ICAM-1 protein levels (a marker of systemic inflammation). Both of these applications relied on longitudinal data, so it is unclear exactly how useful case-control studies will be for mediation because of the importance of establishing the temporal sequence of effects. However, nested case-control studies within biobanks that have multiple stored biospecimens over extended periods of time may provide a way forward.

Establishing the causality of biomarkers (or more precisely, of the underlying biological processes for which they are surrogate measures) requires careful thought because of the potential for uncontrolled confounding and reverse causation. One approach that has been particularly useful is the technique of Mendelian randomization (Davey Smith and Ebrahim, 2003). This is essentially an instrumental variables technique (Greenland, 2000) that uses a gene as a predictor of the biomarker, thereby allowing a test of the causal effect of the biomarker on disease by instead testing for an association between the gene and disease (and between the gene and biomarker). Obviously genes are not influenced by disease, so reverse causation is not an issue. The method relies on the assumption that genes are transmitted at random from parents to offspring and hence are unconfounded (at least within ancestrally homogeneous populations) and on the assumption that the gene has no independent effect on disease ("pleiotropy") other than through the biomarker (Didelez and Sheehan, 2007). These assumptions have not always been carefully validated in applications, but the approach has become an active area of methodological research. For example, Bowden *et al.* (2016) have shown how median estimation can provide efficient and unbiased estimates even if some markers violate the no-pleiotropy assumption but at least half do not; this situation seems likely to hold in GWAS applications. Nevertheless, most genes are only weak instrumental variables, so enormous sample sizes may be needed for precise estimation, and the approach does not provide a clear means of hypothesis testing.

2.6   Inferring causation

Epidemiologists have developed a series of criteria for judging when an inference of causality is warranted from an observed association, of which the most famous are those outlined by Sir Austin Bradford Hill (Bradford Hill, 1965), as described in most epidemiology textbooks: dose-response, temporal sequence, strength, lack of other explanations, consistency across multiple studies, coherence across types of evidence, etc. For the 24th annual Bradford Hill Lecture at the London School of Hygiene & Tropical Medicine, Ioannidis (2016) provided a provocative critique of these criteria, based on his extensive experience in meta-analysis and concluded that experiment and consistency (replication) were the most important, and the temporal sequence was also useful where it could be operationalized; he argued that the other six criteria were either difficult to operationalize, not predictive of causality, or even detrimental. As noted earlier, for a relationship to be causal, exposure must precede disease. This is particularly important in case-control studies to avoid "recall bias" or "reverse causation" (the disease or its treatment influencing exposure rather than exposure causing disease). There is a rapidly growing literature on methods of causal inference. Chapter 6 of this book reviews these concepts and identifies special causal issues for case-control studies.

Ultimately, however, the causal nature of an association is best assessed by controlled experiments, and, where possible, by a randomized controlled trial of a well-defined intervention.

2.7   Future directions

The case-control design has been around for well over a half a century and is one of the major workhorses of epidemiology. It was influential, for example, in establishing smoking as the major cause of lung cancer (Cornfield *et al.*, 1959). The methodology – both design and analysis – is thus well established, although it continues to be refined, as in the emergence of various hybrid designs. More recently, genetics and especially the development of GWASs have provided an impetus for further extensions of the approach. Such developments will doubtless continue to meet the needs of other "omics" studies. For example, there has been growing interest in using similar design and analysis approaches for conducting "environment-wide association studies" (EWAS) (Patel *et al.*, 2010) using high-density metabolomic methods to assay the "exposome" (Wild, 2012) in a manner analogous to the genome. A major challenge here is disentangling the effects of complex mixtures (Dominici *et al.*, 2010), for which a variety of statistical methods have been developed (Billionnet *et al.*, 2012; Sun *et al.*, 2013; Davalos *et al.*, 2017). The kinds of techniques described above (Section 2.5.3) for GWIS may ultimately make it feasible to test for gene-environment-wide interactions across the entire genome and "exposome" (Khoury and Wacholder, 2009; Thomas, 2010; Thomas *et al.*, 2012). However, in conducting such studies, it is important to keep in mind the basic principles underlying the case-control design and to take measures to minimize potentially misleading results from confounding, selection bias, information bias, insufficient power or precision, and misleading inference from multiple comparisons.

Bibliography

Albert, J. H. and Chib, S. (1993). Bayesian analysis of binary and polychotomous response data. *Journal of the American Statistical Association*, **88**, 669–679.

Albert, P. S., Ratnasinghe, D., Tangrea, J., and Wacholder, S. (2001). Limitations of the case-only design for identifying gene-environment interactions. *American Journal of Epidemiology*, **154**, 687–693.

Andrieu, N., Goldstein, A. M., Thomas, D. C., and Langholz, B. (2001). Counter-matching in studies of gene-environment interaction: Efficiency and feasibility. *American Journal of Epidemiology*, **153**, 265–274.

Armstrong, B. G., Whittemore, A. S., and Howe, G. R. (1989). Analysis of case-control data with covariate measurement error: Application to diet and colon cancer. *Statistics in Medicine*, **8**, 1151–1163. Discussion 1165–1166.

Austin, H., Flanders, W. D., and Rothman, K. J. (1989). Bias arising in case-control studies from selection of controls from overlapping groups. *International Journal of Epidemiology*, **18**, 713–716.

Bernstein, J. L., Langholz, B., Haile, R. W., Bernstein, L., Thomas, D. C., Stovall, M.,

Malone, K. E., Lynch, C. F., Olsen, J. H., Anton-Culver, H., Shore, R. E., Boice, Jr., J. D., Berkowitz, G. S., Gatti, R. A., Teitelbaum, S. L., Smith, S. A., Rosenstein, B. S., Børresen-Dale, A. L., Concannon, P., and Thompson, W. D. (2004). Study design: Evaluating gene-environment interactions in the etiology of breast cancer - the WECARE study. *Breast Cancer Research*, **6**, R199–214.

Billionnet, C., Sherrill, D., and Annesi-Maesano, I. (2012). Estimating the health effects of exposure to multi-pollutant mixture. *Annals of Epidemiology*, **22**, 126–141.

Bind, M. A., Vanderweele, T. J., Coull, B. A., and Schwartz, J. D. (2016). Causal mediation analysis for longitudinal data with exogenous exposure. *Biostatistics*, **17**, 122–134.

Bowden, J., Davey Smith, G., Haycock, P., and Burgess, S. (2016). Consistent estimation in Mendelian randomization with some invalid instruments using a weighted median estimator. *Genetic Epidemiology*, **40**, 304–314.

Bradford Hill, A. (1965). The environment and disease: Association or causation? *Journal of the Royal Society of Medicine*, **58**, 295–300.

Breslow, N. E. and Chatterjee, N. (1999). Design and analysis of two-phase studies with binary outcome applied to Wilms tumor prognosis. *Journal of the Royal Statistical Society: Series C (Applied Statistics)*, **48**, 457–468.

Breslow, N. E., Lumley, T., Ballantyne, C. M., Chambless, L. E., and Kulich, M. (2009). Using the whole cohort in the analysis of case-cohort data. *American Journal of Epidemiology*, **169**, 1398–1405.

Cardis, E., Richardson, L., Deltour, I., Armstrong, B., Feychting, M., Johansen, C., Kilkenny, M., McKinney, P., Modan, B., Sadetzki, S., Schuz, J., Swerdlow, A., Vrijheid, M., Auvinen, A., Berg, G., Blettner, M., Bowman, J., Brown, J., Chetrit, A., Christensen, H. C., Cook, A., Hepworth, S., Giles, G., Hours, M., Iavarone, I., Jarus-Hakak, A., Klaeboe, L., Krewski, D., Lagorio, S., Lonn, S., Mann, S., McBride, M., Muir, K., Nadon, L., Parent, M. E., Pearce, N., Salminen, T., Schoemaker, M., Schlehofer, B., Siemiatycki, J., Taki, M., Takebayashi, T., Tynes, T., van Tongeren, M., Vecchia, P., Wiart, J., Woodward, A., and Yamaguchi, N. (2007). The interphone study: Design, epidemiological methods, and description of the study population. *European Journal of Epidemiology*, **22**, 647–664.

Carroll, R. J., Ruppert, D., Stefanski, L. A., and Crainiceanu, C. M. (2006). *Measurement Error in Nonlinear Models: A Modern Perspective*. Chapman & Hall/CRC Press, Boca Raton, FL, 2nd edition.

Casey, G., Conti, D., Haile, R., and Duggan, D. (2013). Next generation sequencing and a new era of medicine. *Gut*, **62**, 920–932.

Chatterjee, N. and Carroll, R. J. (2005). Semiparametric maximum likelihood estimation exploiting gene-environment independence in case-control studies. *Biometrika*, **92**, 399–418.

Cologne, J. B. and Shibata, Y. (1995). Optimal case-control matching in practice. *Epidemiology*, **6**, 271–275.

Cornfield, J. (1951). A method of estimating comparative rates from clinical data. Applications to cancer of the lung, breast, and cervix. *Journal of the National Cancer Institute*, **11**, 1269–1275.

Cornfield, J., Haenszel, W., Hammond, E. C., Lilienfeld, A. M., Shimkin, M. B., and Wynder, E. L. (1959). Smoking and lung cancer: Recent evidence and a discussion of some questions. *Journal of the National Cancer Institute*, **22**, 173–203.

Cox, D. R. and Hinkley, D. V. (1974). *Theoretical Statistics*. Chapman & Hall, London.

Curtis, D. (1997). Use of siblings as controls in case-control association studies. *Annals of Human Genetics*, **61**, 319–333.

Davalos, A. D., Luben, T. J., Herring, A. H., and Sacks, J. D. (2017). Current approaches used in epidemiologic studies to examine short-term multipollutant air pollution exposures. *Annals of Epidemiology*, **27**, 145–153.e1.

Davey Smith, G. and Ebrahim, S. (2003). 'Mendelian randomization': Can genetic epidemiology contribute to understanding environmental determinants of disease? *International Journal of Epidemiology*, **32**, 1–22.

Day, N. E., Byar, D. P., and Green, S. B. (1980). Overadjustment in case-control studies. *American Journal of Epidemiology*, **112**, 696–706.

de Boor, C. (1978). *A Practical Guide to Splines*. Springer-Verlag, New York.

Devlin, B., Roeder, K., and Wasserman, L. (2001). Genomic control, a new approach to genetic-based association studies. *Theoretical Population Biology*, **60**, 155–160.

Didelez, V. and Sheehan, N. (2007). Mendelian randomization as an instrumental variable approach to causal inference. *Statistical Methods in Medical Research*, **16**, 309–330.

Dominici, F., Peng, R. D., Barr, C. D., and Bell, M. L. (2010). Protecting human health from air pollution: Shifting from a single-pollutant to a multipollutant approach. *Epidemiology*, **21**, 187–194.

Flanders, W. D. and Austin, H. (1986). Possibility of selection bias in matched case-control studies using friend controls. *American Journal of Epidemiology*, **124**, 150–153.

Flanders, W. D., DerSimonian, R., and Rhodes, P. (1990). Estimation of risk ratios in case-base studies with competing risks. *Statistics in Medicine*, **9**, 423–435.

Gauderman, W. J., Zhang, P., Morrison, J. L., and Lewinger, J. P. (2013). Finding novel genes by testing G x E interactions in a genome-wide association study. *Genetic Epidemiology*, **37**, 603–613.

Gordis, L. (1982). Should dead cases be matched to dead controls? *American Journal of Epidemiology*, **115**, 1–5.

Greenland, S. (1980). The effect of misclassification in the presence of covariates. *American Journal of Epidemiology*, **112**, 564–569.

Greenland, S. (1988). Statistical uncertainty due to misclassification: Implications for validation substudies. *Journal of Clinical Epidemiology*, **41**, 1167–1174.

Greenland, S. (1990). Randomization, statistics, and causal inference. *Epidemiology*, **1**, 421–429.

Greenland, S. (2000). An introduction to instrumental variables for epidemiologists. *International Journal of Epidemiology*, **29**, 722–729.

Greenland, S. and Robins, J. M. (1985). Confounding and misclassification. *American Journal of Epidemiology*, **122**, 495–506.

Greenland, S. and Thomas, D. C. (1982). On the need for the rare disease assumption in case-control studies. *American Journal of Epidemiology*, **116**, 547–553.

Greenland, S., Thomas, D. C., and Morgenstern, H. (1986). The rare-disease assumption revisited. A critique of "estimators of relative risk for case-control studies". *American Journal of Epidemiology*, **124**, 869–883.

Gusev, A., Bhatia, G., Zaitlen, N., Vilhjalmsson, B. J., Diogo, D., Stahl, E. A., Gregersen, P. K., Worthington, J., Klareskog, L., Raychaudhuri, S., Plenge, R. M., Pasaniuc, B., and Price, A. L. (2013). Quantifying missing heritability at known GWAS loci. *PLoS Genetics*, **9**, e1003993.

Hastie, T. and Tibshirani, R. (1990). *Generalized Additive Models*. Chapman & Hall, London.

Hogue, C. J., Gaylor, D. W., and Schulz, K. F. (1983). Estimators of relative risk for case-control studies. *American Journal of Epidemiology*, **118**, 396–407.

Hsu, L., Jiao, S., Dai, J. Y., Hutter, C., Peters, U., and Kooperberg, C. (2012). Powerful cocktail methods for detecting genome-wide gene-environment interaction. *Genetic Epidemiology*, **36**, 183–194.

Huang, Y.-T. (2015). Integrative modeling of multi-platform genomic data under the framework of mediation analysis. *Statistics in Medicine*, **34**, 162–178.

Huang, Y.-T., Liang, L., Moffatt, M. F., Cookson, W. O., and Lin, X. (2015). iGWAS: Integrative genome-wide association studies of genetic and genomic data for disease susceptibility using mediation analysis. *Genetic Epidemiology*, **39**, 347–356.

Imai, K., Keele, L., and Tingley, D. (2010). A general approach to causal mediation analysis. *Psychological Methods*, **15**, 309–334.

Ioannidis, J. P. A. (2016). Exposure-wide epidemiology: Revisiting Bradford Hill. *Statistics in Medicine*, **35**, 1749–1762.

Kaplan, S., Novikov, I., and Modan, B. (1998). A methodological note on the selection of friends as controls. *International Journal of Epidemiology*, **27**, 727–729.

Kempf, A. M. and Remington, P. L. (2007). New challenges for telephone survey research in the twenty-first century. *Annual Review of Public Health*, **28**, 113–126.

Khoury, M. J. and Wacholder, S. (2009). Invited commentary: From genome-wide association studies to gene-environment-wide interaction studies – challenges and opportunities. *American Journal of Epidemiology*, **169**, 227–230. Discussion 234–235.

Kupper, L. L., McMichael, A. J., and Spirtas, R. (1975). A hybrid epidemiologic study design useful in estimating relative risk. *Journal of the American Statistical Association*, **70**, 524–528.

Langholz, B. and Goldstein, L. (1996). Risk set sampling in epidemiologic cohort studies. *Statistical Science*, **11**, 35–53.

Langholz, B. and Goldstein, L. (2001). Conditional logistic analysis of case-control studies with complex sampling. *Biostatistics*, **2**, 63–84.

Langholz, B. and Thomas, D. C. (1990). Nested case-control and case-cohort sampling: A critical comparison. *American Journal of Epidemiology*, **131**, 169–176.

Langholz, B., Thomas, D. C., Stovall, M., Smith, S. A., Boice, Jr., J. D., Shore, R. E., Bernstein, L., Lynch, C. F., Zhang, X., and Bernstein, J. L. (2009). Statistical methods for analysis of radiation effects with tumor and dose location-specific information with application to the WECARE study of asynchronous contralateral breast cancer. *Biometrics*, **65**, 599–608.

Li, D. and Conti, D. V. (2009). Detecting gene-environment interactions using a combined case-only and case-control approach. *American Journal of Epidemiology*, **169**, 497–504.

Li, R., Boerwinkle, E., Olshan, A. F., Chambless, L. E., Pankow, J. S., Tyroler, H. A., Bray, M., Pittman, G. S., Bell, D. A., and Heiss, G. (2000). Glutathione S-transferase genotype as a susceptibility factor in smoking-related coronary heart disease. *Atherosclerosis*, **149**, 451–462.

Liddell, F. D. K., McDonald, J. C., and Thomas, D. C. (1977). Methods of cohort analysis: Appraisal by application to asbestos mining (with discussion). *Journal of the Royal Statistical Society: Series A. (Statistics in Society)*, **140**, 469–491.

Link, M. W. and Kresnow, M. J. (2006). The future of random-digit-dial surveys for injury prevention and violence research. *American Journal of Preventive Medicine*, **31**, 444–450.

Lubin, J. H., Alavanja, M. C., Caporaso, N., Brown, L. M., Brownson, R. C., Field, R. W., Garcia-Closas, M., Hartge, P., Hauptmann, M., Hayes, R. B., Kleinerman, R., Kogevinas, M., Krewski, D., Langholz, B., Letourneau, E. G., Lynch, C. F., Malats, N., Sandler, D. P., Schaffrath-Rosario, A., Schoenberg, J. B., Silverman, D. T., Wang, Z., Wichmann, H. E., Wilcox, H. B., and Zielinski, J. M. (2007). Cigarette smoking and cancer risk: Modeling total exposure and intensity. *American Journal of Epidemiology*, **166**, 479–489.

Ma, X., Buffler, P. A., Layefsky, M., Does, M. B., and Reynolds, P. (2004). Control selection strategies in case-control studies of childhood diseases. *American Journal of Epidemiology*, **159**, 915–921.

Maclure, M. (1991). The case-crossover design: A method for studying transient effects on the risk of acute events. *American Journal of Epidemiology*, **133**, 144–153.

Manolio, T. A., Collins, F. S., Cox, N. J., Goldstein, D. B., Hindorff, L. A., Hunter, D. J., McCarthy, M. I., Ramos, E. M., Cardon, L. R., Chakravarti, A., Cho, J. H., Guttmacher, A. E., Kong, A., Kruglyak, L., Mardis, E., Rotimi, C. N., Slatkin, M., Valle, D., Whittemore, A. S., Boehnke, M., Clark, A. G., Eichler, E. E., Gibson, G., Haines, J. L., Mackay, T. F., McCarroll, S. A., and Visscher, P. M. (2009). Finding the missing heritability of complex diseases. *Nature*, **461**, 747–753.

Mantel, N. (1973). Synthetic retrospective studies and related topics. *Biometrics*, **29**, 479–486.

Marchbanks, P. A., McDonald, J. A., Wilson, H. G., Burnett, N. M., Daling, J. R., Bernstein, L., Malone, K. E., Strom, B. L., Norman, S. A., Weiss, L. K., Liff, J. M., Wingo, P. A., Burkman, R. T., Folger, S. G., Berlin, J. A., Deapen, D. M., Ursin, G., Coates, R. J., Simon, M. S., Press, M. F., and Spirtas, R. (2002). The NICHD women's contraceptive and reproductive experiences study: Methods and operational results. *Annals of Epidemiology*, **12**, 213–221.

McLaughlin, J. K., Blot, W. J., Mehl, E. S., and Mandel, J. S. (1985). Problems in the use of dead controls in case-control studies: I. General results. *American Journal of Epidemiology*, **121**, 131–139.

Miettinen, O. (1976). Estimability and estimation in case-referent studies. *American Journal of Epidemiology*, **103**, 226–235.

Miettinen, O. S. (1982). Design options in epidemiology research: An update. *Scandinavian Journal of Work, Environment & Health*, **8** (Suppl 1), 1295–1311.

Miettinen, O. S. (1985). *Theoretical Epidemiology: Principles of Occurrence Research in Medicine*. John Wiley & Sons, New York.

Mukherjee, B., Ahn, J., Gruber, S. B., and Chatterjee, N. (2012). Testing gene-environment interaction in large scale case-control association studies: Possible choices and comparisons. *American Journal of Epidemiology*, **175**, 177–190.

Nelson, L. M., Longstreth, Jr., W. T., Koepsell, T. D., and van Belle, G. (1990). Proxy respondents in epidemiologic research. *Epidemiologic Reviews*, **12**, 71–86.

Patel, C. J., Bhattacharya, J., and Butte, A. J. (2010). An environment-wide association study (EWAS) on type 2 diabetes mellitus. *PLoS One*, **5**, e10746.

Pearl, J. (2014). Interpretation and identification of causal mediation. *Psychological Methods*, **19**, 459–481.

Piegorsch, W., Weinberg, C., and Taylor, J. (1994). Non-hierarchical logistic models and case-only designs for assessing susceptibility in population-based case-control studies. *Statistics in Medicine*, **13**, 153–162.

Poole, C. (1986). Exposure opportunity in case-control studies. *American Journal of Epidemiology*, **123**, 352–358.

Prentice, R. L. (1986). A case-cohort design for epidemiologic studies and disease prevention trials. *Biometrika*, **73**, 1–11.

Prentice, R. L. and Breslow, N. E. (1978). Retrospective studies and failure time models. *Biometrika*, **65**, 153–158.

Price, A. L., Patterson, N. J., Plenge, R. M., Weinblatt, M. E., Shadick, N. A., and Reich, D. (2006). Principal components analysis corrects for stratification in genome-wide association studies. *Nature Genetics*, **38**, 904–909.

Pritchard, J. K., Stephens, M., Rosenberg, N. A., and Donnelly, P. (2000). Association mapping in structured populations. *The American Journal of Human Genetics*, **67**, 170–181.

Risch, N. and Merikangas, K. (1996). The future of genetic studies of complex human diseases. *Science*, **273**, 1616–1617.

Robins, J. and Pike, M. (1990). The validity of case-control studies with nonrandom selection of controls. *Epidemiology*, **1**, 273–284.

Robins, J., Greenland, S., and Breslow, N. E. (1986). A general estimator for the variance of the Mantel-Haenszel odds ratio. *American Journal of Epidemiology*, **124**, 719–723.

Rosenbaum, P. R. (1989). Optimal matching for observational studies. *Journal of the American Statistical Association*, **84**, 1024–1032.

Rosenbaum, P. R. and Rubin, D. B. (1985). Constructing a control group using multivariate matched sampling methods that incorporate the propensity score. *The American Statistician*, **39**, 33–38.

Sackett, D. L. (1979). Bias in analytic research. *Journal of Chronic Diseases*, **32**, 51–63.

Satagopan, J. M. and Elston, R. C. (2003). Optimal two-stage genotyping in population-based association studies. *Genetic Epidemiology*, **25**, 149–157.

Shaw, G. L., Tucker, M. A., Kase, R. G., and Hoover, R. N. (1991). Problems ascertaining friend controls in a case-control study of lung cancer. *American Journal of Epidemiology*, **133**, 63–66.

Sheehe, P. R. (1962). Dynamic risk analysis in retrospective matched pair studies of disease. *Biometrics*, **18**, 323–341.

Siegmund, K. D., Langholz, B., Kraft, P., and Thomas, D. C. (2000). Testing linkage disequilibrium in sibships. *The American Journal of Human Genetics*, **67**, 244–248.

Siemiatycki, J. (1989). Friendly control bias. *Journal of Clinical Epidemiology*, **42**, 687–688.

Smith, A. H., Kark, J. D., Cassel, J. C., and Spears, G. F. S. (1977). Analysis of prospective epidemiologic studies by minimum distance case-control matching. *American Journal of Epidemiology*, **105**, 567–574.

Spiegelman, D. and Gray, R. (1991). Cost-efficient study designs for binary response data with Gaussian covariate measurement error. *Biometrics*, **47**, 851–869.

Spielman, R. S., McGinnis, R. E., and Ewens, W. J. (1993). Transmission test for linkage disequilibrium: The insulin gene region and insulin-dependent diabetes mellitus (IDDM). *The American Journal of Human Genetics*, **52**, 506–516.

Sun, Z., Tao, Y., Li, S., Ferguson, K. K., Meeker, J. D., Park, S. K., Batterman, S. A., and Mukherjee, B. (2013). Statistical strategies for constructing health risk models with multiple pollutants and their interactions: Possible choices and comparisons. *Environmental Health*, **12**, 85.

Thomas, D. (2010). Gene-environment-wide association studies: Emerging approaches. *Nature Reviews Genetics*, **11**, 259–272.

Thomas, D. C. (1988). Exposure-time-response relationships with applications to cancer epidemiology. *Annual Review of Public Health*, **9**, 451–482.

Thomas, D. C. (2009). *Statistical Methods in Environmental Epidemiology*. Oxford University Press, Oxford.

Thomas, D. C., Stram, D., and Dwyer, J. (1993). Exposure measurement error: Influence on exposure-disease relationships and methods of correction. *Annual Review of Public Health*, **14**, 69–93.

Thomas, D. C., Casey, G., Conti, D. V., Haile, R. W., Lewinger, J. P., and Stram, D. O. (2009). Methodological issues in multistage genome-wide association studies. *Statistical Science*, **24**, 414–429.

Thomas, D. C., Lewinger, J., Murcray, C. E., and Gauderman, W. J. (2012). Invited commentary: GE-Whiz! Ratcheting gene-environment studies up to the whole genome and the whole exposome. *American Journal of Epidemiology*, **175**, 203–207.

Thompson, W. D. (1990). Nonrandom yet unbiased. *Epidemiology*, **1**, 262–265.

Tian, C., Gregersen, P. K., and Seldin, M. F. (2008). Accounting for ancestry: Population substructure and genome-wide association studies. *Human Molecular Genetics*, **17**, R143–150.

Wacholder, S., McLaughlin, J. K., Silverman, D. T., and Mandel, J. S. (1992a). Selection of controls in case-control studies. I. Principles. *American Journal of Epidemiology*, **135**, 1019–1028.

Wacholder, S., Silverman, D. T., McLaughlin, J. K., and Mandel, J. S. (1992b). Selection of controls in case-control studies. II. Types of controls. *American Journal of Epidemiology*, **135**, 1029–1041.

Wacholder, S., Silverman, D. T., McLaughlin, J. K., and Mandel, J. S. (1992c). Selection of controls in case-control studies. III. Design options. *American Journal of Epidemiology*, **135**, 1042–1050.

Welter, D., MacArthur, J., Morales, J., Burdett, T., Hall, P., Junkins, H., Klemm, A., Flicek, P., Manolio, T., Hindorff, L., and Parkinson, H. (2014). The NHGRI GWAS catalog, a curated resource of SNP-trait associations. *Nucleic Acids Research*, **42**, D1001–1006.

Westreich, D. (2012). Berkson's bias, selection bias, and missing data. *Epidemiology*, **23**, 159–164.

White, J. E. (1982). A two stage design for the study of the relationship between a rare exposure and a rare disease. *American Journal of Epidemiology*, **115**, 119–128.

Wild, C. P. (2012). The exposome: From concept to utility. *International Journal of Epidemiology*, **41**, 24–32.

Witte, J. S., Gauderman, W. J., and Thomas, D. C. (1999). Asymptotic bias and efficiency in case-control studies of candidate genes and gene-environment interactions: Basic family designs. *American Journal of Epidemiology*, **148**, 693–705.

Yu, J., Pressoir, G., Briggs, W. H., Vroh Bi, I., Yamasaki, M., Doebley, J. F., McMullen, M. D., Gaut, B. S., Nielsen, D. M., Holland, J. B., Kresovich, S., and Buckler, E. S. (2005). A unified mixed-model method for association mapping that accounts for multiple levels of relatedness. *Nature Genetics*, **38**, 203–208.

Zaffanella, L., Savitz, D. A., Greenland, S., and Ebi, K. L. (1998). The residential case-specular method to study wire codes, magnetic fields, and disease. *Epidemiology*, **9**, 16–20.

Zeger, S. L., Thomas, D., Dominici, F., Samet, J. M., Schwartz, J., Dockery, D., and Cohen, A. (2000). Exposure measurement error in time-series studies of air pollution: Concepts and consequences. *Environmental Health Perspectives*, **108**, 419–26.

Part II

Classical Case-Control Studies

3

Basic Concepts and Analysis

Barbara McKnight

University of Washington

3.1 Introduction

Case-control studies examine the association between exposures or other lifestyle choices and the risk of disease. When the disease of interest is rare, the case-control study allows us to evaluate these associations using fewer subjects than a follow-up study by over-sampling cases and under-sampling controls from the population. This chapter describes logistic regression analysis of unmatched case-control data, and Chapter 4 describes logistic regression analysis of matched and frequency-matched case-control data. I begin by reviewing several measures of disease occurrence and the association of exposures to disease in the population, showing how different association measures can and cannot be estimated solely from data collected in a case-control study. Sections containing practical advice for the use of logistic regression to analyze unmatched case-control data follow.

3.2 Populations and simple case-control samples

3.2.1 Population measures of disease occurrence

The primary measure of disease occurrence in the population is the age-specific disease incidence rate. For T = the age at disease onset and T_d = the age at death, it measures the instantaneous rate at which disease occurs among living, disease-free members of the population at time t with exposure level x. It is defined by

$$\lambda_x(t) = \lim_{\Delta t \to 0} P(T \in [t, t + \Delta t) \mid T \geq t, T_d \geq t, X = x)/\Delta t.$$

Statistical methods to estimate $\lambda_x(t)$ and draw inferences about its association with putative disease risk factors x based on follow-up time-to-event data are in common use (Cox, 1972; Tanner and Wong, 1983; Yandell, 1983).

Another measure that is sometimes considered is based on the probability individuals develop disease during a certain age or time interval. Following Breslow and Day (1980) I define the risk of disease in a time or age interval from t to $t + \Delta t$, as

$$P_{x, \Delta t}(t) = P(t \leq T < t + \Delta t, T \leq T_d \mid T \geq t, T_d \geq t, X = x),$$

where X measures exposure. The proportion of subjects who develop disease during a cohort study estimates the risk of disease in the study interval. The risk depends not only on the disease incidence rate but also on the death rate among disease-free individuals during the time interval. Over long intervals $[t, t + \Delta t)$, or age or time intervals where the risk of death is high, it is possible that associations with the risk of disease could be due to associations with death; over short intervals, associations with the risk of disease usually approximate associations with disease incidence. When the interval length Δt is short, the disease incidence rate at t for those with $X = x$ can be approximated by $\frac{1}{\Delta t} P_{x, \Delta t}(t)$.

The prevalence of disease, defined as

$$p(t) = P(T \leq t \mid T_d \geq t),$$

is generally not a good measure of disease *occurrence*, as it also measures how well subjects survive disease: a rapidly lethal disease will have low prevalence, but a chronic disease may have high prevalence, even if the incidence rates for the two diseases are the same. For this reason it is important that etiologic case-control studies sample newly diagnosed, "incident" cases. For example, in Rogentine, Jr *et al.* (1972), the association of HLA type A2 and prevalent acute lymphocytic leukemia arose because HLA type is associated with better *survival*, not because it causes leukemia (Rogentine *et al.*, 1973).

3.2.2 Measures of association

There are a number of useful ways to measure the association between exposure and the risk of the disease in the population. The difference between the disease incidence rates in exposed and unexposed individuals, sometimes called the risk difference (RD), is one measure. For $x = 1$ for exposed subjects and $x = 0$ for unexposed subjects it is defined by

$$\mathrm{RD}(t) = \lambda_1(t) - \lambda_0(t).$$

The risk difference is a useful measure when the association of exposure with the actual number of cases or population proportion who would develop disease is of interest, as when estimating the impact of a population intervention like a smoking cessation program. A positive risk difference indicates a positive association between exposure and disease, a negative risk difference indicates a negative association between exposure and disease, and a risk difference of zero indicates no association between exposure and disease.

Another useful measure is the relative risk (RR). It is defined by

$$\text{RR}(t) = \frac{\lambda_1(t)}{\lambda_0(t)},$$

and measures the proportional increase in the disease incidence associated with exposure. A relative risk greater than one indicates a positive association between exposure and disease, a relative risk less than one indicates a negative association between exposure and disease and a relative risk equal to one indicates no association between exposure and disease. Note that both these measures of association can depend on age, t, though they are often assumed to be constant.

A third useful measure is the relative risk difference (RRD). It measures the difference in disease incidence at two different levels of exposure, relative to the incidence rate at some baseline level of exposure, often no exposure. For $\lambda_1(t)$ and $\lambda_2(t)$ denoting incidence at two different levels of exposure, and $\lambda_0(t)$ the incidence at a baseline level of exposure, it is defined by

$$\text{RRD}(t) = \frac{\lambda_1(t) - \lambda_2(t)}{\lambda_0(t)}.$$

When the second level of exposure is the baseline level, $\text{RRD}(t) = \text{RR}(t) - 1$.

3.2.3   The odds ratio in case-control studies

The odds ratio is another useful measure of association; it is defined over an interval of time of length Δt beginning at t by

$$\text{OR}(t, \Delta t) = \frac{P_{1,\Delta t}(t)/(1 - P_{1,\Delta t}(t))}{P_{0,\Delta t}(t)/(1 - P_{0,\Delta t}(t))}.$$

For rare diseases or short Δt it approximates $\text{RR}(t)$ (Cornfield, 1951). Like the relative risk, an odds ratio greater than one indicates a positive association between exposure and disease, an odds ratio less than one indicates a negative association between exposure and disease, and an odds ratio equal to one indicates no association between exposure and disease.

Because case-control studies oversample cases, they do not usually offer an estimate of $P_{x,\Delta t}(t)$ unless case and control sampling probabilities are known (Cornfield, 1951; Scott and Wild, 1986). However, defining $P_{t,\Delta t}(X = x \mid D = d)$ to be the probability that a case ($d = 1$) or a control ($d = 0$) was exposed ($x = 1$) or not ($x = 0$) before being sampled in the age interval $[t, t + \Delta t)$, Cornfield (1951) showed that

$$\frac{P_{t,\Delta t}(X = 1 \mid D = 1)/P_{t,\Delta t}(X = 0 \mid D = 1)}{P_{t,\Delta t}(X = 1 \mid D = 0)/P_{t,\Delta t}(X = 0 \mid D = 0)} = \frac{P_{1,\Delta t}(t)/(1 - P_{1,\Delta t}(t))}{P_{0,\Delta t}(t)/(1 - P_{0,\Delta t}(t))}.$$

Since $P_{t,\Delta t}(X = x \mid D = d)$ can be estimated by the proportions of cases or controls with prior exposure, the data from case-control studies offer a way to estimate the odds ratio and thus the relative risk and relative risk difference over short age or time intervals.

3.2.4 The relative risk difference in case-control studies

The odds ratio and relative risk are multiplicative measures of association. The risk difference and relative risk difference are additive measures. Risk differences cannot be estimated from case-control data without additional information about the population, but the odds ratio approximation to the relative risk can be used to estimate the relative risk difference. Defined over an interval of time of length Δt beginning at t by

$$\text{RRD}(t, \Delta t) = \frac{P_{1,\Delta t}(t)/(1 - P_{1,\Delta t}(t)) - P_{2,\Delta t}(t)/(1 - P_{2,\Delta t}(t))}{P_{0,\Delta t}(t)/(1 - P_{0,\Delta t}(t))},$$

it approximates the relative risk difference, and can be estimated using case-control data.

3.2.5 Logistic model for cohort-study data

Logistic regression is a useful way to estimate odds ratios after adjustment for potential confounding variables. This section expands the definition of $\boldsymbol{x}$ to include not only exposures of interest but also adjustment variables and effect-modifying variables. It describes logistic regression in the very simple situation where all explanatory variables are binary, and the data come from a cohort or follow-up study. Section 3.2.6 extends this to case-control studies, and Chapter 4 extends it to matched case-control studies.

Let $x_E = 1$ for exposed subjects and 0 for unexposed subjects, and $x_A = 1$ for older subjects and 0 for younger subjects. Letting $\boldsymbol{x} = x_E$, Table 3.1 shows how the logistic model

$$\text{logit}(P_{\boldsymbol{x},\Delta t}(t)) = \alpha + \beta x_E \tag{3.1}$$

permits the estimation of the crude odds ratio $\text{OR}(t) = e^{\beta}$ based on regression coefficient estimates, since $\text{logit}(p) = \log[p/(1-p)]$.

TABLE 3.1
Coefficient interpretation in a binary exposure
logistic model (Equation 3.1).

$\text{logit}(P_{\boldsymbol{x},\Delta t}(t))$			
$x_E = 1$	$x_E = 0$	Difference	Odds Ratio
$\alpha + \beta$	α	β	e^{β}

Adding the second variable x_A to the model permits estimation of an age-group-adjusted odds ratio. If $\boldsymbol{x} = (x_E, x_A)$, and

$$\text{logit}(P_{\boldsymbol{x},\Delta t}(t)) = \beta_0 + \beta_A x_A + \beta_E x_E, \tag{3.2}$$

then Table 3.2 shows how e^{β_E} is the age-group-specific odds ratio assumed common to both age groups, also referred to as the age-adjusted odds ratio.

TABLE 3.2
Coefficient interpretation in a binary-exposure, binary-adjustment logistic
model (Equation 3.2).

Age Group	$\text{logit}(P_{\boldsymbol{x},\Delta t}(t))$		Difference	Odds Ratio
	$x_E = 1$	$x_E = 0$		
Younger	$\alpha + \beta_E$	α	β_E	e^{β_E}
Older	$\alpha + \beta_A + \beta_E$	$\alpha + \beta_A$	β_E	e^{β_E}

Table 3.3 categorizes data from the Framingham Heart Study (FHS) (Dawber *et al.*, 1951) by age group, systolic blood pressure (SBP) group at baseline, and whether or not they developed Coronary Heart Disease (CHD) during follow-up.

TABLE 3.3
18-year follow-up data on men age 45-62 from the Framingham Heart Study.

	Age < 55 SBP				Age ≥ 55 SBP			Total
	≥ 165	< 165			≥ 165	<165		
CHD	23	71	94	CHD	21	49	70	164
no CHD	38	278	316	no CHD	24	139	163	479
	61	349	410		45	188	233	
		OR = 2.37					OR = 2.48	

Age-group-specific odds ratios differ slightly, but taking exposure to mean SBP ≥ 165 mmHg when we fit the logistic model in Equation (3.2), we obtain

$$\text{logit}(P_{\boldsymbol{x},\Delta t}(t)) = -1.37 + 0.33x_A + 0.88x_E \qquad (3.3)$$

for an estimated common odds ratio of $e^{0.88} = 2.42$.

We can estimate age-group specific odds ratios by adding an interaction term

$$\text{logit}(P_{\boldsymbol{x},\Delta t}(t)) = \beta_0 + \beta_A x_A + \beta_E x_E + \gamma x_E x_A. \qquad (3.4)$$

The estimates of β_E and γ then become 0.86 and 0.05.

As shown in Table 3.4, a positive sign of γ would tell us that the estimated age-group-specific odds ratio associated with high SBP is greater in the older participants and a negative sign of γ would tell us that the estimated age-group-specific odds ratio associated with high SBP is lower in the older participants. This is an example of "effect modification" by age.

TABLE 3.4
Coefficient interpretation in a binary exposure, binary interaction variable logistic model (Equation 3.4).

Age Group	logit($P_{\boldsymbol{x},\Delta t}(t)$)		Difference	Odds Ratio
	$x_E = 1$	$x_E = 0$		
< 55	$\alpha + \beta_E$	α	β_E	e^{β_E}
≥ 55	$\alpha + \beta_A + \beta_E + \gamma$	$\alpha + \beta_A$	$\beta_E + \gamma$	$e^{\beta_E + \gamma}$

3.2.6   Logistic model for case-control study data

As mentioned in Section 3.2.5, under the case-control design we do not have a direct estimate of $P_{x,\Delta t}(t)$ in the population, but letting

$$S = \begin{cases} 1 & \text{Sampled in the case-control sample,} \\ 0 & \text{Otherwise,} \end{cases}$$

we can estimate the related quantity

$$P_{\boldsymbol{x},\Delta t}^{CC}(t) = P(t \leq T < t + \Delta t \,|\, T \geq t, \boldsymbol{X} = \boldsymbol{x}, S = 1)$$

using sample proportions. Let π denote the ratio of case $(D = 1)$ to control $(D = 0)$ sampling probabilities for population members. Assuming there is no selection bias, π does not depend on exposure, and here we also assume it does not depend on other variables. The ratio π is typically far greater than one, as cases in the population are rare and usually have a much higher probability of being sampled than disease-free controls. The following equations show how logistic models for $P_{\boldsymbol{x},\Delta t}^{CC}(t)$ are related to logistic models for $P_{\boldsymbol{x},\Delta t}(t)$:

$$
\begin{aligned}
\mathrm{logit}(P_{\boldsymbol{x},\Delta t}^{CC}(t)) &= \log\left(\frac{P(D=1\,|\,x_E, x_A, S=1)}{P(D=0\,|\,x_E, x_A, S=1)}\right) \\[2mm]
&= \log\left(\frac{P(D=1, x_E, x_A, S=1)}{P(D=0, x_E, x_A, S=1)}\right) \\[2mm]
&= \log\left(\frac{P(S=1\,|\,x_E, x_A, D=1)\cdot P(D=1\,|\,x_E, x_A)\cdot P(x_E, x_A)}{P(S=1\,|\,x_E, x_A, D=0)\cdot P(D=0\,|\,x_E, x_A)\cdot P(x_E, x_A)}\right) \\[2mm]
&= \log\pi + \mathrm{logit}(P(D=1\,|\,X_E = x_E, X_A = x_A)) \\[2mm]
&= \log\pi + \mathrm{logit}\,(P_{\boldsymbol{x},\Delta t}(t)).
\end{aligned}
$$

Table 3.5 shows that, as for the odds ratio from a 2×2 table, log odds ratio coefficients in logistic models based on $P_{\boldsymbol{x},\Delta t}^{CC}(t)$ from case-control studies have the same interpretations as the analogous coefficients in logistic models for $P_{\boldsymbol{x},\Delta t}(t)$ in cohort studies. It is only the intercept term that does not have a population interpretation, for it depends not only on the baseline risk of disease in the population but also on the often unknown ratio of sampling probabilities, π.

TABLE 3.5
Coefficient interpretation in a binary exposure, binary interaction variable logistic model fit to case-control data.

Age	$\mathrm{logit}(P_{\boldsymbol{x},\Delta t}^{CC}(t))$ $x_E = 1$	$\mathrm{logit}(P_{\boldsymbol{x},\Delta t}^{CC}(t))$ $x_E = 0$	$\mathrm{logit}(P_{\boldsymbol{x},\Delta t}^{CC}(t))$ Difference	Odds Ratio
< 55	$\log\pi + \alpha + \beta_E$	$\log\pi + \alpha$	β_E	e^{β_E}
≥ 55	$\log\pi + \alpha + \beta_A + \beta_E + \gamma$	$\log\pi + \alpha + \beta_A$	$\beta_E + \gamma$	$e^{\beta_E + \gamma}$

This is illustrated in the case-control sample in Table 3.6 from the Framingham data:

TABLE 3.6
Case-control sample from the FHS data given in Table 3.3.

	Age < 55 SBP ≥ 165	< 165			Age ≥ 55 SBP ≥ 165	< 165		Total
CHD	23	71	94	CHD	21	49	70	164
no CHD	17	89	106	no CHD	8	50	58	164
	40	160	200		29	99	128	
			OR $= 1.70$				OR $= 2.68$	

For this sample, the sampling probability ratio is $\frac{1}{164/479} = 2.92$. When the logistic model without interaction is fit to these data, we obtain

$$\text{logit}(P^{CC}_{\boldsymbol{x},\Delta t}(t)) = -0.26 + 0.30x_A + 0.70x_E.$$

The coefficients for x_A and x_E differ from those obtained from the full cohort data in Equation (3.3) due to sampling variability, but the intercept also differs because it estimates the original intercept term plus the log ratio of case to control sampling probabilities: $-1.37 + \log(2.92) = -1.37 + 1.07 = -0.30$.

Prentice and Pyke (1979) showed that maximum likelihood estimates of the log odds ratio coefficients from these models based on case-control data can be obtained by maximizing the likelihood for cohort-study data given in Chapter 2. Standard methods of inference for models fit by maximum likelihood are all available for logistic models fit to case-control data, including Wald-based confidence intervals, and Wald, score, and likelihood ratio tests, as described briefly in Chapter 2.

3.2.6.1   Collapsibility

One sometimes underappreciated aspect of the comparison between crude and stratum-specific odds ratios is that, even when there is no confounding, the stratum-specific odds ratio can have a different value from the crude odds ratio. As shown in Chapter 6, this is because the odds ratio is not a "collapsible" measure of association. The nonlinearity of the function that relates probabilities of disease to odds ratios means that two pairs of exposed and unexposed subjects at equally different probabilities of disease might be related by different odds ratios, because the probability of disease is different between the two pairs. Hypothetical cohort-study data in the Table 3.7, similar to those in Greenland *et al.* (1999b), demonstrate this numerically. The odds ratio is the same in each of the two age strata, but different from the crude odds ratio of 2.25, even though there is no association between age group and systolic blood pressure. This example highlights how whether or not there is a difference between crude and stratum-specific odds ratios in the data should not be used to determine if a variable is a confounder.

TABLE 3.7
Hypothetical data illustrating lack of collapsibility.

	Age < 55 SBP				Age ≥ 55 SBP			Total
	≥ 165	< 165			≥ 165	< 165		
CHD	40	20	60	CHD	80	60	140	200
no CHD	60	80	140	no CHD	20	40	60	200
	100	100	200		100	100	200	
		OR = 2.67					OR = 2.67	

3.3   Logistic models for more general case-control data

3.3.1   Exposures

3.3.1.1   Categorical variables

The logistic model generalizes to account for confounding and effect modification by more complicated variables, and to describe more complicated relationships. One simple extension is an exposure variable with more than two categories. In a case-control study of esophageal cancer conducted in France (Tuyns *et al.*, 1977) and examined in detail by Breslow and Day (1980), four categories of daily consumption of alcohol were considered. Data and estimated odds ratios from two models described below are given in Table 3.8.

TABLE 3.8
Data from the Esophageal Cancer Study (Tuyns *et al.*, 1977) and estimated odds ratios according to two models for exposure.

			Dummy-Variable		Grouped-Linear	
Alcohol (g/day)	Cases	Controls	OR	95% CI	OR	95% CI
0-39	29	386	1.0	(reference)	1.0	(reference)
40-79	75	280	3.6	(2.3, 5.6)	2.8	(2.4, 3.4)
80-119	51	87	7.8	(4.7, 13.0)	8.1	(5.6, 11.7)
120+	45	22	27.2	(14.4, 51.3)	23.1	(13.3, 40.0)

Exposure variables with $K > 2$ categories can be modeled using a set of indicator or "dummy" variables. Here $K = 4$ and we set $x_{E2} = 1$ if 40-79 g/day alcohol, 0 otherwise; $x_{E3} = 1$ if 80-119 g/day alcohol, 0 otherwise; $x_{E4} = 1$ if 120+ g/day alcohol, 0 otherwise; and fit the model

$$\text{logit}(P^{CC}_{\boldsymbol{x},\Delta t}(t)) = \beta_0 + \beta_2 x_{E2} + \beta_3 x_{E3} + \beta_4 x_{E4}.$$

When the categories are ordered as they are here, and a trend of higher or lower risk with higher category is a hypothesis, this can be examined using an ordinal variable $x_E = 1, 2, 3,$ or 4 according as alcohol consumption is 0-39, 40-79, 80-119, or 120+ g/day in a model sometimes referred to as "grouped-linear":

$$\text{logit}(P^{CC}_{\boldsymbol{x},\Delta t}(t)) = \beta_0 + \beta_1 x_E.$$

Formulas for $\text{logit}(P^{CC}_{\boldsymbol{x},\Delta t}(t))$ in Table 3.9 for these two models show how odds ratios comparing different exposure levels are not constrained at all under the indicator variable model, but are assumed to be the same with each transition to a higher category under the ordinal variable model.

TABLE 3.9
Comparison of dummy-variable and grouped-linear exposure models.

	$\text{logit}(P^{CC}_{\boldsymbol{x},\Delta t}(t))$			
	Exposure Level			
Model	0-39 g/day	40-79 g/day	80-119 g/day	120+ g/day
Dummy-Variable	α	$\alpha + \beta_{E2}$	$\alpha + \beta_{E3}$	$\alpha + \beta_{E4}$
Grouped-Linear	$\alpha + \beta_E$	$\alpha + 2\beta_E$	$\alpha + 3\beta_E$	$\alpha + 4\beta_E$

Table 3.8 shows that in the esophageal cancer data, the "grouped-linear" model requires the odds ratio comparing the third to the second group to be somewhat higher than it is for the dummy-variable model, and the other ORs to be somewhat lower. These two models are nested, and a likelihood ratio test comparing them is not statistically significant, so the grouped-linear model is an adequate summary of the dose-response relationship. However, when the prior hypothesis is a trend in risk with increasing category of exposure, it is "closer to the raw data" to present ORs and CIs based on the dummy-variable model, and a P-value for trend based on the ordinal variable model.

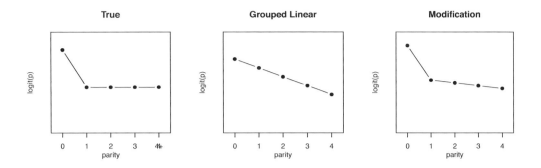

FIGURE 3.1
True and fitted values for parity exposure models.

Occasionally the expected association with any exposure is different from the association with additional exposure. One example is the association of parity with breast cancer risk, where the history of a first full-term pregnancy may be expected to have a larger association with risk than the history of any additional full-term pregnancy beyond the first. A grouped-linear model like the one fit to the esophageal cancer data may not be the best choice. Figure 3.1 shows this for hypothetical data where it is only the first full-term pregnancy that is related to risk. The leftmost panel shows how the log odds of being a case depends on parity; the middle panel shows how the fit of the ordinal parity variable model would lead to the false conclusion that higher parity is related to lower risk.

A small modification of the ordinal variable model can accommodate situations like this. If parity is four or less in the sample, the variables $x_P = 1$ if parity > 0 and 0 if parity is zero, and $x_{P2} = 0$ if parity $= 0$ or 1, 1 if parity $= 2$, 2 if parity $= 3$ and 3 if parity $= 4$ can be used in the model,

$$\text{logit}(P^{CC}_{x,\Delta t}(t)) = \alpha + \beta_1 x_P + \beta_2 x_{P2}. \qquad (3.5)$$

Table 3.10 and the rightmost panel of Figure 3.1 show how this model separates the odds ratio associated with the first full-term pregnancy from the assumed equal odds ratios associated with each additional full-term pregnancy beyond the first. For the hypothetical model, it shows how the modified model comes closer to the "truth."

TABLE 3.10
Parameter interpretation for the modified group-linear exposure model in Equation (3.5).

	$\text{logit}(P^{CC}_{x,\Delta t}(t))$		
	Parity	Parity $-$ 1	Odds Ratio
Parity $= 1$	$\alpha + \beta_1$	α	e^{β_1}
Parity $= 2$	$\alpha + \beta_1 + \beta_2$	$\alpha + \beta_1$	e^{β_2}
Parity $= K > 2$	$\alpha + \beta_1 + K\beta_2$	$\alpha + \beta_1 + (K-1)\beta_2$	e^{β_2}

3.3.1.2 Choice of the reference category

When more than one level of the categorical exposure variable is studied, odds ratios are usually presented relative to a single reference category, as in Table 3.8. Although the reference category most commonly chosen is the no exposure or lowest exposure category, this choice is entirely arbitrary, and it is easy to draw misleading conclusions if the reference category is rare.

The UK National Case-Control Study Group examined the association between oral contraceptive use and the risk of breast cancer among young women (UK National Case-Control Study Group, 1989) (Table 3.11).

TABLE 3.11
Crude odds ratios relating OC use to breast cancer risk from the UK National Case-Control Study Group.

Duration OC Use	Cases	Controls	OR	95% CI
Never Used	67	80	1.00	reference
1 - 48 Months	218	285	0.91	(0.63, 1.32)
49-96 Months	272	247	1.32	(0.91, 1.90)
97+ Months	198	143	1.65	(1.12, 2.44)

Although the odds ratio comparing those who used oral contraceptives for more than eight years to never users was significantly different from one (Table 3.11), it is tempting, though incorrect, to conclude that the odds ratio comparing those who used oral contraceptives for 4 to 8 years to those who used oral contraceptives for four or fewer years is not significantly different from one, since the confidence intervals overlap, and OR estimates for these two groups are within each others' confidence intervals.

The confidence interval widths depend not only on the sample size in the exposure groups but also the sample size in the reference category of never users. Never use is relatively rare in this population, and confidence intervals for odds ratios relative to never users take the smaller amount of information about never users into account. When the larger numbers of women who used oral contraceptives from 49 to 96 months are compared directly to users for one to 48 months the crude odds ratio estimate is 1.44 with a 95% confidence interval (1.13, 1.84) that excludes 1.0.

3.3.1.3 Continuous variables: Linear logistic models

When the exposure variable is continuous, a linear logistic model can be used to examine the evidence for trend in risk with higher exposure. Letting x_E = exposure level, the model $\text{logit}(P_{\boldsymbol{x},\Delta t}^{CC}(t)) = \alpha + \beta x_E$ describes the situation where the comparison of exposure level $x_E + 1$ to level x_E is associated with the same odds ratio, no matter what the value of x_E. Even if this model does not fit exactly, tests of the hypothesis $H_0 : \beta = 0$ are still useful as tests for trend: e^β gives an estimated weighted average odds ratio associated with a one unit higher value of x.

3.3.1.4 Continuous variables: Nonlinear logistic models

Sometimes it is of interest to model the way risk depends on x more finely, to see how odds ratios comparing different levels of exposure depend on the two levels being compared. Figure 3.2 compares several models fit to quantitative exposure data about daily tobacco consumption from the case-control study on esophageal cancer examined by Breslow and

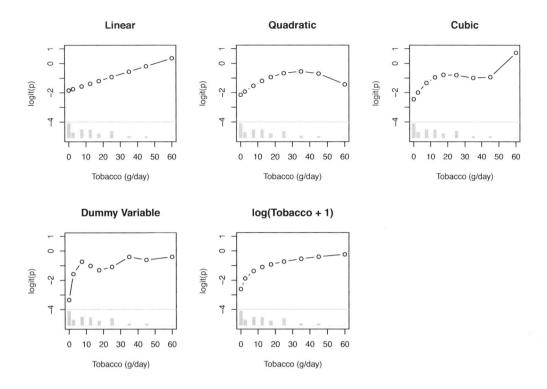

FIGURE 3.2
Comparison of exposure models for the association between tobacco exposure level and esophageal cancer risk.

Day (1980). Gray bar charts at the bottom of each graph give the relative frequency of subjects in each of the tobacco consumption categories. It is easy to see that shape constraints inherent in the linear, quadratic, and cubic models impose forms not entirely consistent with the data. The best fitting smooth model appears to be the log model, and although a likelihood ratio test comparing it to the dummy-variable (DV) model is statistically significant ($\chi_7^2 = 26.83$, P = 0.0004), it is the model that is the least statistically significantly different from the dummy-variable model, of the smooth models considered (Table 3.12). An exploratory analysis of these data with the goal of summarizing the dose-response relationship with a simple model might do well to choose this log model. However, a pre-defined data analysis plan that called for fitting a linear model to examine the trend in risk with amount of exposure would be acceptable.

Results from fitting a nonlinear logistic model to exposure data can be presented as tables of odds ratios comparing different pairs of exposure levels, or as a plot showing how the odds ratio comparing to some standard exposure level depends on exposure. Table 3.12 presents OR estimates from the dummy-variable and log models, comparing all levels of tobacco exposure to none.

The apparent discrepancy in the odds ratios between these two models is due mainly to the difference in the way the two models fit the low and no exposure categories, and the choice of the no exposure category as the reference. Figure 3.3 shows how the choice of a reference category can affect the apparent differences between models. Plots in the

TABLE 3.12
Comparison of DV and log model fits relating
tobacco exposure level to esophageal cancer risk.

Tobacco (g/day)	DV Model OR	DV Model 95% CI	Log model OR	Log model 95% CI
0	1.0	(reference)	1.0	(reference)
2.5	5.9	(1.9, 17.8)	2.1	(1.7, 2.5)
7.5	13.6	(5.1, 36.7)	3.4	(2.5, 4.7)
12.5	10.2	(3.7, 27.9)	4.5	(3.0, 6.6)
17.5	7.6	(2.5, 23.4)	5.4	(3.5, 8.2)
25	9.5	(3.4, 26.7)	6.5	(4.0, 10.5)
35	18.9	(5.6, 64.0)	7.8	(4.6, 13.3)
45	15.3	(4.4, 54.1)	9.0	(5.1, 15.9)
60	18.9	(1.5, 239.5)	10.6	(5.8, 19.5)

top row compare linear, dummy-variable, and log models when the reference category is zero exposure; plots in the bottom row compare the same three models when the reference category is 12.5 g/day of tobacco exposure.

3.3.1.5 Continuous variables: Quantile groups

Sometimes investigators divide subjects into groups based on the values of a continuous exposure variable, as was done in Section 3.3.1.1 for the esophageal cancer case-control study. Advantages of this approach are that odds ratios comparing groups can be presented beside case and control counts, that an explicit functional form for the relationship is not assumed, and that subjects with outlying values of the continuous variable do not exert undue influence on the estimation. A disadvantage can be lower power, due to ignoring within-category differences in risk (Hitchcock, 1966).

Investigators sometimes base the grouping on the quantiles of the exposure distribution, but this is rarely a good idea. If the values of the quantitative exposure vary from study to study because of population or sampling differences, it is best to choose round-number, well-recognized cut-points between groups. When different studies use the same groupings, their results are directly comparable, and it is easy for the reader to evaluate level of risk for different types of individuals. Quantile boundaries are often nonround numbers, and they vary from study to study, making comparison of results difficult.

The only exception to this recommendation is when the largest study-to-study differences in exposure levels are due to the differences in assay, instrument, or other technical method used to quantify the amount of exposure rather than differences in the populations studied. In these cases, subjects with exposures in the top quarter of exposures in the sample may be more comparable across study than subgroups from each study whose exposure level exceeds the same measured value.

3.3.1.6 More than one characteristic of exposure

When more than one characteristic of an exposure is of interest, as it is when examining the effects of dose, duration, and recency of drug exposure, or jointly evaluating how parity and age at first birth are related to risk, the use of logistic models can lead to the mistaken belief that comparisons of exposure values for one characteristic of exposure compared to no exposure can be adjusted for another characteristic. Table 3.13 illustrates the data that are available for a hypothetical drug exposure example, where an × indicates a cell where data are impossible. For any category of drug duration, there is no possible comparison

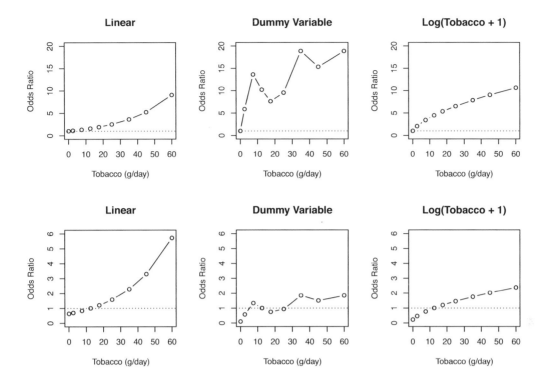

FIGURE 3.3
Effect of reference category on the comparison of exposure models.

between never users and users who used the same dose, and for any category of drug dose, there is no possible comparison between never users and users who used the drug for the same duration.

It is nonetheless possible to fit logistic models that include terms for both dose and duration to data such as these, but careless interpretation of coefficients from these models can lead to false conclusions. From these data, one can make adjusted comparisons among exposed individuals, and comparisons to never users can be made with subjects exposed to *combinations* of the two exposure characteristics (McKnight *et al.*, 1999).

A different but related issue arises in studies where there is good reason to adjust for a total exposure when studying how the levels of components of the total are related to disease risk. In nutritional epidemiology, odds ratios for association between disease and daily average nutrient intake are often adjusted for total daily Kcals consumed. Another example is studying risks associated with pregnancy outcome, adjusted for gravidity.

In dietary studies, when the nutrient exposure of interest provides a large portion of the daily Kcal consumed, care must be exercised in interpreting the results of the analysis (Wacholder *et al.*, 1994). If, adjusted for total Kcal, higher fat consumption is associated with higher disease risk, for example, this may be because fat consumption increases the risk of disease or it may be because some low-fat sources of calories decrease risk.

TABLE 3.13
Data schematic for more than one characteristic of exposure.

		Dose			
		None	Low	Medium	High
	None		×	×	×
	Low	×			
Duration	Medium	×			
	High	×			

3.3.2 Confounding control

Because epidemiologic data are observational, care must be taken to control confounding in the analysis if inferences about causation are to be drawn. Thoughtful descriptions (McNamee, 2003) characterize confounding variables as those that cause exposure in the population and cause disease among the unexposed in the population, or are associated with their causes, but are not themselves results of exposure. Chapter 6 reviews the precise descriptions of the population assumptions necessary to determine if a set of variables is sufficient to control confounding using Directed Acyclic Graphs (DAGs). It shows how case-control sampling can result in data with different associations and independencies than those present in the population. Major practical implications for logistic regression analysis of case-control data are 1) that the choice of confounding variables should be based on assumptions about what is true in the population and not on association or lack of association in the data, and 2) that without supplemental data about the population, only *conditional* causal odds ratios can be estimated.

The conditional causal odds ratio can be interpreted as the measure of association among individuals with like values of the adjustment variables. Under the assumption that all members of each such group have approximately the same risk of disease, this odds ratio is an average causal effect (ACE) (Holland and Rubin, 1987) that because of the assumed homogeneity within groups with like values could be viewed as the average subject-specific odds ratio.

This section will assume that interest centers on the estimation of the conditional causal odds ratio, and that a set of variables sufficient to control confounding has been identified. The paragraphs that follow will give practical suggestions for how to include adjustment for these variables in a logistic regression analysis.

3.3.2.1 Adjustment for confounding using logistic regression

Table 3.2 shows how adding the age-group variable to a simple logistic model can adjust for the possible confounding effect of age-group: age-group-specific odds ratios compare exposed to unexposed individuals in the same age group, and cannot be confounded by associations between age group and disease or age group and exposure. When potential confounding variables are more complicated than the binary age-group variable, more modeling choices

TABLE 3.14

Age-group-specific alcohol exposure data in the
Esophageal Cancer Study.

Age groups		0-79 g/day alcohol $x_E = 0$	80+ g/day alcohol $x_E = 1$	Total
25-34	Controls	106	9	115
	Cases	0	1	1
35-44	Controls	164	26	190
	Cases	5	4	9
45-54	Controls	138	29	167
	Cases	21	25	46
55-64	Controls	139	27	166
	Cases	34	42	76
65-74	Controls	88	18	106
	Cases	36	19	55
75+	Controls	31	0	31
	Cases	8	5	13

are possible, but in general, adding an appropriately specified variable to a logistic model controls its possible confounding effect.

3.3.2.2 Categorical variables

For categorical confounding variables with more than two levels, additional indicators can be added so that there is one for each but one of the groups. The model below shows how this would work for a race/ethnicity variable in a study of individuals with European, African, Asian, or mixed heritage. Letting $x_{Af} = 1$ for those with African heritage and 0 otherwise; $x_{As} = 1$ for those of Asian heritage and 0 otherwise; $x_M = 1$ for those of mixed heritage and 0 otherwise; and $x_E = 1$ for exposed subjects and 0 otherwise, and under the model

$$\text{logit}(P^{CC}_{\boldsymbol{x},\Delta t}(t)) = \alpha_0 + \alpha_{Af}x_{Af} + \alpha_{As}x_{As} + \alpha_M x_M + \beta x_E$$

we have that the heritage-specific odds ratio for the association between exposure and disease is given by e^β in each group.

When the categorical confounding variable is ordinal, a choice must be made. A dummy-variable model like the one given above is acceptable, but the ordinal nature of the variable allows a more parsimonious model. Grouped data from a case-control study of esophageal cancer considered by Breslow and Day (1980) are given in Table 3.14 for six age groups by a binary alcohol exposure variable.

Letting $x_A = 1, 2, 3, 4, 5$, or 6 according as age is 25-34, 35-44, 45-54, 55-64, 65-74, or 75+ years and letting $x_E = 1$ if alcohol consumption was ≥ 80 g/day, 0 otherwise, the grouped-linear model

$$\text{logit}(P^{CC}_{\boldsymbol{x},\Delta t}(t)) = \alpha_0 + \alpha_1 x_A + \beta x_E$$

assumes that the increase in log odds of being a case associated with one higher age group is always the same no matter what two adjacent groups are compared. This may or may not fit the data well, but it is often a reasonable approximation if risk increases or decreases with

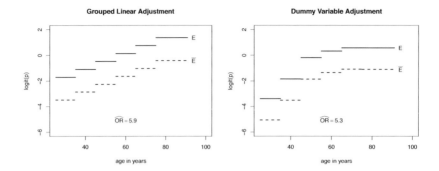

FIGURE 3.4
Comparison of grouped-linear and dummy-variable adjustment for age group. (Drawn lines: exposed; dashed lines: nonexposed.)

higher levels of the ordinal variable. When it does not fit the data well, residual confounding may occur.

As shown for the dummy-variable model in Figure 3.4, in the esophageal cancer data the probability of being a case rises steeply with age in the younger age categories and then levels off. The estimated odds ratio associated with high alcohol exposure based on this grouped-linear adjustment for age group is 5.9, whereas when the dummy-variable model is used to adjust for age group, the estimated odds ratio is 5.3. These estimates are similar, even though a departure from the grouped-linear logistic model for age is evident in these data.

3.3.2.3   Continuous variables

Continuous confounding variables can be included as linear or more complicated terms. As with categorical variables, different modeling choices are available. A linear model is often adequate to recover most of the variability in risk associated with the variable, but as with ordinal categorical variables, model misspecification can fail to remove all confounding by the variable. The top row of Figure 3.5 uses continuous measurements from the esophageal cancer data to compare linear and quadratic adjustment for age in years. Again, despite obvious lack of fit by the linear model, conclusions drawn from the fit of these two models would differ only minimally.

Very occasionally, quadratic models are not sufficient to recover the variation in risk associated with a continuous variable, and more complicated models are required. A simple choice that makes few assumptions is a linear regression spline, which fits a continuous model, assumed linear on the logistic scale between pre-defined cutpoints that were chosen here to be the same as the group boundaries for the grouped data. See Greenland (1995) for details. This model fits similarly to the quadratic model for the esophageal cancer data, and provides a similar odds ratio estimate (bottom row, Figure 3.5).

One advantage to logistic regression modeling is that several confounders can be controlled simultaneously by including them all in the same model. Occasionally interaction terms, formed as products between confounding variables, are required to remove the joint confounding effect of several variables. And sometimes control of a nonconfounder can create confounding as shown in Greenland *et al.* (1999a) and Chapter 6.

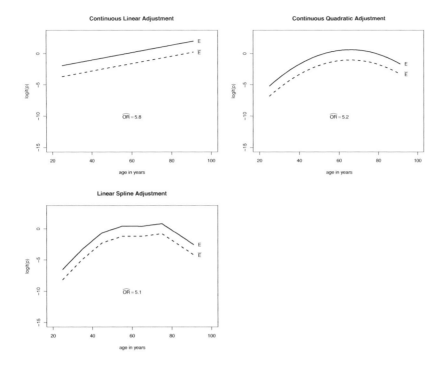

FIGURE 3.5
Comparison of continuous linear, quadratic, and linear spline adjustment for age. (Drawn lines: exposed; dashed lines: nonexposed.)

3.3.2.4 Number of variables

It is possible to include too many adjustment variables in the model even if their joint inclusion does not induce confounding. Maximum likelihood estimation breaks down when, relative to the sample size, the number of coefficients estimated in the logistic regression model is too large. Based on simulation studies, Peduzzi *et al.* (1996) showed that estimates can be biased, with poor precision, and tests can be biased when there are fewer than 10 outcome events per variable. Subsequent simulations by Vittinghoff and McCulloch (2007) showed that in logistic regression there are a number of settings with 5-9 events per variable where there is little bias, and a few settings with 10-14 events per variable where there is important bias. Chapter 4 describes one statistical method, conditional logistic regression, that can solve the bias problem when the number of adjustment variables is large relative to the sample size, and strata of subjects with like values of the adjustment variables can be formed.

3.3.3 Precision variables

In linear regression modeling, including variables that are strongly related to the outcome, sometimes called precision variables, can improve the precision of estimates of association between the variables of interest and the outcome. Robinson and Jewell (1991) showed that the intuition from linear regression does not carry over completely to logistic regression. When a variable strongly related to outcome, but not related to the exposure of interest, is included in a logistic regression model, this can increase the estimated standard error

TABLE 3.15

Breast cancer by family history and induced abortion history.

		Control	Breast Cancer Case
No FH	no IA	601	568
	IA	228	240
First Degree FH	no IA	59	120
	IA	18	43

of the coefficient of the exposure variable. However, because of the noncollapsibility of the odds ratio, adjusting for a variable strongly related to the outcome can also make the odds ratio estimate farther from one and the asymptotic relative efficiency of the test that the adjusted odds ratio is one is greater than one (Neuhaus, 1998). The increase in power is only meaningful, however, when the precision variable is very strongly associated with the outcome.

The strong relationships described in the previous paragraph must hold in the *data* for the adjustment to the increase power. As shown in Chapter 6, associations in the population may not be the same in case-control data. If a potential precision variable X is independent of exposure, so that the $X \rightarrow D \leftarrow E$ Directed Acyclic Graph holds in the population, sampling conditional on case status can create dependency between X and E in the sample, so that X may not meet the requirements for a "precision" variable. Pirinen *et al.* (2012) give an example where including a variable meeting the association criteria in the population, but not the sample, can reduce power in a case-control study.

3.3.4 Effect modification

Additional variables can also be effect modifiers – their values are related to the strength of the association between exposure and disease. Some effect modifiers have such a strong effect that their value determines whether there is an association between exposure and disease. For example, there is no association between dietary phenylalanine and intellectual ability in those without phenylketonuria, but in those with phenylketonuria, the association is strong. In theory it is possible for an effect modifier to have such a strong effect that its value determines the sign of the exposure-disease association.

More often, however, the value of an effect modifying variable is related only to the magnitude of an always-positive or always-negative exposure-disease association. When both associations have the same sign, the choice of the measure of "effect" used to quantify the association can determine whether the variable is an effect modifier. Table 3.15 gives data on the association between prior induced abortion (IA) and incident breast cancer by whether or not the case-control study participant had a first-degree family history (FH) of breast cancer (Daling *et al.*, 1996).

Table 3.16 shows that the estimated crude odds ratios for the association between prior IA and incident breast cancer are very similar in the two FH groups (1.11 versus 1.17). However, because the risk of disease is higher in the group with a first-degree FH, the relative risk difference depends on FH group (0.11 versus 0.38).

Logistic regression provides the modeling framework for examining whether odds ratios are modified by a variable like family history. As shown in Section 3.2.5, letting x_I and x_H be 0-1 indicators for prior induced abortion and family history, respectively, the addition of a product term $x_I x_H$ to the logistic model

$$\text{logit}(P^{CC}_{\boldsymbol{x},\Delta t}(t)) = \beta_0 + \beta_I x_I + \beta_H x_H + \beta_{IH} x_I x_H$$

TABLE 3.16
ORs and OR/RR differences for the breast cancer data.

		OR relative to neither	OR relative to no IA	OR Difference relative to no IA
No FH	no IA	1.00	1.00	0.00
	IA	1.11	1.11	0.11
First Degree FH	no IA	2.15	1.00	0.00
	IA	2.53	1.17	0.38

allows the odds ratio associated with prior induced abortion to depend on family history, and the test of $H_0 : \beta_{IH} = 0$ tests whether there is effect modification on the odds ratio scale. If assessment of effect modification on the additive odds-ratio-difference scale is of interest, it can be examined using the following binomial generalized linear model:

$$\text{logit}(P^{CC}_{\boldsymbol{x}, \Delta t}(t)) = \beta_0 + \log(1 + \beta_I x_I + \beta_H x_H + \beta_{IH} x_I x_H).$$

See Chapter 11 for more details about regression models for measures of association other than the odds ratio.

3.4 Modeling strategy

In logistic regression analysis of case-control data, multiple decisions must be made. A functional form for the exposure-disease relationship must be chosen. Adjustment variables, the functional form of those variables, and possible interactions between those variables must be chosen. The introduction of any effect-modifying, or interaction, variables with exposure must be decided upon.

All these choices are subject to overt or unconscious biases, and there can be strong temptation to make the selections in a way that promotes the statistical significance of the exposure-disease relationship, or confirms prior beliefs of the investigators in some other way (Goldacre and Brown, 2016). For this reason, it is important that the primary analysis of data from a case-control study be conducted according to data analysis plan that was formed before the data were examined. This procedure is common in the analysis of data from randomized clinical trials, but it is not adhered to as frequently as it should be in the analysis of data from case-control studies, and it may be one reason for conflicting results from similar studies in different populations or conducted by different investigators (Breslow, 1999). When the analysis model adheres to the form set out in a pre-specified data analysis plan, the interpretation of the P-value is protected, for it evaluates the likelihood of the observed data under a pre-specified null hypothesis that did not depend upon the data. When the analysis model does not adhere to a pre-specified plan, the P-value is hard to interpret, for at least the details of the hypothesis being tested were suggested by the data.

Case-control studies can be very expensive to complete, and they often collect data on the values of a wealth of exposures and possible adjustment variables. These data can contain important information about un-hypothesized relationships between variables and disease, but associations found by chance in the data may also be due entirely to the variability inherent in sampling, and may not exist in the population. To protect interpretation of the P-value for the primary analyses conducted in a case-control study, but allow the possibility that relationships in the data might suggest other fruitful directions for future study, one useful strategy is to divide analyses into "confirmatory" analyses that will be conducted based on pre-specified plans, and "exploratory" analyses that will be allowed to make decisions based on what is seen in the data. An important distinction then is that the results of confirmatory analyses can be interpreted as confirming or refuting the hypothesis that led to the collection of the data and the primary analysis, while the results of exploratory analyses must be interpreted only as hypothesis generating. General recommendations for each of these two types of logistic regression analyses follow in the next two sections.

3.4.1   Confirmatory analysis

The plan for a confirmatory analysis should specify a functional form for the exposure-disease relationship. Often this will be linear, for quantitative exposure, unless some nonlinear relationship on the logistic scale is pre-hypothesized. Occasionally investigators prefer to group a continuous exposure variable so they can present group-specific odds ratios alongside counts of cases and controls without a pre-hypothesized functional form. Adjustment variables should be chosen a priori, and be included in as fine a form as can be supported by the data.

3.4.2   Exploratory analysis

Exploratory analyses can be modified in response to features of the observed data: choosing a well-fitting smooth model to summarize the dose-response relationship found in the data as, for example, the log model for tobacco exposure in the esophageal cancer data example of Section 3.3.1.4. Usually this model choice should be based on the results of statistical hypothesis tests comparing candidate models or, for nonnested models, a penalized criterion such as AIC or BIC (Hastie *et al.*, 2009). Adjustment for confounding should be based on a pre-hypothesized set of potential confounding variables. Because the odds ratio is not collapsible, the comparison of adjusted and unadjusted odds ratios should not be used to determine whether a variable is a confounder, but if richer models do not alter the odds ratios of interest, the higher-order terms can be omitted and the simpler model retained. Hypothesis testing should not be used to determine what variables to adjust for or their functional form because failure to adjust for a confounder can bias the estimate of the odds ratio even when the confounder is not statistically significantly related to the outcome.

   Even in exploratory analyses, care must be taken not to examine too many variables for possible effect modification. It is best to limit the examination of effect modification to variables for which there is some biological rationale, and to correct for multiple comparisons when concluding whether an observed interaction is statistically significant.

3.5   Summary

Focussing on logistic regression analysis, this chapter has presented key issues in the analysis of unmatched case-control data. It has described how the conditional causal odds ratio is related to the relative risk written in terms of the population disease incidence rates, and has shown how to estimate the conditional causal odds ratio when data on variables sufficient to control confounding are available. It has described several choices for modeling risk as a function of exposure level or as a function of different characteristics of exposure. It has also described several choices for modeling confounding adjustment, and shown how to model effect modification on the multiplicative, odds-ratio scale. Finally, it has given advice about how to approach the analysis, depending on whether the goal of modeling and hypothesis testing is to examine the evidence in favor of a prior hypothesis or to explore the data hoping to suggest new hypotheses.

Bibliography

Breslow, N. E. (1999). Discussion: Statistical thinking in practice. *International Statistical Review*, **67**, 252–255.

Breslow, N. E. and Day, N. E. (1980). *Statistical Methods in Cancer Research. Vol. 1: The Analysis of Case-Control Studies*. IARC, Lyon.

Cornfield, J. (1951). A method of estimating comparative rates from clinical data. Applications to cancer of the lung, breast, and cervix. *Journal of the National Cancer Institute*, **11**, 1269–75.

Cox, D. R. (1972). Regression models and life-tables (with discussion). *Journal of the Royal Statistical Society. Series B (Methodological)*, **34**, 187–220.

Daling, J. R., Brinton, L. A., Voigt, L. F., Weiss, N. S., Coates, R. J., Malone, K. E., Schoenberg, J. B., and Gammon, M. (1996). Risk of breast cancer among white women following induced abortion. *American Journal of Epidemiology*, **144**, 373–380.

Dawber, T. R., Meadors, G. F., and Moore, F. E. (1951). Epidemiological approaches to heart disease: The Framingham study. *American Journal of Public Health*, **41**, 279–286.

Goldacre, B. and Brown, T. (2016). Fixing flaws in science must be professionalized. *Journal of Clinical Epidemiology*, **70**, 267–269.

Greenland, S. (1995). Dose-response and trend analysis in epidemiology: Alternatives to categorical analysis. *Epidemiology*, **6**, 356–365.

Greenland, S., Pearl, J., and Robins, J. M. (1999a). Causal diagrams for epidemiologic research. *Epidemiology*, **10**, 37–48.

Greenland, S., Robins, J. M., and Pearl, J. (1999b). Confounding and collapsibility in causal inference. *Statistical Science*, **14**, 29–46.

Hastie, T., Tibshirani, R., and Friedman, J. (2009). *The Elements of Statistical Learning (2nd edition)*. Springer, New York.

Hitchcock, S. E. (1966). Tests of hypotheses about the parameters of the logistic function. *Biometrika*, **53**, 535–544.

Holland, P. W. and Rubin, D. B. (1987). Causal inference in retrospective studies. *ETS Research Report Series*, **1987**, 203–231.

McKnight, B., Cook, L. S., and Weiss, N. S. (1999). Logistic regression analysis for more than one characteristic of exposure. *American Journal of Epidemiology*, **149**, 984–992.

McNamee, R. (2003). Confounding and confounders. *Occupational and Environmental Medicine*, **60**, 227–234.

Neuhaus, J. M. (1998). Estimation efficiency with omitted covariates in generalized linear models. *Journal of the American Statistical Association*, **93**, 1124–1129.

Peduzzi, P., Concato, J., Kemper, E., Holford, T. R., and Feinstein, A. R. (1996). A simulation study of the number of events per variable in logistic regression analysis. *Journal of Clinical Epidemiology*, **49**, 1373–1379.

Pirinen, M., Donnelly, P., and Spencer, C. C. A. (2012). Including known covariates can reduce power to detect genetic effects in case-control studies. *Nature Genetics*, **44**, 848–851.

Prentice, R. L. and Pyke, R. (1979). Logistic disease incidence models and case-control studies. *Biometrika*, **66**, 403–411.

Robinson, L. D. and Jewell, N. P. (1991). Some surprising results about covariate adjustment in logistic regression models. *International Statistical Review*, **59**, 227–240.

Rogentine, G. N., Trapani, R. J., Yankee, R. A., and Henderson, E. S. (1973). HL-A antigens and acute lymphocytic leukemia: The nature of the HL-A2 association. *Tissue Antigens*, **3**, 470–476.

Rogentine, Jr, G. N., Yankee, R. A., Gart, J. J., Nam, J., and Trapani, R. J. (1972). HL-A antigens and disease: Acute lymphocytic leukemia. *Journal of Clinical Investigation*, **51**, 2420–2428.

Scott, A. J. and Wild, C. J. (1986). Fitting logistic models under case-control or choice based sampling. *Journal of the Royal Statistical Society. Series B (Methodological)*, **48**, 170–182.

Tanner, M. A. and Wong, W. H. (1983). The estimation of the hazard function from randomly censored data by the kernel method. *The Annals of Statistics*, **11**, 989–993.

Tuyns, A. J., Pequignot, G., and Jensen, O. M. (1977). Le cancer de l'œsophage en Ille-et-Vilaine en fonction des niveaux de consommation d'alcool et de tabac. *Bulletin du Cancer*, **64**, 45–60.

UK National Case-Control Study Group (1989). Oral contraceptive use and breast cancer risk in young women. *The Lancet*, **333**, 974–982.

Vittinghoff, E. and McCulloch, C. E. (2007). Relaxing the rule of ten events per variable in logistic and Cox regression. *American Journal of Epidemiology*, **165**, 710–718.

Wacholder, S., Schatzkin, A., Freedman, L. S., Kipnis, V., Hartman, A., and Brown, C. C. (1994). Can energy adjustment separate the effects of energy from those of specific macronutrients? *American Journal of Epidemiology*, **140**, 848–855.

Yandell, B. S. (1983). Nonparametric inference for rates with censored survival data. *The Annals of Statistics*, **11**, 1119–1135.

4

Matched Case-Control Studies

Barbara McKnight

University of Washington

4.1 Introduction

Case-control study investigators sometimes choose to match controls to cases based on the values of suspected confounders or other variables in the designs of their studies. This chapter describes the reasons for matching in the design, several methods for matching, and the statistical methods required to account for matching in logistic regression analysis of matched case-control data.

4.2 Matched designs

4.2.1 Reasons for matching

The primary reasons to match in a case-control study are to improve the precision of adjusted odds ratio estimates, to obtain controls easily, or to control for confounding by unobservable variables that can be assumed to have similar values for subjects in the same matched set. When confounding would bias an unadjusted estimate of the exposure-disease odds ratio, but case and control distributions of the confounders are so different that few cases and controls have the same values of the confounding variables, confounder-adjusted odds ratios comparing cases and controls have low precision. Matching on the confounders will create case and control samples with the same distribution of the confounding variables, which can increase both the precision of adjusted odds ratio estimates and the power of hypothesis tests based on adjusted models (Thomas and Greenland, 1983).

When it is difficult to identify representative samples of controls from the population that gave rise to the cases, and friend, neighbor or family-member controls are easily identified and are suitable members of the source population, matching can facilitate control identification (Wacholder *et al.*, 1992). This type of matching is also implemented when members in the same matched set have similar values of important confounding variables that are not readily observed so that it would otherwise be difficult to adjust for them (Chapter 2). For example, choosing sibling controls and controlling for sibship in the analysis can adjust for a host of unobserved lifestyle and genetic factors that cluster within families.

Matching can increase statistical efficiency even when the matching variable is not a confounder. If the matching variable is causally associated with disease, but not exposure in the population, Chapter 6 note that case-control sampling will create an association between a disease-influencing exposure and the matching variable in the sample. Even though disease status and the matching variable will be marginally unassociated in the matched sample, within subgroups of like exposure, the matching variable will be associated with case status and the crude odds ratio estimate based on the matched sample will be confounded by the failure to control the matching variable (Didelez *et al.*, 2010; Mansournia *et al.*, 2013). In this setting, the adjusted odds ratio estimate will be a large-sample unbiased estimate of the conditional causal odds ratio, and it can be slightly more precise than an adjusted odds ratio based on an unmatched sample (Thomas and Greenland, 1983; Breslow, 1982).

4.2.2   Types of matching

Matching on the basis of one or more observed variables can be carried out on both an individual and grouped basis. In individual-matched studies, each case is matched to one or more controls who have the same or similar values of the matching variables. When there is one such control per case we call the study "pair-matched."

Sometimes it is difficult to find a population control who matches exactly on a variable like age, and an extremely close match is not required to assure comparability. A match within one or two years of age, for example, is often considered close enough for matched sets. Inexact matching is sometimes called "caliper matching" (Rubin, 1976), where the size of the caliper determines how closely controls must be matched to cases on the matching variable.

In a related inexact matching method, controls are required to be in the same five- or ten-year age interval as the case to whom they are matched. In this design, matched sets of cases and controls in the same five-year age interval are exchangeable, and they can be pooled into a single five-year age stratum in the analysis. This is similar to a "frequency-matched" design, where matched controls are not sought for individual cases but instead care is taken to identify a number of controls that is the same multiple (often one) of the number of cases in each category of the grouped matching variable(s).

Occasionally there are a large number of variables on which investigators want to match controls to cases, and it is difficult to find an individually-matched control who matches closely on all variables for each case. In cohort studies, this problem is sometimes addressed by developing a propensity score and matching on it, but as noted in Chapter 6, there are difficulties associated with propensity-score matching in case-control studies, so this strategy will not be considered here. To solve this problem in case-control studies, investigators may decide to loosen matching criteria, either by dropping some of the matching variables or allowing nonexact matches for some of them. Usually residual differences in the values of matching variables within matched sets can still be controlled with covariate adjustment in the logistic regression analysis.

And as mentioned above, when it is difficult to measure or even know all the variables that investigators want to be comparable between cases and controls, one observed variable may sometimes capture all or almost all of the comparability information, as happens when sibling controls are chosen. This type of matching, including sampling friend controls, neighbor controls, or controls from the same clinical practice as the case, is sometimes also performed when it provides ready access to suitable controls, and when there is otherwise no good way to identify all members of the population from which cases arose to sample them in a representative way (Wacholder *et al.*, 1992).

One important characteristic of matched designs is that the distributions of any variables associated with the matching variables are altered in the controls, so the effects of the matching cannot be removed in the analysis without external data on the distribution of matching variables in the population. Because of this, the benefits of matching should be weighed carefully against potential risks, discussed below, when designing a study.

4.2.3 Disadvantages to matching

Although matching in a case-control study can improve confounding control, can improve statistical precision and can make it easier to identify valid population controls, matched control samples may no longer be representative of the control population. If the matching variables are associated in any way with exposure, the distribution of exposure histories in matched controls will be more similar to the distribution in cases than to the distribution among controls in the population, and crude odds ratio estimates based on the matched sample will be biased toward one. The only odds ratio estimates that can be expected to estimate the corresponding population odds ratio without bias are those that are conditional on combinations of matching-variable values. Thus, analysis of data from matched case-control studies must adjust for the matching variables in order to avoid bias, as noted in Chapter 6 and Mansournia *et al.* (2013).

If the matching variables are results of exposure and should not be controlled (Chapters 3 and 6), the adjusted odds ratios that can be estimated unbiasedly from the matched data are not of scientific interest. The only solution to such an "overmatched" study is to obtain information external to the sample about the distribution of the matching variable(s) in the population. This external data could be used to produce an unadjusted odds ratio estimate using standardization methodology as described in Chapter 6 and Rothman *et al.* (2012) based on elements estimated as described in Scott and Wild (1991).

If the matching variables are causally associated with exposure but not disease in the population, and if they are not a result of exposure, the adjusted odds ratio is potentially of scientific interest, but matching on the variable and adjusting for it can reduce the precision of odds ratio estimates compared to crude or adjusted estimates from a similarly-sized unmatched sample (Thomas and Greenland, 1983; Breslow, 1982) and adjustment for these variables is not required to control confounding.

4.3 Adjusted analyses using logistic regression

To begin our examination of adjusted logistic analyses of matched case-control data, consider first the analysis of a frequency-matched case-control study using dummy variable adjustment for the matching variables in logistic regression. Chapter 3 introduced data from the Framingham Heart Study (FHS), a longitudinal cohort study conducted in Framingham, Massachusetts beginning in 1948 to identify risk factors for cardiovascular disease. Table 3.3 gave data on the incidence of coronary heart disease (CHD) during the first 18 years of follow-up among male FHS participants. Subjects counted in Table 3.3 are categorized by whether or not they developed CHD during follow-up, age group (< 55 years versus ≥ 55 years) and systolic blood pressure (SBP) group (< 165 mmHg versus ≥ 165 mmHg). Scientific interest in these data centers on estimating the association between SBP group and CHD incidence, after adjustment for age group. To illustrate the effect of frequency matched sampling, here we draw an age-group frequency-matched case-control sample from the data given in Table 3.3; the sample counts are given in Table 4.1.

TABLE 4.1
Frequency-matched case-control sample from FHS.

	Age < 55 SBP				Age ≥ 55 SBP			Total
	≥ 165	< 165			≥ 165	< 165		
CHD	23	71	94	CHD	21	49	70	164
no CHD	11	83	94	no CHD	9	61	70	164
	34	154	188		30	110	140	
		OR= 2.44				OR $= 2.90$		

Table 3.6 gave counts for an unmatched case-control sample from the data in Table 3.3; in that sample, the total number of controls was equal to the total number of cases. Here, not only is the total number of controls the same as the total number of cases, but because of the frequency matching, the numbers of controls and cases are also the same within each of the two age groups.

As in Section 3.2.1, for $T =$ the age at disease onset and $T_d =$ the age at death, define the risk of disease in an age interval from t to $t + \Delta t$, as

$$P_{\boldsymbol{x}, \Delta t}(t) = P(t \leq T < t + \Delta t, T \leq T_d \,|\, T \geq t, T_d \geq t, \boldsymbol{X} = \boldsymbol{x}),$$

where for each subject the vector $\boldsymbol{X}$ contains exposure measures and any adjustment, precision, and/or effect modifying variables. Further letting

$$S = \begin{cases} 1 & \text{Sampled for case-control study,} \\ 0 & \text{Not sampled for case-control study,} \end{cases}$$

the case-control sample proportions of cases among subjects for whom $\boldsymbol{X} = \boldsymbol{x}$ and $T \in [t, t + \Delta t)$ can be used to estimate the case-control sample analogue of the population risk:

$$P_{\boldsymbol{x}, \Delta t}^{CC}(t) = P(t \leq T < t + \Delta t | T \geq t, \boldsymbol{X} = \boldsymbol{x}, S = 1).$$

Defining $x_A = 1$ for subjects 55 years of age or older and 0 for younger subjects, Section 3.2.6 showed that when an unmatched case-control sample is drawn from the cohort study data, the control sampling probabilities and the sampling probability ratios

$$\pi_{x_A} = \frac{P(S = 1 | D = 1, X_A = x_A)}{P(S = 1 | D = 0, X_A = x_A)}$$

do not depend on age stratum x_A. Because of the frequency matching on age group here, older controls are more likely to be sampled than younger controls and so the ratio of case to control sampling probabilities depends on the age group. Comparing Table 3.3 to Table 4.1 we see that in the younger group ($x_A = 0$) the ratio is $\pi_0 = \frac{1}{94/316} = 3.36$ while in the older group ($x_A = 1$) it is $\pi_1 = \frac{1}{70/163} = 2.33$.

Letting $x_E = 1$ for subjects with SBP $\geq$ 165 mmHg and 0 for subjects with SBP $<$ 165 mmHg, a logistic model written in terms of the population odds ratio associated with SBP $\geq$ 165 mmHg, adjusted for age group, is given by:

$$\text{logit}(P_{\boldsymbol{x},\Delta t}(t)) = \beta_0 + \beta_A x_A + \beta_E x_E. \tag{4.1}$$

By arguments identical to those given in Section 3.2.6, the same logistic model in terms of frequency-matched case-control sample proportions of cases is related to the coefficients in the population logistic model (4.1) via the sampling probability ratios:

$$
\begin{aligned}
\text{logit}(P_{\boldsymbol{x},\Delta t}^{CC}(t)) &= \log \pi_{x_A} + \text{logit}\ (P_{\boldsymbol{x},\Delta t}(t)) \\
&= \log \pi_{x_A} + \alpha + \beta_A x_A + \beta x_E.
\end{aligned}
$$

Table 4.2 shows that because the sampling probability ratios depend on age stratum, the case-control exposure-adjusted log odds ratios comparing older subjects to younger subjects in the same SBP exposure group depend not only on the population odds ratios, but also on the ratios of sampling probabilities: $\beta_A + \log \pi_1 - \log \pi_0$. Because controls have been matched to cases, external information about the sampling probability ratios is required to estimate the population association of the matching variables with disease. When we fit this model to our frequency-matched case-control sample, we obtain:

$$\text{logit}(P_{\boldsymbol{x},\Delta t}^{CC}(t)) = -0.17 - 0.03 x_A + 0.97 x_E,$$

and the coefficient -0.03 of x_A estimates $\beta_A + \log \pi_1 - \log \pi_0$, a quantity that depends on both the population and the sampling design. If we did not have information about the sampling probability ratios π_1 and π_0, we could not recover meaningful information about the population association between age group and the risk of CHD.

TABLE 4.2

$\text{logit}(P_{\boldsymbol{x},\Delta t}^{CC}(t))$ under adjustment model

SBP	Age $<$ 55	Age $\geq$ 55
$<$ 165	$\log \pi_0 + \alpha$	$\log \pi_1 + \alpha + \beta_A$
$\geq$ 165	$\log \pi_0 + \alpha + \beta$	$\log \pi_1 + \alpha + \beta_A + \beta$

Table 4.3 shows that this is also true in the logistic model with interaction:

$$\text{logit}(P_{\boldsymbol{x},\Delta t}^{CC}(t)) = \alpha + \beta_A x_A + \beta x_E + \gamma x_A x_E,$$

where exposure-group specific odds ratios associated with age group also depend on the sampling probability ratios. Table 4.3 also shows that because of the cancellation of sampling probability ratios for exposure-disease odds ratios within age group, the coefficient γ of the interaction term involving x_A still provides the log ratio of age-group-specific odds ratios associated with SBP $\geq$ 165, even though the sample was frequency-matched on x_A.

TABLE 4.3

$\text{logit}(P_{\boldsymbol{x},\Delta t}^{CC}(t))$ under interaction model

SBP	Age $<$ 55	Age $\geq$ 55
$<$ 165	$\log \pi_0 + \alpha$	$\log \pi_1 + \alpha + \beta_A$
$\geq$ 165	$\log \pi_0 + \alpha + \beta$	$\log \pi_1 + \alpha + \beta_A + \beta + \gamma$

These characteristics of coefficient interpretation extend to more complicated logistic models fit to matched case-control data: coefficients of matching variables and combinations of matching variables do not have a population interpretation, but coefficients of unmatched variables and coefficients of interaction terms between unmatched variables and matching variables do have a population interpretation.

4.3.1   Logistic regression analysis of matched data

There are several ways logistic regression can adjust for matching variables and any additional confounders in the analysis of matched data from a case-control study. The type of adjustment variable used depends in part on the nature of the matching in the design. When cases and controls are pair-matched or frequency-matched on the values of a few, observable confounding variables, simple covariate adjustment for the matching variables in a logistic regression model may be adequate to adjust for the matching if the model assumptions are approximately correct. For example, in a case-control study that was pair-matched or frequency matched on age, linear or other continuous-variable adjustment models recommended in Chapter 3 can usually provide unbiased estimates of age-specific odds ratios associated with exposure, and a special "matched analysis" is not required (Pearce, 2016). As long as few adjustment terms are required in the logistic model relative to the sample size, exponentiated exposure-variable coefficient estimates will provide unbiased estimates of the common, conditional causal odds ratios for the association between one-unit differences in the exposure of interest and case status.

When controls are matched to cases on variables intended to account for a number of unobserved confounding variables, as when sibling, friend, or neighborhood controls are chosen, the situation is different. In this type of matching, it is only membership in the unique matched set that is observed, and not the values of all the confounding variables associated with the set membership. The only way to adjust for the confounders in the logistic regression analysis is to include a separate indicator variable for each (but one) of the matched sets. In pair-matched data with $I = \frac{n}{2}$ pairs, this means including $\frac{n}{2} - 1$ separate indicator variables. When many different observed confounding variables must be included in a logistic model, whether or not they were matching variables, the situation is similar: a large number of adjustment variables are required relative to the sample size.

Models with a large number of variables relative to sample size present a challenge to ordinary maximum likelihood estimation: maximum-likelihood estimates of coefficients may be very biased, even in large samples (Neyman and Scott, 1948). An extreme example is given by logistic regression models fit to pair-matched data, where the maximum likelihood estimate of the odds ratio associated with a binary exposure will be close to the square of the true odds ratio in large samples (Breslow and Day, 1980; Pike *et al.*, 1980). The logistic model that adjusts for matched set with indicator variables is the correct model to fit, but an alternative to the maximum likelihood method is needed to estimate the odds ratio of interest without considerable bias.

4.3.2   Conditional logistic regression

The conditional maximum likelihood estimation (CMLE) method provides consistent odds ratio estimates when a large number of strata need to be accounted for with indicator variables in the logistic model. Conditional logistic regression estimation is appropriate for the same model that we might wish to fit with ordinary maximum likelihood methods. It yields large-sample unbiased estimates of odds ratios of interest, but provides no estimates of coefficients associated with matching variables. The usual methods of likelihood-based inference including Wald's tests and associated confidence intervals, score tests and likelihood ratio tests are available, but they are based on an alternative likelihood formed from the conditional probability that the case(s) in each stratum is/are the one(s) associated with their observed covariate values.

As noted in Chapter 2, for $d_j = 1$ if the jth subject is a case and 0 if he or she is a control, the ordinary prospective likelihood maximized when a logistic regression model $\text{logit}(P_{\boldsymbol{x},\Delta t}^{CC}(t)) = \boldsymbol{x}^T\boldsymbol{\theta}$ is fit to case-control data is given by:

$$L(\boldsymbol{\theta}) \propto \prod_{j=1}^{n} \text{expit}(\boldsymbol{x}_j^T\boldsymbol{\theta})^{d_j} (1 - \text{expit}(\boldsymbol{x}_j^T\boldsymbol{\theta}))^{1-d_j} = \prod_{j=1}^{n} \left(\frac{e^{d_j \boldsymbol{x}_j^T\boldsymbol{\theta}}}{1 + e^{\boldsymbol{x}_j^T\boldsymbol{\theta}}} \right).$$

If we distinguish between variables, $x_{S1}, \ldots, x_{SI}$, that indicate stratum or matched set and terms $x_1, \ldots, x_K$ for other explanatory variables including the exposure of interest, we can write the linear predictor as

$$\boldsymbol{x}^T\boldsymbol{\theta} = \alpha_1 x_{S1} + \alpha_2 x_{S2} + \cdots + \alpha_I x_{SI} + \beta_1 x_1 + \cdots + \beta_K x_K$$

and note that this likelihood, generated from the binomial probability that a subject is a case under a prospective-sampling logistic model, is a function of *all* the coefficients, $\boldsymbol{\theta} = (\alpha_1, \ldots, \alpha_I, \beta_1, \ldots, \beta_K)^T$, in the linear predictor $\boldsymbol{x}^T\boldsymbol{\theta}$.

The conditional likelihood is derived from the conditional probability that the case(s) in a stratum is/are the stratum member(s) associated with their observed combination(s) of the explanatory variables, given the combinations of explanatory variable values in each stratum and the total number of cases and controls in each stratum. Re-indexing the case-control indicators for the jth subject in the ith stratum, we let the case-control outcome be defined by

$$d_{ij} = \begin{cases} 1 & \text{case,} \\ 0 & \text{control.} \end{cases}$$

We let J_i be the total number of cases and controls in the ith stratum, and we let x_{kij} be the value of the kth explanatory variable for the jth subject in the ith stratum. Then letting $D_i = \sum_{j=1}^{J_i} d_{ij}$, rewriting $\boldsymbol{x}^T\boldsymbol{\theta} = \boldsymbol{v}^T\boldsymbol{\alpha} + \boldsymbol{w}^T\boldsymbol{\beta}$ for $\boldsymbol{v} = (D_1, \ldots, D_I)^T$, $\boldsymbol{w} = \sum_{i=1}^{I} \sum_{j=1}^{J_i} (x_{1ij}d_{ij}, \ldots, x_{Kij}d_{ij})^T$, $\boldsymbol{\alpha} = (\alpha_1, \ldots, \alpha_I)^T$, and $\boldsymbol{\beta} = (\beta_1, \ldots, \beta_K)^T$, it can be shown (Cox and Snell, 1989; Boos and Stefanski, 2013) that for $c(\boldsymbol{w}, \boldsymbol{v})$ equal to the number of ways the observed d_{ij}s could be assigned within each stratum and still result in the same values of $\boldsymbol{w}$ and $\boldsymbol{v}$, the conditional likelihood for $\boldsymbol{\beta}$ is given by:

$$L_c(\boldsymbol{\beta}) = \frac{c(\boldsymbol{w}, \boldsymbol{v}) \exp\{\boldsymbol{w}^T\boldsymbol{\beta}\}}{\sum_{\boldsymbol{u}} c(\boldsymbol{u}, \boldsymbol{v}) \exp\{\boldsymbol{u}^T\boldsymbol{\beta}\}}.$$

In the case of strata formed by matching M controls to each case, where $\boldsymbol{x}_{i1}$ is the covariate values for the case and $\boldsymbol{x}_{ij}, j = 2, \ldots, J_i \equiv M + 1$ is the covariate values for the $(j-1)$-st control in the ith matched set, this simplifies to (Breslow *et al.*, 1978):

$$\prod_{i=1}^{I} \frac{\exp(\boldsymbol{x}_{i1}^T\boldsymbol{\beta})}{\sum_{j=1}^{M+1} \exp(\boldsymbol{x}_{ij}^T\boldsymbol{\beta})}.$$

For matched pairs it simplifies further to

$$\prod_{i=1}^{I} \frac{\exp\{\boldsymbol{x}_{i1}^T\boldsymbol{\beta}\}}{\exp\{\boldsymbol{x}_{i1}^T\boldsymbol{\beta}\} + \exp\{\boldsymbol{x}_{i2}^T\boldsymbol{\beta}\}} = \prod_{i=1}^{I} \text{expit}\{(\boldsymbol{x}_{i1}^T - \boldsymbol{x}_{i2}^T)\boldsymbol{\beta}\}.$$

Because the probability for each stratum used to generate this likelihood conditions on the stratum's total number of cases and controls, the likelihood does not depend on the parameters α that describe how case status is associated with stratum membership. This is because the conditional probability does not depend on any matching variables used to define the strata. Thus, although indicators for stratum membership are in the logistic model being fit by conditional logistic regression, the procedure does not provide estimates for the coefficients α of the stratum indicator variables. The lack of estimates $\hat{\alpha}$ does not mean that matched-set membership or matching variables have not been controlled by a conditional logistic regression model. It means only that the coefficients of indicators for the matched sets have not been estimated.

Conditional logistic regression requires that strata be formed and that indicators for stratum membership be included in the model. When the bias of ordinary maximum likelihood estimates is due to a large number of quantitative and other adjustment variables that are not stratum indicators, strata based on like values of the adjustment variables must be formed to use the method. Each stratum constructed in this way must contain at least one case and one control for its data to be used. When the formed strata include subjects with dissimilar values for a few of the adjustment variables, residual confounding can be controlled by adding these few variables as adjustment terms (for which a coefficient will be estimated) to the model. These added variables must be viewed solely as adjustment variables. Their coefficient estimates will have no useful population interpretation because some of the variable-case association is accounted for by stratum indicator coefficients α that are not estimated.

For large strata with several cases, maximization of the conditional likelihood can be computationally intensive, but efficient algorithms have been derived (Hirji *et al.*, 1987) and are available in Stata (StataCorp, 2015). An approximate version is available in the `elrm` package in R (R Core Team, 2016; Zamar *et al.*, 2007). The similarity of the conditional likelihood to the partial likelihood used for Cox regression analysis means that approximations (Gail *et al.*, 1981) proposed in that setting can be useful as well. Several statistical packages, including Stata (StataCorp, 2015) and the `survival` package in R (R Core Team, 2016; Therneau, 2015), have procedures that will fit logistic regression models by conditional maximum likelihood and provide inference based on large-sample approximations.

4.3.3   Bias of ordinary MLEs in matched data

Pike *et al.* (1980) and Breslow and Day (1980) show the extent of bias from ordinary, unconditional maximum likelihood estimation (MLE) for matched case-control data with small stratum sizes. For strata formed of one case and one control, in large samples the maximum likelihood estimate of the odds ratio is approximately the square of the correct one. In strata formed of 10 cases and 10 controls, the bias depends on the proportion of subjects who are exposed and the value of the odds ratio, but can be as high as 15% for very large odds ratios.

Figure 4.1 presents simulation results comparing odds ratio estimates from maximum likelihood and conditional likelihood inferences for indicator-variable-adjusted models based on matched case-control samples under two scenarios. In the first scenario, 1 control is matched to 1 case; in the second, 5 controls are matched to 5 cases. In both designs there are 200 cases and 200 controls: with pair matching there are 200 strata and with strata formed of 5 cases and 5 controls there are 40 strata. In the simulations, the probability controls were exposed was 0.3, and the maximum odds ratio relating exposure to matched set was 1.2. With 10 subjects per stratum, the bias in the unconditional maximum likelihood estimate of the odds ratio is minimal, but it is severe for one-to-one matched data. Conditional logistic regression estimates show little bias for either of the two types of data.

This example shows that ordinary maximum-likelihood does not induce large bias in

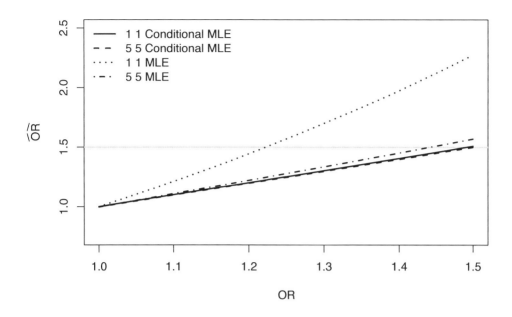

FIGURE 4.1

Average odds ratio estimates over 5000 simulation replications plotted against the true odds ratio. Four curves represent conditional or ordinary maximum likelihood with 1 case and 1 control or with 5 cases and 5 controls in each matching stratum.

frequency-matched data where the matched sets are relatively large. Thus, the bias is not a feature of the matched data, but, rather, results from logistic regression analysis of case-control data when the number of adjustment variables is large (Pearce, 2016).

Figure 4.2 presents the proportion of 5000 replications for which the likelihood or conditional likelihood ratio test rejected the null hypothesis that the odds ratio is one. In pair-matched data, the unconditional likelihood ratio test rejects the null hypothesis far too often when the odds ratio is one, but the conditional likelihood ratio test has the appropriate size. The power of the conditional logistic regression likelihood ratio test for pair-matched data is similar to both conditional and ordinary likelihood ratio tests for the same number of subjects when there are five cases and five controls per stratum.

4.4   Infertility matched case-control study example

These ideas are illustrated by a comparison of model fits to data from a matched case-control study. Trichopoulos *et al.* (1976) studied risk factors for secondary infertility in Athens in the 1970s. Two controls were matched to each case: the controls sought care from the same gynecologic clinic as the case, were the same age, had the same parity, and had a similar level of education. Both cases and controls were queried about a history of both spontaneous

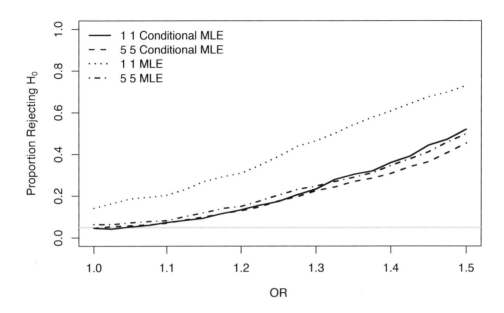

FIGURE 4.2
Estimated size and power of the likelihood ratio test over 5000 simulation replications plotted against the true odds ratio. Four curves represent conditional or ordinary maximum likelihood with 1 case and 1 control or with 5 cases and 5 controls in each matching stratum.

abortion and a history of (illegal) induced abortion. Raw data for the matched sets, sorted by the values of all matching variables but clinic, were listed in the article, and data for all but one subject, a control, who had a history of two or more prior spontaneous and two or more prior induced abortions, are available in the `survival` package (Therneau, 2015) of the R statistical programming language (R Core Team, 2016).

Logistic models with various forms of adjustment for the matching variables were fit to the data by either the maximum likelihood or conditional maximum likelihood methods. Population variation in women's desire to become pregnant means that a history of induced abortions is negatively associated with a history of spontaneous abortions in this population. Infection following prior spontaneous abortion might also lead to secondary infertility. For that reason, it is important to adjust odds ratios associated with history of induced abortion for history of spontaneous abortion. At the time the article was published, no "matched-data" methods were available that could also adjust for a confounding variable, like history of spontaneous abortion, that was not a matching variable. Here, we compare the modern method of conditional logistic regression to other possibilities. All models include the following two indicator variables for history of spontaneous abortion:

$$x_{S1} = \begin{cases} 1 & \text{1 Prior Spontaneous Abortion,} \\ 0 & \text{Otherwise,} \end{cases}$$

$$x_{S2} = \begin{cases} 1 & \text{2+ Prior Spontaneous Abortions,} \\ 0 & \text{Otherwise,} \end{cases}$$

and all contained the following two indicator variables for history of induced abortion:

$$x_{I1} = \begin{cases} 1 & \text{1 Prior Induced Abortion,} \\ 0 & \text{Otherwise,} \end{cases}$$

$$x_{I2} = \begin{cases} 1 & \text{2+ Prior Induced Abortions,} \\ 0 & \text{Otherwise.} \end{cases}$$

The following four models were fit to the data.

Unadjusted: A model that adjusts only for prior spontaneous abortion and includes no adjustment for matched set or matching variables:

$$\text{logit}(P^{CC}_{x,\Delta t}(t)) = \alpha + \beta_{SA1}x_{SA1} + \beta_{SA2}x_{SA2} + \beta_{IA1}x_{IA1} + \beta_{IA2}x_{IA2}.$$

Covariate Adjusted: A model that adds linear adjustment for age and parity, and adjusts for education level with two indicator variables. Letting

x_A = age in years,

x_P = number of prior full-term pregnancies,

$$x_{E1} = \begin{cases} 1 & \text{6 - 11 years education,} \\ 0 & \text{Otherwise,} \end{cases}$$

$$x_{E2} = \begin{cases} 1 & \text{12+ years education,} \\ 0 & \text{Otherwise,} \end{cases}$$

the model is

$$\begin{aligned} \text{logit}(P^{CC}_{x,\Delta t}(t)) = \ & \alpha + \alpha_A x_A + \alpha_P x_P + \alpha_{E1}x_{E1} + \alpha_{E2}x_{E2} + \\ & \beta_{SA1}x_{SA1} + \beta_{SA2}x_{SA2} + \beta_{IA1}x_{IA1} + \beta_{IA2}x_{IA2}. \end{aligned}$$

Matched Set Adjusted: Indicator variables, one for each but one of the 83 matched sets, are included in the model. Letting

$$x_{Mi} = \begin{cases} 1 & i\text{th matched set,} \\ 0 & \text{Otherwise,} \end{cases}$$

the model is

$$\begin{aligned} \text{logit}(P^{CC}_{x,\Delta t}(t)) = \ & \alpha + \alpha_2 x_{M2} + \cdots + \alpha_{83}x_{M83} + \\ & \beta_{SA1}x_{SA1} + \beta_{SA2}x_{SA2} + \beta_{IA1}x_{IA1} + \beta_{IA2}x_{IA2}. \end{aligned}$$

Pooled Matched Set Adjusted: Indicator variables, one for each but one of the 63 strata formed from matched sets with the same values of the age, parity and education variables, are included in the model. Letting

$$x_{PMi} = \begin{cases} 1 & i\text{th pooled matched set,} \\ 0 & \text{Otherwise,} \end{cases}$$

the model is

$$\begin{aligned} \text{logit}(P^{CC}_{x,\Delta t}(t)) = \ & \alpha + \alpha_{PM2}x_{PM2} + \cdots + \alpha_{PM63}x_{PM63} + \\ & \beta_{SA1}x_{SA1} + \beta_{SA2}x_{SA2} + \beta_{IA1}x_{IA1} + \beta_{IA2}x_{IA2}. \end{aligned}$$

All four models were fit by maximum likelihood. The matched set and pooled matched set adjusted models were also fit by conditional maximum likelihood.

Table 4.4 gives odds ratio estimates for the association between prior induced abortion and the risk of secondary infertility from these models. Comparing the unadjusted and covariate adjusted logistic models, we see that covariate adjustment for the matching variables increases the odds ratio estimates. This is likely due to confounding by the matching variables, but some portion of the difference may also be due to the lack of collapsibility of the odds ratio (Chapters 3 and 6). When thorough adjustment for matched set is included in a model fit by maximum likelihood, the estimated odds ratios become extraordinarily high and more highly statistically significantly different from one. This is likely due to the bias introduced by including 83 indicator variables in the model and fitting with maximum likelihood. This bias is ameliorated slightly when only 63 variables, indicating pooled matched sets, replace the matched-set specific indicators.

Conditional logistic regression provides unbiased estimates in models with these indicator variable adjustment models. These odds ratios are lower, similar to each other, and roughly similar to covariate-adjusted odds ratios obtained by maximum likelihood. Results from the covariate-adjusted maximum likelihood fit and either of the conditional maximum likelihood fits all provide a good summary of the information about the association between induced abortion and secondary infertility in these data.

TABLE 4.4

Odds ratio relative to no prior induced abortions, adjusted for age, education, parity, and prior number of spontaneous abortions.

Model	Induced Abortions	OR	95% CI	P-value
MLE Unadjusted	1	1.6	(0.8, 3.2)	1.9×10^{-1}
	2+	2.3	(1, 5.3)	5.6×10^{-2}
MLE Covariate Adjusted	1	3.5	(1.6, 8)	2.5×10^{-3}
	2+	13.4	(4, 44.8)	2.7×10^{-5}
MLE Matched Sets	1	8.3	(2.6, 26.1)	3.2×10^{-4}
	2+	82.9	(12.9, 531.2)	3.1×10^{-6}
MLE Pooled Matched Sets	1	7.0	(2.4, 20.6)	3.9×10^{-4}
	2+	59.0	(10.7, 326.6)	3.0×10^{-6}
CMLE Matched Sets	1	4.0	(1.6, 9.9)	2.8×10^{-3}
	2+	16.8	(4, 70.8)	1.3×10^{-4}
CMLE Pooled Matched Sets	1	3.9	(1.6, 9.5)	3.1×10^{-3}
	2+	17.8	(4.4, 72.4)	5.7×10^{-5}

4.5   Summary

Matching is an attractive option for the design of a case-control study when subjects within a matched set have similar values of important but unobserved confounders, or when matching can increase the conditional causal odds ratio estimate's precision by making case and control distributions of confounding variables the same. Matching can also make identification of suitable controls easier when easy-to-identify subjects like family members, neighbors, or friends can serve as controls.

When case and control distributions of matching variables differ markedly, finding an exact match for some cases may require screening a large number of potential controls. Also, unlike unmatched designs that rely on covariate adjustment alone, a design that matches on variables influenced by exposure cannot be compensated for in the analysis unless stratum-specific sampling probabilities are known. This means that matching variables should be chosen very carefully.

Conditional logistic regression is a flexible method that provides consistent estimates of the conditional causal odds ratio even when adjusting for many variables by stratification. In matched case-control data, it permits adjustment not only for matching variables but also for variables that were not part of the matching and for slight differences between values of imperfectly matched variables.

Bibliography

Boos, D. D. and Stefanski, L. A. (2013). *Essential Statistical Inference: Theory and Methods*. Springer, New York.

Breslow, N. (1982). Design and analysis of case-control studies. *Annual Review of Public Health*, **3**, 29–54.

Breslow, N. E. and Day, N. E. (1980). *Statistical Methods in Cancer Research. Vol. 1: The Analysis of Case-Control Studies*. IARC, Lyon.

Breslow, N. E., Day, N. E., Halvorsen, K. T., Prentice, R. L., and Sabai, C. (1978). Estimation of multiple relative risk functions in matched case-control studies. *American Journal of Epidemiology*, **108**, 299–307.

Cox, D. R. and Snell, E. J. (1989). *Analysis of Binary Data*. CRC Press, 2nd edition.

Didelez, V., Kreiner, S., and Keiding, N. (2010). Graphical models for inference under outcome-dependent sampling. *Statistical Science*, **25**, 368–387.

Gail, M. H., Lubin, J. H., and Rubinstein, L. V. (1981). Likelihood calculations for matched case-control studies and survival studies with tied death times. *Biometrika*, **68**, 703–707.

Hirji, K. F., Mehta, C. R., and Patel, N. R. (1987). Computing distributions for exact logistic regression. *Journal of the American Statistical Association*, **82**, 1110–1117.

Mansournia, M. A., Hernn, M. A., and Greenland, S. (2013). Matched designs and causal diagrams. *International Journal of Epidemiology*, **42**, 860–869.

Neyman, J. and Scott, E. L. (1948). Consistent estimates based on partially consistent observations. *Econometrica*, **16**, 1–32.

Pearce, N. (2016). Analysis of matched case-control studies. *BMJ*, **352**, i969.

Pike, M. C., Hill, A. P., and Smith, P. G. (1980). Bias and efficiency in logistic analyses of stratified case-control studies. *International Journal of Epidemiology*, **9**, 89–95.

R Core Team (2016). *R: A Language and Environment for Statistical Computing*. R Foundation for Statistical Computing, Vienna, Austria.

Rothman, K. J., Greenland, S., and Lash, T. L. (2012). *Modern Epidemiology*. Lippincott Williams & Wilkins, Philadelphia, 3rd edition.

Rubin, D. B. (1976). Multivariate matching methods that are equal percent bias reducing, I: Some examples. *Biometrics*, **32**, 109–120.

Scott, A. J. and Wild, C. J. (1991). Fitting logistic regression models in stratified case-control studies. *Biometrics*, **47**, 497–510.

StataCorp (2015). *Stata Statistical Software: Release 14*. StataCorp LP, College Station, TX.

Therneau, T. M. (2015). *A Package for Survival Analysis in S*. version 2.38.

Thomas, D. C. and Greenland, S. (1983). The relative efficiencies of matched and independent sample designs for case-control studies. *Journal of Chronic Diseases*, **36**, 685–697.

Trichopoulos, D., Handanos, N., Danezis, J., Kalandidi, A., and Kalapothaki, V. (1976). Induced abortion and secondary infertility. *British Journal of Obstetrics and Gynaecology*, **83**, 645–650.

Wacholder, S., Silverman, D. T., McLaughlin, J. K., and Mandel, J. S. (1992). Selection of controls in case-control studies: II. Types of controls. *American Journal of Epidemiology*, **135**, 1029–1041.

Zamar, D., McNeney, B., and Graham, J. (2007). elrm: Software implementing exact-like inference for logistic regression models. *Journal of Statistical Software*, **21**, 1–18.

5

Multiple Case or Control Groups

Barbara McKnight

University of Washington

5.1 Introduction

Case-control studies can sample more than one case group and/or more than one control group for a number of reasons. Sometimes multiple case or control groups may be sampled to examine the robustness of an observed association between exposure and disease. As one example, in a clinic-based study of alcohol consumption and lung cancer, one might use both bone-fracture controls and acne controls to protect against the possibility that, unbeknownst to investigators, one or the other of these conditions is associated with alcohol use. As another example, if the association of prior vasectomy with prostate cancer is stronger for less aggressive disease, this may be because vasectomized men are more likely to be screened and diagnosed, and not because vasectomy causes cancer (Stanford *et al.*, 1999). In addition, when different subtypes of disease lead to different treatment options and have different prognoses, it can be of public health importance to determine whether an exposure is associated with the incidence of all, or only some, subtypes of the disease. For example, Britton *et al.* (2002) compared joint hormone receptor positive and hormone receptor negative breast cancer cases to population controls.

At other times, different types of controls are available for the assessment of different types of exposure. For example, Sherman *et al.* (1988) selected two control groups when studying the association between human papilloma virus (HPV) infection and vulvar cancer: a representative population control group obtained by random digit dialing (RDD) for whom only blood specimens were available for serologic HPV testing, and a more select control group of women who had undergone surgery for benign conditions of the vulva in whom vulvar tissue was also available for HPV DNA testing. Investigators were interested in estimating the odds ratio relating prior history of an ano-genital tumor to case status, but recognized that this association might differ between comparisons of cases to these two control groups. Since prior ano-genital tumors might share risk factors with benign conditions of the vulva, they expected the odds ratio associated with prior tumor comparing cases to the more representative RDD controls to be higher than the odds ratio comparing cases to the less representative group of controls who provided vulvar tissue.

When a study collects data on more than a single case and single control group, modeling the joint relationship between all groups and confounders and exposures of interest offers the possibility of estimating multiple odds ratios and comparing them. By using the data together to fit one model, this procedure might be expected to lead to additional precision compared to sets of pairwise comparisons using logistic models, at the cost of only a few, plausible assumptions. This chapter describes the polytomous logistic regression model that can be fit to multiple-category outcome data in a case-control study, evaluates its advantages and disadvantages compared to pairwise logistic regression analysis of two groups at a time, and describes how constraints on the polytomous model can provide a basis for important scientific inferences.

5.2   Polytomous logistic regression models

The polytomous logistic regression model relates the values of explanatory variables to the probabilities of outcome when the outcome has more than two categories. As is true for logistic regression modeling of binary outcome case-control-study data (Chapter 3), prospective modeling of the probability of outcome has a population interpretation when the data were collected conditional on outcome variable status. This chapter will use simplified notation for these outcome probabilities given below.

For $I > 2$ outcome categories, let $D_j = i, i = 0, \ldots, I - 1$ give the outcome category to which the jth subject belongs, let $S_j = 1$ indicate that the jth subject was sampled for the multiple outcome group study, and $\boldsymbol{x}_j$ be a vector of explanatory variables for the jth subject. Then define the conditional probability of being in the ith outcome group, given explanatory variable vector $\boldsymbol{x}_j$ and having been sampled to be

$$p_i(\boldsymbol{x}_j) = P(D_j = i | \boldsymbol{x}_j, S_j = 1),$$

for $i = 0, \ldots, I - 1$ and $j = 1, \ldots, n$.

When there are more than two outcome categories, arguments by Prentice and Pyke (1979) allow us to use the likelihood drawn from the multinomial distribution of the outcome variable. For simplicity, most of this chapter will focus on the situation, like the vulvar cancer and breast cancer examples, where $I = 3$. The polytomous logistic model relates the values of the explanatory variables $\boldsymbol{x}_j$ to ratios of outcome category probabilities. For a trinomial model ($I = 3$) this involves two equations based on ratios relating two of the outcome group probabilities to a third:

$$\log \frac{p_1(\boldsymbol{x}_j)}{p_0(\boldsymbol{x}_j)} = \alpha^{(1)} + \boldsymbol{x}_j^T \boldsymbol{\beta}^{(1)},$$

$$\log \frac{p_2(\boldsymbol{x}_j)}{p_0(\boldsymbol{x}_j)} = \alpha^{(2)} + \boldsymbol{x}_j^T \boldsymbol{\beta}^{(2)}.$$

As described in Chapter 3, coefficients $\boldsymbol{\beta}$ in these models can be interpreted as log incidence rate ratios or as log odds ratios and they are the same parameters that would be estimated in a binary logistic model comparison that involves only two groups, since the normalizing constants $p_0(\boldsymbol{x}_j) + p_1(\boldsymbol{x}_j)$ and $p_0(\boldsymbol{x}_j) + p_2(\boldsymbol{x}_j)$ would cancel. The choice of which category's probability is numerator or denominator in each equation is arbitrary, but it influences the interpretation of the coefficients $\boldsymbol{\beta}$. In the breast cancer example we might choose the control group in both denominators so that the coefficients $\boldsymbol{\beta}$ are log odds ratios for each of the two diseases relative to control. In the vulvar cancer example, we might choose the case group for both numerators so that the coefficients $\boldsymbol{\beta}$ are log odds ratios for disease relative to each of the two control groups.

With an arbitrary choice of the 0th, first, and second outcome categories, and setting $\alpha^{(0)} = 0$ and $\boldsymbol{\beta}^{(0)} = \boldsymbol{0}$, we can write the outcome probabilities in terms of the explanatory variables in the model parameters:

$$p_i(\boldsymbol{x}_j) = \frac{e^{\alpha^{(i)} + \boldsymbol{x}_j^T \boldsymbol{\beta}^{(i)}}}{e^{\alpha^{(0)} + \boldsymbol{x}_j^T \boldsymbol{\beta}^{(0)}} + e^{\alpha^{(1)} + \boldsymbol{x}_j^T \boldsymbol{\beta}^{(1)}} + e^{\alpha^{(2)} + \boldsymbol{x}_j^T \boldsymbol{\beta}^{(2)}}}$$

for $i = 0, 1, 2$. Letting

$$d_{ij} = \begin{cases} 1 & j\text{th subject is in } i\text{th outcome group,} \\ 0 & \text{otherwise,} \end{cases}$$

the trinomial likelihood function is given by:

$$
\begin{aligned}
L(\boldsymbol{\beta}) \quad &\propto \quad \prod_{j=1}^{n} p_0(\boldsymbol{x}_j)^{d_{1j}} p_1(\boldsymbol{x}_j)^{d_{2j}} p_2(\boldsymbol{x}_j)^{d_{3j}} \\
&= \quad \prod_{j=1}^{n} \frac{e^{d_{1j}(\alpha^{(1)} + \boldsymbol{x}_j^T \boldsymbol{\beta}^{(1)}) + d_{2j}(\alpha^{(2)} + \boldsymbol{x}_j^T \boldsymbol{\beta}^{(2)})}}{1 + e^{\alpha^{(1)} + \boldsymbol{x}_j^T \boldsymbol{\beta}^{(1)}} + e^{\alpha^{(2)} + \boldsymbol{x}_j^T \boldsymbol{\beta}^{(2)}}}.
\end{aligned}
$$

Coefficient estimates are obtained by maximizing this likelihood, and tests of hypothesis, including hypotheses that odds ratios comparing two different case groups to control for a case group to two different control groups are the same, can be formed in the usual way with likelihood ratio, score, or Wald's tests. Many statistical packages, including both Stata (StataCorp, 2015) and R (R Core Team, 2016), have functions or packages that can fit multinomial logistic models. These models can also be fit using an equivalent conditional logistic regression model (Becher, 1991) or an equivalent log-linear model (Fienberg, 2007).

5.2.1 Vulvar cancer example: Two control groups

Table 5.1 gives data provided by Sherman *et al.* (1988) on the association between prior ano-genital tumor and case-control status for in situ vulvar cancer cases, biopsy controls, and controls obtained by random-digit dialing (RDD controls).

Letting $\boldsymbol{x}_j = (x_{Aj}, x_{Tj})$ for

$$x_{Aj} = \begin{cases} 1 & \text{Age} \geq 50, \\ 0 & \text{Otherwise,} \end{cases}$$

$$x_{Tj} = \begin{cases} 1 & \text{Prior AG tumor,} \\ 0 & \text{Otherwise,} \end{cases}$$

and assigning

$$D_j = \begin{cases} 0 & \text{In Situ Vulvar Cancer Case,} \\ 1 & \text{Biopsy control,} \\ 2 & \text{RDD control,} \end{cases}$$

TABLE 5.1

Case-control status for vulvar cancer and two types of controls versus prior or concurrent history of ano-genital tumor, by age group.

		Cancer In Situ	Biopsy Controls	RDD Controls
No History AG tumor	Age < 50	58	65	113
	Age ≥ 50	37	43	97
History AG tumor	Age < 50	20	1	0
	Age ≥ 50	8	4	2

the following polytomous logistic model was fit to these data:

$$\log\left(\frac{p_0(\boldsymbol{x}_j)}{p_1(\boldsymbol{x}_j)}\right) = \alpha^{(1)} + \beta_A^{(1)} x_{Aj} + \beta_T^{(1)} x_{Tj}, \tag{5.1}$$

$$\log\left(\frac{p_0(\boldsymbol{x}_j)}{p_2(\boldsymbol{x}_j)}\right) = \alpha^{(2)} + \beta_A^{(2)} x_{Aj} + \beta_T^{(2)} x_{Tj}. \tag{5.2}$$

Here $e^{\beta_T^{(1)}}$ can be interpreted as the age-group adjusted odds ratio for the association of prior AG tumor with case status when comparing to biopsy controls and $e^{\beta_T^{(2)}}$ can be interpreted as the age-group adjusted odds ratio for the association of prior AG tumor with case status when comparing to RDD controls. In the polytomous model we can compare these two OR estimates and impose the constraint that $\beta_T^{(1)} = \beta_T^{(2)}$ to estimate an assumed common OR and test whether it is, indeed, common to the two comparisons. Table 5.2 gives results from fitting these models to the vulvar cancer data and comparing the fits with a likelihood ratio test. As expected, a prior ano-genital tumor appears much more strongly associated with case status when comparing cases to RDD controls than when comparing cases to biopsy controls. Under the null hypothesis that these two ORs are the same, the estimated OR is intermediate between the two, but we can reject this null hypothesis (P = 0.045).

5.3 Comparison to pairwise logistic regression

Begg and Gray (1984) compared statistical inference using the polytomous logistic regression

TABLE 5.2

Age-group adjusted OR associated with prior ano-genital tumor under constrained and unconstrained models.

Model	Controls	OR	95% CI	$\log(L(\hat{\boldsymbol{\beta}}))$	P-value
Unconstrained	Biopsy	6.4	(2.4, 17.3)	-29.93	
	RDD	31.3	(7.3, 134.5)		
Constrained	Biopsy	13.5	(5.7, 32.0)	-31.94	0.0451
	RDD	13.5	(5.7, 32.0)		

TABLE 5.3
Comparison of polytomous and pairwise logistic
models for the vulvar cancer data.

Controls	Polytomous $\hat{\beta}$	SE	Pairwise Logistic $\hat{\beta}$	SE
Biopsy	1.857	0.506	1.849	0.506
RDD	3.444	0.744	3.413	0.743

model to inferences that could be obtained by making the pairwise comparisons described by each polytomous model equation using separate binary logistic regression models fit to the data on just two of the outcome groups. They found that tests and coefficient estimates from pairwise logistic models are often almost as efficient as inferences from the polytomous logistic model, particularly when there are few outcome categories, the common denominator outcome category has a moderate or high probability, and model coefficients are not large. In the cases they studied, the lowest efficiencies occurred when there were a large number (7-11) of outcome categories, or with fewer categories, when the probability of the baseline category is less than a third and/or odds ratios are large as four or more.

5.3.1 Vulvar cancer example continued

Pairwise logistic models following equations (5.1) and (5.2) were fit to the vulvar cancer data and estimates of coefficients $\beta_T^{(i)}$ and their standard errors for the two estimation procedures are compared in Table 5.3. There is no important difference between the two methods for obtaining estimates in the unconstrained model from these data.

It is not possible to use standard statistical software to estimate the constrained, common odds ratio after separate binary logistic fits of the pairwise models without additional computation. Standard software can be used to make an approximate test of whether the two ORs are different, however: a logistic model can be fit to compare the two compared outcome groups (two control groups in our example) in a binary logistic model. This comparison was performed in the example data by fitting the logistic model in Equation (5.3):

$$\log \left(\frac{p_1(\boldsymbol{x})/(p_1(\boldsymbol{x}) + p_2(\boldsymbol{x}))}{p_2(\boldsymbol{x})/(p_1(\boldsymbol{x}) + p_2(\boldsymbol{x}))} \right) = \alpha^{(3)} + \beta_A^{(3)} x_A + \beta_T^{(3)} x_T. \quad (5.3)$$

The odds ratio for the risk of being a sampled biopsy control associated with a prior AG tumor is estimated to be $e^{\hat{\beta}_T^{(3)}} = 1.70$ from the fit of model (5.3), and results from the likelihood ratio test of whether, adjusted for age group, the two controls have a similar history of AG tumors are similar to the polytomous logistic regression model likelihood ratio test that the odds ratios associated with prior AG tumor are the same ($\chi_1^2 = 4.533$, P = 0.033).

5.4 Advantages of polytomous model

In addition to the situations where the polytomous model offers greater efficiency, the main advantage to polytomous logistic regression over the pairwise comparison of groups using logistic regression is its ability to fit models where coefficients in different equations are constrained to have the same value. In Section 5.2 we estimated an odds ratio associated

TABLE 5.4
First-pass data-presentation table for the
testicular cancer data.

	Cases	Controls
Cryptorchid	32	12
Same Side Only	22	?
Opposite Side Only	5	?
Bilateral	5	2
Not Cryptorchid	286	658
Total	318	670

with prior ano-genital tumor comparing cases to both biopsy and RDD controls under the
constraint that these two odds ratios be the same. This allowed us to perform a likelihood
ratio test of whether the two odds ratios are the same, and to estimate the common odds
ratio. Although this constrained odds ratio model was really only of interest as a null model
to be tested in this example, odds ratios constrained to be the same across polytomous
logistic models can occasionally be of scientific importance, as the next example shows.

5.4.1   Testicular cancer example: Side of cryptorchism

Strader *et al.* (1988) performed a case-control study to examine the association between
cryptorchism and the risk of testicular cancer. One question of scientfic interest was whether
the environment in the undescended testical contributed to increased risk of testicular cancer
or whether there was a more systemic abnormality in cryptorchid men that increased the
risk of cancer. If the testicular environment before surgical correction led to increased risk
of cancer, one would expect the association of cryptorchism with a testicular cancer to
be higher on the same side as the tumor than it is on the opposite side. A risk-increasing
environment could have implications for the recommended age at which cryptorchism should
be surgically corrected. Strader *et al.* (1988)'s case-control study data in Table 5.4 highlights
the difficulty in approaching this question with standard binary logistic regression methods
for case-control study data: although it is clear whether cases' exposures to cryptorchism
are on the same side or the opposite side from their tumors, the same-side/opposite side
dichotomy has no meaning for controls.

This analysis problem was solved by a clever idea from Professor Norman Breslow using
polytomous logistic regression. Recasting the data in terms of left- and right-sided cancers (none was bilateral) and left- and right-sided cryptorchism gives the presentation in
Table 5.5. Here it becomes evident that a polytomous logistic regression model with constraints on the coefficients will allow estimation of odds ratios associated with ipsilateral
and contralateral tumor.

We can let the three outcome category probabilities be denoted by

$$
\begin{aligned}
p_L(\boldsymbol{x}_j) &= P(\text{left-sided case} \mid \boldsymbol{x}_j, S = 1), \\
p_R(\boldsymbol{x}_j) &= P(\text{right-sided case} \mid \boldsymbol{x}_j, S = 1), \\
p_0(\boldsymbol{x}_j) &= P(\text{control} \mid \boldsymbol{x}_j, S = 1)
\end{aligned}
$$

for the *j*th subject, and let the exposure-side indicators for the *j*th subject be given by

$$
x_{Lj} = \begin{cases} 1 & \text{Left-side cryptorchid,} \\ 0 & \text{Otherwise,} \end{cases}
$$

TABLE 5.5

Testicular cancer data by side of tumor and side of
cryptorchism.

	Left Cases	Right Cases	Controls
Cryptorchid	11	21	12
Left side	8	4	3
Right side	1	14	7
Bilateral	2	3	2
Not Cryptorchid	130	156	658

and

$$x_{Rj} = \begin{cases} 1 & \text{Right-side cryptorchid,} \\ 0 & \text{Otherwise.} \end{cases}$$

Note that these explanatory variables are defined for all cases and controls, including those with bilateral cryptorchism.

We consider the following polytomous logistic model:

$$\log \frac{p_L(\boldsymbol{x}_j)}{p_0(\boldsymbol{x}_j)} = \alpha^{(L)} + \beta_I^{(L)} x_{Lj} + \beta_C^{(L)} x_{Rj}, \tag{5.4}$$

$$\log \frac{p_R(\boldsymbol{x}_j)}{p_0(\boldsymbol{x}_j)} = \alpha^{(R)} + \beta_C^{(R)} x_{Lj} + \beta_I^{(R)} x_{Rj}. \tag{5.5}$$

The model given by (5.4) and (5.5) can impose the constraint that the ipsilateral log odds ratios $\beta_I^{(L)} = \beta_I^{(R)}$ and contralateral log odds ratios $\beta_C^{(L)} = \beta_C^{(R)}$ are the same in both equations. We can test this constraint, and in addition we can test whether these two odds ratios are equal to each other, and whether they are one, using standard likelihood-based methods. The Stata statistical package (StataCorp, 2015) has a particularly nice interface for imposing cross-equation constraints in polytomous logistic models.

Odds ratio estimates for fits of various versions of the model given by (5.4) and (5.5) with different constraints imposed are given in Table 5.6 along with the values of likelihood ratio test statistics comparing each model to the unconstrained model. From Table 5.6 we see there is little evidence for departure from the constrained model where sidedness matters only through whether the cryptorchism was on the same or opposite side from the tumor, but there is strong evidence that the ipsilateral odds ratio is higher than the contralateral odds ratio and strong evidence that the ipsilateral OR is greater than 1.

5.5   Extensions

As the example in Section 5.4.1 shows, it can be of interest to compare models that impose cross-equation constraints on the regression coefficients. In studies with many case subtypes, an unconstrained polytomous logistic regression model would include a large number of equations with a large number of regression coefficients. In this setting, Chatterjee (2004) proposed parameterizing regression coefficients in the different polytomous model equations in terms of characteristics of the different disease outcomes as one way to reduce the number

TABLE 5.6
Comparison of unconstrained and constrained models
for the testicular cancer data.

Model	$e^{\beta_I^{(L)}}$	$e^{\beta_I^{(R)}}$	$e^{\beta_C^{(L)}}$	$e^{\beta_C^{(R)}}$	LRT
Unconstrained	10.49	6.60	0.83	2.78	–
Constrained	8.01	8.01	1.59	1.59	1.81
No Contralateral	7.66	7.66	1.00	1.00	2.70
No Ipsilateral	1.00	1.00	1.33	1.33	42.72
All Same	4.45	4.45	4.45	4.45	14.01
All Null	1.00	1.00	1.00	1.00	43.27

of parameters and examine scientifically meaningful hypotheses. The general approach uses variables that define disease outcome characteristics as independent variables in a "second-stage" regression model defining how polytomous logistic regression coefficients for a variable depend on these outcome characteristic variables. He proposes two estimation procedures for the constrained models, a full maximum-likelihood procedure that can be computationally intensive when there are a large number of parameters, and a pseudo-conditional-likelihood method that is much more computationally feasible and is nearly as efficient as maximum likelihood.

The constraints $\beta_I^{(L)} = \beta_I^{(R)} = \beta_I$ and $\beta_C^{(L)} = \beta_C^{(R)} = \beta_C$ used in the example in Section 5.4.1 can be fit in his general framework. Let

$$\boldsymbol{Z}_L = \begin{pmatrix} 1 & 0 \\ 0 & 1 \end{pmatrix} \text{ and } \boldsymbol{Z}_R = \begin{pmatrix} 0 & 1 \\ 1 & 0 \end{pmatrix}.$$

Then we can write

$$\begin{pmatrix} \beta_I^{(L)} \\ \beta_C^{(L)} \end{pmatrix} = \boldsymbol{Z}_L \begin{pmatrix} \beta_I \\ \beta_C \end{pmatrix} \text{ and } \begin{pmatrix} \beta_C^{(R)} \\ \beta_I^{(R)} \end{pmatrix} = \boldsymbol{Z}_R \begin{pmatrix} \beta_I \\ \beta_C \end{pmatrix}.$$

Including intercept terms, this reduces the full, six-parameter model in equations (5.4) and (5.5) to a four-parameter model. Examples in the next subsection give a flavor of additional types of constraints that can be imposed in these models. For numerical examples and more details, the reader is referred to Chatterjee (2004).

5.5.1   Constraint models

Consider a case-control study of invasive breast cancer in women, where breast cancer cases are characterized by whether their tumor is estrogen receptor positive (ER positive), and whether it is progesterone receptor positive (PR positive). The cross-classification of these two binary characteristics yields four types of cases to be compared to controls, and so in the least constrained polytomous logistic model, there would be four equations with four intercepts and four coefficients for each risk factor or adjustment variable in the model given in Equation (5.6):

$$\log \left(\frac{p_i(\boldsymbol{x})}{p_0(\boldsymbol{x})} \right) = \alpha^{(i)} + \boldsymbol{x}^T \boldsymbol{\beta}^{(i)}, \ i = 1, \dots, 4. \tag{5.6}$$

To express cross-equation constraints on these coefficients, we write the regression coefficients in terms of indicators for ER positivity and PR positivity of the tumor. For simplicity,

TABLE 5.7

Four possible types of breast cancer cases
depending on estrogen and progesterone receptor
positivity.

Case group	ER status	PR status	$\beta_E^{(x_{ER}, x_{PR})}$
$i = 1$	negative	negative	$\beta^{(0,0)}$
$i = 2$	negative	positive	$\beta^{(0,1)}$
$i = 3$	positive	negative	$\beta^{(1,0)}$
$i = 4$	positive	positive	$\beta^{(1,1)}$

attention will be restricted to the coefficients $\beta_E^{(i)}$ of a single risk factor of interest, x_E. Let the outcome-characteristic indicators be denoted by

$$x_{ER} = \begin{cases} 1 & \text{ER+,} \\ 0 & \text{Otherwise,} \end{cases}$$

and

$$x_{PR} = \begin{cases} 1 & \text{PR+,} \\ 0 & \text{Otherwise.} \end{cases}$$

Then instead of indexing the four regression coefficients $\beta_E^{(i)}$ of x_E by $i = 1, \ldots, 4$, we might instead index them by the values of x_{ER} and x_{PR}, as shown in Table 5.7.

For the model given in Equation (5.6), the simplest constraint on the coefficients might be that the odds ratio associated with x_E is the same for all four subtypes of disease. This would be expressed as a second-stage model

$$\beta_E^{(x_{ER}, x_{PR})} \equiv \theta. \tag{5.7}$$

Another constraint might allow the odds ratios to differ for the different types of disease, but require that the ratio of exposure-disease odds ratios associated with PR positive disease not depend on whether ER is positive or negative, and vice versa. The second stage model for this multiplicative constraint could be expressed as

$$\beta_E^{(x_{ER}, x_{PR})} = \theta_0 + \theta_{ER} x_{ER} + \theta_{PR} x_{ER}. \tag{5.8}$$

An additional parameter could then be used to measure the distance from the multiplicative model:

$$\beta_E^{(x_{ER}, x_{PR})} = \theta_0 + \theta_{ER} x_{ER} + \theta_{PR} x_{ER} + \theta_{ERPR} x_{ER} x_{PR}, \tag{5.9}$$

and although this "saturated" model is equivalent to the model given in Equation (5.6) with no constraints on coefficients of x_E, the parameterization in Equation (5.9) makes it easier to test whether the multiplicative model in Equation (5.8) holds. In addition, either model could be compared to the model in Equation (5.7) by testing whether all θs except θ_0 are zero. Hypotheses of interest based on constraints like these can be tested using standard likelihood-based methods as was done in the example in Section 5.4.1 with the full multinomial likelihood, or when this would not be computationally feasible, the pseudo-conditional likelihood approach (Chatterjee, 2004) can be used.

5.6 Summary

Case-control studies sometimes sample more than one type of case or more than one type of control to allow for more robust conclusions or to answer specific scientific questions. When there are more than two case status outcome groups, polytomous logistic regression models offer efficient estimates of odds ratios associating exposure with the different types of case and control comparisons. When questions of scientific interest can be expressed as hypothesized constraints on these odds ratios, the polytomous logistic model provides a unified method for examining these questions using case-control data.

Bibliography

Becher, H. (1991). Alternative parameterization of polychotomous models: Theory and application to matched case-control studies. *Statistics in Medicine*, **10**, 375–382.

Begg, C. B. and Gray, R. (1984). Calculation of polychotomous logistic regression parameters using individualized regressions. *Biometrika*, **71**, 11–18.

Britton, J. A., Gammon, M. D., Schoenberg, J. B., Stanford, J. L., Coates, R. J., Swanson, C. A., Potischman, N., Malone, K. E., Brogan, D. J., Daling, J. R., and Brinton, L. A. (2002). Risk of breast cancer classified by joint estrogen receptor and progesterone receptor status among women 20–44 years of age. *American Journal of Epidemiology*, **156**, 507–516.

Chatterjee, N. (2004). A two-stage regression model for epidemiological studies with multivariate disease classification data. *Journal of the American Statistical Association*, **99**, 127–138.

Fienberg, S. E. (2007). *The Analysis of Cross-Classified Categorical Data*. Springer, New York.

Prentice, R. L. and Pyke, R. (1979). Logistic disease incidence models and case-control studies. *Biometrika*, **66**, 403–411.

R Core Team (2016). *R: A Language and Environment for Statistical Computing*. R Foundation for Statistical Computing, Vienna, Austria.

Sherman, K. J., Daling, J. R., Chu, J., McKnight, B., and Weiss, N. S. (1988). Multiple primary tumours in women with vulvar neoplasms: A case-control study. *British Journal of Cancer*, **57**, 423–427.

Stanford, J. L., Wicklund, K. G., McKnight, B., Daling, J. R., and Brawer, M. K. (1999). Vasectomy and risk of prostate cancer. *Cancer Epidemiology, Biomarkers and Prevention*, **8**, 881–886.

StataCorp (2015). *Stata Statistical Software: Release 14*. StataCorp LP, College Station, TX.

Strader, C. H., Weiss, N. S., Daling, J. R., Karagas, M. R., and McKnight, B. (1988). Cryptorchism, orchiopexy, and the risk of testicular cancer. *American Journal of Epidemiology*, **127**, 1013–1018.

6

Causal Inference from Case-Control Studies

Vanessa Didelez

Leibniz Institute for Prevention Research and Epidemiology & University of Bremen

Robin J. Evans

University of Oxford

6.1 Introduction

In this chapter we consider when it is possible to draw causal conclusions from a case-control study. This requires special attention because causal conclusions make stronger claims than ordinary predictions. For instance, it may not be sufficient to note that people with a higher alcohol intake are at a higher risk of stroke; rather, we may wish to establish that if we are able to reduce people's alcohol intake, this will have the *effect* of reducing the number of instances of stroke. In other words, we wish to establish that certain *interventions* in the level of an exposure or in a lifestyle choice will result in improved health, and to quantify the strength of such effects. The core problems of causal inference are therefore to estimate and predict the effects of interventions. For background reading on causality and causal inference, see textbooks and overviews by Hernán and Robins (2018), Pearl (2009), Spirtes *et al.* (2000), Rubin (1974), and Dawid (2015).

Readers may be more familiar with the famous Bradford Hill (BH) criteria for causation (Hill, 2015): strength, consistency, specificity, temporality, biological gradient, plausibility, coherence, experiment, and analogy. These are important in order to strengthen causal conclusions in the wider context of scientific investigations. Here, we take a different, but not entirely unrelated, approach, placing the emphasis on first formally defining a causal effect as the effect of an intervention (related to BH's criterion that experimental evidence strengthens causal conclusions), and considering what problems we face when estimating such an effect with case-control data. It can then be formally investigated how and when the Bradford Hill criteria are sensible for a given causal model and scientific query at hand, e.g., an explicit causal model might postulate a plausible dose-response relation reflecting the biological gradient as well as the assumed underlying mechanism. For a recent critical revision of BH's criteria, see Ioannidis (2016).

Taking this formal approach to causal inference, a key question is that of *identifiability*: does the available data, at least in principle, allow us to consistently estimate the desired causal quantity? If the answer is 'no' then this is typically due to *structural bias*. Here, 'in principle' means the sample size is large enough to get reliable nonparametric estimates of distributions. The term 'structural bias' refers to fundamental problems of design and available information – such as the difficulty in distinguishing a 'real' causal effect from correlation due to an unmeasured common cause – and not to particular choices of parametric models or sampling error.

The effect of specific interventions can most unambiguously be investigated in randomised controlled trials (RCTs). However, there are many reasons to use observational data and in particular case-control studies in practice, such as because the disease under investigation is very rare. In case-control studies, we face the following potential sources of structural bias regarding causal inference:

(1) Case-control studies are necessarily observational, so *confounding* is likely to be present.

(2) Case-control studies are retrospective with sampling being conditional on disease status which means there is also a threat of *selection bias* (Hernán *et al.*, 2004).

(3) A consequence of the retrospective sampling is that methods which depend on, or are sensitive to, the marginal distribution of the outcome cannot be used without some modification, since the required information is not generally available. This is potentially relevant to methods of adjusting for confounding as well as to the identifiability of typical causal effect measures, such as the average causal effect (ACE). An effect measure that is not sensitive to the retrospective sampling is the odds ratio (OR) but its interpretation can be complicated by its noncollapsibility (Greenland *et al.*, 1999).

While confounding is a problem of any observational study and has been widely addressed in the causal inference literature (Hernán and Robins, 2018; Pearl, 1995), points (2) and (3) are more specific to case-control studies and will be the focus of this chapter. Note that retrospective sampling gives rise to further sources of bias, such as recall bias or reverse causation which combines measurement error with potential selection bias as addressed later. We can relate our approach to BH's criteria: 'specificity' is partly about excluding sources of bias, and so ensuring that there is no other likely explanation for an

(a)   (b)

FIGURE 6.1
Directed acyclic graphs representing sampling under (a) an unmatched case-control study; (b) a matched case control study with matching variables C.

association; respecting 'temporality' is especially relevant with case-control data, as seen in the context of recall bias. Note that biases can to some extent be avoided by careful design of a case-control study; in this context we refer the reader to Chapter 2 of this book which describes several case-control design options, outlines classical approaches to analysis, and mentions threats to internal validity. One topic not addressed in the present chapter is causal search, where the aim is to automatically identify a causal structure from case-control data, but see Cooper (1995) and Borboudakis and Tsamardinos (2015).

6.1.1 Basic set-up

Throughout D denotes a binary outcome (disease), with $D = 1$ denoting the cases and $D = 0$ the controls. We write X for the exposure and C for a set of covariates, with respective domains $\mathcal{X}$ and $\mathcal{C}$; in general these may be binary, categorical, or continuous, but for simplicity we will largely restrict ourselves to binary X and categorical C. The index $i = 1, \ldots, n$ is used to indicate different units (e.g., D^i, X^i), but usually this is suppressed. For brevity we will often write (for example) $P(D \mid X)$ instead of $P(D = d \mid X = x)$.

6.1.2 Sampling indicator

It will be important to explicitly formalise aspects of the sampling mechanism, so we introduce a binary indicator S, where $S = 1$ means the unit is present in the sample. It follows that data from a case-control study can usually be regarded as a sample from $P(X, C, D \mid S = 1)$, where the sampling proportion $\tilde{p}_S = P(D = 1 \mid S = 1)$ is often known while the population prevalence $\tilde{p} = P(D = 1)$ may or may not be known. We mainly address methods that do not require knowledge of $\tilde{p}$, but see Section 6.5.

6.1.3 Directed acyclic graphs and conditional independence

We use directed acyclic graphs (DAGs) to express the (structural) assumptions we are willing to make about the joint distribution within the *population*, including how a subset of the population is sampled. For example, in Figure 6.1(a) the sampling variable S only depends on the outcome D, whereas in (b) it also depends on measured covariates due to matching factors in C.

The DAG represents conditional independence constraints on the joint probability distribution over the variables shown as nodes in the graph. In particular, any variable should be conditionally independent of its graphical nondescendants given its graphical parents. (For full details and graphical terminology, see the Appendix.) For random variables A, B, Z we denote the statement "A is conditionally independent of B given Z" by $A \perp\!\!\!\perp B \mid Z$ (Dawid, 1979). This means, for instance, that $P(A \mid B, Z) = P(A \mid Z)$.

For example, in Figure 6.1(a) the variable S only has the parent D, so in the population

$$S \perp\!\!\!\perp (X, C) \mid D; \tag{6.1}$$

in particular this means that $P(X, C \mid D, S = 1) = P(X, C \mid D)$. In contrast, the additional $C \to S$ edge in Figure 6.1(b) means that now we can only assert (from the DAG) that

$$S \perp\!\!\!\perp X \mid (C, D). \tag{6.2}$$

The two conditional independence assumptions (6.1) and (6.2), and the fact that the former implies the latter, will be used many times throughout this chapter.

Note that in a DAG, it is the absence of edges that encodes assumptions; the presence of an edge means merely that we allow the *possibility* of a dependence, not that we claim there necessarily is one. Some independencies cannot be seen graphically; for instance it is common to match such that $D \perp\!\!\!\perp C \mid S = 1$, but this is not represented by the graph.

When we include S in our DAGs we express assumptions about the whole population, those that are sampled as well as those that are not. This could include independencies that 'disappear' when we condition on $S = 1$, i.e., that cannot be observed in the sampled population. We address this phenomenon of *selection* again in the following section.

If the graph implies the existence of conditional independencies in the distribution corresponding to the observed data (in particular conditional on $\{S = 1\}$) then these can be checked empirically. Those not conditional on $\{S = 1\}$ should approximately hold in the controls-only data in the situation of a case-control study with a very rare disease.

6.2 Basic concepts of causal inference

When we are interested in causality, it is helpful to use notation that distinguishes causal concepts, such as the effect of an intervention, from associational ones. There are several frameworks for making this distinction, including potential outcomes (Rubin, 1974), structural equations (Goldberger, 1972), the do($\cdot$)-operator (Pearl, 2009), or a decision theoretic approach (Dawid, 2015) (a hierarchy can be found in Richardson and Robins (2013)); these are further often supplemented by DAGs, or extensions thereof, as a shorthand to illustrate assumptions made (Spirtes *et al.*, 2000; Pearl, 2009). We do not go into the subtle differences between these approaches here (see discussion by Dawid (2000); Didelez and Sheehan (2007b)), but explain the basic ideas that are essentially common to all of them.

6.2.1 Intervention distribution

We use $P(D \mid \mathrm{do}(X = x))$ to denote the distribution of D if X is set to $x \in \mathcal{X}$ by an intervention (Pearl, 2009). If a randomised controlled trial can be carried out, then $P(D \mid \mathrm{do}(X = x))$ can immediately be estimated from the corresponding arm of the trial where $X = x$. The intervention distribution is different from a conditional distribution: $P(D \mid X = x)$ simply denotes the distribution amongst units in which $X = x$ is *observed* to have happened; the two are generally distinct if there are other common causes or *confounders*.

An alternative approach uses *potential outcomes* D_x to denote the disease status when the exposure or treatment X is set to $x \in \mathcal{X}$ by an intervention. In the case of binary X, we have potential outcomes D_1 and D_0; these are sometimes also called *counterfactuals* because we can always only observe either D_1^i or D_0^i but not both for a given unit i. For the purposes of this chapter we consider $P(D \mid \mathrm{do}(X = x))$ as equal to the distribution of the corresponding potential outcome $P(D_x)$, and focus on quantities that are functions of these distributions.

6.2.2 Causal effect and causal null hypothesis

In analogy to a randomised trial, we say that X *has a causal effect on* D if, for two different exposure values $x \neq x'$, the intervention distributions differ: $P(D \mid \mathrm{do}(X = x)) \neq P(D \mid \mathrm{do}(X = x'))$. Accordingly, we formalise the causal null hypothesis as

$$H_0^\emptyset : P(D \mid \mathrm{do}(X = x)) = P(D \mid \mathrm{do}(X = x')) \quad \text{for all } x \neq x'.$$

For simplicity, instead of considering the whole distribution it is common to use causal parameters that contrast particular aspects of the intervention distributions: for instance the difference in means $E(D \mid \mathrm{do}(X = x)) - E(D \mid \mathrm{do}(X = x'))$, also called the *average causal effect* (ACE). When D is binary, the ACE is the causal risk difference.

We also consider *conditional* causal effects, which for some pre-exposure covariates C are functions of $P(D \mid C; \mathrm{do}(X))$. These denote the causal effect that X has on D within a subgroup defined by $C = c$, which may be different from that in a different subgroup $C = c' \neq c$. Similarly a conditional causal null hypothesis (within $C = c$) is given as

$$H_0^{C=c} : P(D = 1 \mid C = c; \mathrm{do}(X = x)) = P(D = 1 \mid C = c; \mathrm{do}(X = x')) \quad \text{for all } x \neq x',$$

and we define the overall absence of conditional causal effects as

$$H_0^C = \bigcap_{c \in \mathcal{C}} H_0^{C=c}.$$

Remarks:

(1) We require C to be pre-exposure so that $P(D \mid C; \mathrm{do}(X))$ corresponds to a quantity that could in principle be estimated from an RCT, where people with $C = c$ are randomised to different values of X; if C only occurs, or is only defined, after randomisation then this would not be possible. Formally, C being pre-exposure means that these covariates cannot be affected by an intervention, i.e., $P(C \mid \mathrm{do}(X)) = P(C)$. Due to the retrospective nature of case-control sampling, measurements of covariates may (possibly unintentionally) be post-exposure, and in fact measurement of exposure may be post-outcome and hence affected by *recall bias*. Such situations may not only affect the interpretation of the causal parameter but also the validity of causal conclusions due to, e.g., selection bias as explained below.

(2) The causal effects we consider, either as functions of $P(D \mid \mathrm{do}(X = x))$ or $P(D \mid C; \mathrm{do}(X = x))$, are *total* effects in the sense that they measure the causal effect of X on D as possibly 'transmitted' via several pathways. For example, if X indicates smoking then this has a direct negative effect on lung function and therefore health; however taking up smoking may also reduce appetite, and therefore affect health indirectly via body mass index. Breaking an effect down into direct and different indirect causal effects requires the conceptual blocking of some pathways by interventions; this is a significant topic of its own and will not be considered any further here (VanderWeele, 2015).

(3) The above null hypotheses obviously depend on the choice of C. In particular it does *not* hold that $H_0^\emptyset \Rightarrow H_0^C$: there could be nonzero effects in subgroups that cancel each other out, so that there is a zero overall effect; this is referred to as *unfaithfulness* (Spirtes et al., 2000). However, for pre-exposure covariates C it does hold that $H_0^C \Rightarrow H_0^\emptyset$, so we can regard H_0^C as more informative than H_0.

Even if we are not only interested in testing a causal null hypothesis, it is worthwhile verifying whether a method of estimation is consistent at the causal null under weaker assumptions than general consistency. Indeed, many methods are still valid at the null, even when misspecified models are used; this is also known as the *null-preservation* property (see Chapter 9 of Hernán and Robins, 2018).

(4) Other notions of causal null hypotheses can be found in the literature. For example, when D is continuous one might simply be interested in equality of the means under two treatments $E(D \mid \mathrm{do}(X = 1)) = E(D \mid \mathrm{do}(X = 0))$. A stronger notion is the *sharp* causal null hypothesis which can only be formulated with potential outcomes as it states that there is no causal effect at an individual level, i.e., $D_1^i - D_0^i = 0$ for all units i. We do not consider this further in the present chapter (Hernán, 2004).

6.2.3   Exchangeability and confounding

In order to explain the problem of confounding, we start with the prospective case. Consider a binary treatment X: randomisation of X creates two a priori *exchangeable* groups; that is, at the time of randomisation, those units with $X = 0$ are entirely comparable to units with $X = 1$ regarding the distribution of any measured or unmeasured factors such as age, lifestyle, socioeconomic background. This exchangeability allows causal inference because any subsequent differences between the groups must be due to the different values of X (Hernán and Robins, 2018, Section 3.2). In observational studies exchangeability cannot be guaranteed, as units observed to have $X = 0$ may well have very different attributes than those observed to have $X = 1$; for example, they might be older, have lower alcohol consumption, or higher income. Intuitively, *confounding* occurs when some of these attributes also affect disease risk; formally this implies $P(D \mid X) \neq P(D \mid \mathrm{do}(X))$ as confounding creates a noncausal association between D and X. Hence we seek to take suitable covariates into account to compensate for the lack of exchangeability. A set C of pre-exposure covariates is *sufficient to adjust for confounding* with respect to the effect of X on D (Dawid, 2002; VanderWeele and Shpitser, 2013) if

$$P(D = d \mid C = c; \mathrm{do}(X = x)) = P(D = d \mid C = c, X = x), \tag{6.3}$$

where $P(D \mid C, X)$ is the observational conditional distribution. The absence of confounding corresponds to $C = \emptyset$. In words (6.3) means that once we condition on C, observing $X = x$ is as if X had been set to x by an intervention, at least as far as the resulting distribution of D is concerned; this is called *conditional exchangeability*. Note that, unless we can compare data from an RCT with an observational study, conditional exchangeability is untestable and needs to be justified with subject matter background knowledge. Using potential outcomes, property (6.3) is expressed as $D_x \perp\!\!\!\perp X \mid C$, and also called *strong ignorability* (Rosenbaum and Rubin, 1983).

As explained in the Appendix, with causal DAGs, property (6.3) can be verified by checking that C *blocks all back-door paths* from X to D (Pearl, 1995). In Figure 6.2(a) the only back-door path is given by $X \leftarrow Z \leftarrow C \rightarrow D$ and this is blocked by any of $\{Z\}$, $\{C\}$, or $\{Z, C\}$, but not by $\emptyset$. Minimal sets satisfying (6.3) can be defined, but as the example shows they are not unique (VanderWeele and Shpitser, 2013). Note that if C satisfies (6.3), it does not necessarily follow that a larger set $B \supset C$ satisfies (6.3), even if B consists only of pre-exposure covariates (Greenland, 2003; VanderWeele and Shpitser, 2013).

Methods of adjusting for confounding typically assume that *positivity* is satisfied:

$$0 < P(X = x \mid C = c) < 1 \quad \text{for all } x, c. \tag{6.4}$$

This means that all exposure values are possible for all values of C. As a counterexample,

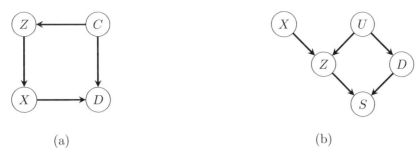

(a)   (b)

FIGURE 6.2
(a) A DAG in which either Z or C alone is sufficient to adjust for confounding. (b) A DAG in which the causal null hypothesis of no effect of X on D holds; including possible ascertainment bias with Z as a symptom.

consider an exposure $X = x_0$ corresponding to two hours of exercise per day; then this is practically impossible to occur for the subgroup of subjects $C = c_0$ who are bedridden. Hence it is not possible to nonparametrically estimate the effect of an intervention $\mathrm{do}(X = x_0)$ for this subgroup as positivity (6.4) is violated.

When C is sufficient to adjust for confounding we have that

$$H_0^C \quad \Leftrightarrow \quad D \perp\!\!\!\perp X \mid C, \tag{6.5}$$

which is immediate from the definition (6.3). This implies that any method for testing $D \perp\!\!\!\perp X \mid C$ can be used to test H_0^C. Furthermore we obtain the intervention distribution as

$$P(D = d \mid \mathrm{do}(X = x)) = \sum_c P(D = d \mid C = c, X = x) P(C = c), \tag{6.6}$$

which is known as *standardisation* (Keiding and Clayton, 2014). This means that when C is sufficient to adjust for confounding, $P(D \mid \mathrm{do}(X))$ is *identified* by (6.6) if we can obtain data from $P(D \mid C, X)$ and $P(C)$, as would be the case in a prospective study with C observed.

However, retrospective data in a case-control study is drawn from $P(D, C, X \mid S = 1)$, and neither $P(D \mid C, X)$ nor $P(C)$ can necessarily be obtained without additional assumptions. We return to this problem in Sections 6.4 and 6.5.

6.2.4   Selection bias

While confounding is the most well known source of bias affecting causal inference from observational data, a different problem is highly relevant in case-control studies: selection bias (Hernán *et al.*, 2004). As a simple toy example, consider two marginally independent variables $A \perp\!\!\!\perp B$ and assume that they both separately affect a third variable Z such that the joint distribution is given by $P(A, B, Z) = P(A)P(B)P(Z \mid A, B)$; graphically we express this as $A \to Z \leftarrow B$. It is easily seen that $P(A, B \mid Z)$ does not factorise, so that $A \not\perp\!\!\!\perp B \mid Z$ in general. Now, assume that Z indicates being sampled; then we find that two quantities that are not associated in the population may very well be associated in the sample if they both affect the probability of being sampled. For example, if A, B indicate the presence of two diseases that are independent in the population, and $Z = 1$ only occurs if either $A = 1$ or $B = 1$, then A and B will be negatively associated in the subset with $Z = 1$. This kind of problem for medical research has been highlighted by Berkson (1946) in the context of sampling cases and controls from one hospital; he demonstrated that people

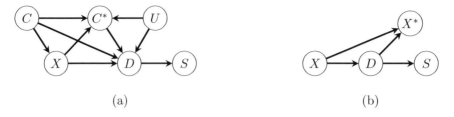

(a)   (b)

FIGURE 6.3
Causal graphs representing forms of recall bias. In (a), some measured covariates C^* are actually recalled after treatment; in (b), we only obtain a measure of exposure after observing the outcome.

who had at least one reason to be in a hospital in the first place are not representative of the population and hence may exhibit 'spurious' associations.

A related example based on Robins (2001) is given in Figure 6.2(b). The DAG shows the null hypothesis of no causal effect of an exposure X (e.g., hormone treatment) on D (e.g., endometrial cancer), and for simplicity there is no confounding affecting X and D. However, exposure may have consequences Z (e.g., bleeding) and subjects with this symptom are more likely to see a doctor. The DAG also expresses that bleeding and cancer may have an unobserved common cause U (e.g., uterine abnormality). In a case-control study, sampling does not only depend on disease status D but also on the presence of symptoms as those are more likely to be found out as cases – this is known as *ascertainment* bias. To confirm this source of possible bias we can apply d-separation to the graph (see Appendix), and find that even though there is a marginal independence $D \perp\!\!\!\perp X$ in the whole population, there is no such independence in the sampled population: $D \not\perp\!\!\!\perp X \mid S$; in addition, this cannot be corrected by stratifying on Z because $D \not\perp\!\!\!\perp X \mid (Z, S)$. The reason for the selection bias here is that when Z affects the probability of being sampled, then X and U become dependent in the sample (as in the earlier toy example we could consider the extreme case where $Z = 1$ if either $X = 1$ or $U = 1$) which creates a noncausal association between X and D. This example illustrates how selection bias can impede identification of the causal null hypothesis (see Section 6.3.1); even if there is a nonzero causal effect of X on D, using DAGs in this way alerts us to the possibility that its estimation might be biased.

6.2.5   Post-exposure covariates and recall bias

An issue closely related to selection bias and the retrospective nature of the sampling is that the actual measurements of covariates and exposure may not follow the intended time ordering (remember BH's criterion of 'temporality'). For example, we may want to adjust for baseline BMI, but are only able to obtain a BMI measurement from after exposure, perhaps because it was taken after first symptoms occurred; alternatively, a subject may try to recall their BMI from before exposure, but may not do so accurately. Similarly, exposure itself may be difficult to retrieve from an objective source, and is instead measured by asking the patient; again, the *recalled* value of exposure may be systematically different for cases and controls.

Let us consider the post-exposure covariate problem first; a possible scenario is depicted in Figure 6.3(a). While the genuine pre-exposure covariate C would be sufficient to adjust for confounding, a post-treatment version of it (C^*) is not. This is due to various issues reflected in certain paths in the DAG: first, the path $X \leftarrow C \rightarrow D$ means there is residual confounding by C, for which C^* cannot adjust; second, the path $X \rightarrow C^* \rightarrow D$ implies that part of the causal effect is transmitted via C^*, so that we should not adjust for it if we desire a total effect for inference; third, the path $C \to C^* \leftarrow U \to D$ means that conditioning on C^* creates a spurious association between the unobserved U and the original C (as in our toy example above) resulting in a new source of residual confounding. Note that one might think that a different reason for conditioning on C^* is the desire to estimate a 'direct' effect of X on D, but again the presence of an unobserved common cause U leads to a noncausal (X, D)-association and hence bias from a selection effect due to $X \to C^* \leftarrow U \to D$; see Aschard *et al.* (2015) for an illustration of this bias in the context of GWAS case-control studies.

Figure 6.3(b) shows the case of the exposure X being affected by recall bias, because the *measured* exposure X^* depends on D; this can occur if $D = 1$ is a negative health outcome and leads patients to search for explanations, and hence exaggerate the actual exposure in their recollection. Nonparametrically, it is impossible to draw causal conclusions based on only D, X^*. If the actual exposure X can be retrieved, we see from the DAG that X^* should be ignored; adjusting for it would lead to a noncausal association because of the selection effect. More generally, there could be other reasons leading to the measured exposure X^* being partly affected by D, suggesting an association which is really due to reverse causation. This can happen, e.g., if both exposure and outcome reflect underlying processes that have developed over time such as cardiovascular problems leading to increased fibrinogen levels instead of the other way around.

6.2.6 Nonparametric identifiability

A case-control study provides data from the observational (i.e., noninterventional) distribution $P(X, C, D \mid S = 1)$. The key problem of *causal inference* is: under what assumptions (if at all) are certain aspects of the intervention distributions $P(D \mid \mathrm{do}(X))$ or $P(D \mid C; \mathrm{do}(X))$ uniquely computable, i.e., *identified*, from $P(X, C, D \mid S = 1)$. For instance in the example of ascertainment bias given earlier, the marginal independence corresponding to a causal null hypothesis cannot be identified from the conditional distribution. We mainly consider *nonparametric identifiability*, relying only on structural assumptions that can be expressed in DAGs (Pearl, 2009), and not particular parametric choices (but see Section 6.5). Moreover, we mainly consider the case of no external information such as the disease prevalence $\tilde{p} = P(D = 1)$, which typically means that besides the causal null hypothesis, only the conditional causal odds ratio (COR) is identified as addressed below.

6.3 Identifying the causal null hypothesis and odds ratios

Let us start by considering the simplest situation. Assume sampling depends on disease status alone (6.1) and there is no confounding, i.e., $P(D \mid \mathrm{do}(X = x)) = P(D \mid X = x)$. Hence, we can identify any causal effect measure if we can obtain $P(D \mid X)$ from $P(X, D \mid S = 1) = P(X \mid D)P(D \mid S = 1)$. However, $P(D \mid X)$ cannot be obtained from $P(X \mid D)$ without additional information such as the disease prevalence $\tilde{p}$ in the population, so that the causal risk difference or risk ratio are not identified. Instead, we can assess from $P(X \mid D)$ whether X and D are independent, and we can compute the (X, D)-OR. Therefore, we start by focusing on approaches to tackle two specific types of causal identification questions: Is there a causal effect of an exposure X on a disease D at all? In other words, can we test a causal null hypothesis? What is the COR describing the causal effect of X on D? It turns out that these questions are closely related and rely on the same assumptions.

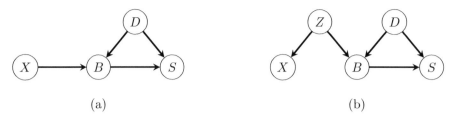

FIGURE 6.4
Examples of possible selection bias: (a) presence in database B directly depends on exposure; (b) case where covariates Z can be found to explain presence in database.

6.3.1   Selection bias and the causal null hypothesis

As alluded to above, if we merely want to know whether X and D are associated at all, it does not matter if we observe data from $P(X \mid D)$ rather than $P(D \mid X)$, because $D \perp\!\!\!\perp X$ can be established by checking that $P(X \mid D) = P(X)$. The problem of testing a causal null hypothesis is similar, except for the need to consider confounding. Due to property (6.5), when C is sufficient to adjust for confounding $H_0^C \Leftrightarrow D \perp\!\!\!\perp X \mid C$, and this independence can be checked using either $P(X, C \mid D)$ or $P(X \mid C, D)$. A case-control study provides data from $P(X, C, D \mid S = 1)$; hence it is sufficient to assume (6.2), so that $P(X, C, D \mid S = 1) = P(X \mid C, D)P(C, D \mid S = 1)$. In fact, assumption (6.2) means that selection bias is ruled out, because it says that the sampling does not, directly or indirectly, depend on both the exposure and the disease status, possibly after taking covariates into account.

As seen in the ascertainment bias example, a graphical 'trick' to check for selection bias is to draw a DAG showing the structural assumptions under the null hypothesis (Hernán *et al.*, 2004; Didelez *et al.*, 2010b; Richardson and Robins, 2013); the latter typically means that there is no directed edge nor directed path from X to D. We can then check graphically whether a set C exists such that each remaining path between X and D is blocked by (C, S); here S needs to be included because the design implies that everything is conditioned on S. If no such set of observable variables C can be found (e.g., when only C^* and not C is available in Figure 6.3(a)), then it is typically impossible (without further information or assumptions) to test the causal null hypothesis. In other situations it may be possible to gather additional information so as to enable valid inference. Consider for example the DAG in Figure 6.4(a). The absence of a directed edge from X to D represents the causal null hypothesis, and for simplicity we assume no confounding. Further, the DAG represents the situation where controls are found in some database (with binary variable B indicating presence in the database), but where exposure leads to under- or over-representation in that database. If these are the only observable variables, then the causal null hypothesis cannot be tested from data conditional on $S = 1$, i.e., it is not identified. However, assume instead the DAG in Figure 6.4(b); this may have been obtained after investigating exactly how subjects get into the database and it is found that a set of covariates Z both explains the presence in the database and predicts exposure X such that $X \perp\!\!\!\perp B \mid Z$. We now find that $S \perp\!\!\!\perp X \mid (Z, D)$. While Z is in this case not needed to adjust for confounding, it does not violate (6.3). Hence, we can test the causal null hypothesis H_0^Z from the sampled data.

For example, suppose B is a register of workers at a nuclear power plant, X is a measure of radiation exposure, and D is an indicator of cancer. Workers may be added to the register either as a precaution based on their level of radiation exposure, or because they have been diagnosed with cancer. This means that selecting individuals from the register for a study may introduce a spurious negative association between X and D, because they are competing explanations for inclusion in the register. However, if precautionary inclusion in the register was based on the individual's role at the plant, Z, as in Figure 6.4(b), then using Z could allow recovery from selection bias.

The question of whether a conditional independence can be tested from a selected sample turns out to be closely related to the question whether the corresponding OR is collapsible. This is therefore addressed next.

6.3.2 Collapsibility of odds ratios

The odds ratio is, first and foremost, a measure of association; in the following section we explore under what assumptions and in what sense it can be used for causal inference. Here we revisit some of its basic properties that will be needed later. We state results below for binary X and D; for generalisation to the nonbinary case see Didelez *et al.* (2010b).

For a binary outcome D and binary exposure X we define the odds ratio OR_{DX} as

$$OR_{DX} = \frac{P(D=1\,|\,X=1)P(D=0\,|\,X=0)}{P(D=0\,|\,X=1)P(D=1\,|\,X=0)}.$$

The OR has a number of (related) properties that render it very useful in case-control studies: (i) it is symmetric: $OR_{DX} = OR_{XD}$; (ii) it is invariant to changes in the marginal distributions of D and X; (iii) it can be used to test independence, since $D \perp\!\!\!\perp X \Leftrightarrow OR_{DX} = 1$. With (i) and (ii) it follows in particular that the OR can be identified based on data from the conditional distribution $P(X\,|\,D)$ even when the sampling proportion of cases $\tilde{p}_S$ is not equal to the population proportion of cases $\tilde{p}$.

We extend the definition to take (a set of) covariates C into account: the conditional odds ratio $OR_{DX}(C = c)$ is given by

$$OR_{DX}(C=c) = \frac{P(D=1\,|\,X=1,C=c)P(D=0\,|\,X=0,C=c)}{P(D=0\,|\,X=1,C=c)P(D=1\,|\,X=0,C=c)}.$$

We write $OR_{DX}(C)$ to refer to the set of all ORs $\{OR_{DX}(C=c), c \in \mathcal{C}\}$. The conditional OR is also symmetric; is invariant to the marginal distributions of $X\,|\,C$ and $D\,|\,C$; and $OR_{DX}(C=c) = 1 \Leftrightarrow D \perp\!\!\!\perp X\,|\,C = c$.

To define collapsibility, assume that C consists of at least two variables C_1, C_2 (each can be a vector). Then $OR_{DX}(C_1, C_2)$ is *collapsible over* C_2 if for all $c_2 \neq c_2'$ and all c_1 in the respective domains

$$OR_{DX}(C_1 = c_1, C_2 = c_2) = OR_{DX}(C_1 = c_1, C_2 = c_2') = OR_{DX}(C_1 = c_1). \tag{6.7}$$

A sufficient condition for property (6.7) is that either $D \perp\!\!\!\perp C_2\,|\,(C_1, X)$ or $X \perp\!\!\!\perp C_2\,|\,(C_1, D)$, and this becomes necessary when C_2 is binary (Whittemore, 1978).

It is interesting to note that in an RCT where X is randomly assigned and hence marginally independent of any covariates C, it is not generally true that $OR_{DX}(C)$ is collapsible over C even when the first equality of (6.7) holds for all of C (i.e., there is no effect modification by C); this is because the marginal independence $X \perp\!\!\!\perp C$ does not help with collapsibility. This may be regarded as a disadvantage of using the OR as a measure of association or effect measure; however, in such a case collapsing over C simply leads to an attenuation towards one (Zeger *et al.*, 1988).

6.3.3   Identification – main results

We define the (conditional) *causal* odds ratio, $COR_{D|X}(C = c)$, for pre-exposure covariates C as

$$COR_{D|X}(C = c) = \frac{P(D = 1 \,|\, C = c; \mathrm{do}(X = 1))P(D = 0 \,|\, C = c; \mathrm{do}(X = 0))}{P(D = 0 \,|\, C = c; \mathrm{do}(X = 1))P(D = 1 \,|\, C = c; \mathrm{do}(X = 0))}.$$

Remarks:

(1) The COR is not symmetric in (X, D), as causality, unlike stochastic dependence, is not symmetric; if X is causal for D then D is not causal for X, i.e., if $COR_{D|X}(C = c) \neq 1$ then $COR_{X|D}(C = c) = 1$.

(2) As noted earlier, even if $COR_{D|X}(C = c) = COR_{D|X}(C = c')$, for all $c \neq c'$, we do not generally have $COR_{D|X}(C) = COR_{D|X}$; the latter is attenuated towards the null. However, $COR_{D|X}(C) \equiv 1$ implies $COR_{D|X} = 1$.

(3) The CORs are straightforward to generalise to nonbinary X, in which case it is common to choose a reference category and compute a set of CORs.

The main implication of Sections 6.3.1 and 6.3.2 is that to test the causal null hypothesis H_0^C and estimate the CORs we need to be able to collapse over S. Throughout we assume that $S \not\perp\!\!\!\perp D \,|\, (C, X)$, i.e., that the sampling is dependent on the outcome variable D as would be the case in any case-control study. Then we have the following result (more general results and proofs are given in Didelez *et al.* (2010b))

Proposition 1 *(i) The conditional odds ratio $OR_{DX}(C, S)$ is collapsible over S if and only if (6.2) holds; hence $OR_{DX}(C, S) = OR_{DX}(C)$. Further, if C is sufficient to adjust for confounding w.r.t. the effect of X on D then the conditional OR is equal to the causal OR, $OR_{DX}(C) = COR_{D|X}(C)$.*
(ii) If (6.2) holds then

$$D \perp\!\!\!\perp X \,|\, C \Leftrightarrow D \perp\!\!\!\perp X \,|\, (C, S = 1),$$

which allows us to test the left-hand side conditional independence even under selection, i.e., conditional on $S = 1$. Further, if C is also sufficient to adjust for confounding of the effect of X on D then testing for independence under selection, $D \perp\!\!\!\perp X \,|\, (C, S = 1)$, is a test of the causal null hypothesis H_0^C.

Remarks:

(1) In Proposition 1, part (ii) is not restricted to the situation of categorical variables so that whatever test statistic seems appropriate given the measurement scales of X, D, C can be used.

(2) In the particular case of binary D and continuous X it is well known that we can consistently estimate the OR using a logistic regression (Prentice and Pyke, 1979). This result, however, relies on the logistic link being correctly specified, while the above results for categorical X and D make no parametric assumptions.

(3) While for a causal interpretation C needs to be sufficient to adjust for confounding, it also needs to contain any matching variables as otherwise (6.2) is unlikely to be satisfied.

(4) Proposition 1 can be generalised in that it is possible that variables that are themselves affected by exposure can sometimes be used to obtain causal conclusions. The key here is that if X affects Z which in turn affects S, it can sometimes be possible to first collapse over S given Z, and subsequently collapse over Z to obtain a COR. The required conditional independence assumptions can again easily be checked graphically on DAGs. An example in the context of retrospective, but not case-control, sampling is given in Didelez *et al.* (2010b); Bareinboim and Pearl (2012) give a complete identification algorithm.

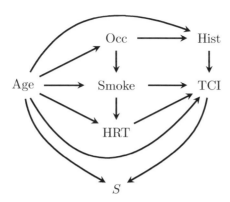

FIGURE 6.5
Example DAG for case-control study on the effect of HRT on TCI; matching is on Age; other covariates: Occupation, Thromboembolic history, Smoking.

Example: Causal effect of HRT on TCI

The above is illustrated with a study of the effect of hormone replacement therapy (HRT) on transient cerebral ischemia (TCI) (Didelez *et al.*, 2010b); note that this is a simplified version of the actual analysis by Pedersen *et al.* (1997). The study is a case-control study matched by age, so that $S \perp\!\!\!\perp HRT \,|\, (Age, TCI)$ but not $S \perp\!\!\!\perp HRT \,|\, TCI$; hence the marginal HRT-TCI OR cannot be consistently estimated as it is not collapsible over S, but the OR conditional on 'age' can consistently be estimated from the sampled data. However, this conditional OR does not necessarily have a causal interpretation unless 'age' is sufficient to adjust for confounding. To examine this, further covariates 'smoking', 'history of thromboembolic disorders' (TH), and 'occupation' were included in a DAG to represent the structural assumptions (Figure 6.5). It can be seen that covariates 'smoking' and 'age' are sufficient to adjust for confounding. Hence the conditional HRT-TCI ORs given these two covariates do have a causal interpretation, and if significantly different from one allow us to reject the causal null hypothesis. For instance the OR of taking oestrogens compared to no HRT was estimated to be just above 2 (pooled over categories of 'smoking' and 'age') which suggests that there is a causal effect of taking oestrogens resulting in higher risk of TCI.

6.4   Reconstructing the joint distribution

In this section, we address the question of when the joint population distribution $P(D, X, C)$ or possibly $P(D \,|\, X, C)$ is identified from a case-control design, i.e., from $P(D, X, C \,|\, S = 1)$. This is especially relevant if we wish to estimate causal effect measures other than conditional ORs, such as unconditional causal risk differences or risk ratios which are more suitable for comparison with results from RCTs. The results of Bareinboim and Tian (2015) and Bareinboim *et al.* (2014) suggest a pessimistic answer to this, as they demonstrate that the conditional distribution $P(Y \,|\, T)$ can be recovered from $P(Y \,|\, T, S = 1)$ if and only if $Y \perp\!\!\!\perp S \,|\, T$; if we take $Y = D$ then this condition will never be satisfied in a case-control

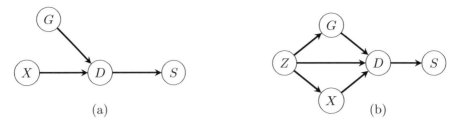

FIGURE 6.6
Examples where independencies allow recovery of joint distributions from data under selection bias: (a) marginal independence of X and G; (b) conditional independence of X and G given Z.

study, where selection S always depends on D by design. Still, we can make some headway if we somewhat relax the definition of 'identifiability' as demonstrated by Evans and Didelez (2015). This is best explained with a small example.

Example: Case-control study with genetic covariate

Assume we are interested in the causal effect of an exposure X (binary or categorical) on disease D and we have additional measurements on genotype G which is *known* to be independent of X in the population, i.e., $X \perp\!\!\!\perp G$. The graphical representation of this marginal independence is via a so-called 'V-structure' where arrows meet head-to-head (at D) with no edge between the parents, X and G, as illustrated in Figure 6.6(a). Such studies are for example carried out to investigate gene-environment interactions (Moerkerke *et al.*, 2010). Further assume that the case-control design is such that $P(X, G, D \mid S = 1) = P(X, G \mid D)P(D \mid S = 1)$. As $X \perp\!\!\!\perp G$, we know that the joint distribution factorises $P(X, G) = P(X)P(G)$; hence we must have

$$\sum_{d=0,1} P(X = x, G = g \mid D = d)P(D = d)$$
$$= \sum_{d=0,1} P(X = x \mid D = d)P(D = d) \sum_{d=0,1} P(G = g \mid D = d)P(D = d)$$

for each value of x, g. This results in (at most) $(|\mathcal{X}| - 1)(|\mathcal{G}| - 1)$ nonredundant equations, each of which is quadratic in the unknown $\tilde{p} = P(D = 1)$ and can have at most two solutions. The true (population) distribution of D must be a solution to each equation, so it is identified up to at most two solutions. We note, however, that the equations become uninformative (i.e., any distribution for D is a solution) if $G \perp\!\!\!\perp D \mid X$ or $X \perp\!\!\!\perp D \mid G$.

General result

The above example demonstrates that if certain marginal independencies (in the population) are known, then we may be able to reconstruct the joint distribution from a conditional one; however, there may be more than one solution, and even infinitely many solutions if there are 'too many' independencies in the population. We call this *generic* identifiability (Evans and Didelez, 2015). Formally, generic k-identifiability means that there are at most k solutions under any true distribution in the model class except possibly for a proper (i.e., lower dimensional) algebraic subset of the model class. The existence of solutions depends on the number of known constraints being at least as large as the number of unknowns, which in an unmatched case-control study would be just one: $\tilde{p}$. The number of constraints in the above example is $(|\mathcal{X}| - 1)(|\mathcal{G}| - 1)$, so if both X and G are binary, there is exactly one constraint.

Entirely general results are difficult to obtain in this context. Here we provide a relatively general result modified from Evans and Didelez (2015) to reflect the situation of a case-control study. Hence, D is binary; we assume that selection is based only on D, so (6.1) and therefore data is available from $P(X, C \mid D)$. The covariates C can be a vector of variables which would correspond to a set of nodes in a DAG.

Proposition 2 *Assume $P(X, C \mid D = d)$, $d = 0, 1$ is given, and the joint population distribution $P(X, C, D)$ obeys a known DAG.*
(i) A necessary (but not sufficient) condition for $P(X, C, D)$ to be generically identifiable is that the DAG contains at least one V-structure.
(ii) If the graphical parents of D are given by $\{X, C\}$, then $P(X, C, D)$ is generically identifiable if at least one constraint is implied on $P(X, C)$ by the DAG.

To illustrate the above result consider the example in Figure 6.6(b) with $C = G \cup Z$. As in Figure 6.6(a) we have a V-structure $X \rightarrow D \leftarrow G$, so property (i) of Proposition 2 is satisfied. The parents of D are G, Z, X, and from the DAG we can read off that $X \perp\!\!\!\perp G \mid Z$ which induces at least one constraint, so property (ii) of Proposition 2 is satisfied and generic identification holds.

Remarks:
(1) Proposition 2 allows causal inference if the causal effect of interest is further identified from $P(X, C, D)$. So for instance when C is sufficient to adjust for confounding we can use the identity (6.6) to compute $P(D \mid \mathrm{do}(X = x))$.

(2) Before quantifying a causal effect, one may first want to test the null hypothesis of no (conditional) causal effect, H_0^C. As noticed before, when the null translates into a conditional independence (or absence of a directed edge in a DAG), this may actually hamper identification. We conjecture that in these cases the null can always be checked directly from a factorisation of $P(X, C \mid D)$ itself; Proposition 1 is an example of this.

(3) When the number of constraints in $P(X, C)$ is larger than one, the model (DAG) itself becomes empirically testable. For instance in Figure 6.6(b) with all variables binary, there are two constraints: $X \perp\!\!\!\perp G \mid Z = z$ for $z = 0, 1$. This yields two equations for one unknown, $\tilde{p}$; so if the two solutions do not agree the model assumptions must be violated.

(4) Once generic identification is established, it is in principle straightforward to fit the model. To perform maximum likelihood estimation we need to maximise the conditional log-likelihood based on $P(X, C \mid D)$, e.g., with the TM algorithm of Edwards and Lauritzen (2001).

(5) Practical problems may occur: if certain associations between (some elements of) C, X, and D are weak, identification becomes unstable. Additionally, if D represents a very rare disease, then the marginal distribution of (X, C) is approximately the same as that for the controls, $P(X, C) \approx P(X, C \mid D = 0)$, so recovering $P(X, C)$ exactly may not lead to substantial new insights. However, the method could be used for sensitivity analyses in such situations.

6.5   Adjusting for confounding

The previous sections addressed nonparametric approaches to causal inference, in that we used only structural assumptions and no external information to obtain identification. These run into practical problems if there are many covariates or some variables are continuous. Hence, we now discuss how popular (semi-)parametric methods for adjusting for confounding with prospective data can be adapted to case-control studies.

For a causal interpretation of the results, we see from the previous sections that we need two assumptions, which we use throughout:

(i) the covariates C are sufficient to adjust for confounding; and

(ii) sampling satisfies (6.2)

so that there is no selection bias and we can collapse over S; note that this typically means that C must contain any covariates used for matching.

6.5.1   Regression adjustment

Regression adjustment simply includes the confounders C into the outcome regression, which means positing a model for $P(D|X,C)$. Note that this results in conditional causal effect measures, which only equal the marginal ones if they are collapsible.

For case-control data, standard theory suggests that, even under retrospective sampling, a correctly specified logistic regression of D on (X,C) consistently estimates the conditional (X,D)-ORs, with only the intercept of that regression distorted due to the sampling proportions being different from the population ones (Prentice and Pyke, 1979). Then, under the assumptions above, the logistic regression coefficients correspond to *conditional* causal (log) ORs. When all variables are categorical and a saturated logistic regression is used, this approach is in fact identical to the one in Section 6.3.3. However, if some of (X,C) are continuous or if higher-order interaction terms are omitted from the logistic regression, this model imposes parametric assumptions on which the validity of the inference rests.

If the logistic regression is misspecified, the approach typically results in biased effect estimates. Unfortunately, this can also happen under the null hypothesis H_0^C, i.e., null-preservation is not guaranteed meaning that the coefficient(s) for the exposure might not be zero under H_0^C if the model is misspecified. One could therefore supplement the analysis by other tests of this null hypothesis along the lines of Proposition 1.

6.5.2   Standardisation

Standardisation is based on equality (6.6), where typically the terms required for the right-hand side are estimated and then plugged in to obtain the left-hand side. This again relies on a parametric model for $P(D \mid X, C)$. However, unlike regression adjustment, standardisation yields the marginal intervention distribution $P(D \mid \mathrm{do}(X))$, from which any marginal causal effect parameters can be computed.

To obtain all ingredients for the right-hand side of (6.6) from case-control data requires additional external information. A number of relevant methods in this context using additional knowledge on the population prevalence $\tilde{p} = P(D = 1)$ are discussed in Persson and Waernbaum (2013). With $\tilde{p}$ we can obtain exact weights to adjust the intercept of the logistic regression model yielding correct predicted values for $P(D = d \mid C = c, X = x)$; further $\tilde{p}$ helps to obtain the case-control weighted distribution of the covariates corresponding to $P(C = c)$. This results in the following estimate of the intervention distribution obtained as weighted average over the covariates

$$\hat{P}(D = 1 \mid \mathrm{do}(X = x))$$
$$= \frac{\tilde{p}}{\#\mathrm{cases}} \sum_{\mathrm{cases}} \mathrm{expit}\, g(x, C_i; \hat{\beta}^*) + \frac{1 - \tilde{p}}{\#\mathrm{controls}} \sum_{\mathrm{controls}} \mathrm{expit}\, g(x, C_i; \hat{\beta}^*)$$

where $g(\cdot)$ is the chosen linear predictor and $\hat{\beta}^*$ is the vector of estimated logistic regression coefficients including the adjusted intercept. The resulting $\hat{P}(D = 1 \mid \mathrm{do}(X = x))$ can then be summarised as marginal causal parameter, such as a marginal COR or risk ratio.

An alternative to adjusting the intercept is to weight the likelihood equations according to the above weights for cases and controls and obtain $\hat{\beta}_w$ as estimated coefficients to be inserted in the above formula instead of $\hat{\beta}^*$. For matched case-control data all of the above estimators can still be applied, but with modified weights that require the prevalence within matching values, i.e., $P(D = 1 \mid M = m)$, where $M \subset C$ are the matching variables (Persson and Waernbaum, 2013). In case that prevalence information is not available (for the un-matched or matched estimators), the authors recommend a sensitivity analysis. Their comparative simulation study suggests that all estimators perform well at finite sample sizes when the logistic regression is correctly specified, but exhibit considerable bias if a misspecified model, e.g., a probit instead of a logit link, is used; sensitivity to misspecified weights is not explored though. Evidently, the same potential lack of null preservation holds as mentioned earlier if the logistic regression is misspecified.

A different approach still relying on $\tilde{p}$ is Targeted Maximum Likelihood estimation (TMLE) (van der Laan, 2008); this additionally exploits the propensity score which we address further below. The TMLE remains consistent if the propensity score is correctly specified even if the logistic regression is not, i.e., it is *doubly robust*.

6.5.3 Propensity scores

For binary exposure, the propensity score is given by $\pi = P(X = 1 \mid C)$; methods for nonbinary exposure exist, but we refrain from going into these here in order to focus on the basic principle. Note that due to assuming positivity (6.4) we have that $0 < \pi < 1$. The propensity score has the property that $X \perp\!\!\!\perp C \mid \pi$, known as *balancing* of the covariates between treatment groups (Rosenbaum and Rubin, 1983). As a consequence, if C is sufficient to adjust for confounding then so is π. The underlying principle can be illustrated with the DAG in Figure 6.2(a), letting $Z = \pi$.

Two related ways of using the propensity score to adjust for confounding with prospective data are by matching or stratification on π, and regression adjustment using the propensity score as covariate in addition to X. Stratification and regression adjustment result in conditional causal effect measures (conditional on π).

A third way of using π is known as inverse probability of treatment weighting (IPTW) (Robins *et al.*, 2000). With prospective data, the method proceeds by re-weighting the sampled units by $\pi_i = P(X = 1 \mid C = c_i)$ if $X_i = 1$ and by $1 - \pi_i = P(X = 0 \mid C = c_i)$ if $X_i = 0$, and then fit a parametric or semi-parametric model for $P(D \mid X)$ on the weighted data. It can be shown that X and C are independent in the weighted sample; IPTW can therefore be thought of as 'removing' any incoming edges from C into X in a causal DAG. Hence, if all models are correctly specified (and under (6.3)), IPTW consistently estimates a *marginal structural model (MSM)*, i.e., a model for $P(D \mid \mathrm{do}(X))$ (Robins *et al.*, 2000). So, like standardisation, IPTW yields marginal causal effect parameters.

In observational studies π is often estimated, typically by fitting a model to $P(X = 1 \mid C)$. However, in a case control setting where everything is conditional on $S = 1$, we do not typically have direct access to data from $P(X = 1 \mid C)$. Månsson *et al.* (2007) provide an overview and comparison of possible approaches for obtaining an estimate of π. In some case-cohort studies, a sub-cohort may be available from which π can consistently be estimated, or if the sampling fraction is known it can exactly be re-weighted; both these approaches result in consistent estimation of a causal effect if the involved models are correctly specified. Other approaches consist of fitting a model for π on the controls only, or on the whole sample; or fitting a model for $P(X = 1 \mid C, D)$ and predicting X for each individual as if they were a control. These last three methods all have the null preserving property that if the model for π is correct they consistently estimate π if X has no effect on D, but they are not consistent otherwise. Estimating π from the controls only is 'nearly' consistent if the disease is very rare. A lack of consistency of the propensity score estimators means that there will be some residual confounding so that we must expect the estimator of the causal effect to be biased. This bias, though small, is confirmed by the simulations of Månsson *et al.* (2007). Further, in finite samples, their simulations suggest that propensity score stratification using the above methods for case-control data sometimes results in an artificial effect modification by the propensity score even under the null and without confounding.

A general issue arising when using the propensity score for stratification or regression adjustment with case-control data is that the outcome model is typically a logistic regression; but as shown in Section 6.3.2 in a DAG such as Figure 6.2(a) with $Z = \pi$, the $OR_{DX}(\pi, C)$ is not collapsible over C as $X \not\perp\!\!\!\perp C \mid (D, \pi)$. Even in the absence of effect modification by C it is possible that $COR_{DX}(\pi)$ is different from $COR_{DX}(C)$. Furthermore, in the presence of effect modification by C, it appears more difficult to interpret $OR_{DX}(\pi)$ meaningfully.

6.6 Instrumental variables

All previous sections relied on the availability of sufficient covariates to control for confounding. Now we consider an approach that can sometimes be employed when this is not the case, i.e., when there is *unobserved* confounding. An *instrumental variable* (IV) can be regarded as 'imperfectly mimicking' randomisation of X when exposure itself cannot be randomised. When the IV is a genetic variant this has become known as Mendelian randomisation (MR) (Davey Smith and Ebrahim, 2003; Didelez and Sheehan, 2007a). Case-control studies play an important role for research into Mendelian randomisation, as the method is often applied in a secondary or meta-analysis, where (some of) the primary analyses were case-control studies. A brief overview of the use of IVs for case-control data is also given in Windmeijer and Didelez (2018).

6.6.1 Definition of instrumental variables

A variable Z is an instrument for the causal effect of an exposure X on an outcome D in the presence of unobserved confounding U under the following three core conditions (Didelez and Sheehan, 2007a).

IV.1: $Z \perp\!\!\!\perp U$, the instrument is independent of the unobserved confounding;
IV.2: $Z \not\perp\!\!\!\perp X$, the instrument and exposure are dependent;
IV.3: $D \perp\!\!\!\perp Z \mid (X, U)$, the outcome is conditionally independent of the instrument.

Here U is such that if it were observed it would be sufficient to adjust for confounding (for simplicity we ignore observed covariates). Note that Z can be vector valued, such as a set of genetic variants obtained from genome wide association studies (GWASs).

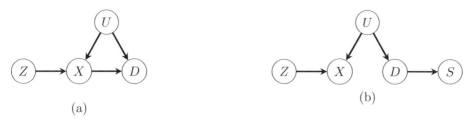

FIGURE 6.7
DAGs representing (a) the IV conditions (prospectively); (b) the IV conditions under the causal null, with a sampling indicator.

The IV assumptions are represented graphically in Figure 6.7(a); it is the absence of any edges between Z and U, as well as between Z and D, that, respectively, implies conditions IV.1 and IV.3. In particular, the assumptions imply that there are no common causes of Z and U, nor of Z and D, which means that we can treat Z in the same way we treat a genuinely randomised quantity; moreover, the only 'input' that Z has into the system is via X, so that we can regard Z as a proxy for randomisation of exposure X. Intuitively, the stronger the dependence between Z and X the better, since this reduces X's susceptibility to being affected by unmeasured variables U; this is expressed in condition IV.2.

An IV can help causal inference in the form of testing and bounding causal quantities, and (under additional assumptions) point estimation. In the following we discuss how to adapt the standard approaches to a case-control setting, where we only observe data from $P(Z, X, D \mid S = 1)$. We assume no matching (we still ignore any observed covariates C), and also that sampling only depends on the outcome: $S \perp\!\!\!\perp (X, U, Z) \mid D$. Together with the IV conditions this implies $P(Z, X, D \mid S = 1) = P(Z, X \mid D)P(D \mid S = 1)$.

6.6.2   Testing the causal null hypothesis with an instrumental variable

With prospective data, we can test for the presence of a causal effect of X on D by testing for an association between Z and D. This is because the only way that Z and D can be associated is via a causal effect of X on D; when we delete the edge from X to D in Figure 6.7(a), the only remaining path $Z \rightarrow X \leftarrow U \rightarrow D$ is unconditionally blocked, so there is no (Z, D)-association. Of course, if the dependence between Z and X (condition IV.2) is only weak relative to the sample size, then this will not be a powerful test.

A small caveat applies to this test if the unobserved confounders U are likely to contain effect modifiers such that the effects in different subgroups have different directions; for example, a treatment which is beneficial for men but harmful for women. These could in principle cancel out exactly, leading to an unfaithful distribution. For many practical situations we consider this to be of minor relevance (Didelez and Sheehan, 2007a).

The null hypothesis (absence of the edge $X \rightarrow D$) under case-control selection is illustrated in Figure 6.7(b). We see that case-control sampling, i.e., conditioning on $S = 1$, produces no association between Z and D under the null as the only path between them is blocked by S. Hence, in analogy to the prospective case, we find that testing $Z \perp\!\!\!\perp D \mid S = 1$ with case-control data is a valid test for causal effect of X on D, where strictly speaking we also assume faithfulness.

As an example consider the analysis of Meleady *et al.* (2003). The data comes from a case-control study and includes homocysteine levels X, cardiovascular disease D (CVD), as well as a genetic IV (the rs1801133 polymorphism) Z with three levels. A χ^2-test of the association between Z and D yields a p-value of 0.357 so no evidence for an association. If Z satisfies the IV conditions this means no evidence for a causal effect of homocysteine on CVD. Note that as this test does not make use of data on the exposure X, it can be carried out using case-control data from, say, a separate study with data on Z and D only.

6.6.3   Instrumental variable estimation

Without additional assumptions, the IV conditions do not generally allow us to identify the causal effect of X on D. However, in the all-discrete case, they impose bounds on the causal effect in the form of minima and maxima for $P(D = 1 \mid do(X = x))$, $x = 0, 1$ (Balke and Pearl, 1994). These bounds are given as simple transformations of the observed relative frequencies and can for example be computed with the Stata command bpbounds. For examples including an application to the above CVD case-control data, see Palmer *et al.* (2011). When applicable, it is recommended to compute the bounds, as they demonstrate what information the data provide without additional parametric constraints.

Point estimation with an IV requires additional parametric assumptions. The simplest case is given by a linear model which gives rise to the *Two-Stage-Least-Square (TSLS)* estimator (Wooldridge, 2010). Even though this is not a suitable assumption in a case-control situation, we mention it here as it has inspired OR estimation which is relevant. Assume that

$$E(D \mid X, U) = \theta X + h(U).$$

Under IV.1-IV.3 it can be shown that $\theta = \mathrm{Cov}(D, Z) / \mathrm{Cov}(X, Z)$, so a consistent estimator $\hat{\theta}_{IV}$ for θ is given by the ratio of the regression coefficient $\hat{\beta}_{D|Z}$ from a regression of D on Z, and $\hat{\beta}_{X|Z}$ of X on Z; that is

$$\hat{\theta}_{IV} = \frac{\hat{\beta}_{D|Z}}{\hat{\beta}_{X|Z}}, \tag{6.8}$$

where Z, X, D are all univariate. More generally, it can be shown that the above is a special case of TSLS, which consists of regressing X on Z to obtain predicted values $\hat{X}$, and then regressing D on $\hat{X}$. From the above, we see that condition IV.2 needs to be strengthened to $\mathrm{Cov}(X, Z) \neq 0$. In fact, when $\mathrm{Cov}(X, Z)$ is close to zero, the TSLS estimator is not only unstable but biased, a phenomenon known as weak-IV bias (Wooldridge, 2010).

Turning to case-control data, note that when we assumed 'no unobserved confounding' in earlier sections of this chapter; targeting an OR as the parameter of interest had the advantage that it often does not require additional information. However, this advantage is lost with IVs and case-control data. If we want to estimate a COR with an IV we still need external information on the sampling proportions or disease prevalence. In the absence of such information, only approximate solutions are available, which we address first.

6.6.3.1   Instrumental variable estimation without external information

Inspired by the linear case where a simple IV estimator of the causal effect is given by the ratio (6.8), it has been suggested to estimate the causal log-OR for the effect of X on D as the ratio of the log-OR between outcome and IV divided by the linear regression coefficient for X on the IV Z, $\beta_{X|Z}$ (Casas *et al.*, 2005):

$$\log OR_{DX} \approx \frac{\log OR_{DZ}}{\beta_{X|Z}}. \tag{6.9}$$

The above has the advantage that OR_{DZ} can be estimated from case-control data, even using a meta-analysis of several such case-control studies; while $\beta_{X|Z}$ can be estimated from the controls only, or from separate studies. This estimator is called *Wald-OR* as such ratios have also been considered in the context of measurement error.

The advantages but also the shortcomings of estimation based on the Wald-OR (6.9) are discussed in Harbord *et al.* (2013). The main points are: it is not consistent either for a population COR or for a conditional COR, even when there is no unobserved confounding. Its justification is as approximation of the causal risk ratio for rare diseases under the assumption that the exposure X has a conditional normal distribution with a specific mean structure (Didelez *et al.*, 2010a). However, the estimator is consistent under the null because, using our earlier reasoning, we expect $OR_{DZ} = 1$ if and only if there is no causal effect. Moreover, Harbord *et al.* (2013) give a number of conditions, some but not all empirically testable, under which the asymptotic bias for estimating the marginal COR is smaller than 10%. In contrast, Didelez *et al.* (2010a) show for the case of a binary exposure, where the normality assumption clearly fails, that in many realistic scenarios the bias can easily be 30% or larger. So, unlike the TSLS-estimator, the performance of the Wald-OR is quite sensitive to the type of exposure distribution.

Using the Wald-OR (6.9) is especially popular in the context of Mendelian randomisation studies because the relations between disease and many genetic factors are easily available from summary data from case-control GWASs, and are in fact often combined in a meta-analytic way to obtain estimates of OR_{DZ}. Moreover, it does not require any assumptions such as knowledge of the disease prevalence. In fact, none of the alternative estimators (addressed below) can be computed when only summary data are available, or without knowledge of the disease prevalence.

Returning to the data from Meleady *et al.* (2003), we find that the log-OR between the genetic variant and CVD is 0.11 (se = 0.077); the linear regression coefficient from a regression of the binary exposure on the genetic factor within the controls is only 0.071 (se = 0.013) indicating a weak instrument; so a rough estimate according to (6.9) would be a COR of 4.73 (95% CI: (0.52; 43.3)). Note that if we used all data for the denominator, instead of only the controls, we would find a linear regression coefficient of 0.082 which would suggest a COR of 3.81 (95% CI: (0.58, 25.1)); the difference in (Z, X)-association for controls compared to the whole sample is due to the selection effect. The very wide confidence intervals are typical for a weak instrument.

6.6.3.2 Instrumental variable estimation using external information

In Mendelian randomisation studies, it is not unrealistic to assume that the population distribution of the gene alleles and hence $E(Z)$ is known. For a *multiplicative structural mean model (MSMM)* (Hernán and Robins, 2006) this is sufficient to estimate the causal risk ratio with an IV from case-control data as shown in Bowden and Vansteelandt (2011). A MSMM assumes

$$\frac{P(D = 1 \mid X, Z)}{P(D = 1 \mid X, Z; \mathrm{do}(X = 0))} = \exp(\psi X), \tag{6.10}$$

so the causal parameter of interest here is the logarithm of the risk ratio ψ, which describes the effect of exposure on the exposed. As an example consider again alcohol consumption: $\exp(\psi X)$ corresponds to the multiplicative reduction in risk of a person who by her own choice would drink an amount X of alcohol, but is forced by an intervention not to drink any.

The MSMM can be fitted using the following estimating equations which remain valid under case-control sampling

$$0 = \sum_i (Z_i - E(Z)) D_i \exp(-\psi X_i),$$

where we see the need to know $E(Z)$. If this is not available but the disease prevalence $\tilde{p}$ in the population is known, then we can instead use the estimate

$$\hat{E}(Z) = \frac{\sum W_i Z_i}{\sum W_i}$$

with weights $W_i = D_i \tilde{p}/\tilde{p}_S + (1 - D_i)(1 - \tilde{p})/(1 - \tilde{p}_S)$, and $\tilde{p}_S = P(D = 1 \mid S = 1)$. The solution to the resulting estimating equations, $\hat{\psi}$, is then a consistent estimator of the logarithm of the causal risk ratio, and its properties as well as formulas for standard errors are detailed in Bowden and Vansteelandt (2011). In contrast, if $\tilde{p}$ is unknown but assumed to be low, $E(Z)$ could be estimated from the controls only; the larger $\tilde{p}$ the more biased the estimator $\hat{\psi}$, though.

In analogy to (6.10), we could also assume a logistic SMM in order to estimate a causal OR describing the effect of exposure on the exposed (Vansteelandt and Goetghebeur, 2003). The estimating equations are more involved and require fitting an associational model for $P(D = 1 \mid X, Z)$ and we refer for the details again to Bowden and Vansteelandt (2011).

A philosophically different approach to combining an IV with case-control sampling has been proposed by Shinohara *et al.* (2012) who target the so-called *principal stratum* causal effect. This approach originates in the context of RCTs with partial compliance and estimates the 'effect of treatment on the compliers'. Again, IV-estimation of this type of causal effect relies on external information on the disease prevalence.

6.7   Conclusions

In conclusion we summarise the main issues of causal inference from case-control data (confounding, selection bias, retrospective sampling), and then discuss the implications for practical analyses.

6.7.1   Summary of main issues

With observational data, including case-control data, confounding poses the biggest threat to the validity of causal conclusions. We have given an intuitive and formal characterisation of when sufficient information to account for confounding is available; causal DAGs and the back-door criterion are useful tools to identify such information. When there is unobserved confounding, instrumental variables provide an alternative if available.

Another danger especially relevant to case-control sampling is selection bias. This can occur when the controls are not truly sampled from the population, but unrepresentative databases are used instead; recall bias and ascertainment bias also fall in this category. The null preservation property is relevant in this context: a method should at least give valid conclusions when the causal null hypothesis is true even if it is potentially biased otherwise; instrumental variables can be exploited in this way. We have also seen the duality between evaluating a causal null hypothesis and a causal odds ratio: selection bias is excluded from inference on both these targets by the same structural assumptions, which can easily be checked on causal DAGs. To construct the DAG and hence to justify these assumptions, a thorough understanding of the sampling process and its implications are crucial.

A third characteristic of case-control studies is that we observe $P(D, X, C \mid S = 1)$, and not the population distribution $P(D \mid X, C)$. However, many standard causal parameters are functions of the latter; marginal causal effects require some information on the covariate distribution $P(C)$ in the population. Such causal effect measures are often chosen with a view to comparison with results from RCTs, as well as to public health decision making. However, we have seen that only conditional causal odds ratios can be obtained from case-control data without external information; further, their interpretation must take noncollapsibility into account. All other methods covered in this chapter require some additional information or are approximative. If certain independencies in the population are known, such as between genetic factors and exposure, these can help to reconstruct the marginal distribution. Knowledge of the disease prevalence $\tilde{p}$ enables standardisation, propensity score methods, IPTW, and IV methods; the distribution within controls can be used to approximate some of the ingredients for these methods when the disease is rare.

In view of the pivotal role of structural assumptions, as well as the possible need for external information which may often only be approximative, it appears that systematic sensitivity analyses are especially relevant to causal inference from case-control data. However, while sensitivity analyses have been considered in a few areas of causal inference, we are not aware of any such work for case-control designs.

6.7.2 Implication for practical analyses of case-control studies

Current practice in epidemiology when faced with case-control data is largely based on logistic regression modelling. As addressed in Section 6.5.1, this enables causal conclusions if the covariates included are sufficient to adjust for confounding, if a conditional causal odds-ratio is the target of inference, and if sources of selection bias, e.g., due to the available database, omitted covariates, recall or ascertainment bias, reverse causation, etc., can be eliminated. When aiming at reliable causal conclusions these assumptions should therefore carefully be addressed and justified, both by empirical evidence and subject matter knowledge; even if their full validity in a given application is doubtful, the source of possible violations and how these might be prevented in future studies or analyses should be clarified (and ideally supplemented by a sensitivity analysis).

We suggest that confidence in and understanding of – and hence critical discussion of – these crucial causal assumptions can always be strengthened by supplementing the analysis with a detailed graphical representation; this should contain the observed variables, relevant unobserved variables, design features, and the known or assumed structural relationships between these in the form of a DAG. While this allows us to graphically verify the assumptions, an important additional benefit of using DAGs is that structural assumptions are made *explicit and transparent* in the first place. When constructing the DAG for a given data situation it is important to justify the absence of further edges or nodes, as these would often result in a violation of assumption or a source of spurious association due to selection (such as if U in Figure 6.3(a) were ignored). Moreover, when addressing the problem of confounding, the user may find it easiest to think about the data generating mechanisms prospectively in order to obtain an appropriate DAG, with careful distinction between pre- and post-exposure covariates based on the way they are measured. Sampling selection would then be addressed by including further nodes and edges relevant to the sampling node S reflecting the study design, and conditioning on the latter. Examples for this were given with Figure 6.2(b) in Section 6.2 showing the problem of ascertainment bias (no adjustment with observed variables results in valid inference), and with Figure 6.5 in Section 6.3.3 illustrating a study on the effect of HRT on TCI (where more than one subset of the covariates allows valid adjustment).

Logistic regression further relies on correct model specification (except in the rare case when a saturated model can be used) and therefore does not satisfy the null-preservation property, but has the advantage of not requiring any extra outside information on disease prevalence. It is therefore important to remember that a valid test for the causal null hypothesis can be obtained under weaker assumptions, either based on Proposition 1 or using an instrument as in Section 6.6.2, and we suggest that any analysis should be complemented by such a test.

In some applications, a logistic regression analysis may be considered too limiting, and this is where the other approaches presented in this chapter may be attractive. This is especially important when the user desires to partly relax some of the assumptions, or to estimate a causal parameter other than a conditional causal odds ratio for example, for better comparability with RCTs. While there are a few examples where alternatives to logistic regression have been applied (Persson and Waernbaum, 2013), more practical analyses are still required to gain a better understanding of their strength and weaknesses. In contrast, there are an increasing number of applications of IV methods for MR studies in case-control settings due to the availability of GWAS data (see references in Harbord *et al.* (2013)). Again, we recommend that such analyses be based on a transparent and well-justified DAG representation of the assumption. As before, this is crucial in order to exclude selection bias by design, or by conditioning on post-IV covariates (Aschard *et al.*, 2015); an explicit consideration of the causal null hypothesis using the IV-outcome association still relies on weaker assumptions, and we again suggest that any IV-analysis should be complemented by such a test.

6.8   Appendix: Directed acyclic graphs

Basic reading for anyone interested in (causal) DAGs are Spirtes *et al.* (2000), Pearl (2009), Dawid (2015), and Hernán and Robins (2018).

Terminology and basics

A *directed acyclic graph* (DAG) $G = (V, E)$ consists of a set of nodes (vertices) V and directed edges E between pairs of distinct nodes, where a single edge $(a, b) \in E$ is represented as $a \to b$. In a DAG there is only at most one type of edge between two nodes. An ordered sequence of distinct nodes $(v_1, \ldots, v_J)$ such that there is an edge in E between any two successive nodes is called a *path*, i.e., $(v_j, v_{j+1}) \in E$ or $(v_{j+1}, v_j) \in E$; if the edges all point in the same direction it is a *directed path*. A DAG is characterised by the assumption that there are no directed paths from one node to itself, i.e., no sequence $a \to \cdots \to a$. A back-door path from a to b is any path that starts with an edge pointing at a, i.e., with $a \leftarrow \cdots b$. Note that this definition is not symmetric in a, b.

If $a \to b$, then a is a *parent* of b, and the set of all *parents* is denoted by pa(b). All nodes $b \in V \backslash \{a\}$ such that there is a directed path from a to b are called *descendants* of a; all others are its *nondescendants*. Each intermediate node $v_j, j = 2, \ldots, J - 1$, on a path $(v_1, \ldots, v_J)$ is either a *collider*, if $\to v_j \leftarrow$, or a *noncollider* in all other cases. Note that the same node can be a collider on one path and a noncollider on another path.

A DAG is associated with a joint distribution of variables represented by the nodes through conditional independencies that correspond to absences of edges in the DAG *(Markov properties)*. First of all, we define that a joint distribution for $X_1 \ldots, X_K$ *factorises* according to a DAG $G = (V, E)$, $V = \{1 \ldots, K\}$ if the pdf/pmf satisfies

$$p(x_1, \ldots, x_K) = \prod_{i \in V} p(x_i | x_{\mathrm{pa}(i)}).$$

Conditional independencies implied by this factorisation can be read off the DAG through 'd-separation', defined next. A path between two nodes a and b is *blocked* by a set $C \subset$

$V\backslash\{a, b\}$ if (i) the path contains a node $v \in C$ that is a noncollider; or (ii) it contains a collider v' such that neither v' nor any descendants of v' are elements of C. Then the sets A and B are *d-separated* by $C \subset V\backslash(A \cup B)$ if all paths between all $a \in A$ and $b \in B$ are blocked by C (see, e.g., Lauritzen (1996) for an equivalent way of reading off separations in a DAG using 'moralisation'). Now, for any distribution that factorises according to a DAG it holds that whenever A and B are d-separated by C then $X_A \perp\!\!\!\perp X_B \,|\, X_C$ (or we also write $A \perp\!\!\!\perp B \,|\, C$). Paths can be blocked by the empty set, e.g., if they contain a collider or if there is no path between two nodes in the first place.

Note that while the factorisation implies that any d-separation corresponds to a conditional independence, the converse is not true. It is possible for a distribution to contain additional conditional or marginal independencies that cannot be seen from the DAG, e.g., due to 'cancellation' of paths. A joint distribution where this does not happen is called *faithful* to the DAG.

Causal DAGs and back-door criterion

A DAG is supplemented with a causal interpretation by demanding that the parents $X_{\mathrm{pa}(a)}$ of a node/variable X_a are its *direct causes* (relative to the given set of nodes/variables X_V). This 'direct cause' requirement means that if we fix $X_{\mathrm{pa}(a)}$ by intervention, manipulations of any other nodes do not have an effect on X_a, while manipulations of any of the parent nodes individually (while holding the other ones fixed) have an effect on X_a (Spirtes *et al.*, 2000). A further requirement is that any 'common cause' of any two variables X_a, X_b must be included in the DAG whether observable or not. While any conditional independencies implied by the DAG involving observable variables can (and should) be checked empirically, these requirements essentially need to be justified based on subject matter knowledge. For example, whether a given set C is sufficient to adjust for confounding, or the IV conditions cannot be (entirely) verified empirically from observational data.

The above definition of a causal DAG can be somewhat relaxed but we will not go into details here. A number of alternative causal interpretations supplementing DAGs with additional or different types of nodes have been proposed (Dawid, 2002; Richardson and Robins, 2013). Another modification common in much of the causality literature is not to represent unobservable variables explicitly as nodes, but to use bi-directed edges $a \leftrightarrow b$ when $a \leftarrow U \rightarrow b$ for an unobservable U; again we do not go into details here (Pearl, 2009).

A popular criterion that is used to find, from a DAG, a set of covariates that is sufficient to adjust for confounding is the *back-door criterion* (Pearl, 1995). This states that given a causal DAG on a set of variables V, we can identify the causal effect of $X \in V$ on $D \in V$ if a set $C \subset V\backslash\{X, D\}$ exists such that C are nondescendants of X and C blocks every back-door path from X to D. The causal effect is then given by (6.6).

Causal DAGs can further be used to check other criteria under which causal effects are identified, leading to different formulae. In fact, a complete characterisation of identification of causal effects can be given. However, this complete characterisation does not cover the case of identification under sampling selection (Bareinboim and Tian, 2015; Bareinboim *et al.*, 2014).

Bibliography

Aschard, H., Vilhjálmsson, B. J., Joshi, A. D., Price, A. L., and Kraft, P. (2015). Adjusting for heritable covariates can bias effect estimates in genome-wide association studies. *The*

American Journal of Human Genetics, **96**, 329 – 339.

Balke, A. and Pearl, J. (1994). Counterfactual probabilities: Computational methods, bounds, and applications. In *Proceedings of the Tenth Annual Conference on Uncertainty in Artificial Intelligence*, pages 46–54. Morgan Kauffman, San Francisco.

Bareinboim, E. and Pearl, J. (2012). Controlling selection bias in causal inference. In *Proceedings of the Fifteenth International Conference on Artificial Intelligence and Statistics*, volume 22 of *Proceedings of Machine Learning Research*, pages 100–108.

Bareinboim, E. and Tian, J. (2015). Recovering causal effects from selection bias. In *Proceedings of the Twenty-Ninth National Conference on Artificial Intelligence*, pages 3475–3481. AAAI Press, Menlo Park, CA.

Bareinboim, E., Tian, J., and Pearl, J. (2014). Recovering from selection bias in causal and statistical inference. In *Proceedings of the 28th National Conference on Artificial Intelligence*, pages 2410–2416. AAAI Press, Menlo Park, CA.

Berkson, J. (1946). Limitations of the application of fourfold table analysis to hospital data. *Biometrics Bulletin*, **2**, 47–53.

Borboudakis, G. and Tsamardinos, I. (2015). Bayesian network learning with discrete case-control data. In *Proceedings of the 31st Conference on Uncertainty in Artificial Intelligence*, pages 151–160. AUAI Press, Arlington, Virginia.

Bowden, J. and Vansteelandt, S. (2011). Mendelian randomization analysis of case-control data using structural mean models. *Statistics in Medicine*, **30**, 678–694.

Casas, J. P., Bautista, L. E., Smeeth, L., Sharma, P., and Hingorani, A. D. (2005). Homocysteine and stroke: Evidence on a causal link from Mendelian randomisation. *The Lancet*, **365**, 224–232.

Cooper, G. F. (1995). Causal discovery from data in the presence of selection bias. In *Proceedings of the Fifth International Workshop on Artificial Intelligence and Statistics*, pages 140–150. Morgan Kaufmann, San Francisco.

Davey Smith, G. and Ebrahim, S. (2003). Mendelian randomization: Can genetic epidemiology contribute to understanding environmental determinants of disease? *International Journal of Epidemiology*, **32**, 1–22.

Dawid, A. P. (1979). Conditional independence in statistical theory (with discussion). *Journal of the Royal Statististical Society, Series B*, **41**, 1–31.

Dawid, A. P. (2000). Causal inference without counterfactuals (with discussion). *Journal of the American Statistical Association*, **95**, 407–448.

Dawid, A. P. (2002). Influence diagrams for causal modelling and inference. *International Statistical Review*, **70**, 161–89.

Dawid, A. P. (2015). Statistical causality from a decision-theoretic perspective. *Annual Review of Statistics and Its Application*, **2**, 273–303.

Didelez, V. and Sheehan, N. A. (2007a). Mendelian randomisation as an instrumental variable approach to causal inference. *Statistical Methods in Medical Research*, **16**, 309–330.

Didelez, V. and Sheehan, N. A. (2007b). Mendelian randomisation: Why epidemiology needs a formal language for causality. In F. Russo and J. Williamson, editors, *Causality and Probability in the Sciences*, volume 5 of *Texts in Philosophy*, pages 263–292. College Publications, London.

Didelez, V., Meng, S., and Sheehan, N. A. (2010a). Assumptions of IV methods for observational epidemiology. *Statistical Science*, **25**, 22–40.

Didelez, V., Kreiner, S., and Keiding, N. (2010b). Graphical models for inference under outcome-dependent sampling. *Statistical Science*, **25**, 368–387.

Edwards, D. and Lauritzen, S. L. (2001). The TM algorithm for maximising a conditional likelihood function. *Biometrika*, **88**, 961–972.

Evans, R. J. and Didelez, V. (2015). Recovering from selection bias using marginal structure in discrete models. In *Proceedings of the 31st Annual Conference on Uncertainty in Artifical Intelligence – Causality Workshop*, pages 46–55. AUAI Press, Corvallis, Oregon.

Goldberger, A. (1972). Structural equation methods in the social sciences. *Econometrica*, **40**, 979–1001.

Greenland, S. (2003). Quantifying biases in causal models: Classical confounding vs collider-stratification bias. *Epidemiology*, **14**, 300–306.

Greenland, S., Robins, J. M., and Pearl, J. (1999). Confounding and collapsibility in causal inference. *Statistical Science*, **14**, 29–46.

Harbord, R. M., Didelez, V., Palmer, T. M., Meng, S., Sterne, J. A. C., and Sheehan, N. A. (2013). Severity of bias of a simple estimator of the causal odds ratio in Mendelian randomization studies. *Statistics in Medicine*, **32**, 1246–1258.

Hernán, M. A. (2004). A definition of causal effect for epidemiological research. *Journal of Epidemiology and Community Health*, **58**, 265–271.

Hernán, M. A. and Robins, J. M. (2006). Instruments for causal inference: An epidemiologist's dream? *Epidemiology*, **17**, 360–372.

Hernán, M. A. and Robins, J. M. (2018). *Causal Inference*. Chapman & Hall/CRC, Boca Raton. Forthcoming.

Hernán, M. A., Hernández-Díaz, S., and Robins, J. M. (2004). A structural approach to selection bias. *Epidemiology*, **15**, 615–625.

Hill, A. B. (2015). The environment and disease: Association or causation? *Journal of the Royal Society of Medicine*, **108**, 32–37.

Ioannidis, J. P. A. (2016). Exposure-wide epidemiology: Revisiting Bradford Hill. *Statistics in Medicine*, **35**, 1749–1762.

Keiding, N. and Clayton, D. (2014). Standardization and control for confounding in observational studies: A historical perspective. *Statistical Science*, **29**, 529–558.

Lauritzen, S. L. (1996). *Graphical Models*. Clarendon Press, Oxford.

Månsson, R., Joffe, M. M., Sun, W., and Hennessy, S. (2007). On the estimation and use of propensity scores in case-control and case-cohort studies. *American Journal of Epidemiology*, **166**, 332–339.

Meleady, R., Ueland, P. M., Blom, H., Whitehead, A. S., Refsum, H., Daly, L. E., Vollset, S. E., Donohue, C., Giesendorf, B., Graham, I. M., Ulvik, A., Zhang, Y., Bjorke Monsen, A.-L., and the EC Concerted Action Project: Homocysteine and Vascular Disease (2003). Thermolabile methylenetetrahydrofolate reductase, homocysteine, and cardiovascular disease risk: The European Concerted Action Project. *The American Journal of Clinical Nutrition*, **77**, 63–70.

Moerkerke, B., Vansteelandt, S., and Lange, C. (2010). A doubly robust test for gene-environment interaction in family-based studies of affected offspring. *Biostatistics*, **11**, 213–225.

Palmer, T. M., Ramsahai, R. R., Didelez, V., and Sheehan, N. A. (2011). Nonparametric bounds for the causal effect in a binary instrumental-variable model. *Stata Journal*, **11**, 345–367.

Pearl, J. (1995). Causal diagrams for empirical research. *Biometrika*, **82**, 669–688.

Pearl, J. (2009). *Causality*. Cambridge University Press, second edition.

Pedersen, A. T., Lidegaard, O., Kreiner, S., and Ottesen, B. (1997). Hormone replacement therapy and risk of non–fatal stroke. *The Lancet*, **350**, 1277–1283.

Persson, E. and Waernbaum, I. (2013). Estimating a marginal causal odds ratio in a case-control design: Analyzing the effect of low birth weight on the risk of type 1 diabetes mellitus. *Statistics in Medicine*, **32**, 2500–2512.

Prentice, R. L. and Pyke, R. (1979). Logistic disease incidence models and case-control studies. *Biometrika*, **66**, 403–411.

Richardson, T. S. and Robins, J. M. (2013). Single world intervention graphs (SWIGs): A unification of the counterfactual and graphical approaches to causality. *Working Paper No.128*. Center for Statistics and the Social Sciences of the University of Washington.

Robins, J. M. (2001). Data, design and background knowledge in etiologic inference. *Epidemiology*, **11**, 313–320.

Robins, J. M., Hernán, M. A., and Brumback, B. (2000). Marginal structural models and causal inference in epidemiology. *Epidemiology*, **11**, 550–560.

Rosenbaum, P. R. and Rubin, D. B. (1983). The central rôle of the propensity score in observational studies for causal effects. *Biometrika*, **70**, 41–55.

Rubin, D. B. (1974). Estimating causal effects of treatments in randomized and nonrandomized studies. *Journal of Educational Psychology*, **66**, 688–701.

Shinohara, R. T., Frangakis, C. E., Platz, E., and Tsilidis, K. (2012). Designs combining instrumental variables with case-control: Estimating principal strata causal effects. *The International Journal of Biostatistics*, **8**, 1–21.

Spirtes, P., Glymour, C., and Scheines, R. (2000). *Causation, Prediction and Search*. MIT Press, Cambridge, Massachusetts, second edition.

van der Laan, M. J. (2008). Estimation based on case-control designs with known prevalence probability. *The International Journal of Biostatistics*, **4**, Issue 1, Article 17.

VanderWeele, T. J. (2015). *Explanation in Causal Inference: Methods for Mediation and Interaction*. Oxford University Press.

VanderWeele, T. J. and Shpitser, I. (2013). On the definition of a confounder. *The Annals of Statistics*, **41**, 196–220.

Vansteelandt, S. and Goetghebeur, E. (2003). Causal inference with generalized structural mean models. *Journal of the Royal Statistical Society, Series B*, **65**, 817–835.

Whittemore, A. S. (1978). Collapsibility of multidimensional contingency tables. *Journal of the Royal Statististical Society, Series B*, **40**, 328–340.

Windmeijer, F. and Didelez, V. (2018). IV methods for binary outcomes. In G. Davey Smith, editor, *Mendelian Randomization: How genes can reveal the biological and environmental causes of disease*. Oxford University Press. Forthcoming.

Wooldridge, J. M. (2010). *Econometric Analysis of Cross Section and Panel Data*. MIT Press, Cambridge, Massachusetts.

Zeger, S. L., Liang, K.-Y., and Albert, P. S. (1988). Models for longitudinal data: A generalized estimating equation approach. *Biometrics*, **44**, 1049–1060.

7

The Case-Crossover Study Design in Epidemiology

Joseph A. "Chris" Delaney
University of Washington

Samy Suissa
McGill University & Jewish General Hospital, Montreal

7.1 Introduction

The effects of exposures to agents, either ingested or environmental, on humans are estimated most reliably from randomized controlled trials. These effects have a direct causal interpretation since randomization accounts for both observed and unobserved confounding (Hernán and Robins, 2006). There are, however, numerous situations when observational studies are necessary to study exposure associations. Sometimes this occurs in the context of rare events, which would require extremely large trials to detect an association. Often, information on an adverse event may not be available in previous clinical trials and conducting new trials is both lengthy and expensive. In other cases, the exposure is not ethically amenable to experimentation and thus cannot be the object of randomization. Finally, the population studied in clinical trials is generally highly selected and researchers may wish to determine if the results in the trial population can be generalized to other portions of the population (Mills *et al.*, 2006).

The estimates of epidemiological associations derived from observational data are, however, vulnerable to unmeasured or unknown confounding factors, associated with both the exposure and the outcome. A particularly serious type of unmeasured confounding in pharmacoepidemiology is confounding by indication (Miettinen, 1983; Walker, 1996). It has also been referred to as channeling bias since one such mechanism is when the treating physician directs specific drugs to patients based on their underlying risk profile (Petri and Urquhart, 1991; Blais *et al.*, 1996; Delaney *et al.*, 2008). In many cases, the information required in order to correct for drug channeling is not present in either clinical or administrative study databases (Suissa and Garbe, 2007).

In environmental epidemiology, studies often involve very small increases in risk that can be clinically meaningful and exposures that are precisely measured. For example, small changes in ambient air pollution are associated with very small increases in the absolute rate of asthma exacerbations (Gleason *et al.*, 2014; Yamazaki *et al.*, 2014), often resulting in small relative risks of the order of 1.05. While the risk of an asthma attack for any one person is very low, this very small increase in risk, when averaged across an entire city, can be of significant public health importance. However, whether this slight increase in risk is real or due to unmeasured confounding factors is always a concern in these studies, so that study designs which can offer strong protection against such confounding are necessary.

Several approaches have been developed to address the potential bias due to unmeasured confounders, including the use of within-subject study designs. In these designs, that are only applicable in rather specific situations, each participant is compared to himself or herself with respect to an epidemiological exposure. Because of their matched nature, these designs automatically correct for all time-invariant measured and unmeasured confounders. Several variations of within-subject designs have been developed including the case-crossover design (Maclure, 1991), the focus of this chapter, as well as the case-time-control design (Suissa, 1995), and the self-controlled case-series design (Farrington, 1995; see also Chapter 22). This chapter will describe the case-crossover design and discuss its applications in situations where the exposure is external (e.g., environmental) and where the exposure is internal or endogenous (e.g., pharmaceutical medications).

7.2   The case-crossover design

The case-crossover study design was first introduced to epidemiology in 1991 by Maclure (1991). It was devised to assess the relationship between transient exposures and acute adverse outcomes. In the case-crossover design, participants serve as their own matched controls, with the controls being the same participant in prior time periods. Given a transient exposure with stable incidence over time, the case-crossover approach uses the contrast in the exposure prevalence just before an event (case) with that at other time points in the participant's history (controls) to estimate an odds ratio of the association. The case-crossover design is used to study short-term exposures that trigger acute outcomes and not the long-term consequences of chronic exposures.

Early examples of case-crossover studies include the effects of episodes of heavy physical exertion on the risk of myocardial infarction (Mittleman *et al.*, 1993) and of cellular phone use on the risk of motor vehicle crashes (Redelmeier and Tibshirani, 1997). These are clear situations where the exposure is evidently transient and the outcome is an acute event.

The upper panel of Figure 7.1 depicts the underlying model of transient exposures and acute risk. Note that the magnitude of the risk does not vary with increasing exposure but the figure illustrates the fact that the duration of the transient exposures can vary. This model can be well characterized by the corresponding two-step function that is shown in the lower panel of Figure 7.1. The relative magnitudes of these two steps represent the rate ratio to be estimated. A graphical illustration of the case-crossover study design is shown in Figure 7.2. The time windows, each of width W, are used to determine the periods over which assessment of exposure occurs. In this example of the case-crossover design, there are two control periods, although a larger number of control periods can be used to increase the study power and improve the precision of the estimates. For instance, the Barbone *et al.* (1998) study on the risk of motor vehicle crash with benzodiazepines used 18 control periods, one day per week, selected from the 18 weeks preceding the case's time window.

The case-crossover design can be quite powerful yet depends on strong assumptions, such as the transient exposure having stable prevalence over time. Indeed, the case-crossover

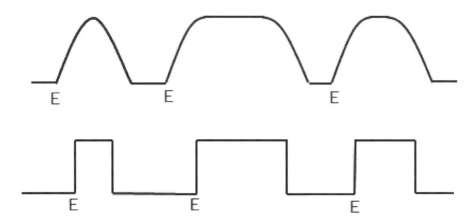

FIGURE 7.1
The underlying model of transient exposures and acute risk used in the case-crossover study. The upper figure shows our conceptual understanding of changes in risk and the lower figure shows the way that the case-crossover design represents this risk.

design will yield biased estimates if there are time trends in the exposure in the source population (Suissa, 1995; Greenland, 1996). When the acute outcome event does not affect future exposures and is not irreversible, accounting for linear time trends in the exposure can be handled using bi-directional sampling of control person-moments, where exposure is sampled both before and after the outcome (Lumley and Levy, 2000). While the use of bi-directional sampling is often feasible in environmental epidemiology, this is often an unsound approach when the outcome will influence future exposure (as with an adverse medication effect). When the outcome may influence the exposure then these designs should only use control periods prior to the event. To control for time trends without bi-directional sampling, the case-time-control (Suissa, 1995) and the case-case-time-control designs (Wang *et al.*, 2011) have been proposed as an extension to the case-crossover design. These designs use control participants to estimate (and remove) the spurious association due to underlying exposure time trends, either using control participants without events (case-time-control) or control periods from future cases (case-case-time-control).

7.2.1 The key assumptions

For a case-crossover design to provide a valid analysis it must clearly meet the following assumptions, in decreasing order of importance:

1. *Transient exposure.* The exposure must change over the same time frame as the units of the time windows. Some exposures, like snow shoveling, fit this paradigm well, as there is considerable period to period variability in this activity (Hammoudeh and Haft, 1996). Other exposures, like a chronic medication or a constant level of an environmental toxin, are poor fits for this study design. Lack of variability in exposure will lead to invalid results.

2. *Acute outcome.* A clear date of onset is needed to define the case time win-

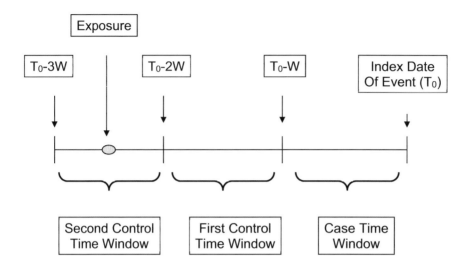

FIGURE 7.2
The case-crossover study design used in the warfarin and GI Bleed example in Section 7.3.2. The event occurs at an index date (T_0) and the periods for assessing exposure are dependent on the width of the time window (W).

dow; otherwise, exposure misclassification could occur. The best events are clear changes of state (like a cardiovascular event or an asthma exacerbation) that can be precisely dated.

3. *No underlying time trends.* The exposure must not be changing in incidence over time or else results will reflect that underlying time trend. The consequences of not meeting this assumption can be mitigated if there is an independent measure of the underlying time trend (case-time-control) or if bidirectional sampling is feasible.

4. *Constant effect.* The effect of exposure on the outcome must be of the same magnitude with each new exposure episode, while the incidence of the outcome under no exposure must be constant and equal with every new episode of no exposure.

5. *Outcome does not influence future exposures.* This is required for bidirectional sampling. Without this assumption the investigator can only use the time periods prior to the outcome event to identify control person-moments.

6. *No unmeasured time-varying confounders.* While the case-crossover design protects against confounders that do not change with time, it cannot account for time-varying confounders unless they are known and measured, in which case statistical adjustment is possible (Lumley and Levy, 2000).

7.2.2 Statistical analysis

Case-crossover designs are typically analyzed using conditional logistic regression to account for matched data, as participant's exposures are compared to exposures at previous time points. This approach assumes an underlying hazard rate λ_{i0} for participant i that is constant across the study periods. The epidemiological exposure modifies this underlying hazard rate and, following Janes *et al.* (2005a), we can model the hazard rate of participant i at time t for exposure status x_{it} as (Janes *et al.*, 2005a,b):

$$\lambda_i(t, x_{it}) = \lambda_{i0} \exp(x_{it}\beta).$$

This assumption of a constant baseline hazard (λ_{i0}) is appropriate for some types of outcomes such as myocardial infarction or death, which may have stable rates over short time periods. They may not be appropriate for other types of outcomes, where the underlying hazard may change quickly over time (e.g., nosocomial infections) and it may be difficult to verify which category an outcome falls into without additional information.

Following Janes *et al.* (2005a), we present the estimating equation as for conditional logistic regression. Let t_{i0} be the event time (or event time window) of participant i, and let W_i be the set of times corresponding to the event time and to the previous time windows. Then the contribution to the estimating equation for participant i is

$$U_i(\beta) = x_{it_{i0}} - \sum_{s \in W_i} x_{is} \frac{\exp(x_{is}\beta)}{\sum_{r \in W_i} \exp(x_{ir}\beta)}.$$

The estimating equation for all n participants is

$$U(\beta) = \sum_{i=1}^{n} U_i(\beta)$$

and the estimate of the log relative hazard (or log rate ratio) is the value $\hat{\beta}$ that satisfies $U(\hat{\beta}) = 0$. The estimate of the risk ratio is $\exp(\hat{\beta})$. It is possible to model exposure history by including lags in the hazard function (Janes *et al.*, 2005b).

The use of the conditional logistic regression estimating equation does not yield consistent estimates in the presence of 'overlap bias' (Janes *et al.*, 2005a). However, 'overlap bias' is only a problem when the exposure pattern is the same for all of the participants in the study, such as in the study of environmental effects (Janes *et al.*, 2005a) and is likely to be small. In areas like pharmacoepidemiology, under reasonable assumptions, 'overlap bias' should be symmetrically distributed around zero and, therefore, should not contribute bias (Lumley and Levy, 2000).

The conditional logistic regression estimates from a case-crossover study will also be affected by autocorrelation when participants are exposed continuously for extensive periods of time. Clearly, exposure in one time window will predict exposure in the next time window when there is a long term treatment. The effect of this autocorrelation is to reduce the number of discordant exposure patterns observed among participants. The consequence on the estimates is the same as overmatching would have in a matched case-control study, namely it will reduce the power to find associations and decrease the precision of the estimates (Lumley and Levy, 2000).

7.3   Two illustrative applications

We explore two contexts of the use of the case-crossover design. One is a hypothetical example, in environmental epidemiology, where the assumptions for this approach will likely work quite well. The other is a previously published example from pharmacoepidemiology, where the challenges of the case-crossover design can be well illustrated.

7.3.1   Environmental epidemiology

There have been several studies that used the case-crossover design for environmental exposures (Mittleman *et al.*, 1993; Janes *et al.*, 2005a,b; Elkind *et al.*, 2011; Suissa *et al.*, 2013; Gleason *et al.*, 2014). An informative example of an environmental epidemiology application is asthma and ozone levels in Gleason *et al.* (2014). The hypothesis was that certain environment agents (specifically ozone, fine particulate matter, and four different pollen types) would be associated with emergency room visits for pediatric asthma. To illustrate how the assumptions would apply, let's consider how the case-crossover assumptions applied to this example:

1. *Transient exposure.* While there may be periods of higher and lower levels of these environmental agents, there is day to day variation that allows comparison between case and control periods. The continuous exposure measurements permitted one to use changes in the levels of these pollutants to estimate the risk of emergency room visits for pediatric asthma.

2. *Acute outcome.* Emergency room visits for pediatric asthma are an important health outcome and can be specifically timed based on medical records. This is clearly an acute outcome.

3. *No underlying time trends.* These respiratory irritants may have time trends but this problem can be corrected with bi-directional sampling, as used by Gleason *et al.* (2014), because the event does not influence atmospheric levels.

4. *Constant effect.* Subsequent episodes of high levels of atmospheric respiratory irritants are likely to have similar associations with pediatric asthma and the same child could have additional asthma episodes upon future exposures to respiratory irritants, making this a plausible assumption.

5. *Outcome does not influence future exposures.* Environmental toxin levels can be measured even after a fatal emergency room visit for pediatric asthma, so this assumption is clearly met.

6. *No unmeasured time-varying confounders.* There were some possible time-varying confounders in this example. Gleason *et al.* (2014) controlled for holiday, school-in-session indicator, and 3-day moving average for temperature and relative humidity. It is unverifiable if this was the complete list of possible exposures or if the adjustment eliminated all possible residual confounding.

In this example, the relevant time window is likely the day, although the authors did explore lagged exposures. These assumptions will also apply to other studies of natural or artificial environment where the exposures change quickly, and these changes may trigger events. Here most of the assumptions of a case-crossover design are met. In the cases where the case-crossover assumptions are not clearly met, there may be reasonable approaches to handle these deviations (statistical adjustment, bidirectional sampling).

7.3.2 Pharmacoepidemiology

A useful example of a pharmacoepidemiology application is the association of warfarin with gastro-intestinal bleeding (GI Bleed) events in Delaney and Suissa (2009). To illustrate how the assumptions would apply, we can examine the case-crossover assumptions in this context.

1. *Transient exposure.* This assumption is often violated in medication examples. Warfarin can be given either as a short-term, acute treatment or as a long-term therapy. So it is possible that the study can meet the short-term exposure requirement, but we need to look at prescription patterns to know for sure. If we misclassify chronic use as acute use, we will bias the rate ratio towards the null (Hebert *et al.*, 2007). In some cases chronic use can be accounted for by using a very long time window for assessing exposure (Wang *et al.*, 2004), but that may cause problems with assumption 3 and is likely better handled using a control group (Hallas *et al.*, 2016).

2. *Acute outcome.* A severe GI Bleed is an acute event that results in immediate care. This assumption is met here.

3. *No underlying time trends.* Drug usage will change in prevalence over time, due to factors like new research, alternative treatments, new guidelines, and direct to customer marketing. In this example, as in others, we need to look at the trend in the source population to be sure drug usage is constant. We can see in Delaney *et al.* (2007) that the authors checked, and this assumption was not met.

4. *Constant effect.* Warfarin is tested over time to ensure that the anticoagulation effect is stable over time.

5. *Outcome does not influence future exposures.* This is almost never true for drug studies, as a major, acute event is likely to change therapy. This means that bi-directional sampling is not possible in this type of example.

6. *No unmeasured time-varying confounders.* There are plausible time-varying confounders in this setting. Examples could be the use of over-the-counter drugs or the onset of an infection during the periods under study, both of which information may not be captured in administrative or clinical databases (Suissa and Garbe, 2007).

7.3.2.1 Data source and analysis

The data used for the illustration linking warfarin with gastro-intestinal bleeding were from the United Kingdom's Clinical Practice Research Database (CPRD) (Walley and Mantgani, 1997). This example was selected specifically because the results could be compared to those from roughly comparable randomized controlled trials of warfarin (in terms of exposure duration and effective dosing). Briefly, all first-ever cases of gastrointestinal (GI) bleed recorded in the CPRD from 2000 through 2005 were identified. All participants had at least 3 years of clinical data in the CPRD at the time of this first GI bleed, with this date being the index date (T_0). The characteristics of this GI bleed case series have been previously reported (Delaney *et al.*, 2007).

Drug exposure was defined by prescriptions for warfarin issued by general practitioners. Because warfarin doses are often adjusted dynamically during the time period covered by a single prescription (Frazee and Chomo, 2003; Glazer *et al.*, 2007), duration is often not recorded or can be unreliable. The most frequent recorded durations for prescriptions are 28 or 30 days, although some are listed as being intended to cover 90 days, so that 30

TABLE 7.1

The sensitivity of estimates of the effect of warfarin exposure on the rate of gastrointestinal bleeding to different time-window definitions for the case-crossover study design, with each exposure time-window (W) matched to two control time-windows. Data from the United Kingdom's Clinical Practice Research Datalink, 2000 to 2005.

Exposure	Case Person-Moments	Control Person-Moments	Rate Ratio	95% Confidence Interval
Case-crossover with exposure window $W = 30$ **days**				
Reference (unexposed)	3855	7706	1.00	Reference
Warfarin Use	173	350	0.98	0.74 to 1.28
Case-crossover with exposure window $W = 90$ **days**				
Reference (unexposed)	3734	7480	1.00	Reference
Warfarin Use	294	576	1.60	1.14 to 2.23
Case-crossover with exposure window $W = 180$ **days**				
Reference (unexposed)	3690	7517	1.00	Reference
Warfarin Use	338	539	3.39	2.57 to 4.97
Case-crossover with exposure window $W = 1$ **year**				
Reference (unexposed)	3664	7485	1.00	Reference
Warfarin Use	364	571	3.57	2.22 to 5.05
Case-crossover with one-year lag in exposure window $W = 30$ **days**				
Reference	3855	7755	1.00	Reference
Warfarin Use	173	301	1.29	1.00 to 1.67
Case-time-control with exposure window $W = 1$ **year**				
Reference	3855	7706	1.00	Reference
Warfarin Use	173	350	1.72	1.08 to 2.43

days was used as the primary time window span. A participant was operationally defined as exposed if given at least one prescription of warfarin during this 30-day time window (the risk period). The two time periods immediately prior to the 30-day risk period were selected as control periods. We also examined the sensitivity of the parameter estimates to altering the risk and control periods to 90, 180 days, and 1 year.

To accommodate the assumption of transiency of exposure, we restricted the analysis to participants with a low prescription intensity, based on previous evidence that chronic exposures to a drug may lead to estimates that are biased towards the null (Hebert *et al.*, 2007). Chronic use of warfarin was defined as more than three prescriptions in the past year (Glazer *et al.*, 2007), excluding prescriptions in the 30-day case window. Another analytical option to account for some participants being on long-term warfarin therapy is the introduction of lags between the exposure windows. We illustrated using one-year lags with the risk period as the 30 days before the event. We then defined the two control periods as being 30-day time windows lagged 1 year before the index date. Finally, to account for time trends in warfarin use, we identified 40,171 age, practice, and index date matched controls, all of whom had no event at the time that they were matched to cases, choosing the 1-year time window to better illustrate this phenomenon. The case-time-control design was then used to adjust the case-crossover estimate for these time trends, using bootstrapping to estimate confidence intervals.

.

TABLE 7.2
The sensitivity of estimates of the effect of warfarin exposure on the rate of
gastrointestinal bleeding to stratification based on past level of prescription intensity for
warfarin. The time window used to measure warfarin exposure is 30 days. Data from the
United Kingdom's Clinical Practice Research Datalink, 2000 to 2005.

Exposure Classification	Case Person-Moments	Control Person-Moments	Rate Ratio	95% Confidence Interval
Stratified case-crossover				
Reference	3855	7706	1.00	Reference
Warfarin Use	173	350	0.98	0.74 to 1.28
Transient (1 to 3 Rx in past years)	30	29	2.59	1.42 to 4.74
Frequent (4 to 6 Rx in past years)	143	321	0.75	0.56 to 1.02

7.3.2.2 Results

There were 4028 cases of GI bleed, of which 4.3% had received warfarin in the 30 days
prior to the diagnosis. In Table 7.1 we show that, using a 30-day time window, we found
no increase in risk of GI bleed when the participant was exposed to warfarin (RR: 0.98;
95% CI: 0.74 to 1.28). The risk was seen to increase with longer time-windows. Between
2000 and 2005, the number of warfarin prescriptions issued increased faster than the rate
of enrollment in the CPRD. This time trend based on a one-year time window to define
exposure showed a significant increase in the use of warfarin over the study period among
controls (rate ratio 2.07; 95 CI: 1.71 to 2.52), due to time trends alone. Correcting for this
time trend using the case-time-control design yielded an estimate of the association between
warfarin and GI bleeds (RR 1.72; 95% CI: 1.08 to 2.43). We also observed an increase in
risk of GI bleed among warfarin users when the control periods were lagged (RR 1.29; 95%
CI: 1.00 to 1.67).

Table 7.2 shows the effect of stratifying the participants based on the intermittency of
warfarin therapy. Among participants who did not meet our definition of chronic users, the
stratified case-crossover design found an increase in the risk of GI bleed among participants
exposed to warfarin (RR 2.59; 95% CI: 1.42 to 4.74).

7.3.2.3 Comparison with randomized controlled trials

A meta-analysis of randomized controlled trials of warfarin provides a plausible size of the
association with bleeding risk (Lip and Edwards, 2006). The RR estimated from the meta-
analysis of similar duration randomized controlled trials was 2.2 (95% CI: 1.7 to 2.7) across
roughly 2 years (trials ranged from 1.2 to 2.3 years). We can compare it with different
estimates from the case-crossover design (with all participants having 3 years of follow-up,
giving similar duration of treatments to the ranges seen in the trials) and treating to similar
levels of effect (warfarin is dosed based on a patient's biological response to the drug, so very
widely varying doses will be required for the same level of therapy in different patients).

It is evident that the association is dependent on the exposure window chosen, ranging
from no association to a large adverse association. Some of these differences might be due
to underlying time trends in warfarin use introducing different degrees of bias in different scenarios. Since the randomized trials are comparable in effective dose and duration,
they give a reasonable gold standard estimate, albeit slightly attenuated by the intention
to treat analysis. If one had to give the best observational estimate possible, the 30-day

exposure window with stratification would be the most logical choice. But with complex drug exposures (like warfarin) the case-crossover design is not the ideal analytic approach and perhaps a different design is best. It should be noted that there are other medication exposures (Suissa *et al.*, 2010) where the assumptions of the case-crossover design are well met and estimates are not as sensitive to design assumptions as with warfarin.

7.4   Discussion

The case-crossover design automatically controls for unmeasured time-invariant confounders, making it a very attractive study design for epidemiology studies where it is difficult to use randomization to control for unmeasured confounding (Maclure, 2007; Consiglio *et al.*, 2013). This is a major advantage for applications like environmental epidemiology, where there are many difficult to measure features of the natural and artificial environment that may act as important confounders for specific participants in a study. However, despite the potential advantages of the case-crossover study design, it is likely that the core assumptions of the case-crossover method are not always addressed in a wide range of important areas in epidemiology.

The case-crossover study design has been used to estimate drug effects in a wide range of pharmacoepidemiology studies, such as Ray *et al.* (1992); Barbone *et al.* (1998); Confavreux *et al.* (2001); Etienney *et al.* (2003); Smeeth *et al.* (2004); Corrao *et al.* (2005); Gislason *et al.* (2006); Brookhart *et al.* (2007); Orriols *et al.* (2013); Fournier *et al.* (2015); Leach *et al.* (2015); Strom *et al.* (2015). Outcomes have tended to be acute events such as motor vehicle crashes (Hebert *et al.*, 2007; Barbone *et al.*, 1998; Orriols *et al.*, 2013), death (Gislason *et al.*, 2006), and myocardial infarction (Smeeth *et al.*, 2004; Gislason *et al.*, 2006). Exposures have typically been a pharmacological agent given for short time periods, such as vaccines (Confavreux *et al.*, 2001), antibiotics (Aberra *et al.*, 2005; Suissa *et al.*, 2010), and psychotropic medication prescriptions (Barbone *et al.*, 1998; Orriols *et al.*, 2013; Leach *et al.*, 2015).

Despite its advantages, the case-crossover design presents a number of challenges when used in pharmacoepidemiology. For instance, it has been shown that the presence of long-term treatment can introduce bias, as well as reduce power. Hebert *et al.* (2007) showed, in a study of the effect of benzodiazepine use on the risk of motor vehicle crash, that including patients who filled a large number of benzodiazepine prescriptions over the one-year period used to measure control exposure introduced a large bias towards the null. For large numbers of prescriptions in the control year (eight or more), the point estimate of the associated risk of motor vehicle crash was protective (rate ratio (RR) 0.81; 95% CI: 0.62 to 1.06). This contrasts with the very significant positive association (RR 1.57; 95% CI: 1.05 to 2.33) among patients with the more transient usage of 0 to 4 prescriptions in the control year, which more nearly met the design assumptions. In general, for any exposure, a lack of discordant exposures in the control periods for the case-crossover design can be a threat to study validity. On the other hand, Wang *et al.* (2004) investigated situations when this design can be used to study prolonged drug exposures and insidious outcomes.

The warfarin example is particularly daunting as some drugs, such as warfarin or benzodiazepines, may be given either as a chronic or acute treatment. This is in contrast to drugs only given for chronic treatment (that always violate case-crossover assumptions) or drugs given only for acute treatment (which may be reasonable exposures for use with a case-crossover design). We saw that the estimates obtained from our case-crossover example are sensitive to improperly specifying the exposure time window. The consequence of the inability to use the data to determine the ideal time window is that one either generates a biased estimate (by picking a single time window) or needs to report a family of estimates, which may cover a wide variation in the strength and significance of the association. While the estimates from the case-crossover approach in our warfarin and GI bleed example may appear low when compared to the results of randomized controlled trials, many participants are likely to have been exposed for shorter time periods than the study windows can capture. The participants with very short exposure times are actually past users and not current users during some case periods in which the analysis counted the participant as exposed. The resulting exposure misclassification would have been the most influential on the estimates based on the longest exposure time windows.

The length of the ideal time window for assessing drug exposure is unknown and will vary between drugs. An exposure time window that is too long or too short may introduce exposure misclassification, which may adversely impact the estimate derived from a case-crossover approach. In the absence of substantive knowledge, sensitivity analyses may be useful in identifying the most appropriate time window. But it is difficult to verify that the selected time window is, in fact, the most appropriate, or even if there is a single appropriate time window. Nevertheless, while it is well known that exposure misclassification introduces bias (van Staa *et al.*, 1994), Greenland (1996) showed that the impact of this misclassification is more severe in the case-crossover or case-time-control setting, as compared to the case-control setting. The impact of this exposure misclassification was visible in the illustrative example where the estimates obtained from the case-crossover and case-time-control designs actually showed a stronger bias towards the null (compared to the estimate obtained from randomized controlled trials) than was observed with a nested case-control approach (Delaney *et al.*, 2007). This is consistent with Greenland (1996) and suggests that this should also be considered when interpreting associations derived from a case-crossover study.

In general, when the different indications to prescribe a drug lead to a mixture of short- and long-term use, this issue of exposure misclassification is likely to be especially severe. Ideally, one would pick an exposure, such as antibiotics, where the typical indication is for a transient exposure (Suissa *et al.*, 2010). This heterogeneity in the length of exposure is true of many drug exposures, including warfarin, and this makes other designs more attractive for medications with variable exposure lengths. With warfarin, guidelines suggest that participants with some medical conditions, such as atrial fibrillation, may require continuous or lifetime therapy. In contrast, recommendations for other indications are that therapy should be for only 3 months. This means that, unless one can separate participants based on indication, any study of warfarin use will be a mixture of both long- and short-term users, making the approach of Hebert *et al.* (2007) appealing.

In summary, the case-crossover design inherently removes the biasing effects of unmeasured, time-invariant confounding factors from the estimated rate ratio, but is sensitive to several assumptions, namely: that the exposure is transient, the outcome is acute, and that there are no exposure time trends. If time periods after the outcome are to be used, then the outcome needs to be independent of the exposure and the design is still subject to time-varying confounding. Finally, the optimal time windows can be challenging to define and may require careful approaches, especially with chronic use medications (Hallas *et al.*, 2016). However, when these assumptions are satisfied, even approximately, the case-crossover design can be a powerful study design, with much less susceptibility to confounding than traditional observational study designs.

Ethical Review: Ethical review for the data used in the illustration was done by the Independent Scientific Advisory Committee of the CPRD.

Funding: The study used in the illustration was funded by the Canadian Institutes of Health Research (CIHR) and the Canadian Foundation for Innovation. Samy Suissa is the recipient of the James McGill Chair award.

Bibliography

Aberra, F. N., Brensinger, C. M., Bilker, W. B., Lichtenstein, G. R., and Lewis, J. D. (2005). Antibiotic use and the risk of flare of inflammatory bowel disease. *Clinical Gastroenterology and Hepatology*, **3**, 459–465.

Barbone, F., McMahon, A. D., Davey, P. G., Morris, A., Reid, I. C., McDevitt, D. G., and MacDonald, T. M. (1998). Association of road-traffic accidents with benzodiazepine use. *Lancet*, **352**, 1331–1336.

Blais, L., Ernst, P., and Suissa, S. (1996). Confounding by indication and hospitalization over time: The risks of beta 2-agonists. *American Journal of Epidemiology*, **144**, 1161–1169.

Brookhart, M. A., Patrick, A. R., Schneeweiss, S., Avorn, J., Dormuth, C., Shrank, W., van Wijk, B. L., Cadarette, S. M., Canning, C. F., and Solomon, D. H. (2007). Physician follow-up and provider continuity are associated with long-term medication adherence: A study of the dynamics of statin use. *Archives of Internal Medicine*, **167**, 847–852.

Confavreux, C., Suissa, S., Saddier, P., Bourdès, V., Vukusic, S., and the Vaccines in Multiple Sclerosis Study Group (2001). Vaccinations and the risk of relapse in multiple sclerosis. *New England Journal of Medicine*, **344**, 319–326.

Consiglio, G. P., Burden, A. M., Maclure, M., McCarthy, L., and Cadarette, S. M. (2013). Case-crossover study design in pharmacoepidemiology: Systematic review and recommendations. *Pharmacoepidemiology and Drug Safety*, **22**, 1146–1153.

Corrao, G., Zambon, A., Faini, S., Bagnardi, V., Leoni, O., and Suissa, S. (2005). Short-acting inhaled beta-2-agonists increased the mortality from chronic obstructive pulmonary disease in observational designs. *Journal of Clinical Epidemiology*, **58**, 92–97.

Delaney, J. A. and Suissa, S. (2009). Case-crossover designs in pharmacoepidemiology. *Statistical Methods in Medical Research*, **18**, 53–65.

Delaney, J. A., Opatrny, L., Brophy, J. M., and Suissa, S. (2007). Interactions between anti-thrombotic drugs and the risk of gastro-intestinal haemorrhage. *Canadian Medical Association Journal*, **177**, 347–351.

Delaney, J. A., Opatrny, L., Brophy, J. M., and Suissa, S. (2008). Confounding in database pharmacoepidemiology studies. *Epidemiology*, **19**, 360–361.

Elkind, M. S., Carty, C. L., O'Meara, E. S., Lumley, T., Lefkowitz, D., Kronmal, R. A., and Longstreth, Jr., W, T. (2011). Hospitalization for infection and risk of acute ischemic stroke: The Cardiovascular Health Study. *Stroke*, **42**, 1851–1856.

Etienney, I., Beaugerie, L., Viboud, C., and Flahault, A. (2003). Non-steroidal anti-inflammatory drugs as a risk factor for acute diarrhea: A case crossover study. *Gut*, **52**, 260–263.

Farrington, C. P. (1995). Relative incidence estimation from case series for vaccine safety evaluation. *Biometrics*, **51**, 228–235.

Fournier, J. P., Azoulay, L., Yin, H., Montastruc, J. L., and Suissa, S. (2015). Tramadol use and the risk of hospitalization for hypoglycemia in patients with noncancer pain. *JAMA Internal Medicine*, **175**, 186–193.

Frazee, L. A. and Chomo, D. L. (2003). Duration of anticoagulant therapy after initial idiopathic venous thromboembolism. *Annals of Pharmacotherapy*, **37**, 1489–1496.

Gislason, G. H., Jacobsen, S., Rasmussen, J. N., Rasmussen, S., Buch, P., Friberg, J., Schramm, T. K., Abildstrom, S. Z., Køber, L., Madsen, M., and Torp-Pedersen, C. (2006). Risk of death or reinfarction associated with the use of selective cyclooxygenase-2 inhibitors and nonselective nonsteroidal anti-inflammatory drugs after acute myocardial infarction. *Circulation*, **113**, 2906–2913.

Glazer, N. L., Dublin, S., Smith, N. L., French, B., Jackson, L. A., Hrachovec, J. B., Siscovick, D. S., Psaty, B. M., and Heckbert, S. R. (2007). Newly detected atrial fibrillation and compliance with antithrombotic guidelines. *Archives of Internal Medicine*, **167**, 246–252.

Gleason, J. A., Bielory, L., and Fagliano, J. A. (2014). Associations between ozone, PM2.5, and four pollen types on emergency department pediatric asthma events during the warm season in New Jersey: A case-crossover study. *Environmental Research*, **132**, 421–429.

Greenland, S. (1996). Confounding and exposure trends in case-crossover and case-time-control designs. *Epidemiology*, **7**, 231–239.

Hallas, J., Pottegård, A., Wang, S., Schneeweiss, S., and Gagne, J. J. (2016). Persistent user bias in case-crossover studies in pharmacoepidemiology. *American Journal of Epidemiology*, **184**, 761–769.

Hammoudeh, A. J. and Haft, J. I. (1996). Coronary-plaque rupture in acute coronary syndromes triggered by snow shoveling. *New England Journal of Medicine*, **335**, 2001.

Hebert, C., Delaney, J. A., Hemmelgarn, B., Lévesque, L. E., and Suissa, S. (2007). Benzodiazepines and older drivers: A comparison of pharmacoepidemiological study designs. *Pharmacoepidemiology and Drug Safety*, **16**, 845–849.

Hernán, M. A. and Robins, J. M. (2006). Estimating causal effects from epidemiological data. *Journal of Epidemiology and Community Health*, **60**, 578–586.

Janes, H., Sheppard, L., and Lumley, T. (2005a). Case-crossover analyses of air pollution exposure data: Referent selection strategies and their implications for bias. *Epidemiology*, **16**, 717–726.

Janes, H., Sheppard, L., and Lumley, T. (2005b). Overlap bias in the case-crossover design, with application to air pollution exposures. *Statistics in Medicine*, **24**, 285–300.

Leach, M. J., Pratt, N. L., and Roughead, E. E. (2015). Psychoactive medicine use and the risk of hip fracture in older people: A case-crossover study. *Pharmacoepidemiology and Drug Safety*, **24**, 576–582.

Lip, G. Y. and Edwards, S. J. (2006). Stroke prevention with aspirin, warfarin and ximelagatran in patients with non-valvular atrial fibrillation: A systematic review and meta-analysis. *Thrombosis Research*, **118**, 321–333.

Lumley, T. and Levy, D. (2000). Bias in the case-crossover design: Implications for studies of air pollution. *Environmetrics*, **11**, 689–704.

Maclure, M. (1991). The case-crossover design: A method for studying transient effects on the risk of acute events. *American Journal of Epidemiology*, **133**, 144–153.

Maclure, M. (2007). 'Why me?' versus 'why now?' – differences between operational hypotheses in case-control versus case-crossover studies. *Pharmacoepidemiology and Drug Safety*, **16**, 850–853.

Miettinen, O. S. (1983). The need for randomization in the study of intended effects. *Statistics in Medicine*, **2**, 267–271.

Mills, N., Metcalfe, C., Ronsmans, C., Davis, M., Lane, J. A., Sterne, J. A., Peters, T. J., Hamdy, F. C., Neal, D. E., and Donovan, J. L. (2006). A comparison of socio-demographic and psychological factors between patients consenting to hospitalization and those selecting treatment (the ProtecT study). *Contemporary Clinical Trials*, **27**, 413–419.

Mittleman, M. A., Maclure, M., Tofler, G. H., Sherwood, J. B., Goldberg, R. J., and Muller, J. E. (1993). Triggering of acute myocardial infarction by heavy physical exertion. Protection against triggering by regular exertion. Determinants of Myocardial Infarction Onset Study Investigators. *New England Journal of Medicine*, **329**, 1677–1683.

Orriols, L., Wilchesky, M., Lagarde, E., and Suissa, S. (2013). Prescription of antidepressants and the risk of road traffic crash in the elderly: A case-crossover study. *British Journal of Clinical Pharmacology*, **76**, 810–815.

Petri, H. and Urquhart, J. (1991). Channeling bias in the interpretation of drug effects. *Statistics in Medicine*, **10**, 577–581.

Ray, W. A., Fought, R. L., and Decker, M. D. (1992). Psychoactive drugs and the risk of injurious motor vehicle crashes in elderly drivers. *American Journal of Epidemiology*, **136**, 873–883.

Redelmeier, D. A. and Tibshirani, R. J. (1997). Association between cellular-telephone calls and motor vehicle collisions. *New England Journal of Medicine*, **336**, 453–458.

Smeeth, L., Thomas, S. L., Hall, A. J., Hubbard, R., Farrington, P., and Vallance, P. (2004). Risk of myocardial infarction and stroke after acute infection or vaccination. *New England Journal of Medicine*, **351**, 2611–2618.

Strom, B. L., Schinnar, R., Karlawish, J., Hennessy, S., Teal, V., and Bilker, W. B. (2015). Statin therapy and risk of acute memory impairment. *JAMA Internal Medicine*, **175**, 1399–1405.

Suissa, L., Fortier, M., Lachaud, S., Staccini, P., and Mahagne, M. H. (2013). Ozone air pollution and ischaemic stroke occurrence: A case-crossover study in Nice, France. *BMJ Open*, **3**, e004060.

Suissa, S. (1995). The case-time-control design. *Epidemiology*, **6**, 248–253.

Suissa, S. and Garbe, E. (2007). Primer: Administrative health databases in observational studies of drug effects-advantages and disadvantages. *Nature Clinical Practice Rheumatology*, **3**, 725–732.

Suissa, S., Dell'Aniello, S., and Martinez, C. (2010). The multitime case-control design for time-varying exposures. *Epidemiology*, **21**, 876–883.

van Staa, T. P., Abenhaim, L., and H., L. (1994). A study of the effects of exposure misclassification due to the time-window design in pharmacoepidemiologic studies. *Journal of Clinical Epidemiology*, **47**, 183–189.

Walker, A. M. (1996). Confounding by indication. *Epidemiology*, **7**, 335–336.

Walley, T. and Mantgani, A. (1997). The UK General Practice Research Database. *Lancet*, **350**, 1097–1099.

Wang, P. S., Schneeweiss, S., Glynn, R. J., Mogun, H., and Avorn, J. (2004). Use of the case-crossover design to study prolonged drug exposures and insidious outcomes. *Annals of Epidemiology*, **14**, 296–303.

Wang, S., Linkletter, C., Maclure, M., Dore, D., Mor, V., Buka, S., and Wellenius, G. A. (2011). Future cases as present controls to adjust for exposure trend bias in case-only studies. *Epidemiology*, **22**, 568–574.

Yamazaki, S., Shima, M., Yoda, Y., Oka, K., Kurosaka, F., Shimizu, S., Takahashi, H., Nakatani, Y., Nishikawa, J., Fujiwara, K., Mizumori, Y., Mogami, A., Yamada, T., and Yamamoto, N. (2014). Association between PM2.5 and primary care visits due to asthma attack in Japan: Relation to Beijing's air pollution episode in January 2013. *Environmental Health and Preventive Medicine*, **19**, 172–176.

8

Small Sample Methods

Jinko Graham and Brad McNeney

Simon Fraser University

Robert Platt

McGill University

8.1   Introduction

8.1.1   Challenges posed by small samples

This chapter reviews small-sample methods for inference of odds ratios in logistic regression models for case-control data. In logistic regression, the maximum likelihood estimator (MLE) of the regression parameters is biased away from zero, particularly when the number of parameters is large compared to the sample size (Heinze and Schemper, 2002). In addition, the first-order normal approximation to the distribution of the MLE becomes unreliable in small samples (e.g., Mehta and Patel, 1995). These two factors lead to biased likelihood-based tests and point and interval estimators in small samples. Another problem in small or sparse data sets is nonexistence of the MLE due to separation (Albert and Anderson, 1984). By "separation," we mean that there is a linear combination of the covariates that perfectly distinguishes cases from controls. When there is separation in the data set, the likelihood does not have a maximum and so the MLE does not exist.

Separation is illustrated in the following example. Herbst *et al.* (1971) sought to identify exposures that might explain a cluster of vaginal cancers in young women in Boston in the late 1960's. This was the first study to identify maternal treatment with diethylstilbesterol (DES) as a risk factor for vaginal cancer in exposed daughters. The study follows a matched case-control design. Using hospital records, patients were matched to four controls based on birth date and type of room (ward versus private). The matching was intended to reflect socioeconomic factors. The data on DES and five other exposures are summarized in Table 8.1.

Separation occurs in these data because we can define a threshold for the DES covariate that separates the cases from the controls, in particular, coding DES exposure as 0 for nonexposed and 1 for exposed, $DES \leq 0$ for all controls and $DES \geq 0$ for all cases. Such separation is termed quasi-complete by Albert and Anderson (1984), in contrast to complete separation when the inequalities are strict. A standard conditional logistic regression analysis of these data with the `clogit()` function of the `survival` package in R and DES as the only covariate reports convergence of the likelihood after 21 iterations but warns that the DES coefficient has not converged.

This chapter reviews alternatives to standard likelihood inference based on large-sample approximations. Although these methods offer improved inference in small samples, they cannot completely overcome the limitations of small or sparse data sets. Studies with small or sparse data sets are inherently less robust than larger studies. For example, small data sets have limits on the ability to adjust for covariates, and changes in only a few data points can lead to substantial changes in the inference.

8.1.2   Notation and likelihoods

To describe the methods of this chapter in more detail we establish notation. Several parametrizations of case-control likelihood for unmatched data have appeared in the literature (e.g., Prentice and Pyke, 1979; Breslow and Day, 1980; Qin and Zhang, 1997). We use the parametrization of Qin and Zhang (1997), in terms of the vector of log odds ratio parameters, $\boldsymbol{\beta}$, and the distribution of covariates in controls, $g(\mathbf{x}) = P(\mathbf{x}|D = 0)$, where $\mathbf{x}$ is an observed vector of covariates. The model for covariate data sampled in an unmatched case-control study is

$$
\begin{aligned}
P(\mathbf{x}|D=0) &= g(\mathbf{x}), \\
P(\mathbf{x}|D=1) &= c(\boldsymbol{\beta}, g) \exp(\mathbf{x}^T \boldsymbol{\beta}) g(\mathbf{x}),
\end{aligned}
\tag{8.1}
$$

TABLE 8.1

Data on cases and controls in the Herbst *et al.* study, reconstructed from their Table 2. Odds ratios are estimated without regard to matching.

Exposure	Level	Cases	Controls	OR
DES	yes	7	0	NA
	no	1	32	
maternal smoking	yes	7	21	3.57
	no	1	11	
prior bleeding	yes	3	1	16.5
	no	5	31	
prior pregnancy loss	yes	6	5	14.6
	no	2	27	
breast-feeding	yes	3	3	5.45
	no	5	29	
Inter-uterine X-ray	yes	1	4	1.0
	no	7	28	

where $c(\boldsymbol{\beta}, g)$ is a normalizing constant. We refer to this as the *unstratified model*.

Suppose the n_0 controls are indexed by $i = 1, \ldots, n_0$ and the n_1 cases by $i = n_0 + 1, \ldots, n$ for $n = n_0 + n_1$. Let $\mathbf{x}_i$ denote the covariate data on the ith individual. Then the likelihood is

$$
\begin{aligned}
L(\boldsymbol{\beta}, g) &= \prod_{i=1}^{n_0} P(\mathbf{x}_i | D = 0) \times \prod_{i=n_0+1}^{n} P(\mathbf{x}_i | D = 1) \\
&= \prod_{i=1}^{n_0} g(\mathbf{x}_i) \times \prod_{i=n_0+1}^{n} c(\boldsymbol{\beta}, g) \exp(\mathbf{x}_i^T \boldsymbol{\beta}) g(\mathbf{x}_i) \\
&= [c(\boldsymbol{\beta}, g)^{n_1}] \left[\prod_{i=1}^{n} g(\mathbf{x}_i) \right] \left[\exp \left(\sum_{i=n_0+1}^{n} \mathbf{x}_i^T \boldsymbol{\beta} \right) \right].
\end{aligned}
\tag{8.2}
$$

For matched data sampled from I population strata, in which each case defines his/her own stratum, the model is in terms of the vector $\boldsymbol{\beta}$, assumed to be common across all strata, and the covariate distributions in each stratum, $g_i(\mathbf{x}) = P(\mathbf{x} | D = 0, \text{stratum } i)$. The model for covariate data sampled in a matched case-control study is

$$
\begin{aligned}
P(\mathbf{x} | D = 0, \text{stratum } i) &= g_i(\mathbf{x}); \quad i = 1, \ldots, I, \\
P(\mathbf{x} | D = 1, \text{stratum } i) &= c(\boldsymbol{\beta}, g_i) \exp(\mathbf{x}^T \boldsymbol{\beta}) g_i(\mathbf{x}); \quad i = 1, \ldots, I,
\end{aligned}
\tag{8.3}
$$

where $c(\boldsymbol{\beta}, g_i)$ is a normalizing constant and i indexes the I strata. We refer to this as the *stratified model*. Index cases within each matched set by $j = 0$ and controls by $j = 1, \ldots, M_i$. Let $\mathbf{x}_j^i$ denote the covariate data on the jth individual in the ith matched set. Let $\mathbf{g}$ denote the collection of covariate distributions in controls, $\mathbf{g} = (g_1, \ldots, g_I)$. Then the likelihood is

$$
\begin{aligned}
L(\boldsymbol{\beta}, \mathbf{g}) &= \prod_{i=1}^{I} P(\mathbf{x}_0^i | D = 1, \text{stratum } i) \prod_{j=1}^{M_i} P(\mathbf{x}_j^i | D = 0, \text{stratum } i) \\
&= \prod_{i=1}^{I} c(\boldsymbol{\beta}, g_i) \exp(\mathbf{x}_0^{iT} \boldsymbol{\beta}) g_i(\mathbf{x}_0^i) \prod_{j=1}^{M_i} g_i(\mathbf{x}_j^i) \\
&= \left[\prod_{i=1}^{I} c(\boldsymbol{\beta}, g_i) \right] \left[\prod_{i=1}^{I} \prod_{j=0}^{M_i} g_i(\mathbf{x}_j^i) \right] \left[\exp\left(\sum_{i=1}^{I} \mathbf{x}_0^{iT} \boldsymbol{\beta} \right) \right]. \quad (8.4)
\end{aligned}
$$

8.1.3 Prospective likelihoods for case-control data

With case-control or "retrospective" sampling, the number of cases is fixed by the design and covariates are random. Under "prospective" sampling, disease status is random and covariates are considered nonrandom and fixed by design. Prentice and Pyke (1979) showed that the maximum likelihood estimator of the odds ratios under retrospective sampling can be obtained by maximizing a likelihood of the same form as a prospective likelihood:

$$
\begin{aligned}
L_U(\alpha^*, \boldsymbol{\beta}) &= \prod_{i=1}^{n_0} \frac{1}{1 + \exp(\alpha^* + \mathbf{x}_i^T \boldsymbol{\beta})} \times \prod_{i=n_0+1}^{n} \frac{\exp(\alpha^* + \mathbf{x}_i^T \boldsymbol{\beta})}{1 + \exp(\alpha^* + \mathbf{x}_i^T \boldsymbol{\beta})} \\
&= \prod_{i=1}^{n} \frac{\exp(d_i(\alpha^* + \mathbf{x}_i^T \boldsymbol{\beta}))}{1 + \exp(\alpha^* + \mathbf{x}_i^T \boldsymbol{\beta})}. \quad (8.5)
\end{aligned}
$$

Here d_i is a binary disease status indicator for the ith subject, and $\alpha^* = \alpha + \log(n_1/n_0) - \log[P(D = 1)/P(D = 0)]$, where α is the intercept term in the logistic regression model for $P(D = 1|\mathbf{x})$, and $P(D = 1)$ and $P(D = 0)$ are the population probabilities of having and not having the disease, respectively. Thus, α^* is the logistic regression intercept, α, shifted by the difference between the log odds, $\log(n_1/n_0)$, of being a case under the sampling design, and the log odds, $\log[P(D = 1)/P(D = 0)]$, of being a case in the population (Scott and Wild, 2001).

We can also express α^* as $\alpha^* = \log c(\boldsymbol{\beta}, g) + \log(n_1/n_0)$. To see why, re-write equation (8.1) with the prospective model

$$
P(D = 1|\mathbf{x}) = \frac{\exp(\alpha + \mathbf{x}^T \boldsymbol{\beta})}{1 + \exp(\alpha + \mathbf{x}^T \boldsymbol{\beta})}
$$

and Bayes rule to obtain

$$
g(\mathbf{x}) = P(\mathbf{x}|D = 0) = \frac{1}{1 + \exp(\alpha + \mathbf{x}^T \boldsymbol{\beta})} \cdot \frac{P(\mathbf{x})}{P(D = 0)}
$$

and

$$
c(\boldsymbol{\beta}, g) \exp(\mathbf{x}^T \boldsymbol{\beta}) g(\mathbf{x}) = P(\mathbf{x}|D = 1) = \frac{\exp(\alpha + \mathbf{x}^T \boldsymbol{\beta})}{1 + \exp(\alpha + \mathbf{x}^T \boldsymbol{\beta})} \cdot \frac{P(\mathbf{x})}{P(D = 1)}.
$$

Taking the ratio of these two equations gives

$$
\frac{c(\boldsymbol{\beta}, g) \exp(\mathbf{x}^T \boldsymbol{\beta}) g(\mathbf{x})}{g(\mathbf{x})} = \exp(\alpha + \mathbf{x}^T \boldsymbol{\beta}) \frac{P(D = 0)}{P(D = 1)},
$$

which leads to $\log c(\boldsymbol{\beta}, g) = \alpha - \log[P(D=1)/P(D=0)]$. Thus,

$$\alpha^* = \alpha - \log[P(D=1)/P(D=0)] + \log(n_1/n_0) = \log c(\boldsymbol{\beta}, g) + \log(n_1/n_0).$$

Qin and Zhang (1997) have shown that the likelihood (8.5) may be viewed as a profile likelihood for retrospective data, obtained as follows. First, over-parameterize the retrospective likelihood (8.2) by including α^* as a parameter. Second, form a profile likelihood function of $(\alpha^*, \boldsymbol{\beta})$ by maximizing over g for fixed values of $(\alpha^*, \boldsymbol{\beta})$, taking into account the constraints on the parameters $(\alpha^*, \boldsymbol{\beta}, g)$. The resulting profile likelihood is as given in equation (8.5).

An analogous argument can be applied to show that the stratified likelihood

$$
\begin{aligned}
L_S(\boldsymbol{\alpha}^*, \boldsymbol{\beta}) &= \prod_{i=1}^{I} \frac{\exp(\alpha_i^* + \mathbf{x}_0^{iT}\boldsymbol{\beta})}{1 + \exp(\alpha_i^* + \mathbf{x}_0^{iT}\boldsymbol{\beta})} \prod_{j=1}^{M_i} \frac{1}{1 + \exp(\alpha_i^* + \mathbf{x}_j^{iT}\boldsymbol{\beta})} \\
&= \prod_{i=1}^{I} \prod_{j=0}^{M_i} \frac{\exp(d_{ij}(\alpha_i^* + \mathbf{x}_j^{iT}\boldsymbol{\beta}))}{1 + \exp(\alpha_i^* + \mathbf{x}_j^{iT}\boldsymbol{\beta})}
\end{aligned}
\tag{8.6}
$$

arises as a profile likelihood derived from the stratified retrospective likelihood (8.4). In (8.6) d_{ij} is a binary disease status indicator for the jth individual in the ith matched set, $\boldsymbol{\alpha}^* = (\alpha_1^*, \ldots, \alpha_I^*)$ and

$$\alpha_i^* = \alpha_i + \log(1/M_i) - \log[P(D=1|\text{stratum } i)/P(D=0|\text{stratum } i)],$$

where α_i is the ith stratum effect in the stratified logistic regression model for $P(D = 1|\mathbf{x}, \text{stratum } i)$, and $P(D = 1|\text{stratum } i)$ and $P(D = 0|\text{stratum } i)$ are the probabilities of having and not having the disease in the ith stratum, respectively. The key differences from the unstratified argument are that (i) the retrospective likelihood (8.4) is over-parameterized by a *vector* of "stratum effects" $\alpha_1^*, \ldots, \alpha_I^*$ and (ii) the profile likelihood function of $(\boldsymbol{\alpha}^*, \boldsymbol{\beta})$ is obtained by maximizing over the *vector* of distribution functions $\mathbf{g} = (g_1, \ldots, g_I)$, taking into account the constraints on all parameters.

A consequence of re-casting profile retrospective likelihoods as prospective likelihoods is that any penalized likelihood method derived for prospective data may be interpreted as a penalized profile likelihood method for retrospective data (see Sections 8.4 and 8.5). However, the probability distribution of the data under retrospective sampling may suggest alternate penalty terms (Section 8.5).

8.1.4 Inference of the parameters of interest

Small or sparse sample inference is typically focused on a limited number of model parameters, with all others considered nuisance parameters. In the unstratified model, the distribution g of covariates in controls is considered a nuisance parameter, and in the stratified model the vector $\mathbf{g}$ of distributions functions is a nuisance parameter. In addition, the vector $\boldsymbol{\beta}$ of log odds ratio parameters may be partitioned into $(\boldsymbol{\beta}_1, \boldsymbol{\beta}_2)$ with $\boldsymbol{\beta}_1$ of interest and $\boldsymbol{\beta}_2$ a nuisance.

Nuisance parameters may be eliminated from the likelihood by conditioning on sufficient statistics (Cox, 1970). While conditioning allows computation of exact conditional distributions, it often leads to a loss of information and efficiency from ignoring part of the likelihood. However, the conditional maximum likelihood estimator, or CMLE, of the log odds ratio has the smallest variance among all estimators defined as the root of an estimating equation (Godambe, 1976). This optimality arises from conditioning on the sufficient statistic for the nuisance parameter.

An alternative to conditioning is to maximize the full likelihood over the nuisance parameters to form a profile likelihood for the parameters of interest. Though maximum profile likelihood inference focuses attention on the parameters of interest, it is really just maximum likelihood inference where the maximization has been broken down into two steps, one to maximize over the nuisance parameters and a second to maximize over the parameters of interest. When the model is a logistic regression, maximum likelihood estimates are biased away from zero (Firth, 1993), and such bias can result in tests with larger-than-nominal level and confidence intervals with lower-than-nominal coverage. Furthermore, the bias increases in the number of nuisance parameters (Heinze and Schemper, 2002). Bias of maximum profile likelihood inference may be reduced by penalizing the profile likelihood; i.e., multiplying the profile likelihood by a function centred at the origin (Barndorff-Nielsen, 1983; Firth, 1993). Doing so has the effect of shifting the location of the maximum towards the origin and reducing the bias of the MLE.

8.1.5 Methods discussed in this chapter

The inference methods we discuss in this chapter can be classified as either conditional or penalized profile likelihood approaches. In particular, we review (i) exact inference based on conditional likelihoods (Section 8.2) and approximate exact inference (Section 8.3) and (ii) penalized profile likelihood methods, derived *via* higher-order approximations to the distribution of estimators and test statistics (Section 8.4), or other considerations such as bias-reduction or prior distributions on the regression coefficients (Section 8.5). In Section 8.6 we give tentative recommendations based on simulation studies that compare the different methods. Simulations are discussed in an online Supplementary Materials document that is available from the Handbook website. The online supplementary materials for this chapter also include R code for most analyses.

8.2 Exact conditional inference

8.2.1 Motivation

Asymptotic or large-sample inference can be unreliable when the sample size is small or the data sparse. A familiar example is the chi-squared test of association in a 2×2 contingency table of case-control status versus a binary exposure. It is well known that the test is only reliable when the expected counts for cells in the data table are sufficiently large (e.g., ≥ 5; Campbell, 2007).

Fisher's exact test (Fisher, 1934) is an alternative based on the conditional distribution of cell counts given the table margins. This conditional distribution depends on the unknown odds ratio, and reduces to a hypergeometric distribution under the null hypothesis of no disease-exposure association (Breslow and Day, 1980). The test of association uses the conditional distribution as a test statistic. The p-value is the sum of conditional probabilities over data with probability as or more extreme (i.e., smaller) than the observed data (Fisher, 1934). No assumptions are made about sample size or sparsity of the data. This section reviews analogous methods for logistic regression under models that are stratified or unstratified (i.e., for matched or unmatched controls).

8.2.2 Methods

Conditional inference is based on the distribution of the sufficient statistic for the parameters of interest, given the sufficient statistic for the nuisance parameters (Cox, 1970). Conditioning on sufficient statistics for nuisance parameters eliminates them from the likelihood. Conditional logistic regression (see Chapter 4 of this Handbook) is an example of *approximate conditional inference* based on large-sample approximations. By contrast, *exact conditional inference* is based on exact finite-sample distributions.

Fisher's exact test is an example of exact conditional inference. Conditioning on the table margins eliminates the nuisance parameter, which is the probability of exposure in controls (Agresti, 1992). The conditional likelihood depends only on the odds ratio parameter of interest. Under the null hypothesis that the odds ratio is one, the conditional likelihood is known, and probabilities from this known distribution are used to calculate p-values. No approximations are made.

8.2.2.1 Conditional distributions

We present the distributions used for exact conditional inference from both matched and unmatched case-control data. For future reference in Section 8.4, we include the distributions needed for joint inference of the entire log odds ratio parameter $\boldsymbol{\beta}$ [equations (8.7) and (8.9) below], though exact inference typically focuses on one particular component of $\boldsymbol{\beta}$, treating all other components as nuisance parameters [equations (8.8) and (8.10)].

For inference from unmatched case-control data, we use the unstratified model of equation (8.1). Let $\mathbf{X}_i$ be the random covariate vector for individual i and $\mathbf{x}_i$ be the vector of observed values. Let $d_i = 1$ if individual i has the disease and 0 otherwise. Let $\mathbf{T}_{\boldsymbol{\beta}}$ be the sufficient statistic for $\boldsymbol{\beta}$ and $\mathbf{t}_{\boldsymbol{\beta}}$ be its observed value. Then $\mathbf{T}_{\boldsymbol{\beta}} = \sum_{i=1}^{n} d_i \mathbf{X}_i$. Similarly, let $\mathbf{T}_g$ be the sufficient statistic for g. $\mathbf{T}_g$ is the unordered collection of observed covariate vectors, or, equivalently, the empirical distribution of covariate vectors. For inference of $\boldsymbol{\beta}$, we use the conditional distribution of $\mathbf{T}_{\boldsymbol{\beta}}$ given $\mathbf{T}_g$ which varies over permutations of the disease-status vector $\mathbf{d} = (d_1, \ldots, d_n)$ and has the form

$$f(\mathbf{t}_{\boldsymbol{\beta}} | \mathbf{t}_g; \boldsymbol{\beta}) = \frac{C(\mathbf{t}_{\boldsymbol{\beta}}) \exp\left(\mathbf{t}_{\boldsymbol{\beta}}^T \boldsymbol{\beta}\right)}{\sum_{\tilde{\mathbf{t}}_{\boldsymbol{\beta}}} C(\tilde{\mathbf{t}}_{\boldsymbol{\beta}}) \exp\left(\tilde{\mathbf{t}}_{\boldsymbol{\beta}}^T \boldsymbol{\beta}\right)}, \tag{8.7}$$

where $C(\tilde{\mathbf{t}}_{\boldsymbol{\beta}})$ is the number of vectors $\tilde{\mathbf{d}} = (\tilde{d}_1, \ldots, \tilde{d}_n)$ consisting of n_0 zeroes and n_1 ones such that $\sum_{i=1}^{n} \tilde{d}_i \mathbf{x}_i = \tilde{\mathbf{t}}_{\boldsymbol{\beta}}$, and the sum in the denominator is over all $\tilde{\mathbf{t}}_{\boldsymbol{\beta}}$ that can be obtained in this way.

If a particular component $\boldsymbol{\beta}_1$ of $\boldsymbol{\beta} = (\boldsymbol{\beta}_1, \boldsymbol{\beta}_2)$ is of interest, the appropriate conditional distribution for inference is that of $\mathbf{T}_{\boldsymbol{\beta}_1} = \sum_{i=1}^{n} d_i \mathbf{X}_{i1}$ given $\mathbf{T}_g$ and $\mathbf{T}_{\boldsymbol{\beta}_2} = \sum_{i=1}^{n} d_i \mathbf{X}_{i2}$, where $\mathbf{X}_i = (\mathbf{X}_{i1}, \mathbf{X}_{i2})$ is partitioned similarly to $\boldsymbol{\beta}$. The conditional distribution varies over permutations of $\mathbf{d}$ constrained to give the observed value of $\mathbf{T}_{\boldsymbol{\beta}_2}$ and is of the form

$$f(\mathbf{t}_{\boldsymbol{\beta}_1} | \mathbf{t}_{\boldsymbol{\beta}_2}, \mathbf{t}_g; \boldsymbol{\beta}_1) = \frac{C(\mathbf{t}_{\boldsymbol{\beta}_1}, \mathbf{t}_{\boldsymbol{\beta}_2}) \exp\left(\mathbf{t}_{\boldsymbol{\beta}_1}^T \boldsymbol{\beta}_1\right)}{\sum_{\tilde{\mathbf{t}}_{\boldsymbol{\beta}_1}} C(\tilde{\mathbf{t}}_{\boldsymbol{\beta}_1}, \mathbf{t}_{\boldsymbol{\beta}_2}) \exp\left(\tilde{\mathbf{t}}_{\boldsymbol{\beta}_1}^T \boldsymbol{\beta}_1\right)}, \tag{8.8}$$

where $C(\tilde{\mathbf{t}}_{\boldsymbol{\beta}_1}, \mathbf{t}_{\boldsymbol{\beta}_2})$ is the number of vectors $\tilde{\mathbf{d}}$ consisting of n_0 zeroes and n_1 ones such that $\sum_{i=1}^{n} \tilde{d}_i \mathbf{x}_{i1} = \tilde{\mathbf{t}}_{\boldsymbol{\beta}_1}$ and $\sum_{i=1}^{n} \tilde{d}_i \mathbf{x}_{i2} = \mathbf{t}_{\boldsymbol{\beta}_2}$, and the sum in the denominator is over all $\tilde{\mathbf{t}}_{\boldsymbol{\beta}_1}$ that can be obtained in this way.

For inference from matched case-control data we use the stratified model of equation (8.3). Let $\mathbf{X}_j^i$ be the random covariate vector for individual j in the ith matched set and $\mathbf{x}_j^i$ be the vector of observed values. Recall that the vector of stratum-specific covariate

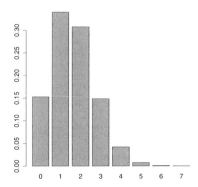

FIGURE 8.1
Conditional distribution for inference of the DES effect, β_1, when $\beta_1 = 0$.

distributions in controls is $\mathbf{g} = (g_1, \ldots, g_I)$. Let $d_{ij} = 1$ if the jth subject in the ith matched set is diseased and 0 otherwise. Now, $\mathbf{T}_{\boldsymbol{\beta}} = \sum_{i=1}^{I} \sum_{j=0}^{M_i} d_{ij} \mathbf{X}_j^i$. Let $\mathbf{T}_{\mathbf{g}}$ be the sufficient statistic for $\mathbf{g}$. $\mathbf{T}_{\mathbf{g}}$ is the unordered collection of observed covariates within each matched set, or, equivalently, a vector whose ith element, $\mathbf{T}_{g_i}$, is the empirical distribution of covariate vectors from matched set i. For inference of $\boldsymbol{\beta}$, we use the conditional distribution of $\mathbf{T}_{\boldsymbol{\beta}}$ given $\mathbf{T}_{\mathbf{g}}$. This distribution varies over permutations of the disease-status vectors $\mathbf{d}^i = (d_{i0}, \ldots, d_{iM_i})$ within each matched set and is of the form

$$f(\mathbf{t}_{\boldsymbol{\beta}}|\mathbf{t}_{\mathbf{g}}; \boldsymbol{\beta}) = \frac{C(\mathbf{t}_{\boldsymbol{\beta}}) \exp\left(\mathbf{t}_{\boldsymbol{\beta}}^T \boldsymbol{\beta}\right)}{\sum_{\tilde{\mathbf{t}}_{\boldsymbol{\beta}}} C(\tilde{\mathbf{t}}_{\boldsymbol{\beta}}) \exp\left(\tilde{\mathbf{t}}_{\boldsymbol{\beta}}^T \boldsymbol{\beta}\right)}, \tag{8.9}$$

where $C(\tilde{\mathbf{t}}_{\boldsymbol{\beta}})$ is the number of vectors $\tilde{\mathbf{d}} = (\tilde{\mathbf{d}}^1, \ldots, \tilde{\mathbf{d}}^I)$ with each sub-vector $\tilde{\mathbf{d}}^i = (\tilde{d}_{i0}, \ldots, \tilde{d}_{iM_i})$ consisting of M_i zeroes and a single one, such that $\sum_{i=1}^{I} \sum_{j=0}^{M_i} \tilde{d}_{ij} \mathbf{x}_j^i = \tilde{\mathbf{t}}_{\boldsymbol{\beta}}$. The sum in the denominator is over all $\tilde{\mathbf{t}}_{\boldsymbol{\beta}}$ that can be obtained in this way.

When β_1 is of interest, the appropriate conditional distribution for inference is that of $\mathbf{T}_{\boldsymbol{\beta}_1} = \sum_{i=1}^{I} \sum_{j=0}^{M_i} d_{ij} \mathbf{X}_{j1}^i$ given $\mathbf{T}_{\mathbf{g}}$ and $\mathbf{T}_{\boldsymbol{\beta}_2} = \sum_{i=1}^{I} \sum_{j=0}^{M_i} d_{ij} \mathbf{X}_{j2}^i$, where $\mathbf{X}_j^i = (\mathbf{X}_{j1}^i, \mathbf{X}_{j2}^i)$ is partitioned similarly to $\boldsymbol{\beta} = (\boldsymbol{\beta}_1, \boldsymbol{\beta}_2)$. The conditional distribution varies over permutations within each matched set of the subvectors $\mathbf{d}^i$ that give the observed value of $\mathbf{T}_{\boldsymbol{\beta}_2}$ and is of the form

$$f(\mathbf{t}_{\boldsymbol{\beta}_1}|\mathbf{t}_{\boldsymbol{\beta}_2}, \mathbf{t}_{\mathbf{g}}; \beta_1) = \frac{C(\mathbf{t}_{\boldsymbol{\beta}_1}, \mathbf{t}_{\boldsymbol{\beta}_2}) \exp\left(\mathbf{t}_{\boldsymbol{\beta}_1}^T \beta_1\right)}{\sum_{\tilde{\mathbf{t}}_{\boldsymbol{\beta}_1}} C(\tilde{\mathbf{t}}_{\boldsymbol{\beta}_1}, \mathbf{t}_{\boldsymbol{\beta}_2}) \exp\left(\tilde{\mathbf{t}}_{\boldsymbol{\beta}_1}^T \beta_1\right)}, \tag{8.10}$$

where $C(\tilde{\mathbf{t}}_{\boldsymbol{\beta}_1}, \mathbf{t}_{\boldsymbol{\beta}_2})$ is the number of $\tilde{\mathbf{d}} = (\tilde{\mathbf{d}}^1, \ldots, \tilde{\mathbf{d}}^I)$ such that $\sum_{i=1}^{I} \sum_{j=0}^{M_i} \tilde{d}_{ij} \mathbf{x}_{j1}^i = \tilde{\mathbf{t}}_{\boldsymbol{\beta}_1}$ and $\sum_{i=1}^{I} \sum_{j=0}^{M_i} \tilde{d}_{ij} \mathbf{x}_{j2}^i = \mathbf{t}_{\boldsymbol{\beta}_2}$.

In the DES example with adjustment for maternal smoking, we have the covariate vectors $\mathbf{X}_j^i = (X_{j1}^i, X_{j2}^i)$. Here X_{j1}^i is coded as 1 if individual j in matched set i is DES-exposed and 0 otherwise, and the variable X_{j2}^i is coded as 1 for mothers who smoke and 0 otherwise. The sufficient statistic T_{β_1} is a count of DES-exposed cases, with observed value 7. The sufficient statistic T_{β_2} is a count of the number of cases whose mothers smoke, with observed value 7. The conditional distribution for T_{β_1} under the null hypothesis that $\beta_1 = 0$ is shown in Figure 8.1.

The permutation distributions described above are for exact conditional inference from "retrospective" case-control data, in which the number of cases is fixed by the design and covariates are random. Conveniently, these distributions also arise for exact conditional inference from "prospective" data, in which disease status is random and the covariates are considered nonrandom and fixed by the design. Models for prospective data include the same parameters of interest as models for retrospective data, but different nuisance parameters. In both models the parameters of interest are the log odds ratios $\boldsymbol{\beta}$ or a sub-vector $\boldsymbol{\beta}_1$ of $\boldsymbol{\beta} = (\boldsymbol{\beta}_1, \boldsymbol{\beta}_2)$. The nuisance parameter in the model for prospective data is an intercept term, or a vector of stratum effects if sampling is stratified. The nuisance parameter in the model for retrospective data is a single covariate distribution, or a vector of stratum-specific covariate distributions if matching is used. However, accounting for the design and conditioning on the sufficient statistic for the nuisance parameter yields equivalent permutation distributions for inference of the parameters of interest. For example, for exact conditional inference of $\boldsymbol{\beta}$ from prospective data, we have fixed covariate values (i.e., a fixed empirical distribution $\mathbf{t}_g$) by design, and we condition on the sufficient statistic, n_1, for the nuisance intercept parameter. The resulting permutation distribution (e.g., Mehta and Patel, 1995, equation 5) is the same as $f(\mathbf{t}_{\boldsymbol{\beta}}|\mathbf{t}_g; \boldsymbol{\beta})$ in equation (8.7), obtained for retrospective data. In the retrospective case we have a fixed number of cases, n_1, by the case-control design and condition on the sufficient statistic, $\mathbf{t}_g$, for the nuisance distribution function g. The practical importance of obtaining the same permutation distribution under prospective and retrospective sampling is that methods and software developed for inference from prospective data can be applied to retrospective (case-control) data. We return to this point in Section 8.2.3.

8.2.2.2 Hypothesis testing

We focus on inference of $\boldsymbol{\beta}_1$ from a matched case-control study; i.e, on inference based on the conditional distribution $f(\mathbf{t}_{\boldsymbol{\beta}_1}|\mathbf{t}_{\boldsymbol{\beta}_2}, \mathbf{t_g}; \boldsymbol{\beta}_1)$ in equation (8.10). Inference of $\boldsymbol{\beta}_1$ from unmatched case-control data is obtained by replacing $f(\mathbf{t}_{\boldsymbol{\beta}_1}|\mathbf{t}_{\boldsymbol{\beta}_2}, \mathbf{t_g}; \boldsymbol{\beta}_1)$ with $f(\mathbf{t}_{\boldsymbol{\beta}_1}|\mathbf{t}_{\boldsymbol{\beta}_2}, \mathbf{t}_g; \boldsymbol{\beta}_1)$ from equation (8.8). Under the null hypothesis, $H_0 : \boldsymbol{\beta}_1 = \mathbf{0}$, the conditional distribution (8.10) reduces to

$$f(\mathbf{t}_{\boldsymbol{\beta}_1}|\mathbf{t}_{\boldsymbol{\beta}_2}, \mathbf{t_g}; \boldsymbol{\beta}_1 = \mathbf{0}) = \frac{C(\mathbf{t}_{\boldsymbol{\beta}_1}, \mathbf{t}_{\boldsymbol{\beta}_2})}{\sum_{\tilde{\mathbf{t}}_{\boldsymbol{\beta}_1}} C(\tilde{\mathbf{t}}_{\boldsymbol{\beta}_1}, \mathbf{t}_{\boldsymbol{\beta}_2})}.$$

For example, the null distribution for testing the DES effect conditional on maternal smoking is shown in Figure 8.1.

The p-values for the test of $H_0 : \boldsymbol{\beta}_1 = \mathbf{0}$ versus $H_1 : \boldsymbol{\beta}_1 \neq \mathbf{0}$ are the probability of seeing a value of a test statistic as or more extreme than the observed value under the conditional distribution. Possible test statistics in exact conditional inference include the conditional probabilities and conditional scores tests (Mehta and Patel, 1995). For the conditional probabilities test, the test statistic is the null conditional probability $P_0(\mathbf{T}_{\boldsymbol{\beta}_1}) = f(\mathbf{T}_{\boldsymbol{\beta}_1}|\mathbf{t}_{\boldsymbol{\beta}_2}, \mathbf{t_g}; \boldsymbol{\beta}_1 = \mathbf{0})$ and the critical region is all $\tilde{\mathbf{t}}_{\boldsymbol{\beta}_1}$ with probability $P_0(\tilde{\mathbf{t}}_{\boldsymbol{\beta}_1})$ as small or smaller than $P_0(\mathbf{t}_{\boldsymbol{\beta}_1})$. Formally, with critical region

$$\mathcal{R}_P(\mathbf{t}_{\boldsymbol{\beta}_1}) = \{\tilde{\mathbf{t}}_{\boldsymbol{\beta}_1} : P_0(\tilde{\mathbf{t}}_{\boldsymbol{\beta}_1}) \leq P_0(\mathbf{t}_{\boldsymbol{\beta}_1})\}, \tag{8.11}$$

the p-value is

$$\sum_{\tilde{\mathbf{t}}_{\boldsymbol{\beta}_1} \in \mathcal{R}_P(\mathbf{t}_{\boldsymbol{\beta}_1})} f(\tilde{\mathbf{t}}_{\boldsymbol{\beta}_1}|\mathbf{t}_{\boldsymbol{\beta}_2}, \mathbf{t_g}; \boldsymbol{\beta}_1 = \mathbf{0}).$$

For example, the observed number of DES exposed cases is $t_{\boldsymbol{\beta}_1} = 7$. From the null distribution (Figure 8.1 and Table 8.2) we see that the value $\tilde{t}_{\boldsymbol{\beta}_1} = 7$ has the lowest probability. Therefore the critical region is $\mathcal{R}_P(7) = \{7\}$ and the p-value is $f(7|t_{\boldsymbol{\beta}_2}, \mathbf{t_g}; \boldsymbol{\beta}_1 = 0) = 5.3 \times 10^{-5}$.

TABLE 8.2
Conditional probabilities, $P_0(\tilde{t}_{\beta_1})$, and scores, $S_0(\tilde{t}_{\beta_1})$, in the DES
example.

$\tilde{t}_{\beta_1}$	0	1	2	3	4	5	6	7
$P_0(\tilde{t}_{\beta_1})$	0.153	0.340	0.307	0.149	0.043	0.008	0.001	0.000
$S_0(\tilde{t}_{\beta_1})$	2.161	0.314	0.122	1.587	4.707	9.484	15.916	24.005

For the conditional scores test, the test statistic is the null conditional score statistic

$$S_0(\mathbf{T}_{\boldsymbol{\beta}_1}) = (\mathbf{T}_{\boldsymbol{\beta}_1} - \boldsymbol{\mu}_1)^T \boldsymbol{\Sigma}_1^{-1} (\mathbf{T}_{\boldsymbol{\beta}_1} - \boldsymbol{\mu}_1),$$

where $\boldsymbol{\mu}_1$ is the mean and $\boldsymbol{\Sigma}_1$ is the variance of $\mathbf{T}_{\boldsymbol{\beta}_1}$ under the null conditional distribution
$f(\mathbf{t}_{\boldsymbol{\beta}_1} | \mathbf{t}_{\boldsymbol{\beta}_2}, \mathbf{t_g}; \boldsymbol{\beta}_1 = \mathbf{0})$. The critical region is

$$\mathcal{R}_S(\mathbf{t}_{\boldsymbol{\beta}_1}) = \{\tilde{\mathbf{t}}_{\boldsymbol{\beta}_1} : S(\tilde{\mathbf{t}}_{\boldsymbol{\beta}_1}) \geq S(\mathbf{t}_{\boldsymbol{\beta}_1})\} \tag{8.12}$$

and the p-value is

$$\sum_{\tilde{\mathbf{t}}_{\boldsymbol{\beta}_1} \in \mathcal{R}_S(\mathbf{t}_{\boldsymbol{\beta}_1})} f(\tilde{\mathbf{t}}_{\boldsymbol{\beta}_1} | \mathbf{t}_{\boldsymbol{\beta}_2}, \mathbf{t_g}; \boldsymbol{\beta}_1 = \mathbf{0}).$$

For the DES example, the possible values of $S_0(\tilde{t}_{\beta_1})$ are shown in Table 8.2. The critical
region is $\mathcal{R}_S(7) = \{7\}$, so the p-value from the conditional scores test is the same as for the
conditional probabilities test.

8.2.2.3 Estimation

We discuss interval estimation before point estimation because interval estimation follows
directly from hypothesis testing. The most obvious approach to constructing a confidence
interval is to invert a two-sided exact conditional hypothesis test, but this can result in a
noninterval confidence region (see Supplementary Materials). Instead, for scalar β_1, Mehta
and Patel (1995) suggest an interval estimator, $(\beta_1^-(\alpha), \beta_1^+(\alpha))$, with level $1 - \alpha$ confidence
obtained by combining one-sided confidence limits as follows. The lower limit, $\beta_1^-(\alpha)$, is the
solution to $R(\beta_1^0; t_{\beta_1}) = \alpha/2$, where

$$R(\beta_1^0; t_{\beta_1}) = \sum_{\tilde{t}_{\beta_1} \geq t_{\beta_1}} f(\tilde{t}_{\beta_1} | \mathbf{t}_{\boldsymbol{\beta}_2}, \mathbf{t_g}; \beta_1^0) \tag{8.13}$$

is the area from the observed t_{β_1} to the right under the conditional distribution assuming
$H_0 : \beta_1 = \beta_1^0$. For the DES example, $t_{\beta_1} = 7$ and the function $R(\beta_1^0; 7)$ is shown in Figure 8.2.
From the figure we see that the value $\beta_1^-(0.05) = 1.426$ for a 95% confidence interval because
$R(1.426, 7) = 0.05/2$.

The upper confidence limit, $\beta_1^+(\alpha)$, solves

$$L(\beta_1^0; t_{\beta_1}) = \alpha/2, \tag{8.14}$$

where

$$L(\beta_1^0; t_{\beta_1}) = \sum_{\tilde{t}_{\beta_1} \leq t_{\beta_1}} f(\tilde{t}_{\beta_1} | \mathbf{t}_{\boldsymbol{\beta}_2}, \mathbf{t_g}; \beta_1^0) \tag{8.15}$$

is the area from t_{β_1} to the left under the conditional distribution assuming $H_0 : \beta_1 = \beta_1^0$. In
the DES example, a solution $\beta_1^+(\alpha)$ to equation (8.14) does not exist because $t_{\beta_1} = 7$ is the
maximum possible value, $t_{\beta_1}^{\max}$, of the support of the conditional distribution. As a function

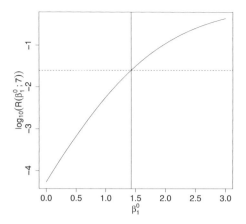

FIGURE 8.2

Log_{10} of $R(\beta_1^0; 7)$ in the DES example. The dashed horizontal line is at $R(\beta_1^0; 7) = 0.025$. The dashed vertical line is at $\beta_1^0 = \beta_1^-(0.05) = 1.426$.

of t_{β_1}, $L(\beta_1^0; t_{\beta_1})$ is the cumulative distribution function of the conditional distribution. Thus, $L(\beta_1^0; 7) = L(\beta_1^0; t_{\beta_1}^{\max}) = 1$ for *all* values of β_1^0 and so is never equal to $\alpha/2$ for any α. The convention is to set $\beta_1^+(\alpha) = \infty$. Analogously, we set $\beta_1^-(\alpha) = -\infty$ when t_{β_1} is the minimum possible value of the support of the conditional distribution.

Point estimates may be obtained by conditional maximum likelihood (CMLE); that is, by maximizing the appropriate conditional likelihood function. For example, in a matched case-control study, estimates of β_1 may be obtained by maximizing equation (8.10) as a function of β_1. However, when there is separation, and the sufficient statistic t_{β_1} takes on its maximum or minimum possible value, the conditional likelihood does not have a maximum (Mehta and Patel, 1995) and the CMLE does not exist. Figure 8.3 shows this for the DES example.

When the CMLE does not exist we use a median unbiased estimator (MUE). An estimator $\tilde{\beta}_1$ is median unbiased if $P(\tilde{\beta}_1 \leq \beta_1) \geq 1/2$ and $P(\tilde{\beta}_1 \geq \beta_1) \leq 1/2$ (e.g., Read, 1985). Intuitively, the idea is that the estimator is as likely to overestimate the target as it is to underestimate it. The MUE can be written in terms of confidence interval endpoints $\beta_1^-(\alpha)$ and $\beta_1^+(\alpha)$ for $\alpha = 1$ (Hirji *et al.*, 1989; Mehta and Patel, 1995). When the CMLE does not exist, one of the confidence interval endpoints is infinite. In this case, the MUE is taken to be the finite endpoint of the confidence interval. For instance, in the DES example, $\beta_1^+(1) = \infty$ and the MUE is $\beta_1^-(1) = 3.19$.

8.2.3 Implementation and application

The computational challenge for inference of $\boldsymbol{\beta}_1$ is to enumerate the support and probability mass function (pmf) of the conditional distribution of $\mathbf{T}_{\boldsymbol{\beta}_1}$ given $(\mathbf{t}_{\boldsymbol{\beta}_2}, \mathbf{t}_g)$ for unmatched data in equation (8.8) or given $(\mathbf{t}_{\boldsymbol{\beta}_2}, \mathbf{t_g})$ for matched data in equation (8.10). Hirji *et al.* (1987) develops an efficient algorithm for computing these conditional pmfs. Their algorithm is implemented in the commercial software package LogXact (Cytel Inc., 2015).

LogXact has a standard point-and-click interface reminiscent of other statistical packages such as JMP. The logistic regression interface allows users to highlight variables in a list of variables, and then add them as the response variable, the stratum variable, or as a

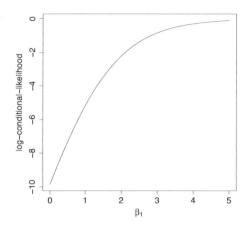

FIGURE 8.3
Log-conditional likelihood for the DES effect.

covariate in the model. The package was designed for analysis of data sets from prospective designs, where disease status is random and covariates are nonrandom and fixed by design. By contrast, case-control studies are retrospective, with the number of cases and controls fixed by design and random covariates. As discussed at the end of Section 8.2.2.1, exact conditional inference from both retrospective and prospective data is based on the same permutation distribution provided the prospective model includes the appropriate nuisance intercept or stratum effects. That is, users with unmatched case-control data should ensure that the logistic regression model for disease status includes an intercept term (the default) and users with matched case-control data should include the matched sets as a stratum variable.

Though LogXact was developed to implement exact inference, the default is large-sample maximum-likelihood inference. This default was chosen to avoid surprising the user with the long run times that are sometimes necessary for exact inference. When the user opts for exact inference, the output includes CMLEs, MUEs, exact interval estimates, and exact tests. To our knowledge, exact logistic regression has not yet been implemented in freely available software.

We illustrate with an application of LogXact to the DES data set to infer the DES effect adjusted for maternal smoking. We perform both an unmatched analysis, ignoring the matching, and a matched analysis. For an unmatched analysis we specify a model that includes an intercept and model terms for DES and maternal smoking. We obtain a conditional probabilities test p-value for the DES effect of 1.5×10^{-6}, a MUE of 4.549, and a 95% confidence interval of $(2.432, \infty)$. For the matched analysis, we create a categorical variable that identifies the matched set membership of each subject and select this variable as the "Stratum" variable in the program's logistic regression interface. We then specify model terms for DES and maternal smoking. We obtain a conditional probabilities test p-value of 1.28×10^{-5}, a MUE of 3.190, and a 95% confidence interval of $(1.425, \infty)$. It is interesting that the MUE of the log odds ratio from the unmatched analysis is greater than the MUE from the matched analysis, since unmatched analyses of matched data tend to give conservative estimates of log odds ratios (Breslow and Day, 1980, p. 271).

8.2.4 Limitations

The point estimator of the regression parameter of interest from exact logistic regression is biased (Heinze and Schemper, 2002). However, the main limitations of exact logistic regression are the computation required and conservative inference, in which hypothesis tests tend to have size less than the nominal level. Computationally, the limiting factor is the computer memory required to store the support of the conditional distribution. To quote the LogXact manual (Cytel Inc., 2015, Section G.2, page 798): "The type of logistic regression problem one can expect to solve by exact methods has a maximum of 7 covariates (all binary), 300 observations and 200 covariate patterns."

Exact inference tends to be conservative because of the discreteness of the exact conditional distributions (e.g., Agresti, 2013, Section 7.3.7). The discreteness arises because the conditional distribution has relatively few support points due to the constraints imposed by conditioning. Thus, to control the size of the test, we may need to use a rejection region with less than nominal level, which reduces power. Conditioning constraints can be particularly restrictive when conditioning on a covariate that takes many different values, leading to few permutations of the disease-status vector that are consistent with the observed value of the sufficient statistic. Reducing the covariate to a coarser set of values may help. For example, a continuous variable such as age could be categorized into 5- or 10-year categories. However, this approach is unsatisfactory because it loses covariate information.

Another approach to reducing conservativeness is to use mid-p-values. For example, the mid-p-value for the conditional probabilities test of $H_0 : \boldsymbol{\beta}_1 = \mathbf{0}$ is

$$\sum_{\tilde{\mathbf{t}}_1 : P_0(\tilde{\mathbf{t}}_{\boldsymbol{\beta}_1}) < P_0(\mathbf{t}_{\boldsymbol{\beta}_1})} f(\tilde{\mathbf{t}}_{\boldsymbol{\beta}_1} | \mathbf{t}_{\boldsymbol{\beta}_2}, \mathbf{t_g}; \boldsymbol{\beta}_1 = \mathbf{0}) + (1/2) f(\mathbf{t}_{\boldsymbol{\beta}_1} | \mathbf{t}_{\boldsymbol{\beta}_2}, \mathbf{t_g}; \boldsymbol{\beta}_1 = \mathbf{0}). \tag{8.16}$$

Compared to the conventional p-value,

$$\sum_{\tilde{\mathbf{t}}_1 : P_0(\tilde{\mathbf{t}}_{\boldsymbol{\beta}_1}) \leq P_0(\mathbf{t}_{\boldsymbol{\beta}_1})} f(\tilde{\mathbf{t}}_{\boldsymbol{\beta}_1} | \mathbf{t}_{\boldsymbol{\beta}_2}, \mathbf{t_g}; \boldsymbol{\beta}_1 = \mathbf{0}),$$

we see that the mid-p-value in equation (8.16) uses only half of the probability of the observed value of the test statistic, while the conventional p-value uses all of it. Thus mid-p-values are smaller than conventional p-values and are therefore less conservative. Simulation studies (e.g., Heinze and Puhr, 2010) have demonstrated that hypothesis tests based on mid-p-values are more powerful than tests based on conventional p-values, and that confidence intervals obtained by inverting mid-p-value tests achieve nominal coverage.

We illustrate mid-p-values with the DES data set. Rather than make inference of the effect of DES exposure after adjusting for maternal smoking, we could make inference of the effect of maternal smoking after adjusting for DES exposure. The conditional null distribution for such inference is a pmf with probability mass 0.2 at $\tilde{t}_{\beta_1} = 6$ and 0.8 at $\tilde{t}_{\beta_1} = 7$. If we observe $t_{\beta_1} = 6$, the conventional p-value is $f(6|t_{\boldsymbol{\beta}_2}, \mathbf{t_g}; \beta_1 = 0) = 0.2$. If we observe $t_{\beta_1} = 7$, the conventional p-value is $f(6|t_{\boldsymbol{\beta}_2}, \mathbf{t_g}; \beta_1 = 0) + f(7|t_{\boldsymbol{\beta}_2}, \mathbf{t_g}; \beta_1 = 0) = 1$. By contrast, a mid-p-value for $t_{\beta_1} = 6$ is $(1/2)f(6|t_{\boldsymbol{\beta}_2}, \mathbf{t_g}; \beta_1 = 0) = 0.1$ and for $t_{\beta_1} = 7$ it is $f(6|t_{\boldsymbol{\beta}_2}, \mathbf{t_g}; \beta_1 = 0) + (1/2)f(7|t_{\boldsymbol{\beta}_2}, \mathbf{t_g}; \beta_1 = 0) = 0.6$. These mid-p-values are less conservative (i.e., smaller) than the conventional p-values.

The maternal smoking example illustrates that discreteness can prevent meaningful inference altogether. For example, a level 5% test of the maternal smoking effect, based on either the p-value or mid-p-value, has zero power because it is impossible to reject the null hypothesis at the 5% level. In the most extreme case of discreteness, $\mathbf{d}$ is the only configuration of disease-status indicators that gives the observed value of $\mathbf{t}_{\boldsymbol{\beta}_2}$. In this case, the support of the conditional distribution of $\mathbf{T}_{\boldsymbol{\beta}_1}$ is a single point, namely the observed value of $\mathbf{t}_{\boldsymbol{\beta}_1}$; i.e., the conditional distribution is *degenerate*.

8.3   Approximate exact conditional inference

8.3.1   Motivation

Hypothesis tests and confidence intervals for exact logistic regression of $\boldsymbol{\beta}_1$ (Section 8.2) are based on the conditional distributions $f(\mathbf{t}_{\boldsymbol{\beta}_1}|\mathbf{t}_{\boldsymbol{\beta}_2}, \mathbf{t}_g; \boldsymbol{\beta}_1)$ for unmatched data given in equation (8.8) and $f(\mathbf{t}_{\boldsymbol{\beta}_1}|\mathbf{t}_{\boldsymbol{\beta}_2}, \mathbf{t_g}; \boldsymbol{\beta}_1)$ for matched data given in equation (8.10). As already noted, the support of these conditional distributions can sometimes be too large to enumerate in computer memory. In such case, we may resort to approximate exact logistic regression. Throughout Section 8.3, we focus on approximate exact inference of the log odds ratio $\boldsymbol{\beta}_1$ from *unmatched* case-control data. We briefly discuss inference from matched case-control data in Section 8.3.4.

Approximate exact inference from unmatched case-control data relies on Monte Carlo approximation of the probabilites that define the p-values and confidence limits. For example, the p-value from the conditional scores test can be approximated by the proportion of observations, drawn from $f(\mathbf{t}_{\boldsymbol{\beta}_1}|\mathbf{t}_{\boldsymbol{\beta}_2}, \mathbf{t}_g; \boldsymbol{\beta}_1 = \mathbf{0})$, that fall in the critical region

$$\mathcal{R}_S(\mathbf{t}_{\boldsymbol{\beta}_1}) = \{\tilde{\mathbf{t}}_{\boldsymbol{\beta}_1} : S_0(\tilde{\mathbf{t}}_{\boldsymbol{\beta}_1}) \geq S_0(\mathbf{t}_{\boldsymbol{\beta}_1})\},$$

where $S_0(\mathbf{t}_{\boldsymbol{\beta}_1}) = (\mathbf{t}_{\boldsymbol{\beta}_1} - \boldsymbol{\mu}_1)^T \boldsymbol{\Sigma}_1^{-1}(\mathbf{t}_{\boldsymbol{\beta}_1} - \boldsymbol{\mu}_1)$ is the conditional scores statistic, $\boldsymbol{\mu}_1$ is the mean, and $\boldsymbol{\Sigma}_1$ is the variance of the sufficient statistic $\mathbf{T}_{\boldsymbol{\beta}_1}$ under $f(\mathbf{t}_{\boldsymbol{\beta}_1}|\mathbf{t}_{\boldsymbol{\beta}_1}, \mathbf{t}_g; \boldsymbol{\beta}_1 = \mathbf{0})$. Rather than sampling from $f(\mathbf{t}_{\boldsymbol{\beta}_1}|\mathbf{t}_{\boldsymbol{\beta}_2}, \mathbf{t}_g; \boldsymbol{\beta}_1 = \mathbf{0})$, we may sample from $f(\mathbf{y}|\mathbf{t}_{\boldsymbol{\beta}_2}, \mathbf{t}_g; \boldsymbol{\beta}_1 = \mathbf{0})$, where $\mathbf{y}$ is a finer summary of the disease status than $\mathbf{t}_{\boldsymbol{\beta}_1}$ (Mehta *et al.*, 2000; Forster *et al.*, 2003; Zamar *et al.*, 2007). This alternate sampling strategy works because probabilities of $\mathbf{t}_{\boldsymbol{\beta}_1}$ can be obtained from probabilities of $\mathbf{y}$.

8.3.2   Monte Carlo

The definition of $\mathbf{Y}$ is conditional on $\mathbf{t}_g$, the empirical distribution of the covariates. The empirical distribution $\mathbf{t}_g$ consists of the q unique values of the covariates, denoted $\mathbf{x}_{(1)}, \ldots, \mathbf{x}_{(q)}$, and the number of copies $m_1, \ldots, m_q$ of each. Let the random variable Y_j be the number of cases with the jth unique covariate vector value and define $\mathbf{Y} \equiv (Y_1, \ldots, Y_q)$. Let $\mathbf{y} = (y_1, \ldots, y_q)$ be the observed value of $\mathbf{Y}$. We may think of $\mathbf{y}$ as a summary of the disease-status vector $\mathbf{d}$, in which we have tallied the number of cases having each unique value of $\mathbf{x}$. Thus

$$\sum_{j=1}^{q} y_j \mathbf{x}_{(j)} = \sum_{i=1}^{n} d_i \mathbf{x}_i = (\mathbf{t}_{\boldsymbol{\beta}_1}, \mathbf{t}_{\boldsymbol{\beta}_2}),$$

so that $\mathbf{t}_{\boldsymbol{\beta}_1}(\mathbf{y}) = \sum_j y_j \mathbf{x}_{(j)1}$ and $\mathbf{t}_{\boldsymbol{\beta}_2}(\mathbf{y}) = \sum_j y_j \mathbf{x}_{(j)2}$ are functions of $\mathbf{y}$, where $(\mathbf{x}_{(j)1}, \mathbf{x}_{(j)2})$ is the partition of $\mathbf{x}_{(j)}$ matching the partition $(\boldsymbol{\beta}_1, \boldsymbol{\beta}_2)$ of $\boldsymbol{\beta}$.

Analogous to equation (8.8), the distribution of $\mathbf{Y}$ given $(\mathbf{t}_{\boldsymbol{\beta}_2}, \mathbf{t}_g)$ is

$$f(\mathbf{y}|\mathbf{t}_{\boldsymbol{\beta}_2}, \mathbf{t}_g; \boldsymbol{\beta}_1) = \frac{C'(\mathbf{y}) \exp\left(\mathbf{t}_{\boldsymbol{\beta}_1}(\mathbf{y})^T \boldsymbol{\beta}_1\right)}{\sum_{\tilde{\mathbf{y}}} C'(\tilde{\mathbf{y}}) \exp\left(\mathbf{t}_{\boldsymbol{\beta}_1}(\tilde{\mathbf{y}})^T \boldsymbol{\beta}_1\right)},$$

where $C'(\mathbf{y}) = \prod_{j=1}^{q} \binom{m_j}{y_j}$, $\tilde{\mathbf{y}} = (\tilde{y}_1 \ldots, \tilde{y}_q)$ is a vector of counts that satisfy the constraints:

$$
\begin{aligned}
0 \leq \tilde{y}_j \leq m_j; \; j = 1, \ldots, q \\
\textstyle\sum_{j=1}^{q} \tilde{y}_j = n_1 \\
\mathbf{t}_{\boldsymbol{\beta}_2}(\tilde{\mathbf{y}}) \equiv \textstyle\sum_{j=1}^{q} \tilde{y}_j \mathbf{x}_{(j)2} = \mathbf{t}_{\boldsymbol{\beta}_2},
\end{aligned}
\tag{8.17}
$$

and the sum in the denominator is over all such $\tilde{\mathbf{y}}$. Recall that m_j is the number of subjects with unique covariate value $\mathbf{x}_{(j)}$ and n_1 is the number of cases.

The probabilities that define p-values and confidence limits for β_1 are based on its sufficient statistic $\mathbf{T}_{\beta_1}$. For example, the p-value, p_S, for the conditional scores test is the conditional probability of the critical region $\mathcal{R}_S(\mathbf{t}_{\beta_1})$ under the null hypothesis $H_0 : \beta_1 = \mathbf{0}$; specifically,

$$p_S = \sum_{\tilde{\mathbf{t}}_{\beta_1} \in \mathcal{R}_S(\mathbf{t}_{\beta_1})} f(\tilde{\mathbf{t}}_{\beta_1} | \mathbf{t}_{\beta_2}, \mathbf{t}_g; \beta_1 = \mathbf{0}),$$

where $\mathcal{R}_S(\mathbf{t}_{\beta_1}) = \{\tilde{\mathbf{t}}_{\beta_1} : S_0(\tilde{\mathbf{t}}_{\beta_1}) \geq S_0(\mathbf{t}_{\beta_1})\}$. Probabilities of $\mathbf{t}_{\beta_1}$ can be written as probabilities of $\mathbf{y}$. For example,

$$p_S = \sum_{\tilde{\mathbf{y}} \in \mathcal{R}_S(\mathbf{y})} f(\tilde{\mathbf{y}} | \mathbf{t}_{\beta_2}, \mathbf{t}_g; \beta_1 = \mathbf{0}),$$

where $\mathcal{R}_S(\mathbf{y})$ is the set of $\tilde{\mathbf{y}}$ that satisfy the constraints in (8.17) and, in addition, give values $\mathbf{t}_{\beta_1}(\tilde{\mathbf{y}})$ of the sufficient statistic that are in the critical region $\mathcal{R}_S(\mathbf{t}_{\beta_1})$. We can thus estimate p_S by the proportion of $\tilde{\mathbf{y}}$ sampled from $f(\mathbf{y} | \mathbf{t}_{\beta_2}, \mathbf{t}_g; \beta_1 = \mathbf{0})$ that fall in $\mathcal{R}_S(\mathbf{y})$.

The simplest approach to sampling $\mathbf{Y}$ from $f(\mathbf{y} | \mathbf{t}_{\beta_2}, \mathbf{t}_g; \beta_1)$ is "rejection" sampling (Mehta *et al.*, 2000). Samples are first drawn from $f(\mathbf{y} | \mathbf{t}_g; \beta_1)$, without regard to the sufficient statistic $\mathbf{t}_{\beta_2}$. Samples not satisfying this constraint are discarded. According to the authors, although this approach requires minimal computer memory, it rejects samples too often, leading to long computing times.

To avoid long computing times, these authors propose an algorithm that samples directly from $f(\mathbf{y} | \mathbf{t}_{\beta_2}, \mathbf{t}_g; \beta_1)$. The first step is to construct a compact representation of the support of $f(\mathbf{y} | \mathbf{t}_{\beta_2}, \mathbf{t}_g; \beta_1)$ as a layered network of arcs and nodes. Recall that the vector $\mathbf{y}$ has as its jth element the number of cases with the jth unique covariate vector, $\mathbf{x}_{(j)}$, and that there are q unique covariate vectors. At layer j of the network ($j = 1, \ldots, q$), an arc represents the jth element, $\tilde{y}_j$, of the sampled $\tilde{\mathbf{y}}$ and nodes contain the partial sums $\sum_{k=1}^{j} \tilde{y}_k$ and $\sum_{k=1}^{j} \tilde{y}_k \mathbf{x}_{(k)2}$, which track how the number of cases and $\mathbf{t}_{\beta_2}$ accumulate through the layers, respectively. During network construction, nodes at layer j that are incompatible with the constraints, $\sum_{k=1}^{q} \tilde{y}_j = n_1$ and $\sum_{k=1}^{q} y_j \mathbf{x}_{(j)2} = \mathbf{t}_{\beta_2}$, are pruned. Incompatibility means that there are no possible $\tilde{y}_{j+1}, \ldots, \tilde{y}_q$ that would lead to a $\tilde{\mathbf{y}}$ that satisfies both constraints. Paths through the resulting network represent all $\tilde{\mathbf{y}}$ that satisfy the constraints. An illustration of an example network can be found in Mehta *et al.* (2000, Figure 1).

Once the network that represents the support has been created, the next step is to superpose sampling weights that allow sampling of paths according to the target distribution. Sampling a path can be achieved by randomly selecting an arc to follow at each node visited during a pass through the network. Mehta *et al.* (2000) develop a recursive algorithm to calculate sampling weights for each arc such that randomly following arcs according to their weights produces a realization from $f(\mathbf{y} | \mathbf{t}_{\beta_2}, \mathbf{t}_g; \beta_1)$. Although the resulting algorithm samples without rejection, the construction of the network can exhaust computer memory. The memory limitations of the Monte Carlo approach prompted development of Markov chain Monte Carlo approaches (Forster *et al.*, 2003; Zamar *et al.*, 2007). These are discussed in the next section.

8.3.3 Markov chain Monte Carlo

Markov chain Monte Carlo (MCMC) is an interative approach to sampling from a target distribution, which in our case is $f(\mathbf{y} | \mathbf{t}_{\beta_2}, \mathbf{t}_g; \beta_1)$. Starting from an initial state, say $\mathbf{y}^0$, we propose a new value, $\mathbf{y}^*$. The proposal is either accepted or rejected. If accepted, $\mathbf{y}^*$

becomes the next in our sample, $\mathbf{y}^1$. If rejected we set $\mathbf{y}^1 = \mathbf{y}^0$. The process of proposing new realizations and then either accepting or rejecting them is repeated for a large number, N, of iterations. The acceptance probability is chosen so that, for large N, the sequence $\mathbf{y}^1, \mathbf{y}^2, \ldots, \mathbf{y}^N$ behaves like a sample from the target distribution. The key advantage of Markov chain Monte Carlo (MCMC) algorithms over the Monte Carlo algorithm of Mehta *et al.* (2000) is that they do not require a complete enumeration of the sample space of $f(\mathbf{y}|\mathbf{t}_{\beta_2}, \mathbf{t}_g; \boldsymbol{\beta})$. We discuss an algorithm due to Forster *et al.* (2003) and the modifications of Zamar *et al.* (2007).

Forster *et al.* (2003) start from an initial $\mathbf{y}^0$ that satisfies the constraints (8.17), and then generates proposals that also satisfy the constraints and differ only in a few entries from the current value. Specifically, at iteration $k+1$, the algorithm proposes $\mathbf{y}^* = \mathbf{y}^k + s \cdot \mathbf{v}$, where (i) $\mathbf{y}^k = (y_1^k, \ldots, y_q^k)$ is the current value of the vector of counts for cases with each unique covariate vector, (ii) for a user-defined integer r, $\mathbf{v}$ is a vector of integers of length q from the set

$$\mathbf{V}_r = \left\{ \mathbf{v} : \sum_{j=1}^q |v_j| \leq r, v_j \text{ integer and coprime for } j = 1, \ldots, q; \sum_{j=1}^q v_j = \sum_{j=1}^q v_j \mathbf{x}_{(j)} = 0 \right\},$$

and (iii) s is an integer such that

$$0 \leq y_j^k + s v_j \leq m_j; \ j = 1, \ldots, q. \tag{8.18}$$

There are thus two components to a proposal, $\mathbf{v}$ and s, where $\mathbf{v}$ is in $\mathbf{V}_r$ and s satisfies (8.18). The set of all proposals arising from the current $\mathbf{y}^k$ consists of all possible values of $\mathbf{y}^* = \mathbf{y}^k + s \cdot \mathbf{v}$.

Further details about the constraints that define $\mathbf{V}_r$ are as follows. The constraint $\sum_{j=1}^q |v_j| \leq r$ restricts $\mathbf{V}_r$ to a "ball" of radius r. If r is too large, $\mathbf{V}_r$ may be too large to enumerate. On the other hand, if r is too small, the algorithm can only make small changes in the $\mathbf{y}$-values and will "mix" poorly, requiring a long run to adequately explore the sample space. The requirement that the v_i be coprime (i.e., they have no common factor) is so that the scalar multiplier s can be uniquely identified from the perturbation, $s \cdot \mathbf{v}$, of $\mathbf{y}^k$. The constraints $\sum_j v_j = \sum_j v_j \mathbf{x}_{(j)2} = 0$ ensure that $\mathbf{y}^* = \mathbf{y}^k + s \cdot \mathbf{v}$ satisfies the constraints on the number of cases and the sufficient statistic $\mathbf{t}_{\beta_2}$ in (8.17).

Proposals, $\mathbf{y}^*$, are sampled from a distribution that is proportional to the target distribution, but only over the proposal neighbourhood defined by the possibilities for $s \cdot \mathbf{v}$. This sampling strategy leads to an algorithm that always accepts its proposals (Forster *et al.*, 2003). However, when $s = 0$ the proposal does not actually change the current $\mathbf{y}$ value, and so the algorithm is not guaranteed to move at each iteration.

Though the algorithm avoids enumeration of the entire sample space, it does require enumeration of $\mathbf{V}_r$. To enumerate $\mathbf{V}_r$, the authors first enumerate the larger set

$$\mathbf{V}_r' = \left\{ \mathbf{v} : \sum_{j=1}^q |v_j| \leq r, \ v_j \text{ integer and coprime for } j = 1, \ldots, q \right\},$$

and then keep only those $\mathbf{v}$ that satisfy the constraints $\sum_j v_j = \sum_j v_j \mathbf{x}_{(j)} = 0$. However, since the size of $\mathbf{V}_r'$ grows rapidly with the length, q, of $\mathbf{y}$, enumeration can be impractical (Zamar *et al.*, 2007). To accommodate data sets with many unique covariate values (i.e., large q), Zamar *et al.* (2007) implement an extension with the following two differences:

1. They sample from a subset $\mathbf{V}_r^A$ of $\mathbf{V}_r$ whose vectors satisfy the additional constraint that $0 \leq |v_j| \leq m_i$ for all $1 = 1, \ldots, q$. This improves mixing, because vectors for which some $|v_i| > m_i$ will only satisfy $0 \leq s v_j \leq m_i$ for $s = 0$.

TABLE 8.3

Exact and approximate exact MUEs, 95% confidence intervals, and p-values for the DES effect, adjusted for maternal smoking.

Method	MUE	95% CI	p-value
Unmatched analyses:			
exact (LogXact)	4.55	$(2.43, \infty)$	1.5×10^{-6}
MC appx. exact (LogXact)	NA	$(2.48, \infty)$	0
MCMC appx. exact (`elrm`)	4.97	$(2.62, \infty)$	0
Matched analyses:			
exact (LogXact)	3.19	$(1.42, \infty)$	1.3×10^{-5}
MC appx. exact (LogXact)	NA	$(1.08, \infty)$	8.6×10^{-7}
MCMC appx. exact (`elrm`)	2.70	$(1.22, \infty)$	1.1×10^{-4}

2. They sample vectors uniformly from $\mathbf{V}_r^A$ without enumerating a larger set $\mathbf{V}_r'$ or storing $\mathbf{V}_r^A$. Details on how to sample uniformly from $\mathbf{V}_r^A$ are given in Zamar (2006).

8.3.4 Implementation and application

We illustrate these ideas using the DES data set, with matching ignored, to infer the DES effect adjusted for maternal smoking. We compare results from approximate methods to those from exact logistic regression in LogXact as described in Section 8.2.

The Monte Carlo method of Mehta *et al.* (2000) is also implemented in LogXact, as an option of the program's logistic regression interface. Estimates are based on the default of 10,000 Monte Carlo samples. LogXact did not return an MUE for these data, though the documentation suggests that it should, in general. The confidence interval and hypothesis test p-value are close to those from the exact analysis (Table 8.3).

The MCMC method of Zamar *et al.* (2007) has been implemented in the `elrm` R package. Information on running `elrm` is given in the Supplementary Materials. Estimates based on 1 million MCMC replicates (Table 8.3) are close to the true values obtained from LogXact.

For approximate exact inference, we have focused on unmatched case-control data, but analysis of matched data is also possible. With matched data, users must specify stratum effects in their logistic regression model to account for the matched design, as discussed in Section 8.2. Exact and Monte Carlo approximate exact analysis results from LogXact are shown in Table 8.3. Approximate exact results are based on 10,000 Monte Carlo samples. As already noted for the exact analyses, for these data the MUE of the log odds ratio from the unmatched analysis is greater than the MUE from the matched analysis, contrary to the tendency of unmatched analyses of matched data that tend to give conservative estimates (Breslow and Day, 1980). Results from `elrm` based on 1 million MCMC replicates (Table 8.3) are reasonably close to the true values obtained from LogXact.

8.3.5 Limitations

Approximate methods were developed to avoid the problem of running out of computer memory when enumerating the support of the conditional distribution. The trade-off is that they can require long runs to provide accurate approximations. Thus, approximate exact inference shares all the strengths and weaknesses of exact conditional inference, with the added worry about the precision of Monte Carlo approximations. The primary limitation of exact methods is that the conditional distributions used for inference can be highly discrete, leading to poor resolution of tail probabilities and conservative p-values. The higher-order methods discussed in the next section use continuous distributions that avoid the discreteness of exact distributions.

8.4 Higher-order and other approximations

8.4.1 Motivation

Section 8.2 described methods for exact conditional inference in exponential families. It is well known that the unconditional estimator is biased for the conditional parameters (Breslow, 1981). When the number of nuisance parameters is large, computation can be very complex, and sometimes intractable.

In settings when exact conditional inference is intractable and numerical approximations to the conditional likelihood (Section 8.3) are computationally infeasible, theoretical approximations to the conditional likelihood may be the only feasible option. Several approximations, typically involving higher-order expansions of the conditional likelihood, have been developed. In this section we provide an overview of these methods and describe the most commonly used saddlepoint approximation.

Daniels (1954) developed the saddlepoint approximation. The Edgeworth expansion of the likelihood is a power-series based expansion of the density. The Edgeworth expansion has been shown to have poor quality approximations in the tails of the distribution. The saddlepoint approximation uses a modification of the Edgeworth expansion to generate an approximate conditional estimator.

Since saddlepoint and other higher-order approximations are based on power-series expansions of the likelihood, they have the potential advantage over exact methods of being continuous in the tails.

Strawderman and Wells (1998) describe saddlepoint and higher-order approximations in this problem, and provide extensive comparison to exact methods.

8.4.2 Theory

Given $X_1, \ldots, X_n$ independent and identically distributed with expectation $E(X_i) = \mu$, variance $\text{Var}(X_i) = \sigma^2$, and cumulants κ_r, the Edgeworth expansions for the density and cumulative distribution function of

$$S_n^* = \frac{\sum (X_i - \mu)}{\sigma \sqrt{n}}$$

are given by

$$f_{S_n^*}(s) = \phi(s) \left\{ 1 + \frac{\rho_3 H_3(s)}{6\sqrt{n}} + \frac{\rho_4 H_4(s)}{24n} + \frac{\rho_3^2 H_6(s)}{72n} + O(n^{-3/2}) \right\}$$

and

$$F_{S_n^*}(s) = \Phi(s) - \phi(s) \left\{ 1 + \frac{\rho_3 H_2(s)}{6\sqrt{n}} + \frac{\rho_4 H_3(s)}{24n} + \frac{\rho_3^2 H_5(s)}{72n} + O(n^{-3/2}) \right\},$$

where $\phi(s)$ and $\Phi(s)$ are the density and cumulative distribution function of the standard normal distribution, $\rho_r = \kappa_r/\sigma^r$, and $H_i(s)$ is the ith Hermite polynomial evaluated at s (Daniels, 1954).

The saddlepoint approximation to $f_{S_n^*}(s)$ can be derived in two ways. The first derivation, which gives the method its name, involves writing the density as the inverse Fourier transform of the characteristic function. The contour of integration of this expression can be deformed so that it passes through a saddlepoint. For large sample sizes, the integrand is negligible outside the immediate neighbourhood of the saddlepoint. An expression for the density can be derived by expanding around the saddlepoint.

The second derivation, due to Daniels, involves "tilting" the Edgeworth expansion. The density of interest is multiplied by an exponential form, and then an Edgeworth expansion taken on this modified density. The expanded modified density is divided back by the exponential form.

For conditional densities, Barndorff-Nielsen and Cox (1979) derived the double saddlepoint approximation, in which the numerator and denominator of the conditional density are approximated by separate saddlepoint expansions. The problem simplifies considerably in the generalized linear model. Barndorff-Nielsen (1983) derived the likelihood for the double saddlepoint approximation in the generalized linear model, which he termed the modified profile likelihood. For a generalized linear model with parameter $\boldsymbol{\theta} = (\boldsymbol{\theta}_1, \boldsymbol{\theta}_2)$ and sufficient statistics $\mathbf{T}_1$ and $\mathbf{T}_2$ for $\boldsymbol{\theta}_1$ and $\boldsymbol{\theta}_2$ respectively, the modified profile likelihood for $\boldsymbol{\theta}_1$ conditional on the estimated $\hat{\boldsymbol{\theta}}_2$ is given by

$$L_{MP}(\boldsymbol{\theta}_1; \mathbf{t}_1 | \mathbf{T}_2 = \mathbf{t}_2) = |I_{22}(\boldsymbol{\theta}_1, \hat{\boldsymbol{\theta}}_2(\boldsymbol{\theta}_1))|^{1/2} L_P(\boldsymbol{\theta}_1, \hat{\boldsymbol{\theta}}_2(\boldsymbol{\theta}_1)), \tag{8.19}$$

where $L_P(\boldsymbol{\theta}_1, \hat{\boldsymbol{\theta}}_2(\boldsymbol{\theta}_1))$ is the profile likelihood, and $I_{ij}(\boldsymbol{\theta}_1, \boldsymbol{\theta}_2)$ is the i, jth block of the information matrix.

8.4.2.1 Likelihood

In the stratified (matched) case-control setting, the modified profile likelihood, or double saddlepoint, approximation to the exact conditional likelihood can be derived in a straightforward way. Assuming the same $\boldsymbol{\beta}$ and separate intercepts α_i for each table/cluster, Levin (1990) and Platt (1998) showed the following.

The profile (unconditional) likelihood is given in equation (8.6). To maximize the profile likelihood, one can solve the score equation for α_i^*, $i = 1, \ldots, I$, as a function of $\boldsymbol{\beta}$, and plug the corresponding $\hat{\alpha}_i^*(\boldsymbol{\beta})$ into the likelihood, leaving

$$L_P(\boldsymbol{\beta}) = \prod_{i=1}^{I} \prod_{j=0}^{M_i} \frac{\exp(d_{ij}(\hat{\alpha}_i^*(\boldsymbol{\beta}) + \mathbf{x}_j^{iT}\boldsymbol{\beta}))}{1 + \exp(\hat{\alpha}_i^*(\boldsymbol{\beta}) + \mathbf{x}_j^{iT}\boldsymbol{\beta})} \tag{8.20}$$

which can be maximized for $\boldsymbol{\beta}$. This profile likelihood has poor asymptotic properties in most settings. $\hat{\boldsymbol{\beta}}_P$, the estimator derived by maximizing $L_P(\boldsymbol{\beta})$, is biased if $I \to \infty$ as $n \to \infty$; this is inevitable given that each case forms his or her own stratum.

The modified profile likelihood $L_{MP}(\boldsymbol{\beta}|M_1, \ldots, M_I, t_1, \ldots, t_I)$ is then given by

$$L_{MP}(\boldsymbol{\beta}|M_1, \ldots, M_I, t_1, \ldots, t_I) \propto \prod_{i=1}^{I} \prod_{j=0}^{M_i} \frac{\exp(d_{ij}(\hat{\alpha}_i^*(\boldsymbol{\beta}) + \mathbf{x}_j^{iT}\boldsymbol{\beta}))}{1 + \exp(\hat{\alpha}_i^*(\boldsymbol{\beta}) + \mathbf{x}_j^{iT}\boldsymbol{\beta})} |I_\alpha(\boldsymbol{\beta}, \hat{\alpha}(\boldsymbol{\beta}))|^{1/2} \tag{8.21}$$

where M_i and t_i are the number of controls in set i, and the sufficient statistic for α_i^*, respectively.

8.4.2.2 Estimation

The modified profile likelihood (double saddlepoint) estimator can be derived either by straightforward maximization or by solving a score equation. Levin (1990) suggested a correction to the saddlepoint likelihood, score statistic and information statistic, to improve the performance near $\boldsymbol{\beta} = 0$. This correction replaces the power $\frac{1}{2}$ in equation (8.21) with $\frac{1}{2}(1 + M_i)/(1 + M_I - 1)$. Levin's correction has the effect that the modified profile likelihood and its first derivative agree with those of the exact conditional likelihood.

8.4.2.3 Hypothesis testing

Higher-order approximations give a natural tail probability approximation (Pierce and Peters, 1992). For scalar β and a test of $H_0 : \beta = \beta_0$ the tail probability is given by

$$P(T_1 \leq t | \mathbf{T}_2, \beta_0) \doteq \Phi \left(w + \frac{1}{w} \left\{ \log \rho - \log(w/z) \right\} \right). \tag{8.22}$$

Here T_1 is the sufficient statistic for β, $\mathbf{T}_2$ is the sufficient statistic for $\boldsymbol{\alpha}$, and

$$w = \text{sign} \left(\hat{\beta} - \beta_0 \right) \left\{ 2 \left[\ell_P(\hat{\beta}) - \ell_P(\beta_0) \right] \right\}^{1/2},$$

where $\ell_P(\hat{\beta})$ is the logarithm of (8.20). Further

$$z = (\hat{\beta} - \beta_0) \sqrt{I(\hat{\beta})_{11.2}} ,$$

where $I(\hat{\beta})_{11.2} = -\partial^2 \ell_P(\beta)/\partial \beta^2$, and

$$\rho = \left\{ \frac{|I(\hat{\beta}, \hat{\boldsymbol{\alpha}}(\hat{\beta}))_{22}|}{|I(\beta_0, \hat{\boldsymbol{\alpha}}(\beta_0))_{22}|} \right\}^{1/2} ,$$

where I_{22} is the component of the information matrix corresponding to the α_i^*.

If the covariates x_j^i are binary, the statistic T_1 will be integer-valued and we may improve the approximation (8.22) by modifying the value of z as described in Pierce and Peters (1992, section 4). Bedrick and Hill (1992) demonstrated the properties of higher-order tail probability approximations via simulation.

8.4.3 Other approximations

McCullagh (1984) developed approximations to the mean and variance of the noncentral hypergeometric distribution, which can be used to perform approximate conditional inference on the common odds ratio in a series of matched sets.

Let X be a noncentral hypergeometric random variable with log odds ratio parameter β, sample sizes n and m, total number of successes t, and total sample size $N = m + n$ (i.e., from a single 2×2 table). Estimators of the mean and variance of X satisfy the equations

$$\tilde{\mu}(m - t + \tilde{\mu}) + \tilde{v} = e^\beta \left\{ (t - \mu)(n - \mu) + \tilde{v} \right\}, \tag{8.23}$$

and

$$\tilde{v} = \frac{N}{N-1} \left\{ \frac{1}{\tilde{\mu}} + \frac{1}{t - \tilde{\mu}} + \frac{1}{n - \tilde{\mu}} + \frac{1}{m - t + \tilde{\mu}} \right\}^{-1}. \tag{8.24}$$

With estimates $\tilde{\mu}_i$ and $\tilde{v}_i$, $i = 1, \ldots, I$, an estimator for the odds ratio parameters discussed in this chapter can be derived using Newton-Raphson algorithms for generalized linear models. Breslow and Cologne (1986) demonstrated the properties of this estimator under a variety of settings and showed that it has reasonable properties. Platt, Leroux, and Breslow used this approximation to conduct meta-regression (Platt *et al.*, 1998).

TABLE 8.4
Results of saddlepoint analysis for Ille-et-Vilaine data. Log
odds ratio regression.

	Exact	**Uncond.**	**McCull.**	**SP (Corr.)**
Intercept	1.7026	1.7047	1.7027	1.7027
SE(Int.)	0.1998	0.2009	0.2002	0.1998
Age	-0.1255	-0.1260	-0.1255	-0.1255
SE(Age)	0.1878	0.1890	0.1883	0.1878

TABLE 8.5
Results of saddlepoint analysis for Ille-et-Vilaine data. Common OR.

	Exact	**Uncond.**	**McCull.**	**SP (Corr.)**
Intercept	1.6584	1.6699	1.6584	1.6584
SE(Int.)	0.1888	0.1899	0.1891	0.1890
95% CI	(1.273,2.049)	(1.300,2.044)	(1.273,2.049)	(1.282,2.029)

8.4.4 Implementations and application

Platt (1998) re-analyzed the data on esophageal cancer in the French department of Ille-et-Vilaine originally examined by Breslow and Day (1980). These data consisted of 200 cases of esophageal cancer diagnosed between January 1972 and April 1974 and 775 adult male controls. Subjects were stratified by age, and the alcohol consumption variable dichotomized. This gave rise to six 2×2 tables. The parameter of interest was the common odds ratio for alcohol consumption, controlling for the stratification factor age.

Tables 8.4 and 8.5 present two analyses of the Ille-et-Vilaine data. In both analyses, the parameter of interest is the odds ratio for esophageal cancer with alcohol consumption (dichotomized into high and low). Table 8.4 gives an analysis using log odds ratio regression where the log odds ratio for a given table is of the form $\beta_0 + \beta_1(x - 3.5)$ where x corresponds to age group, $x = 1, \ldots, 6$. Table 8.5 presents an analysis of the same data using a common odds ratio for alcohol consumption. For the common odds ratio problem, tail probability approximations enable the calculation of 95% confidence intervals. In both cases, the saddlepoint inference results are essentially identical to the exact conditional inference results.

8.4.5 Limitations

Higher-order approximations have some advantages over other methods, but have limitations that should be acknowledged. While higher-order approximations give tail probabilities that overcome the discrete nature of exact conditional methods, and point estimation performs well in many situations, they are approximations and biased (sometimes substantially) in small samples. Correction terms are helpful for asymptotic unbiasedness. Finally, given the ease of computation of approximate exact methods (Section 8.3), the need for these methods may be limited.

8.5 Bias-reduced and other penalized maximum likelihood approaches

8.5.1 Introduction

The maximum likelihood estimator (MLE) of the parameter $\boldsymbol{\theta}$ may be obtained by finding the root of the score function, $U(\boldsymbol{\theta})$, defined to be the derivative of the log-likelihood, $\log L(\boldsymbol{\theta})$. Firth (1993) proposed a modified score function for exponential family models and showed that the estimator defined as its root has reduced bias compared to the MLE. To describe Firth's modification, we establish notation. Let $i(\boldsymbol{\theta})$ be the Fisher information in the sample, defined to be the negative expected value of the derivative of $U(\boldsymbol{\theta})$. Further, let $b(\boldsymbol{\theta})$ be the bias of the MLE $\hat{\boldsymbol{\theta}}$ when $\boldsymbol{\theta}$ is the value of the parameter that generates the data. For exponential family models, the bias can be expanded as $b(\boldsymbol{\theta}) = b_1(\boldsymbol{\theta})/n + b_2(\boldsymbol{\theta})/n^2 + \cdots$ for a series of kth order bias terms $b_k(\boldsymbol{\theta})$; $k = 1, 2, \ldots$. Firth's modified score function is $U^*(\boldsymbol{\theta}) = U(\boldsymbol{\theta}) - i(\boldsymbol{\theta})b_1(\boldsymbol{\theta})/n$ and the estimator, $\boldsymbol{\theta}^*$, is its root. Firth shows that $\boldsymbol{\theta}^*$ eliminates the first-order bias of the MLE; i.e., the bias of $\boldsymbol{\theta}^*$ may be expressed as $b^*(\boldsymbol{\theta}) = b_2^*(\boldsymbol{\theta})/n^2 + b_3^*(\boldsymbol{\theta})/n^3 + \cdots$ for a series of bias terms $b_k^*(\boldsymbol{\theta})$; $k = 2, 3, \ldots$. He suggests that the estimator is approximately normally distributed with variance $i(\boldsymbol{\theta})^{-1}$, where $\boldsymbol{\theta}$ is the parameter value that generated the data. The variance can be estimated by $I(\boldsymbol{\theta}^*)^{-1}$, where $I(\boldsymbol{\theta}^*)$ is the observed Fisher information evaluated at $\boldsymbol{\theta}^*$.

Firth's estimator $\boldsymbol{\theta}^*$ can also be described as a maximum penalized-likelihood estimator. The penalized likelihood is $L_p(\boldsymbol{\theta}) \propto L(\boldsymbol{\theta})\sqrt{|i(\boldsymbol{\theta})|}$, obtained by multiplying the likelihood $L(\boldsymbol{\theta})$ by the Jeffreys prior for $\boldsymbol{\theta}$ (Jeffreys, 1946). The Jeffreys prior is proportional to $\sqrt{|i(\boldsymbol{\theta})|}$, the square-root of the determinant of the Fisher information in the sample and is therefore data dependent. For logistic regression models, the Jeffreys prior for the vector of regression coefficients $\boldsymbol{\theta}$ is unimodal, with mode at the origin, and is symmetric about the origin in the sense that $\sqrt{|i(\boldsymbol{\theta})|} = \sqrt{|i(-\boldsymbol{\theta})|}$ (Chen *et al.*, 2008).

When applied to logistic regression for prospective data, the approach has become known as Firth logistic regression. In this case, $\boldsymbol{\theta}$ is comprised of an intercept α and log odds ratio parameters $\boldsymbol{\beta}$. Firth shows that penalization by the Jeffreys prior has the desirable effect of shrinking the upwardly biased MLE towards the origin. The shrinkage estimator always exists, even when the MLE does not exist in the case of separation. In contrast, "corrective" estimators which subtract an estimate of the bias from the MLE exist only if the MLE does. Alternate penalties have been proposed (e.g., Gelman *et al.*, 2008; Greenland and Mansournia, 2015) offering more or less shrinkage than the Jeffreys prior.

In this section, we discuss Firth and related penalized-likelihood estimators for case-control data. Firth logistic regression applied to case-control data can be viewed as a penalized-*profile*-likelihood approach, because the prospective likelihood is a profile likelihood for retrospective data (Section 8.1.3). However, the penalty term now lacks Firth's justification, because the Fisher information and first-order bias terms are expectations under different probability distributions. In the case-control setting, the expectations are with respect to $P(\mathbf{x}|D)$, the distribution of covariates given disease status while, in the prospective setting, expectations are with respect to $P(D|\mathbf{x})$. Thus, Firth logistic regression for case-control data remains to be justified.

The parametrization of the model for case-control data includes a covariate distribution function (unmatched data) or multiple covariate distribution functions (matched data) which are, in general, infinite-dimensional parameters. It is not clear how to extend Firth's approach, developed for finite-dimensional parameters, to the infinite-dimensional setting. One approach is to first eliminate the covariate distribution(s) by conditioning on their sufficient statistics, and then penalize the resulting conditional likelihood. This is the approach taken by Heinze and Puhr (2010) for matched case-control data. We are not aware of a similar bias-reduced estimator for unmatched case-control data, perhaps because the conditional likelihood for unmatched data involves a sum over all possible permutations of the cases and controls that is computationally expensive to evaluate even for moderate sample sizes (Breslow and Day, 1980, p. 205). Rather than conditioning, Zhang (2006) uses a profile-likelihood approach to eliminate the covariate distribution for unmatched data, applying a Firth-like correction to the score function obtained by differentiating the profile log-likelihood.

We next discuss methods for unmatched and matched case-control data, respectively. For unmatched data, we begin with Zhang's approach and then discuss application of Firth logistic regression and the penalized logistic regression estimators of Greenland and Mansournia (2015) to case-control data. For matched case-control data, we discuss Firth logistic regression applied to a model that includes stratum effects for the matched sets and Heinze and Puhr's approach, which we call Firth *conditional* logistic regression.

8.5.2 Methods

8.5.2.1 Unmatched case-control data

Zhang's approach is based on the profile likelihood in equation (8.5). The MLE is the root of the profile score function of $(\alpha^*, \boldsymbol{\beta})$, which is the derivative of the corresponding log-profile-likelihood. Let $\boldsymbol{\theta} = (\alpha^*, \boldsymbol{\beta})$ and $U_p(\boldsymbol{\theta})$ be the profile score function. Zhang proposes a Firth-like modification, $U_p(\boldsymbol{\theta}) - i_p(\boldsymbol{\theta})b_1(\boldsymbol{\theta})/n$, of the profile score function, where the information term $i_p(\boldsymbol{\theta})$ is minus the expected derivative of the profile score function, and $b_1(\boldsymbol{\theta})$ is the first-order bias of the MLE of $\boldsymbol{\theta}$. However, as expectations, both $i_p(\boldsymbol{\theta})$ and $b_1(\boldsymbol{\theta})$ depend on the unknown covariate distribution, g, that generated the data, and so cannot be evaluated. Let $\hat{i}_p(\boldsymbol{\theta})$ and $\hat{b}_1(\boldsymbol{\theta})$ be the information and bias terms of the profile log-likelihood for $\boldsymbol{\theta}$ with g replaced by $\hat{g}_{\boldsymbol{\theta}}$, the distribution that maximizes the likelihood for fixed $\boldsymbol{\theta}$. Then the modified profile score function, $U_p^*(\boldsymbol{\theta}) = U_p(\boldsymbol{\theta}) - \hat{i}_p(\boldsymbol{\theta})\hat{b}_1(\boldsymbol{\theta})/n$, can be evaluated for given $\boldsymbol{\theta}$. The estimator is the root of $U_p^*(\boldsymbol{\theta})$, denoted $\boldsymbol{\theta}_p^*$, which we label the Zhang logistic regression estimator. In parallel with Firth logistic regression, one can integrate $U_p^*(\boldsymbol{\theta})$ and exponentiate to obtain a penalized profile likelihood; thus, Zhang logistic regression can also be viewed as a penalized profile likelihood approach.

An alternative to Zhang's approach for estimating $\boldsymbol{\beta}$ is to apply Firth logistic regression for prospective data, ignoring the case-control sampling design, and then extract $\boldsymbol{\beta}^*$ from $\boldsymbol{\theta}^*$. Zhang notes that his estimator $\boldsymbol{\beta}_p^*$ is different from $\boldsymbol{\beta}^*$ *except* when the design is balanced in terms of the number of cases and controls. However, in simulations with large (Ma *et al.*, 2013) and small (Supplementary Materials) sample sizes, both Zhang and Firth logistic regression gave very similar point estimates and standard errors, even for unbalanced case-control data sets with 1 : 4 case:control ratios.

Greenland and Mansournia (2015) instead propose a penalty term that is the product of independent log-$F(m, m)$ distributions for each regression parameter, other than the intercept. As m increases, each prior distribution becomes more concentrated about zero, increasing the amount of shrinkage. Greenland and Mansournia recommend against penalizing α^*, which is rarely in a neighbourhood of zero. Although there is no simple rule-of-thumb for choosing m, these authors suggest reporting analyses under the minimal log-$F(1, 1)$ penalty and other more concentrated priors with higher m.

Conveniently, penalization by a log-$F(m, m)$ prior can be achieved with standard GLM software through data augmentation, as follows. For each covariate, we add one observation of $m/2$ successes and $m/2$ failures (allowing for $m/2$ to be noninteger), and a single row to

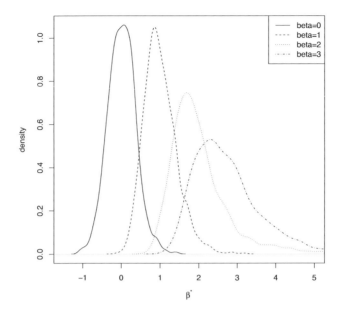

FIGURE 8.4

Density estimates of the distribution of the Firth logistic regression estimator, β^*, from simulations of data sets of 10 cases and 40 controls. We simulated 1000 replicate data sets with a single covariate having a standard normal distribution in controls. The covariate effect sizes were $\beta = 0$, 1, 2, or 3.

the design matrix comprised of all zeroes, except for a single one at the index of the covariate being penalized. Analyzing the augmented data set with ordinary logistic regression gives the penalized estimates and standard errors (Greenland and Mansournia, 2015).

Inference from penalized profile likelihood approaches can be based on Wald statistics. However, for small or sparse data sets, such Wald-based confidence intervals can have poor coverage properties, due to a breakdown in the normal approximation, particularly for large effect sizes. For example, Figure 8.4 shows density estimates of the distribution of the Firth estimator, β^*, in simulations of case-control data sets comprised of a single covariate measured in 10 cases and 40 controls. The distribution of the estimator becomes increasingly skewed to the right as β increases.

For prospective data, Heinze and Schemper (2002) recommend inference based on penalized-likelihood ratio statistics rather than Wald statistics. Let β_k be the kth component of $\boldsymbol{\theta}$. The test statistic for $H_0 : \beta_k = \beta_{k0}$ is twice the log of the ratio of two penalized likelihood values, one at the maximizer over the entire parameter space Θ, and the other at the maximizer over the null hypothesis-restricted subset $\{\boldsymbol{\theta} \in \Theta : \beta_k = \beta_{k0}\}$. The penalized-likelihood ratio statistic is assumed to have an approximate chi-squared distribution on one degree of freedom (Heinze and Schemper, 2002). The test can be inverted to give confidence intervals. Limited simulations with case-control data (results not shown) suggest that interval estimates based on penalized-likelihood ratio statistics achieve nominal coverage, within simulation error, whereas those based on Wald statistics do not.

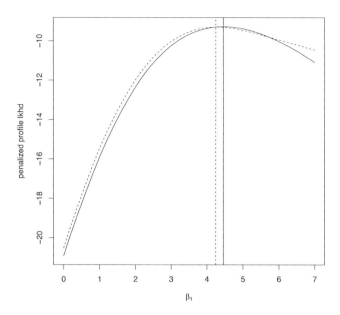

FIGURE 8.5
Penalized profile likelihoods for the DES effect using the penalty derived by saddlepoint approximation (solid curve) or by Firth's approach (dashed curve). The corresponding maximum penalized-profile-likelihood estimators are indicated by vertical lines.

8.5.2.2 Matched case-control data

Heinze and Puhr (2010) discuss several Firth-type approaches to estimation from matched case-control data. One of the possibilities is stratified Firth logistic regression. That is, we penalize the stratified prospective likelihood $L_S(\boldsymbol{\alpha}^*, \boldsymbol{\beta})$ in equation (8.6) by $|I(\boldsymbol{\alpha}^*, \boldsymbol{\beta})|^{1/2}$, where $I(\boldsymbol{\alpha}^*, \boldsymbol{\beta})$ is the observed Fisher information from the prospective model. The penalty term $|I(\boldsymbol{\alpha}^*, \boldsymbol{\beta})|^{1/2}$ is of similar form to the penalty $|I_{\boldsymbol{\alpha}^*}(\hat{\boldsymbol{\alpha}}^*(\boldsymbol{\beta}), \boldsymbol{\beta})|^{1/2}$ in the modified profile likelihood of Section 8.4, derived through saddlepoint approximation (saddlepoint-penalized likelihood). However, the profile likelihoods being penalized are slightly different. The saddlepoint approach penalizes $L_P(\boldsymbol{\beta}) = L_S(\hat{\boldsymbol{\alpha}}^*(\boldsymbol{\beta}), \boldsymbol{\beta})$, the stratified likelihood $L_S(\boldsymbol{\alpha}^*, \boldsymbol{\beta})$ with $\boldsymbol{\alpha}^*$ profiled out, whereas the Firth approach penalizes $L_S(\boldsymbol{\alpha}^*, \boldsymbol{\beta})$. Figure 8.5 shows the Firth- and saddlepoint-penalized profile likelihoods for the DES effect. Though the two curves are very similar, the Firth-penalized likelihood estimate is shrunken slightly more toward the origin than the saddlepoint-penalized likelihood for these data. Indeed, in our simulations (see Supplementary Materials), we find that the Firth estimator is consistently shrunk more toward the origin than the saddlepoint estimator.

Though Heinze and Puhr discuss stratified Firth logistic regression for matched case-control data, they ultimately recommend a Firth *conditional* logistic regression approach that maximizes a conditional likelihood penalized by an empirical version of its Jeffreys prior. The conditional likelihood, $L_c(\boldsymbol{\beta})$, is given in our equation (8.9). This is the conditional probability of the sufficient statistic, $\mathbf{T}_{\boldsymbol{\beta}}$, for $\boldsymbol{\beta}$, given the sufficient statistic, $\mathbf{T}_{\mathbf{g}}$, for the covariate distributions $\mathbf{g}$. The Jeffreys prior is proportional to $\sqrt{|i_c(\boldsymbol{\beta})|}$, where the conditional Fisher information in the sample, $i_c(\boldsymbol{\beta})$, is minus the expected value of the second

TABLE 8.6
Estimates, standard errors, and 95% confidence intervals for
the DES effect, adjusted for maternal smoking, from the
different penalized profile likelihood approaches. For
comparison, exact logistic regression (unmatched) and exact
conditional logistic regression (matched) MUEs and
confidence intervals are shown.

Method	Est.	Std. err.	95% CI
Unmatched analyses:			
Zhang	5.334	1.629	NA
Firth	5.336	1.647	(2.889,10.25)
log-$F(1,1)$	5.625	1.690	(2.922,10.63)
log-$F(2,2)$	4.508	1.294	(2.330, 7.73)
exact	4.549	NA	(2.432, ∞)
Matched analyses:			
Firth	4.096	1.289	(2.152,8.322)
Firth cond'l	3.569	1.291	(1.720,8.331)
exact	3.190	NA	(1.425, ∞)

derivative of $\log L_c(\boldsymbol{\beta})$. The empirical Jeffreys prior is obtained by replacing $i_c(\boldsymbol{\beta})$ by the *observed* Fisher information in the sample, denoted $I_c(\boldsymbol{\beta})$. The penalized conditional likelihood is then $L_c^*(\boldsymbol{\beta}) = L_c(\boldsymbol{\beta})\sqrt{|I_c(\boldsymbol{\beta})|}$. Heinze and Puhr recommend tests and confidence intervals derived from penalized-likelihood ratio statistics, analogous to those in Heinze and Schemper (2002).

8.5.3   Implementation and application

8.5.3.1   Unmatched case-control data

For Zhang logistic regression, we implemented the point estimator and standard errors in R. For Firth logistic regression, we used the `logistf()` function from the `logistf` R package (Heinze *et al.*, 2013). For log-$F(m,m)$ penalized logistic regression, we implemented the estimator, standard errors and penalized-profile-likelihood confidence intervals using the data augmentation approach discussed above and the `glm()` function in R.

We applied the Zhang, Firth, log-$F(1,1)$, and log-$F(2,2)$ penalized logistic regression estimators to the DES data, ignoring the matching and adjusting for the effect of maternal smoking. The results are presented in Table 8.6. The Zhang and Firth estimates and standard errors are very similar. In terms of shrinkage of the point estimate towards zero, the log-$F(1,1)$ penalty shrinks the least, the Zhang and Firth penalties shrink slightly more, and the log-$F(2,2)$ penalty shrinks the most. As expected, the standard errors and confidence interval widths are ordered inversely to the amount of shrinkage, with log-$F(1,1)$ having the largest spreads, Zhang/Firth next, and log-$F(2,2)$ the smallest.

8.5.3.2   Matched case-control data

For stratified Firth logistic regression we used the `logistf()` function from the `logistf` package. For Firth conditional logistic regression we used the `coxphf` R package (Heinze and Ploner, 2002; Ploner and Heinze, 2015) for penalized proportional hazards regression (G. Heinze, personal communication).

We applied stratified Firth logistic regression and Firth conditional logistic regression to the DES data, accounting for the matching and adjusting for the effect of maternal smoking.

The results are presented in Table 8.6, along with those of exact conditional logistic regression, for comparison. Of the two Firth approaches, the Firth conditional logistic regression estimate is the closest to the estimate from exact conditional logistic regression, presumably because both the exact and Firth conditional estimators are based on conditional distributions that eliminate the stratum effects.

8.5.4 Limitations

In Firth logistic regression, the penalty is designed to reduce bias under prospective sampling. In contrast, the penalty in Zhang logistic regression is designed to reduce bias under retrospective sampling and is therefore better justified for application to case-control data. Under case-control sampling, the penalties in both Firth and Zhang logistic regression correspond to data-dependent prior distributions, whereas log-$F(m, m)$ penalties are data-independent. In the Bayesian paradigm, a data-dependent prior distribution may be viewed as an approximation to a data-independent prior distribution that depends on some unknown parameter that has been estimated from the data. From the Bayesian standpoint, one problematic aspect of both Firth and Zhang logistic regression is that the identity of the data-independent priors being approximated is unclear (Greenland and Mansournia, 2015). While there is no formal justification for applying Firth logistic regression to case-control data, it appears to perform well in practice for small samples (Supplementary Materials). However, confidence intervals based on large-sample approximations to Wald statistics can perform badly for both Firth and Zhang logistic regression when applied to small case-control samples. Instead, we recommend confidence intervals based on penalized-likelihood-ratio statistics, which outperformed Wald-based intervals in our own limited simulations and the simulation investigations of others (Heinze and Schemper, 2002; Heinze and Puhr, 2010). More work is required to theoretically justify the application of Firth logistic regression to case-control data and assess its limitations.

8.6 Conclusions

There are numerous challenges with small samples, including the following: the finite-sample bias of the MLE can be substantial; large-sample approximate distributions used for inference may be unreliable; and standard ML inference may not be possible due to separation. We have reviewed inference methods for both unmatched and matched case-control designs that address some of these challenges. The methods can be classified as either exact conditional, including approximate exact conditional, or penalized likelihood.

In the Supplementary Materials we review simulation studies conducted by Heinze and Schemper (2002) and Heinze and Puhr (2010), and detail our own limited simulations. For sample sizes of 100 or less, the broad conclusions from these simulations is that penalized maximum likelihood methods are preferred over exact conditional and standard ML methods. For unmatched data, we found that log-$F(2, 2)$-penalized likelihood inference performed best of all methods considered in terms of absolute bias and MSE of the point estimator, as well as power. Another attractive feature of log-$F(m, m)$-penalized methods is that they can be implemented with standard logistic regression software through data augmentation. For matched data, penalized methods are preferable to exact and standard ML methods, but within the class of penalized methods results are inconclusive. The inconclusive results suggest the need for additional simulation studies to compare performance among existing penalized methods, as well as the potential for developing new penalized methods for matched case-control data based on log-$F(m, m)$ priors.

Bibliography

Agresti, A. (1992). A survey of exact inference for contingency tables. *Statistical Science*, **7**, 131–153.

Agresti, A. (2013). *Categorical Data Analysis*. John Wiley & Sons, Hoboken, 3rd edition.

Albert, A. and Anderson, J. A. (1984). On the existence of maximum likelihood estimates in logistic regression models. *Biometrika*, **71**, 1–10.

Barndorff-Nielsen, O. E. (1983). On a formula for the distribution of the maximum likelihood estimator. *Biometrika*, **70**, 343–365.

Barndorff-Nielsen, O. E. and Cox, D. R. (1979). Edgeworth and saddle-point approximations with statistical applications. *Journal of the Royal Statistical Society: Series B (Statistical Methodology)*, **41**, 279–312.

Bedrick, E. and Hill, J. (1992). An empirical assessment of saddlepoint approximations for testing a logistic regression parameter. *Biometrics*, **48**, 529–544.

Breslow, N. E. (1981). Odds ratio estimators when the data are sparse. *Biometrika*, **68**, 73–84.

Breslow, N. E. and Cologne, J. (1986). Methods of estimation in log odds ratio regression models. *Biometrics*, **42**, 949–954.

Breslow, N. E. and Day, N. E. (1980). *Statistical Methods for Cancer Research: Volume 1 – The Analysis of Case-Control Data*. IARC Scientific Publications, Lyon.

Campbell, I. (2007). Chi-squared and Fisher-Irwin tests of two-by-two tables with small sample recommendations. *Statistics in Medicine*, **26**, 3661–3675.

Chen, M.-H., Ibrahim, J. G., and Kim, S. (2008). Properties and implementation of Jeffreys's prior in binomial regression models. *Journal of the American Statistical Association*, **103**, 1659–1664.

Cox, D. R. (1970). *The Analysis of Binary Data*. Methuen, London.

Cytel Inc. (2015). *LogXact 11 Manual*. Cambridge, MA.

Daniels, H. (1954). Saddlepoint approximations in statistic. *Annals of Mathematical Statistics*, **25**, 631–650.

Firth, D. (1993). Bias reduction of maximum likelihood estimates. *Biometrika*, **80**, 27–38.

Fisher, R. A. (1934). *Statistical Methods for Research Workers*. Oliver and Boyd, Edinburgh, 5th edition.

Forster, J. J., McDonald, J. W., and Smith, P. W. (2003). Markov chain Monte Carlo exact inference for binomial and multinomial logistic regression models. *Statistics and Computing*, **13**, 169–177.

Gelman, A., Jakulin, A., Pittau, M. G., and Su, Y.-S. (2008). A weakly informative default prior distribution for logistic and other regression models. *The Annals of Applied Statistics*, **2**, 1360–1383.

Godambe, V. P. (1976). Conditional likelihood and unconditional optimum estimating equations. *Biometrika*, **63**, 277–284.

Greenland, S. and Mansournia, M. A. (2015). Penalization, bias reduction, and default priors in logistic and related categorical and survival regressions. *Statistics in Medicine*, **34**, 3133–3143.

Heinze, G. and Ploner, M. (2002). SAS and SPLUS programs to perform Cox regression without convergence problems. *Computer Methods and Programs in Biomedicine*, **67**, 217–223.

Heinze, G. and Puhr, R. (2010). Bias-reduced and separation-proof conditional logistic regression with small or sparse data sets. *Statistics in Medicine*, **29**, 770–777.

Heinze, G. and Schemper, M. (2002). A solution to the problem of separation in logistic regression. *Statistics in Medicine*, **21**, 2409–2419.

Heinze, G., Ploner, M., Dunkler, D., and Southworth, H. (2013). *logistf: Firth's bias reduced logistic regression*. R package version 1.21.

Herbst, A. L., Ulfelder, H., and Poskanzer, D. C. (1971). Adenocarcinoma of the vagina. *New England Journal of Medicine*, **284**, 878–881.

Hirji, K. F., Mehta, C. R., and Patel, N. R. (1987). Computing distributions for exact logistic regression. *Journal of the American Statistical Association*, **82**, 1110–1117.

Hirji, K. F., Tsiatis, A. A., and Mehta, C. R. (1989). Median unbiased estimation for binary data. *The American Statistician*, **43**, 7–11.

Jeffreys, H. (1946). An invariant form for the prior probability in estimation problems. *Proceedings of the Royal Society of London A: Mathematical, Physical and Engineering Sciences*, **186**, 453–461.

Levin, B. (1990). The saddlepoint correction in conditional logistic likelihood analysis. *Biometrika*, **77**, 275–285.

Ma, C., Blackwell, T., Boehnke, M., and Scott, L. J. (2013). Recommended joint and meta-analysis strategies for case-control association testing of single low-count variants. *Genetic Epidemiology*, **37**, 539–550.

McCullagh, P. (1984). On the elimination of nuisance parameters in the proportional odds model. *Journal of the Royal Statistical Society: Series B (Statistical Methodology)*, **46**, 250–256.

Mehta, C. R. and Patel, N. R. (1995). Exact logistic regression: Theory and examples. *Statistics in Medicine*, **14**, 2143–2160.

Mehta, C. R., Patel, N. R., and Senchaudhuri, P. (2000). Efficient Monte Carlo methods for conditional logistic regression. *Journal of the American Statistical Association*, **95**, 99–108.

Pierce, D. and Peters, D. (1992). Practical use of higher order asymptotics for multiparameter exponential families. *Journal of the Royal Statistical Society: Series B (Statistical Methodology)*, **54**, 701–737.

Platt, R. W. (1998). Estimation using the modified profile likelihood in log odds ratio regression analysis. *Communications in Statistics: Simulation and Computation*, **27**, 905–920.

Platt, R. W., Leroux, B., and Breslow, N. E. (1998). Generalized linear mixed models for meta-analysis. *Statistics in Medicine*, **17**, 643–654.

Ploner, M. and Heinze, G. (2015). *coxphf: Cox regression with Firth's penalized likelihood*. R package version 1.11.

Prentice, R. L. and Pyke, R. (1979). Logistic disease incidence models and case-control studies. *Biometrika*, **66**, 403–411.

Qin, J. and Zhang, B. (1997). A goodness-of-fit test for logistic regression models based on case-control data. *Biometrika*, **84**, 609–618.

Read, C. B. (1985). Median unbiased estimator. In S. Kotz and N. L. Johnson, editors, *Encyclopedia of Statistical Sciences*, volume 5, pages 424–426. John Wiley, New York.

Scott, A. J. and Wild, C. J. (2001). Maximum likelihood for generalised case-control studies. *Journal of Statistical Planning and Inference*, **96**, 3–27.

Strawderman, R. L. and Wells, M. T. (1998). Approximately exact inference for the common odds ratio in several 2×2 tables. *Journal of the American Statistical Association*, **93**, 1294–1307.

Zamar, D. (2006). *Markov Chain Monte Carlo Exact Inference for Logistic Regression*. Master's thesis, Simon Fraser University, Burnaby, BC, Canada.

Zamar, D., McNeney, B., and Graham, J. (2007). elrm: Software implementing exact-like inference for logistic regression models. *Journal of Statistical Software*, **21**, 1–18.

Zhang, B. (2006). Bias-corrected maximum semiparametric likelihood estimation under logistic regression models based on case-control data. *Journal of Statistical Planning and Inference*, **136**, 108–124.

9

Power and Sample Size for Case-Control Studies

Mitchell H. Gail

National Cancer Institute

Sebastien Haneuse

Harvard University

9.1   Introduction

9.1.1   General considerations

Protocols for case-control studies usually require a statistical calculation of the required sample size and power of the proposed study. To some this may seem to be a perfunctory exercise. However, in order to compute power or required sample size, one must understand the objectives of the study, the measurements to be used, the hypotheses to be tested, and the planned statistical analysis. Indeed, one can often learn a lot about the proposed study by reading the section on sample size first.

Case-control studies are usually designed to test for an association between an exposure, X, and dichotomous disease outcome, D, where $D = 1$ for a case and $D = 0$ for a noncase

TABLE 9.1
Cross-classification of disease
status D and dichotomous
exposure X.

Exposure	Disease status	
	$D = 0$	$D = 1$
$X = 0$	N_{00}	N_{01}
$X = 1$	N_{10}	N_{11}

(control). They can also be used to estimate the strength of the association between X and D, often expressed as the logarithm of the odds ratio,

$$\beta = \log \left[\frac{P(D = 1|\ X = x + 1)P(D = 0|\ X = x)}{P(D = 0|\ X = x + 1)P(D = 1|\ X = x)} \right]$$

$$= \log \left[\frac{P(X = x + 1|\ D = 1)P(X = x|\ D = 0)}{P(X = x + 1|\ D = 0)P(X = x|\ D = 1)} \right].$$

When X takes on values 0 and 1, the data can be summarized as in Table 9.1 and the maximum likelihood estimate is

$$\widehat{\beta} = \log \left(\frac{N_{11}N_{00}}{N_{01}N_{10}} \right).$$

This is true whether the data arose from a cohort study in which N_{0+} and N_{1+} are fixed by design or from a case-control study in which the number of controls, N_{+0}, and the number of cases, N_{+1}, are fixed (Cornfield, 1951). Exact conditional inference on β can be obtained by conditioning on all the margins of the table (Fisher's "exact" test; Cox (1970)). Large-sample inference on β from case-control data is the same as if a cohort design had been used; however inference on the logistic intercept is not the same (Prentice and Pyke, 1979).

One possible objective of the case-control study is to estimate β with a required degree of precision. Because the sample size determines the variance of $\widehat{\beta}$, a criterion like $\sqrt{\mathrm{Var}(\widehat{\beta})} \leq c$ will only be satisfied with large enough samples of cases and controls. A second objective might be to test the null hypothesis of $\beta = \beta_0$. Hereafter, we will be interested in the null hypothesis of no association, i.e., $H_0 : \beta = 0$. The power, γ, of a statistical test of the null hypothesis is the probability, under the alternative hypothesis, that the test will lead to rejection of the null hypothesis at significance level α. Sample size is often chosen to assure the power equals or exceeds a certain value; we will often use $\gamma = 0.9$. Although sample sizes are sometimes chosen to achieve a desired precision (Lemeshow *et al.*, 1988), we will focus on the calculation of sample sizes needed to achieve a fixed level of power, γ.

Why is it important to calculate power? Such a calculation can reveal whether the experiment has a good chance of providing statistically significant evidence of the hypothesized association, $\beta \neq 0$. If the power is small, the investigator should not proceed, because the experiment is unlikely to achieve its objective. If the hypothesis is worth pursuing, it is worth redesigning the study and if necessary increasing sample size to achieve acceptable power. In this chapter we will describe some simple ways to estimate power as well as more sophisticated techniques that more accurately estimate power in the presence of complicating factors, such as confounding and measurement error. But even the simpler methods can often reveal whether an experiment is futile.

Another reason for designing a study with sufficient power concerns its contribution to the literature. As pointed out in Table I of Peto *et al.* (1976), the probability that a statistically significant result truly represents a nonnull association is an increasing function of the study's power. A small study with p-value of, say, 0.01 is not as convincing as a larger similarly designed study with p-value of 0.01. This can be seen from a Bayesian calculation of positive predictive value (PPV) of the statistically significant result:

$$\text{PPV} = \frac{\pi\gamma}{\pi\gamma + (1-\pi)\alpha},$$

where π is the prior probability that $\beta \neq 0$.

9.1.2 Power calculations

In order to calculate required sample size, one needs to specify the proposed test statistic, α, γ, and the hypothesized nonnull parameter, θ. In Section 9.1.1, $\theta = \beta$, but θ could refer to any one-dimensional parameter of interest, such as the expected value of a score. Choosing θ requires subject matter knowledge to understand how strong the association needs to be to have practical importance. The proposed θ should also be consistent with other data that might be available concerning this exposure and disease outcome. Sample size varies inversely with θ^2 and is thus highly dependent on θ [see equations (9.1) and (9.2)].

If the parameter of interest, θ, is one-dimensional, as in the examples above, the test statistic is often asymptotically equivalent to a test with critical region

$$T > Z_{1-\alpha}\widehat{\sigma}_0 n^{-1/2},$$

where $Z_{1-\alpha} = \Phi^{-1}(1-\alpha)$ is the $(1-\alpha)$th quantile of the standard normal distribution, n is the sample size (explained further below), and $n^{1/2}T$ is normally distributed with null mean 0 and null variance σ_0^2, which is consistently estimated by $\widehat{\sigma}_0^2$. Under the alternative hypothesis ($\theta > 0$), T is normally distributed with mean θ and variance σ_θ^2/n. Then the power is approximately

$$\gamma = P_\theta(T > Z_{1-\alpha}\sigma_0 n^{-1/2}) = 1 - \Phi\left\{\frac{(Z_{1-\alpha}\sigma_0 n^{-1/2} - \theta)}{\sigma_\theta n^{-1/2}}\right\}.$$

Inverting this equation, we obtain the sample size formula:

$$n = \frac{\{-\Phi^{-1}(1-\gamma)\sigma_\theta + Z_{1-\alpha}\sigma_0\}^2}{\theta^2} = \frac{\{Z_\gamma\sigma_\theta + Z_{1-\alpha}\sigma_0\}^2}{\theta^2}. \tag{9.1}$$

If, instead, the critical region is

$$T > Z_{1-\alpha}\widehat{\sigma}_\theta n^{-1/2},$$

where $\widehat{\sigma}_\theta^2$ is a consistent estimate for σ_θ^2, then the sample size is given by

$$n = \frac{\sigma_\theta^2 \{Z_\gamma + Z_{1-\alpha}\}^2}{\theta^2}. \tag{9.2}$$

We are evaluating two different test statistics, depending on whether one used critical value $Z_{1-\alpha}\widehat{\sigma}_0 n^{-1/2}$ or $Z_{1-\alpha}\widehat{\sigma}_\theta n^{-1/2}$. These test statistics both have size α, but their powers and required sample sizes usually differ. These calculations are for a one-sided alternative, $\theta > 0$. Many journals require two-sided tests, which can be accommodated by setting the previous α to $\alpha/2$. Equations (9.1) and (9.2) are equal for the comparison of two populations of normally distributed variables with equal variances $\sigma_0^2 = \sigma_\theta^2 = \sigma^2$, in which case $n\theta^2/\sigma^2$ is called the noncentrality of the corresponding chi-square test. In Section 9.3 we specialize these formulas for case-control studies, where n is the number of cases plus controls.

We will assume that tests are based on asymptotically normally distributed statistics in this chapter. If exact conditional tests are used with small samples, there is usually some loss of power compared to unconditional tests. Power calculations are available for exact conditional tests (Gail and Gart, 1973); see also Cytel Studio®10 (Cytel Inc., 2012).

The remainder of this chapter is organized as follows. In Section 9.2 we introduce an example to motivate sample size calculations and to provide realistic distributions for power calculations based on simulations. In Section 9.3, we consider unmatched case-control designs and give sample size formulas derived within the framework of logistic regression for various types of exposures. Sample size calculations are also presented for logistic models with adjustment for confounders. These calculations require additional information regarding the joint distributions of exposure and confounders and the strength of the confounders' effects on disease outcome. We also discuss tests for interactions within the unconditional logistic framework. Section 9.4 describes simple methods for matched case-control data. Other factors influence required sample size, including measurement error in exposures (Section 9.5), missing data (Section 9.6), and control for multiplicity in discovery studies (Section 9.7). Although analytic approaches, such as illustrated in Section 9.3 are often sufficient, simulation methods to estimate power are more flexible and can handle more realistic complexities of case-control design (Section 9.8). Some comments on software (Section 9.9) precede a brief discussion (Section 9.10).

9.2   Population-based case-control study of breast cancer in Poland

Women with incident breast cancer (cases) aged 20-74 years and diagnosed between 2000 and 2003 in Warsaw or Łódź were compared to controls who were frequency matched to cases on city and 5-year age group and sampled using the Polish Electronic System, which has demographic data on all residents of Poland (Garcia-Closas *et al.*, 2006). We use data from the 1,968 cases and 2,162 controls with complete information on age, education level (0=none, 1=completed elementary school, 2=some high school, 3=completed high school, 4=training after high school, 5=some college, 6=graduated college, 7=post-graduate/professional), age at first birth (years), age at menarche (years), history of a biopsy for benign breast disease (0=0, 1=at least one), family history of breast cancer (0=0, 1=at least one female relative), and body mass index (BMI in kg/m^2).

The means and standard deviations of risk factor values are shown in Table 9.2 separately for cases and controls. The ages are similar because of frequency matching. Increased risk is associated with higher educational level, delayed first birth, early age at menarche, previous benign breast biopsy, and family history. Increasing BMI is protective in these data, in both women under age 50 and women aged 50 or more (Section 9.8.3), whereas other studies have found that increased BMI is protective in pre- but not post-menopausal women.

The estimated variances, covariances, and correlations for the risk factors are presented separately for cases and controls in Table 9.3. Higher education level is positively correlated with age at first birth and benign breast biopsy, and inversely correlated with age, age at menarche, and BMI. We will use these data to motivate and compare sample size calculations.

TABLE 9.2
Means and standard deviations (SD) of risk factor levels in cases and controls in the Polish breast cancer study, together with log odds ratio (OR) estimates, standard error (SE) estimates, and p-values from separate univariate logistic regressions.

Risk factor	Cases $(n_1=1,968)$		Controls $(n_0=2,162)$		Estimated log OR (SE)	Two-sided p-value
	Mean	SD	Mean	SD		
Age (yrs)[†]	55.7	9.94	55.9	9.98	-0.020 (0.031)	0.519
Education (0-7)	3.4	1.76	2.9	1.60	0.169 (0.019)	<0.001
Age 1st birth (yrs)	24.5	4.61	23.6	4.22	0.220 (0.036)	<0.001
Age menarche (yrs)[‡]	13.5	1.71	13.7	1.72	-0.061 (0.018)	0.001
Benign biopsy (0,1)	0.10	0.30	0.06	0.25	0.485 (0.115)	<0.001
Family history (0,1)	0.11	0.31	0.06	0.23	0.678 (0.118)	<0.001
BMI (kg/m^2)[‡]	27.4	5.38	28.0	5.33	-0.116 (0.029)	<0.001

[†] log odds ratio for a 10-year contrast

[‡] log odds ratio for a 5-unit contrast

TABLE 9.3
Variances, covariances (above the diagonal), and correlations (below the diagonal) for the cases and controls in the Polish breast cancer data.

Cases	Age	Education	Age first birth	Age menarche	Benign biopsy	Family history	BMI
Age	98.5	-2.53	-2.75	3.22	-0.15	0.12	16.1
Education	-0.15	3.09	2.61	-0.31	0.05	0.01	-1.50
Age first birth	-0.06	0.32	21.3	0.22	0.06	0.00	-1.85
Age menarche	0.19	-0.10	0.03	2.91	0.00	0.01	-0.17
Benign biopsy	-0.05	0.09	0.04	0.00	0.09	0.01	-0.14
Family history	0.04	0.02	0.00	0.02	0.06	0.10	0.02
BMI	0.30	-0.16	-0.08	-0.02	-0.84	0.01	29.0

Controls	Age	Education	Age first birth	Age menarche	Benign biopsy	Family history	BMI
Age	99.6	-3.01	-1.81	1.91	-0.03	0.11	11.5
Education	-0.19	2.56	2.18	-0.32	0.05	0.02	-1.46
Age first birth	-0.04	0.32	17.8	0.44	0.05	0.01	-3.12
Age menarche	0.11	-0.12	0.06	2.95	-0.02	0.00	-0.32
Benign biopsy	-0.01	0.14	0.05	-0.04	0.06	0.01	-0.04
Family history	0.05	0.06	0.01	0.07	0.08	0.05	0.05
BMI	0.22	-0.17	-0.14	-0.03	-0.03	0.04	28.4

9.3 Unmatched case-control study: Sample size for logistic models

9.3.1 A single exposure covariate

In this section, we study methods to analyze a single exposure X that may be binary, ordinal, or continuous, so long as the logit of disease probability is linear in X. In unmatched case-control studies, a random sample of cases from the source population is compared to a random sample of controls from the population. The controls in the Polish study were matched to cases and are therefore slightly older than a simple random sample of controls. We ignore this feature in this section, realizing that estimates of age effects are biased toward 0. There is a vast literature on sample size calculations to cover the cases of dichotomous exposure, as for example in Chapter 7 of Breslow and Day (1987), and logit-linear exposure models for ordered categorical exposures or continuous exposures for this design (McKeown-Eyssen and Thomas, 1985; Lubin *et al.*, 1988; Novikov *et al.*, 2010). We can cover all these cases by considering the logistic model:

$$\text{logit}\{P(D = 1 \mid X)\} = \beta_0 + \beta X. \tag{9.3}$$

If $X = 0$ or 1 then $\exp(\beta)$ is the dichotomous odds ratio. If $X = 0, 1, \ldots, K$, then $\exp(\beta)$ is the odds ratio increase per category for $K + 1$ ordered categories. If X is continuous, the $\exp(\beta)$ is the odds ratio per unit increase in X. We consider four tests of the null hypothesis $\beta = 0$, two based on the Wald statistics and two based on score tests.

From Prentice and Pyke (1979), we know that the maximum likelihood estimate $\widehat{\beta}$ has variance:

$$\text{Var}[\widehat{\beta}] = \left(\mathcal{I}_{\beta\beta} - \mathcal{I}_{\beta\beta_0} \mathcal{I}_{\beta_0\beta_0}^{-1} \mathcal{I}_{\beta_0\beta} \right)^{-1},$$

where

$$\mathcal{I} = \left[\begin{array}{cc} \mathcal{I}_{\beta_0\beta_0} & \mathcal{I}_{\beta\beta_0} \\ \mathcal{I}_{\beta_0\beta} & \mathcal{I}_{\beta\beta} \end{array} \right]$$

is minus the retrospective expectation of the Hessian of the log-likelihood for a cohort study. Note, however, that: (1) the intercept $\widehat{\beta}_0$ is consistent for the intercept in the case-control population, but not the general population; (2) the variance of $\widehat{\beta}_0$ is not obtained from $\mathcal{I}$ alone; and (3) the "expectation" is with respect to the retrospective sampling. This complicates the calculation of $\sigma_{\widehat{\beta}}^2 = n\text{Var}[\widehat{\beta}]$. Nonetheless, if we test the null hypothesis $\beta = 0$ with $\widehat{\beta} > Z_{1-\alpha}\widehat{\sigma}_{\widehat{\beta}} n^{-1/2}$, where n is the total number of cases plus controls, $1 - \alpha = 0.975$, and $Z_{0.975} = 1.96$ corresponds to a two-sided 0.05 level test, we can use equation (9.2). If we also calculate $\sigma_0^2 = n\text{Var}_0[\widehat{\beta}]$, we can use equation (9.1) corresponding to the test $\widehat{\beta} > Z_{1-\alpha}\widehat{\sigma}_0 n^{-1/2}$.

To compute $\text{Var}[\widehat{\beta}]$ for sample size calculations we need to know the distribution $F(x)$ of X in the source population and the conditional probability of disease in the general population, $P^*(D = 1|x)$. If we know the disease prevalence in the general population, π, we can equate it to

$$\pi = \int P^*(D = 1 \mid x) \, dF(x) = \int \frac{\exp(\beta_0^* + \beta x)}{1 + \exp(\beta_0^* + \beta x)} \, dF(x), \tag{9.4}$$

where $\beta_0^* = \beta_0 - \log(\text{case sampling fraction}) + \log(\text{control sampling fraction})$ is the logistic intercept in the source population, which is usually smaller than β_0. If F, β and π are known, then (9.4) can be solved for β_0^*, yielding P^*. The distribution of X in cases is

$$F_1(x) = \pi^{-1} \int_{-\infty}^{x} P^*(D = 1 \mid u) \, dF(u)$$

and that in the controls is

$$F_0(x) = (1 - \pi)^{-1} \int_{-\infty}^{x} P^*(D = 0 \mid u) \, dF(u).$$

Let $\lambda = n_1/n$ be the proportion of cases in the case-control sample. Thus the ratio of controls to cases is

$$\frac{n_0}{n_1} = \frac{n - n_1}{n_1} = \frac{1}{\lambda} - 1 = \frac{1 - \lambda}{\lambda}.$$

From the retrospective sampling, the information matrix $\mathcal{I}$ has components:

$$\mathcal{I}_{\beta_0\beta_0} = n\left\{\lambda\int P(D=1|\ x)P(D=0|\ x)\ dF_1(x)\right.$$
$$\left. + (1-\lambda)\int P(D=1|\ x)P(D=0|\ x)\ dF_0(x)\right\}, \qquad (9.5)$$

$$\mathcal{I}_{\beta_0\beta} = n\left\{\lambda\int xP(D=1|\ x)P(D=0|\ x)\ dF_1(x)\right.$$
$$\left. + (1-\lambda)\int xP(D=1|\ x)P(D=0|\ x)\ dF_0(x)\right\}, \qquad (9.6)$$

$$\mathcal{I}_{\beta\beta} = n\left\{\lambda\int x^2P(D=1|\ x)P(D=0|\ x)\ dF_1(x)\right.$$
$$\left. + (1-\lambda)\int x^2P(D=1|\ x)P(D=0|\ x)\ dF_0(x)\right\}. \qquad (9.7)$$

Expressions (9.5) – (9.7) are needed to compute $\mathrm{Var}[\widehat{\beta}]$ away from the null to apply equations (9.1) or (9.2). However, at the null hypothesis $\beta=0$,

$$P(D=1|x) = P(D=1) = \lambda = 1 - P(D=0|x),$$

and

$$\mathcal{I}_{\beta_0\beta_0} = n\lambda(1-\lambda),$$
$$\mathcal{I}_{\beta_0\beta} = n\lambda(1-\lambda)\{\lambda\int x\ dF_1(x) + (1-\lambda)\int x\ dF_0(x)\} \equiv n\lambda(1-\lambda)\bar{\mu}_1,$$
$$\mathcal{I}_{\beta\beta} = n\lambda(1-\lambda)\{\lambda\int x^2\ dF_1(x) + (1-\lambda)\int x^2\ dF_0(x)\} \equiv n\lambda(1-\lambda)\bar{\mu}_2.$$

The variance of $\widehat{\beta}$ is given by $(\mathcal{I}_{\beta\beta} - \mathcal{I}_{\beta\beta_0}\mathcal{I}_{\beta_0\beta_0}^{-1}\mathcal{I}_{\beta_0\beta})^{-1}$.

Expressions (9.5) – (9.7) simplify for a rare disease for which

$$F_0(x) \approx F(x), \quad P^*(D=1|\ X) \approx \exp(\beta_0^* + \beta X), \quad P^*(D=0|\ X) \approx 1$$

and

$$F_1(x) \approx \int_{-\infty}^{x} \exp(\beta u)\ dF(u)\ /\ \int_{-\infty}^{\infty} \exp(\beta u)\ dF(u)$$
$$\equiv m_F^{-1}(\beta)\int_{-\infty}^{x} \exp(\beta u)\ dF(u), \qquad (9.8)$$

where $m_F(\beta)$ is the moment generating function of F. Hence

$$\mathcal{I}_{\beta_0\beta_0} \approx n\left\{\lambda m_F^{-1}(\beta)\int \exp(\beta x)P(D=1|\ x)P(D=0|\ x)\ dF(x)\right.$$
$$\left. + (1-\lambda)\int P(D=1|\ x)P(D=0|\ x)\ dF(x)\right\},$$

$$\mathcal{I}_{\beta_0\beta} \approx n \left\{ \lambda m_F^{-1}(\beta) \int x \exp(\beta x) P(D=1|\ x) P(D=0|\ x)\ dF(x) \right.$$

$$\left. + (1-\lambda) \int x P(D=1|\ x) P(D=0|\ x)\ dF(x) \right\},$$

$$\mathcal{I}_{\beta\beta} \approx n \left\{ \lambda m_F^{-1}(\beta) \int x^2 \exp(\beta x) P(D=1|\ x) P(D=0|\ x)\ dF(x) \right.$$

$$\left. + (1-\lambda) \int x^2 P(D=1|\ x) P(D=0|\ x)\ dF(x) \right\}.$$

The previous discussion pertains to the Wald statistic $\widehat{\beta} \left\{ \mathrm{Var}[\widehat{\beta}] \right\}^{-1/2}$. An alternative widely used test is based on the score:

$$\mathcal{U}_\beta = \sum_{i=1}^{n} X_i \left\{ D_i - P(D=1|\ X_i) \right\}.$$

In view of the retrospective sampling, the expectation of the score is

$$\begin{aligned} \mathrm{E}[\mathcal{U}_\beta] &= n \left\{ \lambda \mathrm{E}[X_i(1 - P(D=1|\ X_i))|\ D_i=1] \right. \\ &\qquad \left. - (1-\lambda)\mathrm{E}[X_i(P(D=1|\ X_i))|\ D_i=0] \right\} \\ &= n \left\{ \lambda \int x(1 - P(D=1|\ x))\ dF_1(x) \right. \\ &\qquad \left. - (1-\lambda) \int x P(D=1|\ x)\ dF_0(x) \right\}. \end{aligned} \qquad (9.9)$$

The variance of the score is

$$\mathrm{Var}[\mathcal{U}_\beta] = \mathcal{I}_{\beta\beta} - \mathcal{I}_{\beta\beta_0} \mathcal{I}_{\beta_0\beta_0}^{-1} \mathcal{I}_{\beta_0\beta}.$$

At the null hypothesis:

$$\mathcal{U}_{\beta:\beta=0} = \sum_{i=1}^{n_1} X_i(1-\lambda) - \sum_{i=n_1+1}^{n} X_i \lambda,$$

where the first n_1 observations are cases and the next $n_0 = n - n_1$ are controls. The null variance is

$$\mathrm{Var}(\mathcal{U}_{\beta:\beta=0}) = n\lambda(1-\lambda)(\bar{\mu}_2 - \bar{\mu}_1^2). \qquad (9.10)$$

Dividing by $n\lambda(1-\lambda)$, we obtain the equivalent statistic for testing the null hypothesis:

$$T = \frac{\mathcal{U}_{\beta:\beta=0}}{n\lambda(1-\lambda)} = \overline{X}_{\mathrm{cases}} - \overline{X}_{\mathrm{controls}}, \qquad (9.11)$$

the difference in mean exposures. For use in expression (9.1),

$$\sigma_0^2 = n\mathrm{Var}_0(T) = \frac{\bar{\mu}_2 - \bar{\mu}_1^2}{\lambda(1-\lambda)}, \qquad (9.12)$$

and

$$\sigma_\theta^2 = \frac{n\mathrm{Var}[\mathcal{U}_\beta]}{\{n\lambda(1-\lambda)\}^2} = \frac{\mathcal{I}_{\beta\beta} - \mathcal{I}_{\beta\beta_0} \mathcal{I}_{\beta_0\beta_0}^{-1} \mathcal{I}_{\beta_0\beta}}{n\{\lambda(1-\lambda)\}^2}. \qquad (9.13)$$

Note, use of expression (9.2) only requires the variance in equation (9.13).

Now we consider some special cases for the distributions F. Suppose X is binary with outcomes 0 or 1, and that $P(X = 1) = \mu$. The probability that $X = 1$ in cases is:

$$
\begin{aligned}
\mu_1 &= \frac{\mu P^*(D = 1|\ X = 1)}{\mu P^*(D = 1|\ X = 1) + (1 - \mu)P^*(D = 1|\ X = 0)} \\[2mm]
&= \frac{\mu\{1 + \exp(-\beta_0^* - \beta)\}^{-1}}{\mu\{1 + \exp(-\beta_0^* - \beta)\}^{-1} + (1 - \mu)\{1 + \exp(-\beta_0^*)\}^{-1}},
\end{aligned}
$$

while the probability that $X = 1$ in the controls is:

$$
\begin{aligned}
\mu_0 &= \frac{\mu P^*(D = 0|\ X = 1)}{\mu P^*(D = 0|\ X = 1) + (1 - \mu)P^*(D = 0|\ X = 0)} \\[2mm]
&= \frac{\mu\{1 + \exp(\beta_0^* + \beta)\}^{-1}}{\mu\{1 + \exp(\beta_0^* + \beta)\}^{-1} + (1 - \mu)\{1 + \exp(\beta_0^*)\}^{-1}}.
\end{aligned}
$$

For use in equations (9.1) or (9.2), $\theta = \mathrm{E}[T] = \mu_1 - \mu_0$. Note, if the disease is rare then

$$
\exp(\beta_0^* + \beta x) \ll 1, \quad \mu_1 \approx \frac{\mu \exp(\beta)}{\mu \exp(\beta) + 1 - \mu} \quad \text{and} \quad \mu_0 \approx \mu.
$$

Thus,

$$
\frac{T}{\{\widehat{\mathrm{Var}}[T]\}^{1/2}} = \frac{T}{\{\widehat{\sigma}_0^2/n\}^{1/2}} = \frac{\overline{X}_{\text{cases}} - \overline{X}_{\text{controls}}}{[\widehat{\mu}(1 - \widehat{\mu})\{(n\lambda)^{-1} + \{n(1 - \lambda)\}^{-1}\}]^{1/2}}
$$

is the familiar test statistic for a difference in two proportions, where $\widehat{\mu}$ is the proportion with $X = 1$ in the combined cases and controls. To compute the sample size from the corresponding equation (9.1), however, we require σ_θ^2 given by expression (9.13). Because F_1 and F_0 are each Bernoulli distributions with known respective probabilities μ_1 and μ_0, σ_θ^2 can be calculated from the information matrix given by expressions (9.5)–(9.7).

If $X = 0, 1, 2, \ldots, K$ for $K + 1$ categories with respective probabilities $\rho_0, \rho_1, \ldots, \rho_K$ that define the distribution F, one can perform similar calculations to compute the mean and variances for T, and the variance of the per category log odds ratio β.

If X is normally distributed with mean 0 and variance τ^2 in the general population and if the disease is rare, then F_0 is Normal$(0, \tau^2)$ and, from expression (9.8), F_1 is Normal$(\beta\tau^2, \tau^2)$. Hence, for the score statistic:

$$
\theta = \mathrm{E}[T] = \mathrm{E}[\overline{X}_{\text{cases}} - \overline{X}_{\text{controls}}] = \beta\tau^2 - 0 = \beta\tau^2.
$$

If the disease is rare, the null variance of T is

$$
n^{-1}\tau^2\{\lambda^{-1} + (1 - \lambda)^{-1}\} = \tau^2\{n\lambda(1 - \lambda)\}^{-1} = n^{-1}\sigma_0^2.
$$

Under the alternative, the mixed case-control population has mean $\lambda\beta\tau^2$ and variance $\{\tau^2 + \beta^2\tau^4\lambda(1 - \lambda)\}$. Hence,

$$
n^{-1}\sigma_\theta^2 = \{\tau^2 + \beta^2\tau^4\lambda(1 - \lambda)\}\{n\lambda(1 - \lambda)\}^{-1}.
$$

To illustrate these ideas, suppose we wanted to detect a log odds ratio $\beta = 0.3$ (or odds ratio $\exp(\beta) = 1.35$) for the association of the presence of benign breast disease with breast cancer. The prevalence of benign breast disease in controls, which approximates that in the general population, is 0.06475 in the Polish population. Assuming equal numbers of cases and controls (i.e., $\lambda = 0.5$), we calculate the sample size required to attain power 0.9 ($Z_\gamma = 1.2816$) with a two-sided 0.05 level test ($Z_{1-\alpha} = 1.96$) from equations (9.1) and (9.2) applied to the logistic model. The required total sample sizes n (cases plus controls) for the Wald tests are, respectively, 6,790 and 6,863. For the score tests, they are 6,775 and 6,702. Because the Polish study had $n = 4,130$ cases plus controls, its power was only about 0.71 to detect an odds ratio of 1.35 for benign breast disease. Note that required sample size depends on the precise test statistic used.

Suppose instead one wished to detect an association with BMI, measured on a continuous scale. In the Polish control data, the mean BMI was 28.0, with standard deviation 5.33. The variable $X =$(BMI-28)/5.33 therefore has mean 0 and variance 1 in the Polish population. Suppose we want to detect a positive association of X with breast cancer risk, with log odds per unit increase in X of $\beta = 0.08$. A unit increase in X corresponds to a 5.33 BMI unit increase; a 3 unit increase in X corresponds to an odds ratio of $\exp(3\beta) = 1.27$ for a three standard deviation increase in BMI. This odds ratio is similar to the association found in a study of US women aged 50 years and over (Pfeiffer *et al.*, 2013). Assuming $\lambda = 0.5$, we calculated the sample sizes required for power 0.90 for the Wald test as 6,570 and 6,589, respectively, from equations (9.1) and (9.2). For the score test, the sample sizes were 6,566 and 6,547, respectively. Inverting equation (9.1) for the Wald test, we found that the Polish study had power about 0.73 to detect a log odds of 0.08 per standard deviation increase in BMI.

By changing λ in these equations, one can allow for unequal numbers of cases and controls. With two controls per case (i.e., $\lambda = 1/3$), the sample size required to detect an odds ratio of 1.35 for benign breast disease with a score test based on equation (9.1) is $n = 7,555$, instead of 6,775 with equal numbers of cases and controls. Although the total sample size is larger with $\lambda = 1/3$, the number of cases required is $7,555/3 = 2,519$ instead of $6,775/2 = 3,388$.

McKeown-Eyssen and Thomas (1985) and Lubin *et al.* (1988) discussed sample sizes for score tests like equation (9.11) for a single possibly continuous exposure.

9.3.2 Adjustment for confounders

Suppose there is a single confounder X_1, and that we want to estimate the effect of an exposure X_2 while adjusting for X_1 by fitting the model:

$$\text{logit}\{P(D = 1|\ X_1, X_2)\} = \beta_0 + \beta_1 X_1 + \beta_2 X_2. \tag{9.14}$$

A Wald test of $H_0 : \beta_2 = 0$ requires the maximum likelihood estimate, $\widehat{\beta}_2$, and an estimate of its variance

$$\text{Var}[\widehat{\beta}_2] = \left(\mathcal{I}_{\beta_2,\beta_2} - \mathcal{I}_{\beta_2,\beta_0\beta_1}\mathcal{I}_{\beta_0\beta_1\beta_0\beta_1}^{-1}\mathcal{I}_{\beta_0\beta_1,\beta_2}\right)^{-1},$$

where, for example, $\mathcal{I}_{\beta_0\beta_1,\beta_2}$ is the sub-matrix of elements of the information matrix that correspond to cross-derivatives with respect to β_2 and β_0 or β_1. The score statistic,

$$
\begin{aligned}
\mathcal{U}_{\beta_2:\beta_2=0} &= \sum_{i=1}^{n_1} X_{2i}\{1 - P(D_i = 1|\ X_{1i}; \widehat{\beta}_0, \widehat{\beta}_1, \beta_2 = 0)\} \\
&\quad - \sum_{i=n_1+1}^{n} X_{2i}P(D_i = 1|\ X_{1i}; \widehat{\beta}_0, \widehat{\beta}_1, \beta_2 = 0),
\end{aligned}
\tag{9.15}
$$

requires maximum likelihood estimates $\widehat{\beta}_0$, $\widehat{\beta}_1$ obtained under the null hypothesis $\beta_2 = 0$. Its variance,

$$\text{Var}[\mathcal{U}_{\beta_2:\beta_2=0}] = \mathcal{I}_{\beta_2,\beta_2} - \mathcal{I}_{\beta_2,\beta_0\beta_1}\mathcal{I}_{\beta_0\beta_1\beta_0\beta_1}^{-1}\mathcal{I}_{\beta_0\beta_1,\beta_2},$$

is estimated by plugging in these estimates of β_0, β_1 and $\beta_2 = 0$. These ideas generalize to multiple confounders. The nonnull expectation of $\mathcal{U}_{\beta_2:\beta_2=0}$ is:

$$
\begin{aligned}
\mathrm{E}\left[\mathcal{U}_{\beta_2:\beta_2=0}\right] &= n\left[\lambda \int x_2\{1 - P(D_i = 1|\ x_1, x_2; \widehat{\beta}_0, \widehat{\beta}_1, \beta_2 = 0)\}\ dF_1(x_1, x_2)\right.\\
&\quad\left. - (1 - \lambda) \int x_2 P(D_i = 1|\ x_1, x_2; \widehat{\beta}_0, \widehat{\beta}_1, \beta_2 = 0)\ dF_0(x_1, x_2)\right]\\
&= n\theta.
\end{aligned}
$$

An essential difficulty in allowing for confounders is that one needs to know the joint distribution of X_1 and X_2 in the general population as well as the parameters β_0, β_1 and β_2. It is often a challenge just to specify the value of β_2 under the alternative and the marginal distribution of X_2. But more is needed to compute power while adjusting for a covariate X_1. If, for example, X_1 and X_2 have a bivariate normal distribution, analytic formulas, analogous to expressions (9.5)–(9.7), can be used to compute the required information matrix. Often, however, there will be both discrete and continuous covariates. If pilot data are available from the joint distribution of X_1 and X_2 in the general population, or if the disease is rare and data from controls in a previous case-control study are available, one can use the empirical joint distribution $\widehat{F}(x_1, x_2)$ to compute sample sizes by substituting $\widehat{F}(x_1, x_2)$ in place of F in previous calculations.

We digress to make the formulas needed to account for confounding more general, so that they will apply to other situations, such as tests for interaction. Let $\mathbf{X}$ be a vector of covariates and $\widehat{F}$ be its empirical distribution in the general population, or if disease is rare, in a random sample of nondiseased subjects. Corresponding distributions in cases and controls are assumed to have point masses at the mass points of $\widehat{F}$ but are reweighed according to

$$
d\widehat{F}_1(\mathbf{x}) = \frac{1}{\pi}P^*(D = 1|\ \mathbf{x})\ d\widehat{F}(\mathbf{x})
$$

and

$$
d\widehat{F}_0(\mathbf{x}) = \frac{1}{1 - \pi}P^*(D = 0|\ \mathbf{x})\ d\widehat{F}(\mathbf{x}),
$$

where

$$
\mathrm{logit}\{P^*(D = 1|\mathbf{X} = \mathbf{x})\} = \beta_0^* + \boldsymbol{\beta}^T\mathbf{x},
$$

$\boldsymbol{\beta}$ is a p-dimensional vector corresponding to the p components of $\mathbf{X}$, and the disease prevalence in the population implicitly defines β_0^* via equation (9.4) with $\widehat{F}$ in place of F.

The integrals in the revised equations (9.4), (9.5)-(9.7), and (9.9), extended to multivariate $\mathbf{X}$, become weighted sums over the points of support of $\widehat{F}$. Once the multivariate information matrix has been estimated, sample sizes for Wald tests or score tests can be computed. This computational approach can also be used even if there is an analytic form for the joint distribution, F. Rather than compute integrals, one can approximate them by taking a large random sample from F and proceeding as above.

As an example with confounding, suppose we want to test for an association of breast cancer with benign breast disease, adjusting for education level, a strong risk factor (Table 9.2) that has correlation 0.135 with benign breast disease (Table 9.3). We used $\beta_1 = 0.126$ per education category and $\beta_2 = 0.3$ for presence of benign breast disease. Assuming the disease probability in the general population was 0.01, we estimated $\widehat{\beta}_0^* = -5.0043$. The expected score equations in retrospective sampling generated from $\widehat{F}$ have solutions $\beta_0 = -0.4092$, $\beta_1 = 0.126$, and $\beta_2 = 0.3$ in the absence of constraints on β_2. Under the (false) null model, the solutions are $\beta_0 = -0.4072$, $\beta_1 = 0.133$, and $\beta_2 = 0$. Note that these estimates are not obtained by fitting case-control data but are simply solutions to the expected score equations given the true parameters and $\widehat{F}$. Both unconstrained ($\mathcal{I}$) and constrained ($\mathcal{I}_0$) estimates of the information matrix can be calculated given these parameters and $\widehat{F}$. The values of $\mathrm{Var}[n^{1/2}\widehat{\beta}_2]$ are $\sigma_0^2 = 56.86$ with the constraint and $\sigma_\theta^2 = 58.33$ without. Sample sizes for Wald tests from equations (9.1) and (9.2) are, respectively, 6,742 and 6,810. The expected value of the score test under the alternative is 0.005223, and the variances are $\sigma_0^2 = 0.01759$ and $\sigma_\theta^2 = 0.01714$, leading to sample size estimates 6,705 from equation (9.1) and 6,602 from equation (9.2). Recall that the corresponding sample size estimates without adjustment for confounding were 6,790, 6,863, 6,775, and 6,702. Thus, adjustment for confounding decreased required sample sizes slightly, regardless of the test used.

Lubin and Gail (1990) treated score tests for an exposure in the context of a multivariable logistic model, both for cohort and for case-control studies. They showed, for example, how to compute the sample size required to detect a quadratic deviation from a linear trend in exposure dose on the logistic scale. Such sample sizes are often much larger than required to detect the main or linear effect.

There is a related literature on sample sizes for the Wald test for cohort studies with adjustment for confounding in logistic models. Whittemore (1981) gave approximations for multivariate $\mathbf{X}$ from the exponential family under the rare disease assumption. These approximations do not apply to case-control data, however, because the disease is not rare in the case-control sample and sampling is retrospective. Demidenko (2007), not relying on the rare disease assumption, recommended the logistic calculations for the Wald test using equation (9.2) under the alternative, claiming that this was common practice for testing. His calculations were for prospective cohort data, however, not retrospective sampling.

9.3.3   Tests for interaction

Power calculations for tests for interactions can be accommodated in the previous multivariate framework. Consider the logistic model:

$$\mathrm{logit}\{P(D = 1|\ X_1, X_2)\} = \beta_0 + \beta_1 X_1 + \beta_2 X_2 + \beta_3 X_1 X_2. \tag{9.16}$$

One can test the interaction parameter $\beta_3 = 0$ by regarding $X_3 = X_1 X_2$ as a third covariate and proceeding as above. This would allow one to test for interactions while adjusting for main effects, as is appropriate, and possibly for other covariates in an expanded model. In the previous example, suppose the true model also included a negative interaction $\beta_3 = -0.1$. We might ask how large a sample is needed to detect this interaction. Proceeding as above, we found $\beta_0^* = -4.9733$ for the source population, and in the case-control data, $\beta_0 = -0.3782$. Under the constraint $\beta_3 = 0$ the other parameters were $\beta_0 = -0.3579$, $\beta_1 = 0.1192$, and $\beta_2 = -0.06877$. The expected value of the score for β_3 was -0.004177. The variances for $\widehat{\beta}_3$ were $\sigma_0^2 = 24.18$ and $\sigma_\theta^2 = 23.79$ leading to required sample sizes for the Wald test of 25,158 from equation (9.1) and 24,994 from equation (9.2). The corresponding variances for the score test were $\sigma_0^2 = 0.04135$ and $\sigma_\theta^2 = 0.04204$, leading to sample sizes 25,070 and 25,321 from equations (9.1) and (9.2). The sample sizes required to detect interactions are often at least four times larger than required for main effects, as for example in Figure 7.4 in Breslow and Day (1987).

The usual logistic analysis is valid for arbitrary joint distributions of factors X in the source population. Suppose there are two dichotomous risk factors. Extending the notation in Table 9.1 so that the subscripts refer, respectively, to X_1, X_2, and D, an estimate of the interaction on the logistic scale is

$$\widehat{\beta}_3 = \log\left(\frac{N_{111}N_{100}}{N_{101}N_{110}}\right) - \log\left(\frac{N_{011}N_{000}}{N_{001}N_{010}}\right).$$

The variance of $\widehat{\beta}_3$ has two components, one for $X_1 = 1$ and one for $X_1 = 0$. If, however, X_1 and X_2 are independent in the source population, as might be true for example if X_1 denoted the presence of a mutation and X_2 was an indicator for alcohol consumption, then for a rare disease $\log(N_{100}N_{010}/N_{110}N_{000}) \approx 0$ and $\widehat{\beta}_3$ simplifies to:

$$\widehat{\beta}_3 = \log\left(\frac{N_{111}N_{001}}{N_{101}N_{011}}\right).$$

This "case-only" estimate of interaction has only one component of variance and is more efficient (Piegorsch *et al.*, 1994), but it depends on the independence assumption. The number of cases required for such a case-only analysis depends on β_3 and on the joint distribution of X_1 and X_2 among cases, but standard sample size formulas for a single 2×2 table can be used. Chatterjee and Carroll (2005) show how to increase efficiency for interactions for full logistic regression of case-control data under the assumption of independence of X_1 and X_2 (also see Chapter 24).

9.4 Matched designs

Suppose that in the general population individuals have matching factors M that fall into strata $s \in \{1, \ldots, S\}$ and exposures X, and that:

$$\text{logit}\{P(D = 1 \mid M = s, X)\} = \beta_{0s} + \beta X. \tag{9.17}$$

Suppose we sample a case with $M = s$ and select a control at random from this matching stratum. We are told that the exposures of these two subjects were X_1 and X_0, but not told which exposure corresponded to the case. The conditional probability that the case had exposure X_1 given that there was one case and one control, and that the two exposures were X_1 and X_0, is (Cox, 1970):

$$\rho = \frac{\exp\{\beta(X_1 - X_0)\}}{1 + \exp\{\beta(X_1 - X_0)\}}.$$

Hence conditionally on the matching and that there is a discord, the outcome that the case has exposure X_1 is Bernoulli with probability $\rho = 0.5$ under the null hypothesis $\beta = 0$. If X takes values 0 or 1, then under the alternative, the probability that the case has exposure $X_1 = 1$ is $\rho = \exp(\beta)/\{1 + \exp(\beta)\}$. Now letting X_1 and X_0 correspond to the case and control exposures, respectively, we count the number of matched case-control pairs that fall into each of the four cells defined by (X_1, X_0). We use only the counts in the discordant cells $(1,0)$ and $(0,1)$ to perform a McNemar test of the null hypothesis. Letting W be the number of the T discordant pairs in which $X_1 = 1$ and $X_0 = 0$ we can use the binomial distribution for W to compute the number of discordant pairs, T, required to have power γ to reject the null hypothesis $\beta = 0$ (or $\rho = 0.5$) against an alternative $\beta \neq 0$. The corresponding normal approximation for the required T can be computed from equation (9.1) as

$$T = \frac{\left[Z_\gamma \{\rho(1-\rho)\}^{1/2} + Z_{1-\alpha} \{0.5 \times 0.5\}^{1/2}\right]^2}{(\rho - 0.5)^2},$$

with $\alpha/2$ in place of α for two-sided tests.

It is a challenge to estimate the total number of pairs N required to yield T discordant pairs. If we had pilot data, we could estimate the proportion of discordant pairs and estimate N for the main study by dividing T by this proportion. Typically we do not have such pilot data, however. The expected value of T is

$$\mathrm{E}[T] = N \int \{P(X = 1|\ D = 1, M = s)P(X = 0|\ D = 0, M = s) \qquad (9.18)$$
$$+ P(X = 0|\ D = 1, M = s)P(X = 1|\ D = 0, M = s)\}\ dF_M(s),$$

where F_M is the distribution of the matching factor over the S strata. If we could compute equation (9.18) we could estimate N by dividing the required T by the coefficient of N in equation (9.18). If M were conditionally independent of X given D, then the coefficient would be

$$P(X = 1|\ D = 1)P(X = 0|\ D = 0) + P(X = 0|\ D = 1)P(X = 1|\ D = 0). \qquad (9.19)$$

Expression (9.19) can be regarded as an approximation that replaces the expectation of a function in equation (9.18) by the function of the component expectations (Breslow and Day, 1987). If we know $P(X = 1|\ D = 0)$ and β, and if we ignore matching, we can compute

$$P(X = 1|\ D = 1)$$

$$= \frac{P(X = 1|\ D = 0)}{P(X = 0|\ D = 0)} \times \frac{\exp(\beta)}{1 + \{P(X = 1|\ D = 0)/P(X = 0|\ D = 0)\}\exp(\beta)}$$

and substitute these quantities in expression (9.19) to obtain the needed divisor.

A more accurate calculation is possible if we assume that we know the correlation between $P(X = 1|\ D = 1, M)$ and $P(X = 1|\ D = 0, M)$. In particular, the integral in expression (9.18) can be re-expressed as:

$$\mathrm{E}[P(X = 1|\ D = 1, M)] + \mathrm{E}[P(X = 1|\ D = 0, M)]$$
$$- 2\mathrm{Cov}[P(X = 1|\ D = 1, M), P(X = 1|\ D = 0, M)]$$
$$- 2\mathrm{E}[P(X = 1|\ D = 1, M)]\mathrm{E}[P(X = 1|\ D = 0, M)],$$

where the expectations and the covariance are over the distribution of M. For a given $P(X = 1|\ D = 0)$ and β, Dupont (1988) calculated the required sample size if the correlation above is known and also allowed multiple matched controls for each case.

In nested case-control sampling of a cohort study, a case that arises at a time t is matched to a random sample of J cohort members from the risk set at time t (see Chapters 16 and 18). Near the null hypothesis, the relative efficiency comparing $J : 1$ matching to an infinite number of controls is $J/(J+1)$ (Ury, 1975). This ratio also holds for unmatched case-control studies with J times as many controls as cases (Gail *et al.*, 1976). This ratio suggests that it rarely pays to choose more than 5 controls per case for testing the null hypothesis. However, for estimation of nonnull log odds ratios, precision can be gained with larger values of J in nested case-control designs (Breslow *et al.*, 1983).

Another consideration affecting the matched case-control sample size calculations is that the pool of potential controls may not be large enough to assure that each case is matched to a control (McKinlay, 1974). A case that is not matched to a control contributes nothing to the matched analysis, resulting in a loss of power.

Although matching may offer more complete control for confounding than regression methods, the statistical efficiency of the matched design is similar to the unmatched design, both for testing main effects of exposure and for detecting interactions (Smith and Day, 1984; Breslow and Day, 1987).

9.5 Misclassification and measurement error

Measurement error in an exposure distorts estimates of odds ratios in case-control studies (Chapter 10). We usually assume that case-control status is known without error, but that exposure assessment is subject to measurement error. If X is the true exposure and W is the exposure measurement that is subject to error, we say that the measurement error is "nondifferential" if the distribution of W is conditionally independent of D given X. If so, substituting W for X in the logistic regression (9.3) yields attenuated estimates of β, but the expectation of the estimate at the null hypothesis $\beta = 0$ remains 0. If the measurement error is differential, as for example if cases tend to recall higher values of exposure than controls, then estimates based on W are subject to "recall bias" (Coughlin, 1990), and nonnull estimates of β can result, even when $\beta = 0$. In such circumstances, the size of the test of the null hypothesis is above nominal levels, and power calculations are not warranted. If measurement error afflicts covariate measurements, residual confounding can result, and, again, power calculations are not warranted. We confine attention, therefore, to nondifferential error.

The "classical" nondifferential error model for a continuous exposure, X, is

$$W = X + \epsilon$$

where ϵ has mean 0 and variance ξ^2 and is independent of X and D. Given X, W is independent of D. It follows that $\mathrm{E}[W|D] = \mathrm{E}[X|D]$ and $\mathrm{Var}[W|D] = \mathrm{Var}[X|D] + \xi^2$. If X is normal with mean 0 and variance τ^2 in the general population, and if the disease is rare, it follows from calculations in Section 9.1.2 that the noncentrality parameter for the test based on

$$\frac{\{\overline{X}_{\text{cases}} - \overline{X}_{\text{controls}}\}^2}{\tau^2 \{n\lambda(1-\lambda)\}^{-1}}$$

is

$$\frac{\{\beta\tau^2\}^2}{\tau^2 \{n\lambda(1-\lambda)\}^{-1}}.$$

If we use W in place of X, then the noncentrality is

$$\frac{\{\beta\tau^2\}^2}{(\tau^2 + \xi^2)\{n\lambda(1-\lambda)\}^{-1}}.$$

Hence the ratio of the sample size required from using W compared to using X is

$$\frac{\tau^2 + \xi^2}{\tau^2} = \{\mathrm{Corr}[W, X]\}^{-2}$$

where $\mathrm{Corr}[W, X]$ is the correlation between W and X. The relative efficiency of using W compared to using X is $\{\mathrm{Corr}[W, X]\}^2$ which is the same as the asymptotic relative efficiency for prospective models measured with error (Lagakos, 1988).

Suppose X is dichotomous and that $P(W = 1| X = 1) = \xi_{sens}$ and $P(W = 0| X = 0) = \xi_{spec}$ are the sensitivity and specificity of W with respect to the gold standard X, both in cases and controls. Then $P(W = 1| D = 1)$ is

$$P(X = 1| D = 1)\xi_{sens} + P(X = 0| D = 1)(1 - \xi_{spec}),$$

and $P(W = 1| D = 0)$ is

$$P(X = 1| D = 0)\xi_{sens} + P(X = 0| D = 0)(1 - \xi_{spec}).$$

Using a two-sided 0.05 level Wald test for the log odds ratio for X with equation (9.2) and equal numbers of cases and controls, we estimated $n = 470$ cases plus controls were needed to detect an odds ratio of 2 with power 0.9 and $P(X = 1|D = 0) = 0.2$. If instead we used W and assumed the sensitivity and specificity were both 0.9, then $P(W = 1| D = 0) = 0.26$, $P(W = 1| D = 1) = 0.367$, the odds ratio for W is 1.648, and $n = 802$. Thus even a small amount of misclassification can lead to large increases in required samples size.

Other types of measurement error, such as Berkson error, or error factors that multiply covariates require specialized treatment (Chapter 10).

9.6   Missing data

Covariate information may be missing by design, as in two-phase case-control studies (Chapters 12 and 17) or for reasons uncontrolled by the investigator. In the latter instance, one sometimes uses "complete case" analyses, whereby only cases and controls with complete covariate information are analyzed. Sample size calculations for complete case analyses only require dividing the sample size for a study without missing data by the fraction expected to have complete data. However, complete case analysis may lead to severe loss of information if there is appreciable missing data, and the complete case analysis yields biased results unless the probability of missingness factors into a term that depends on D and a term that depends on covariates (Vach and Blettner, 2005). More principled methods for handling missing covariates such as imputation, the mean score method, and maximum likelihood depend on a missing at random (MAR) assumption, namely the probability of missing a covariate depends only on the measured disease status and other measured covariate(s), and not on the missing covariate itself (Vach and Blettner, 2005). In order to estimate sample sizes that accommodate such procedures, one needs to lay out in advance what procedure will be used, and also specify the amount and pattern of missingness for various covariates. This specification is itself a daunting task, and the corresponding analytical approaches to sample size calculations do not appear to have been developed. However, if the sampling and analysis specifications, including missingness mechanism, are well defined, simulations can be used to compute required sample sizes (Section 9.8).

The simulation approach has been used for power calculations, when missingness is by design, as in a two-phase case-control study (Haneuse *et al.*, 2011). For the two-phase design, the amount and pattern of missingness are subject to control by the investigator, and the analytical options can be defined. Thus power can be estimated by simulating a well-defined sampling and analysis process (Section 9.8).

9.7   Multiple comparisons

To this point, we have assumed that there is a single parameter of interest. This is entirely appropriate for a confirmatory study of a well-defined hypothesis. However, some studies are exploratory and examine many hypotheses. For example, genome-wide association studies compare genotypes of single nucleotide polymorphisms (SNPs) in cases versus controls. Letting $X \in \{0, 1, 2\}$ denote the number of minor alleles of a SNP, one can estimate the log odds ratio per allele β with equation (9.3) and test $H_0 : \beta = 0$. If there are $m = 500,000$ SNPs to be tested, we need to adjust for multiple comparisons to control the rate of false positive results. For example, even if no SNPs are associated with the disease, we would expect that 25,000 SNPs would have "statistically significant" associations if we used the critical value for a single 0.05 level test.

The most common way to account for multiple comparisons is to use the Bonferroni adjusted significance level $\alpha_B = \alpha/m$, where α is the family-wise significance level. In the SNP example, $\alpha_B = 0.05/500,000 = 10^{-7}$. Standard sample size calculations can be performed as in Section 9.3, except the two-sided significance level is now $\alpha_B/2 = 5 \times 10^{-8}$. With this significance level, the probability that one or more SNPs is declared statistically significant under the null hypothesis of no SNP associations is $\alpha = 0.05$ or less. One might think that sample size requirements would increase rapidly with m. If we use tests corresponding to equation (9.2), the ratio of the Bonferroni adjusted sample size to the unadjusted sample size for a single test is:

$$\frac{(Z_\gamma + Z_{1-\alpha_B/2})^2}{(Z_\gamma + Z_{1-\alpha/2})^2}.$$

Let $Z_\gamma = 1.282$, corresponding to $\gamma = 0.9$, and let $\alpha = 0.05$. Then for values $m =$1, 2, 5, 10, 100, 1,000, 10,000, 100,000, 500,000, and 1,000,000, the ratios of required sample sizes are, respectively 1, 1.18, 1.42, 1.59, 2.16, 2.71, 3.25, 3.79, 4.15, and 4.31. Thus, the required sample size increases slowly with m. In particular, the sample size needs only to be quadrupled to accommodate nearly 500,000 multiple comparisons.

A less stringent criterion than family-wise control of the significance level is afforded by control of the false discovery rate (FDR) (Benjamini and Hochberg, 1995). The FDR estimates the probability that the null hypothesis is true given that the statistical test rejected the null hypothesis. In the case where a fraction π_0 of the parameters are null and a fraction $1-\pi_0$ have the same nonnull value, θ, "power" calculations for FDR can be related to standard power calculations (Jung, 2005). For FDR we define "power" as γ_{FDR}, the ratio of the expected number of rejections by FDR criteria among the nonnull parameters divided by the total number of nonnull parameters, $m(1 - \pi_0)$. If we want to control the FDR at level p_{FDR} with FDR power γ_{FDR}, we can compute the required n from equation (9.2) with

$$\alpha_{FDR} = \gamma_{FDR} \times \frac{1 - \pi_0}{\pi_0} \times \frac{p_{FDR}}{1 - p_{FDR}}$$

replacing α and γ_{FDR} replacing γ (Jung, 2005). For two-sided tests, we use $\alpha_{FDR}/2$ in equation (9.2). A problematic aspect of this calculation is the need to specify π_0. For example, what proportion of SNPs have null associations with a given disease? For illustration, assume $\pi_0 = 0.9999$ and set $\gamma_{FDR} = 0.9$. If we want on average no more than a fraction $p_{FDR} = 0.05$ of the FDR rejections to be false positives, then with a two-sided test we use

$$\frac{\alpha_{FDR}}{2} = \frac{1}{2} \times 0.9 \times \frac{0.0001}{0.9999} \times \frac{0.05}{0.95} = 2.4 \times 10^{-6}$$

in equation (9.2). Noting that with the Bonferroni correction

$$\frac{\alpha_B}{2} = \frac{1}{2} \times \frac{0.05}{500,000} = 5 \times 10^{-8}$$

and with $\gamma = 0.9$, the ratio of the Bonferroni adjusted sample size to the FDR adjusted sample size is:

$$\frac{n_B}{n_{FDR}} = \frac{(Z_{0.9} + Z_{1-5 \times 10^{-8}})^2}{(Z_{0.9} + Z_{1-2.4 \times 10^{-6}})^2} = 1.27.$$

Thus compared to FDR control at $p_{FDR} = 0.05$, Bonferroni adjustment requires 27% larger sample size to achieve family-wise control of significance at $\alpha = 0.05$. If we had guessed $\pi_0 = 0.999$ instead of 0.9999, then

$$\frac{\alpha_{FDR}}{2} = \frac{0.9}{2} \times \frac{0.001}{0.999} \times \frac{0.05}{0.95} = 2.4 \times 10^{-5},$$

and the sample size ratio would have been 1.52. This illustrates that sample size calculations for FDR depend on π_0, about which little may be known, in addition to the nonnull parameters of interest. Sample size calculations for FDR have also been extended to allow for the nonnull parameters to have a nondegenerate distribution (Jung, 2005; Liu and Hwang, 2007).

9.8 Simulations for more realistic power estimation

As researchers prepare grant proposals, they need to describe statistical challenges that they may face, such as confounding bias, the potential for missing data, and covariate misclassification or measurement error. Furthermore, the statistical design and analysis plan should outline how to address these challenges. For example if it is anticipated that a key covariate will be missing for some study participants the analysis plan may outline the use of inverse-probability weighting (Seaman and White, 2013) or multiple imputation (White *et al.*, 2011).

In principle, power calculations should also reflect these challenges and proposed solutions. In practice, however, researchers often rely on power calculations (including those presented in previous sections of this chapter) that are based on relatively simple data gathering designs and analysis methods. As a result there is a strong potential for a disconnect between the power calculations reported in the proposal and the realities of the study. On the one hand, the simplified power calculations may underestimate the actual power of the study. While having too much power may not be a bad thing, an implication is that greater resources are being devoted to the study than are necessary. On the other hand, if the reported power overestimates the actual power of the study, then the ultimate success of the study in detecting an exposure effect is threatened from the outset.

Thus researchers should align their calculations with the realities of the anticipated data and analysis as much as possible. One approach is to conduct a Monte Carlo or simulation study (Haneuse *et al.*, 2012). In the remainder of this section we outline a general framework for conducting simulation-based power calculations for case-control studies and illustrate the method with three examples based on the Polish breast cancer study.

9.8.1 A general simulation framework for case-control studies

One fundamental conceptual challenge in the development of sample size/power methods for case-control studies is that the design is *retrospective* whereas the risk model of interest is typically *prospective*; that is, exposures/confounders are random, conditional on disease status. The following general-purpose algorithm overcomes this challenge. Letting X denote the exposure of interest and $\{Z_1, \ldots, Z_p\}$ a collection of confounders that will (ultimately) be adjusted for:

(a) Construct a large "population" of N individuals with joint exposure/confounder distribution $P(X, Z_1, \ldots, Z_p)$. That is, construct a data set consisting of $\{X_i, Z_{i,1}, \ldots, Z_{i,p}\}$ for $i = 1, \ldots, N$.

(b) Given $\{\beta_0^*, \beta_x, \beta_{z_1}, \ldots, \beta_{z_p}\}$, calculate $\pi_i = P(D_i = 1)$ for all N individuals.

(c) For each individual, generate a random draw from a Bernoulli(π_i) distribution.

(d) Identify the N_1 cases in the population who have $D = 1$ and the N_0 noncases with $D = 0$ (note, $N_0 + N_1 = N$).

(e) Randomly sample n_0 individuals from the N_0 noncases and n_1 from the N_1 cases, and "record" their exposure/confounder values.

(f) Fit the model of interest and record whether or not the null hypothesis (i.e., $H_0 : \beta_x = 0$) is rejected.

(g) Repeat steps (c)-(f) *Rep* times.

Finally, power is estimated as the percent of *Rep* instances where the null hypothesis $H_0 : \beta_x = 0$ is rejected. Since *Rep* is finite, the simulation-based estimate is subject to uncertainty, often referred to as Monte Carlo Error (MCE). In the following examples, all results are based on *Rep* $= 5,000$. Koehler *et al.* (2009) describe various techniques for characterizing MCE as well as strategies for determining the value of *Rep* that yields a pre-specified desired precision.

9.8.2 Example 1: A single confounder

We begin with a hypothetical study to investigate the association between family history of breast cancer (FH) and risk of breast cancer. In this Example 1, we suppose that the eventual analysis adjusts for a single confounder, Z. Examples 2 and 3 are more realistic in that they consider multiple confounders and missclassification.

Following Section 9.8.1, we initially constructed a large population ($N = 100,000$) with the observed prevalence of family history among the controls in the Polish data (5.7%). We then generated Z as a Normal($\Delta, 1^2$) for those subjects with FH $= 0$ and a Normal($-\Delta, 1^2$) for those with FH $= 1$. Note, increasing the value of Δ increases the degree of association between FH and Z; in the following we considered values $\Delta = 0.10, 0.25$, and 0.50.

We then conducted two separate simulation studies to estimate power to detect a log odds ratio between family history and breast cancer of 0.61. The first simulation, labeled the "naïve simulation," was based on the model:

$$\text{logit}\{P(D = 1| \text{ FH})\} = \beta_0^* + \beta_x \text{FH}. \qquad (9.20)$$

That is, for each of *Rep* $= 5,000$ repetitions, we generated outcomes based on model (9.20) with $\beta_x = 0.61$, drew a balanced case-control sample of size n, fit model (9.20) but with intercept β_0, and recorded whether the null hypothesis $H_0 : \beta_x = 0$ was rejected. The second simulation, labeled here as the "realistic simulation," followed the same process but used the model

$$\text{logit}\{P(D = 1| \text{ FH}, Z)\} = \beta_0^* + \beta_x \text{FH} + \beta_z Z \qquad (9.21)$$

for both the data generation as well as for evaluating the null hypothesis $H_0 : \beta_x = 0$, but with intercept β_0. As in the naïve simulation, β_x was again set to 0.61, while β_z was set to $\log(2)$. For both simulations the value of β_0^* was specified so that the overall prevalence of $D = 1$ was 0.10.

Figure 9.1(a) presents estimated power as a function of case-control size, n. The solid curve presents estimated power from the naïve simulation based on (9.20) while the dotted/dashed curves present estimated power from the realistic simulation based on model (9.21) for a range of values for Δ. Since the solid curve is above each of the dotted/dashed curves, the naïve simulation overestimates statistical power to detect $\beta_x = 0.61$. In particular, while the solid curve suggests that $n = 1,300$ will be sufficient to obtain 80% power,

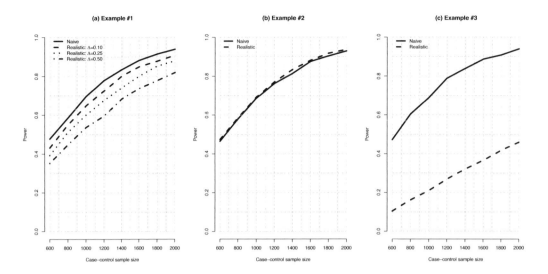

FIGURE 9.1

Estimated power curves for detecting $\beta_x = 0.61$ as the effect of family history in a hypothetical balanced case-control study for breast cancer in Poland. Panel (a) considers the control of a single continuous confounder (Example 1); panel (b) considers the control of multiple confounders based on the observed covariates in the Polish breast cancer data (Example 2); panel (c) additionally considers potential recall bias in the measurement of family history (Example 3).

the more realistic simulation suggests that one would actually need $n = 1,400$, $n = 1,600$ or $n = 1,900$ depending on the strength of association between Z and family history (as measured here by Δ). Consequently, in this instance, planning the study on the basis of a naïve approach to sample size calculations would have the potential to seriously undermine its potential success.

Finally, we emphasize that the "true" numerical value of β_x was the same in both simulations. As such the differences in the power estimates cannot be attributed to the fact that β_x in model (9.20) is marginal with respect to Z, whereas β_x in model (9.21) is conditional with respect to Z. Rather the difference arises because naïvely basing sampling size calculations on model (9.20) corresponds to a form of model misspecification with respect to the magnitude and direction of impact of confounding. Haneuse *et al.* (2012) refer to this phenomenon as *structural misspecification* and provide additional discussion of its potential consequences.

9.8.3   Example 2: Multiple confounders

While Example 1 considers the impact of a single continuous adjustment variable, here we consider the setting in which the main analyses will adjust for multiple confounders. Specifically, building on the observed data in the Polish breast cancer study, we suppose that the model that will eventually be fit will adjust for education (Edu), age at first birth (AFB), benign breast disease (BBD), and BMI, with the latter included as separate terms according to whether the subject was at least 50 years of age:

$$\text{logit}\{P(D=1)\} \;=\; \beta_0^* + \beta_1\text{FH} + \beta_2\text{Edu} + \beta_3\text{AFB} + \beta_4\text{BBD}$$
$$+ \beta_5\text{BMI}\times\text{I}_{\text{age}<50} + \beta_6\text{BMI}\times\text{I}_{\text{age}\geq50}. \tag{9.22}$$

Simulations require specification of the regression coefficients and the joint distribution of the covariates. Since these may not be readily available, it would be tempting to base the calculations on model (9.20), the naïve model of Example 1.

To conduct realistic simulations, we drew samples with replacement from the observed joint covariate distribution among the controls in the Polish data to construct a population of size $N = 100,000$ individuals. Binary outcomes were generated on the basis of model (9.22) with $(\beta_1, \beta_2, \beta_3, \beta_4, \beta_5, \beta_6)$ set to $(0.61, 0.13, 0.12, 0.31, -0.22, -0.03)$, which are the values obtained from a fit of the model to the original data, and β_0^* was set to yield overall prevalence 0.10. Given a set of simulation outcomes, a case-control sample was drawn following steps (d) and (e) in Section 9.8.1, the model (9.22) fit, and a record kept of whether the null hypothesis $H_0 : \beta_1 = 0$ was rejected.

Figure 9.1(b) presents the estimated power curves from the two simulations. The power curves for the naïve analysis and fully adjusted analysis are essentially equivalent, unlike in Example 1. A possible reason why the naïve anaysis is adequate is that the adjustment variables are only weakly associated with family history (Table 9.3).

9.8.4 Example 3: Exposure misclassification

Here we assume the family history data are misclassified because subjects have imperfect recall. We assume the same type of misclassification in cases and controls ("nondifferential" error), which induces less severe and more predictable bias than differential recall bias (Coughlin, 1990). In the statistical analysis section of a grant proposal, details regarding potential misclassification should be laid out, as well as the strategy to adjust for it. Often, however, researchers will base power calculations on the naïve model (9.20) that ignores both confounding and exposure misclassification.

To obtain a more realistic power estimate, our simulation used: (i) the "true" risk model (9.22); (ii) a misclassified version of family history; and (iii) an analysis that accounts for misclassification. For (i) we used the same data generating mechanism as in Example 2. For (ii) we assumed that 90% of those with a truly positive family history are classified as having a positive family history (90% sensitivity), regardless of disease status, and 90% of those with a truly negative family history are classified as family history-negative (90% specificity), regardless of disease status. The recall error is thus "nondifferential" (see Chapter 10). Finally, for the analyses (iii) we used an approach proposed by Lyles and Lin (2010) in which one first estimates the negative and positive predictive values for the true family history status using the observed data and investigator-supplied values for sensitivity and specificity. Subsequently, these predictive values are used as weights in fitting the model of interest. Lyles and Lin (2010) suggest jackknife estimates of standard errors. In our simulations we confirmed that this approach yielded unbiased estimates and confidence intervals with nominal coverage rates.

Figure 9.1(c) presents estimated power from the naïve model (solid line) and realistic model (dashed line). The naïve calculation indicates that a sample size of $n = 1,200$ would provide 80% power to detect $\beta_1 = 0.61$. This sample size yields power less than 30% according to the realistic model. By extrapolating the dashed curve linearly, one finds that more than $n = 3,300$ cases plus controls are needed to attain 80% power. A calculation as in Section 9.3 that ignored confounding and misclassification indicated that $n = 1,254$ cases plus controls are needed for $\gamma = 0.8$, whereas adjustment for misclassification as in

Section 9.5 yielded $n = 3,610$, in reasonable agreement with the more principled estimates based on simulations that take both confounding and misclassification into account.

9.8.5 Elicitation of inputs

To perform realistic power calculations, researchers need to specify more input parameters than required for naïve calculations. Researchers may have access to pilot data to characterize the joint distribution of the covariates and to produce plausible values for parameters that are not of central interest but are required for data generation, such as the regression coefficients that quantify the relationship between confounders and the outcome. Absent pilot data, Haneuse *et al.* (2012) proposed a two-stage strategy in which researchers initially conduct comprehensive simulations based on hypothetical scenarios to provide broad guidance on the potential success of the study. Then, if the study is initiated, the sample size calculations are updated on the basis of the observed distribution of the covariates and observed associations between the confounders and the outcome. In following this strategy, one should not update the value of the regression parameter for which power is being calculated. Doing so, without appropriate adjustments, could inflate type I error.

9.9 Software

Throughout this chapter we have focused on the theoretical aspects of sample size/power calculations, together with resources available to researchers in publications. Researchers also have access to online software for performing these calculations, including the versatile PS software available at `https://biostat.mc.vanderbilt.edu/` (Dupont and Plummer, 1990), as well as the `Power 3.0` program which calculates sample size for cohort and unmatched case-control studies, including calculations for interactions, and is available at `https://dceg.cancer.gov/tools/design/power`. In addition, the Comprehensive R Archive Network (CRAN; `https://cran.r-project.org/`) hosts a number of useful contributed packages for the statistical programming language R (R Core Team, 2016), including: `epiR` for unmatched and matched case-control studies; `powerGWASinteraction` for case-control studies of candidate genes and genome-wide association studies; and `osDesign` which implements the simulation-based strategy of Section 9.8.1. An additional package specifically tailored to genetic epidemiology is `CGEN`, which is available at the Bioconductor package repository (`https://bioconductor.org/`). Finally, the functions used to perform the sample size calculations presented in Section 9.3 have been implemented in the R package `samplesizelogisticcasecontrol` (available at CRAN), while the code written specifically for the calculations performed in Section 9.8 is available from the co-author Haneuse's personal website. A related publication (Gail and Haneuse, 2017) gives R code for the simulations in this paper and also illustrates the inputs for analytical calculations with `samplesizelogisticcasecontrol`.

9.10 Discussion

We have briefly surveyed methods for case-control sample size calculations, but the literature contains many papers that treat topics we did not address, such as sample sizes for exact conditional tests. Our aim was to stress the importance of these calculations in determining the feasibility of a study and to indicate how sample size needs to be tailored to the study design and to the planned method of analysis. For unmatched designs, we have illustrated general approaches based on unconditional logistic regression.

Often the analytical sample size calculations outlined here will be sufficient to determine the feasibility of a study. However, more realistic calculations may be needed to refine the design and to take into account features such as control for confounding, measurement error, and missing data. Although analytical approaches to sample size calculation for some of these subtleties are possible (e.g., Sections 9.3.2, and 9.5), the simulation method (Section 9.8) is more flexible and frees the investigator to try to define the particular characteristics of a study that need special treatment. The challenge then becomes understanding the sampling and subtleties of a study well enough to simulate the data, including features such as missingness or measurement error. Often, such modeling requires the joint distribution of true exposures, confounders, error-prone exposure measurements and missingness probabilities. Simplified joint models and sensitivity analyses may assist in developing a range of plausible sample size requirements. However, pilot data from the study are ideal for learning about these joint distributions and for developing realistic models from which to simulate the case-control data (Haneuse *et al.*, 2012). Such data can also be used with analytical calculations, as illustrated for confounding in Section 9.3.2.

Sample size calculations are an important aspect of protocol development, and a serious effort to calculate sample size should facilitate communication between the statistician and other scientific colleagues. Is the study designed to discover new associations or to test a specific hypothesis? What specific sampling design is planned (e.g., unmatched, matched, one phase, two phases) and what are the main confounders that need to be controlled? Is the exposure measurement the best possible, or is it subject to measurement error compared to some better measurement? What is the smallest exposure effect one wishes to reliably detect, or are there special features of the dose-response curve, such as curvature, that one wishes to demonstrate? What is the planned analysis to test for exposure effects, interactions, or dose-response features? Only with a good understanding of such issues can the statistician compute required sample sizes, assess feasibility, and help refine the protocol.

9.11   Acknowledgements

We thank Dr. Montserrat Garcia-Closis for access to data from the case-control study of breast cancer in Poland. Dr. Gail was supported by the Intramural Research Program of the Division of Cancer Epidemiology and Genetics, National Cancer Institute. Dr. Haneuse was supported by the National Institutes of Health grant R-01 HL094786.

Bibliography

Benjamini, Y. and Hochberg, Y. (1995). Controlling the false discovery rate: A practical and powerful approach to multiple testing. *Journal of the Royal Statistical Society. Series B*, **57**, 289–300.

Breslow, N. E. and Day, N. E. (1987). *Statistical Methods in Cancer Research, Volume II:*

The Design and Analysis of Cohort Studies. International Agency for Research on Cancer, Lyon.

Breslow, N. E., Lubin, J. H., Marek, P., and Langholz, B. (1983). Multiplicative models and cohort analysis. *Journal of the American Statistical Association*, **78**, 1–12.

Chatterjee, N. and Carroll, R. J. (2005). Semiparametric maximum likelihood estimation exploiting gene-environment independence in case-control studies. *Biometrika*, **92**, 399–418.

Cornfield, J. (1951). A method of estimating comparative rates from clinical data: Applications to cancer in the lung, breast, and cervix. *Journal of the National Cancer Institute*, **11**, 1269–1275.

Coughlin, S. (1990). Recall bias in epidemiologic studies. *Journal of Clinical Epidemiology*, **43**, 87–91.

Cox, D. R. (1970). *The Analysis of Binary Data*. Methuen and Company, London.

Demidenko, E. (2007). Sample size determination for logistic regression revisited. *Statistics in Medicine*, **26**, 3385–3397.

Dupont, W. D. (1988). Power calculations for matched case-control studies. *Biometrics*, **44**, 1157–1168.

Dupont, W. D. and Plummer, W. D. (1990). Power and sample size calculations: A review and computer program. *Controlled Clinical Trials*, **11**, 116–128.

Gail, M. and Gart, J. (1973). The determination of sample sizes for use with the exact conditional test in 2x2 comparative trials. *Biometrics*, **29**, 441–448.

Gail, M., Williams, R., Byar, D., and Brown, C. (1976). How many controls? *Journal of Chronic Diseases*, **29**, 723–731.

Gail, M. H. and Haneuse, S. (2017). Power and sample size for multivariate logistic modeling of unmatched case-control studies. *Statistical Methods in Medical Research*, Doi: 10.1177/0962280217737157. [Epub ahead of print].

Garcia-Closas, M., Brinton, L. A., Lissowska, J., Chatterjee, N., Peplonska, B., Anderson, W., Szeszenia-Dabrowska, N., Bardin-Mikolajczak, A., Zatonski, W., Blair, A., *et al.* (2006). Established breast cancer risk factors by clinically important tumour characteristics. *British Journal of Cancer*, **95**, 123–129.

Haneuse, S., Saegusa, T., and Lumley, T. (2011). osDesign: An R package for the analysis, evaluation, and design of two-phase and case-control studies. *Journal of Statistical Software*, **43**, Issue 11.

Haneuse, S., Schildcrout, J., and Gillen, D. (2012). A two-stage strategy to accommodate general patterns of confounding in the design of observational studies. *Biostatistics*, **13**, 274–288.

Jung, S.-H. (2005). Sample size for FDR-control in microarray data analysis. *Bioinformatics*, **21**, 3097–3104.

Koehler, E., Brown, E., and Haneuse, S. (2009). On the assessment of Monte Carlo error in simulation-based statistical analyses. *The American Statistician*, **63**, 155–162.

Lagakos, S. W. (1988). Effects of mismodelling and mismeasuring explanatory variables on tests of their association with a response variable. *Statistics in Medicine*, **7**, 257–274.

Lemeshow, S., Hosmer, D. W., and Klar, J. (1988). Sample size requirements for studies estimating odds ratios or relative risks. *Statistics in Medicine*, **7**, 759–764.

Liu, P. and Hwang, J. T. G. (2007). Quick calculation for sample size while controlling false discovery rate with application to microarray analysis. *Bioinformatics*, **23**, 739–746.

Lubin, J. and Gail, M. (1990). On power and sample size for studying features of the relative odds of disease. *American Journal of Epidemiology*, **131**, 552–566.

Lubin, J., Gail, M., and Ershow, A. (1988). Sample size and power for case-control studies when exposures are continuous. *Statistics in Medicine*, **7**, 363–376.

Lyles, R. and Lin, J. (2010). Sensitivity analysis for misclassification in logistic regression via likelihood methods and predictive value weighting. *Statistics in Medicine*, **29**, 2297–2309.

McKeown-Eyssen, G. E. and Thomas, D. C. (1985). Sample size determination in case-control studies: The influence of the distribution of exposure. *Journal of Chronic Diseases*, **38**, 559–568.

McKinlay, S. M. (1974). The expected number of matches and its variance for matched-pair designs. *Applied Statistics*, **23**, 372–383.

Novikov, I., Fund, N., and Freedman, L. S. (2010). A modified approach to estimating sample size for simple logistic regression with one continuous covariate. *Statistics in Medicine*, **29**, 97–107.

Peto, R., Pike, M., Armitage, P., Breslow, N. E., Cox, D. R., Howard, S. V., Mantel, N., McPherson, K., Peto, J., and Smith, P. G. (1976). Design and analysis of randomized clinical trials requiring prolonged observation of each patient. I. Introduction and design. *British Journal of Cancer*, **34**, 585–612.

Pfeiffer, R., Park, Y., Kreimer, A., Lacey, Jr., J., Pee, D., Greenlee, R., Buys, S., Hollenbeck, A., Rosner, B., Gail, M., *et al.* (2013). Risk prediction for breast, endometrial, and ovarian cancer in white women aged 50 years or older: Derivation and validation from population-based cohort studies. *PLoS Medicine*, **10**, e1001492.

Piegorsch, W., Weinberg, C., and Taylor, J. (1994). Non-hierarchical logistic models and case-only designs for assessing susceptibility in population-based case-control studies. *Statistics in Medicine*, **13**, 153–162.

Prentice, R. L. and Pyke, R. (1979). Logistic disease incidence models and case-control studies. *Biometrika*, **66**, 403–411.

R Core Team (2016). *R: A Language and Environment for Statistical Computing*. R Foundation for Statistical Computing, Vienna.

Seaman, S. R. and White, I. R. (2013). Review of inverse probability weighting for dealing with missing data. *Statistical Methods in Medical Research*, **22**, 278–295.

Smith, P. G. and Day, N. E. (1984). The design of case-control studies: The influence of confounding and interaction effects. *International Journal of Epidemiology*, **13**, 356–365.

Ury, H. K. (1975). Efficiency of case-control studies with multiple controls per case: Continuous or dichotomous data. *Biometrics*, **31**, 643–649.

Vach, W. and Blettner, M. (2005). Missing data in epidemiologic studies. In P. Armitage and T. Colton, editors, *Encyclopedia of Biostatistics*. Wiley, Chichester, 2nd edition.

White, I. R., Royston, P., and Wood, A. M. (2011). Multiple imputation using chained equations: Issues and guidance for practice. *Statistics in Medicine*, **30**, 377–399.

Whittemore, A. S. (1981). Sample size for logistic regression with small response probability. *Journal of the American Statistical Association*, **76**, 27–32.

10

Measurement Error and Case-Control Studies

Raymond J. Carroll

Texas A&M University & University of Technology Sydney

10.1 Background on measurement error and its effects

10.1.1 Preparatory comments

Illuminating discussion of measurement error in case-control studies recently appeared in Chapter 9 of Keogh and Cox (2014); see also Chapter 5 of Gustafson (2004) for a more detailed treatment. There are book-length treatments about general measurement error models; see Gustafson (2004), Carroll *et al.* (2006), Buonaccorsi (2010), the former in particular dealing with the case of binary exposures. Our purpose here is not to review in detail the entire field of measurement error modeling (that would take another book!), but we will give the necessary background. We note that if there is measurement error in the exposure, there can be many consequences, including biases in relative risk estimates, loss of statistical power, and, especially, in the case of two or more predictors measured with error, erroneous conclusions even with an infinite sample size; see Section 10.1.3 below.

A particularly vexing issue with measurement error in case-control studies, one which is typically not of major concern in prospective cohort studies, is that the measurement error can be *differential*, i.e., it can depend upon the response. This is especially the case when the error-prone reported exposure is based on self-report. For example, consider a case-control study of nutrition and cancer, where a subject's diet in cases is measured after cancer diagnosis. It may well be the case that the cases recall their previous true exposures with a different error structure than the controls, leading to differential error.

In what follows, we will use the generic term *measurement error* to mean that a true exposure is not observed, either because it is misclassified in the case of discrete variables, or via a continuous perturbation as arises for continuous variables. We will sometimes use the term *misclassification* as well.

10.1.2   The triple whammy of measurement error

We will describe a few preliminary concepts about measurement error in this section that pertain to cohort data. Many of them apply equally to case-control data, and where necessary will translate them to the case-control context later.

Here we say that the true, *univariate* exposure is X_*, the exposure measured with error is W, the covariates/confounders measured without error is $\mathbf{Z}$, and the predictors in the model are $\mathbf{X} = (X_*, \mathbf{Z})$. The response is D. We emphasize that we are considering only univariate X_*. For a multivariate exposure $\mathbf{X}_*$, the methods to correct for bias caused by measurement error are the same as in what follows, but the effects of that error, especially on hypothesis testing for whether components of $\mathbf{X}_*$ are statistically significant predictors of D, are much more complex; see Chapter 10 of Carroll *et al.* (2006) for a full chapter devoted to this topic, and also page 274 of Buonaccorsi (2010).

In the general literature, there is a model for D given $\mathbf{X}$, and while the model can be complex, here we write it as

$$E(D|\mathbf{X}) = m(\alpha + \mathbf{X}^{\mathrm{T}}\boldsymbol{\beta}).$$

Logistic regression is the prime example in case-control studies, where $m(\cdot) = \mathrm{expit}(\cdot)$, the logistic distribution function.

There are a number of features about measurement error, called the *triple whammy* by Carroll *et al.* (2006).

- Measurement error causes bias in the estimation of $\boldsymbol{\beta}$.

- It also causes a loss of statistical power. The greater the measurement error, the harder it will be to detect whether the covariates, and particularly the exposure, are significant predictors of the outcome.

- It causes a severe loss of features. For example, suppose X_* is uniformly distributed on the interval $[-2, 2]$. Suppose that the mean is $\sin(2X_*)$ and the variance $\sigma_\epsilon^2 = 0.10$. In the top panel of Figure 10.1, we plot 200 simulated observations from such a model that indicate quite clearly the sinusoidal aspect of the regression function. However, suppose that instead of observing X_*, we observe W, normally distributed with mean X_* but with variance 4/9. Thus, what we observe is not X_*, but an unbiased estimate of it, W. In the bottom panel of Figure 10.1, we plot the observed data D versus W. Note that the sinusoid is no longer evident and the main feature of the data, the sinusoid, has been *hidden*.

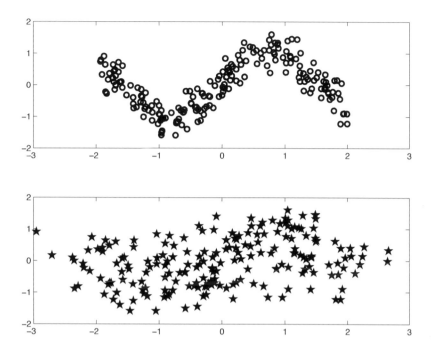

FIGURE 10.1
Illustration of the bias, loss of power, and masking of features caused by measurement error in predictors. Top panel regression on the true covariate. Bottom panel regression on the observed covariate.

10.1.3 Hypothesis testing

Most of the measurement error literature makes the assumption that the measurement error is *nondifferential*, by which we mean technically that, given $\mathbf{X}$, D and W are independent. This can be thought of loosely as that *if you could observe* $\mathbf{X}$, W *would not be an independent predictor of* D. More difficult cases are described in Gustafson (2004) and Buonaccorsi (2010). With nondifferential error, W is often called a *surrogate* for X_*. In the nondifferential case, when X_* is scalar, tests of the hypothesis

$$H_0 : D \text{ and } X_* \text{ are independent given } \mathbf{Z} \tag{10.1}$$

are valid even when W is substituted for X_*. This only holds for a univariate X_*, and is not true for testing single components of a multivariate $\mathbf{X}_*$. However, because of the second feature of the triple whammy, such a test has much less statistical power than if X_* had been observed.

However, and not very well known, tests of

$$H_0 : D \text{ and } \mathbf{Z} \text{ are independent given } X_* \tag{10.2}$$

can be invalid, in the sense that they have a higher than desired Type I error rate. Chapter 3.3 of Carroll *et al.* (2006) shows an example of this in the case that $\mathbf{Z}$ is a binary, for an unbalanced one-way analysis of covariance, unbalanced in the sense that the distribution of

X_* is different in the two groups formed by the values of $\mathbf{Z}$. The issue is also described in detail in Chapter 10 of Carroll *et al.* (2006).

10.1.4 Correcting for bias and the critical components needed

Because of the bias induced by measurement error, measurement error analyses attempt to correct that bias, so that the analyst is actually estimating the parameters of intrinsic interest. In addition, a measurement error analysis is aimed at making correct inferences. No matter what the measurement error analysis, there are two *critical components*:

- The *measurement error model*, i.e., how are W and $\mathbf{X} = (X_*, \mathbf{Z})$ related?

- The *covariate model*, i.e., how is X_* related to $\mathbf{Z}$?

There is an alternative viewpoint, exemplified in case-control studies by equation (5.14) of Gustafson (2004), wherein a model for the distribution of X_* given $(\mathbf{Z}, D)$ is specified.

For example, consider the case that the true exposure is a continuous variable. The so-called *classical measurement error model* has that

$$W = X_* + V_c, \tag{10.3}$$

and it is typically taken that V_c is independent of $(X_*, \mathbf{Z})$, and also that the covariate model has X_* related to $\mathbf{Z}$ through a linear regression. The *Berkson model* turns (10.3) around, so that

$$X_* = W + V_b, \tag{10.4}$$

where V_b is independent of $(W, \mathbf{Z})$. There are also combinations of the classical and Berkson models (see Reeves *et al.*, 1998; Mallick *et al.*, 2002; Li *et al.*, 2007), which have been used particularly in radiation epidemiology.

Given the critical components of the measurement error model, there are a host of statistical methods that correct for the bias caused by measurement error, and also all correct inferences. Some methods are regression calibration (the standard for linear, logistic and Cox regression), SIMEX (Cook and Stefanski, 1994; Stefanski and Cook, 1995; Carroll *et al.*, 2006), instrumental variables, maximum likelihood, etc.

10.1.5 Regression calibration

Because it is so broadly used in linear, logistic and Cox regression, and because case-control studies are generally based on an underlying logistic regression, it is worth here describing the regression calibration (approximate) method for logistic regression. We do so in its simplest form: the books mentioned at the start of this chapter give all the theoretical details anyone would want to see. The algorithm is simple: replace X_* by an estimate of the regression of X_* on $(W, \mathbf{Z})$, then use either theory or the bootstrap for inferences.

We focus on rare diseases, since case-control studies are so often about rare diseases. Then the logistic regression model is

$$P(D = 1 | X_*, \mathbf{Z}) = \text{expit}(\alpha + X_* \beta_1 + \mathbf{Z}^{\mathrm{T}} \boldsymbol{\beta}_2).$$

A well-known approximation for rare diseases is that

$$P(D = 1 | X_*, \mathbf{Z}) \approx \exp(\alpha + X_* \beta_1 + \mathbf{Z}^{\mathrm{T}} \boldsymbol{\beta}_2).$$

TABLE 10.1

Invasive cervical cancer ($D = 1$) and measures of herpes simplex virus type 2: truth = X_*, error-prone = W. See Section 10.2.

	D	X_*	W	Count
Complete Data				
	1	0	0	13
	1	0	1	3
	1	1	0	5
	1	1	1	18
	0	0	0	33
	0	0	1	11
	0	1	0	16
	0	1	1	16
Incomplete Data				
	1		0	316
	1		1	375
	0		0	701
	0		1	535

Now if model (10.3) holds with $X_* = \gamma_0 + \mathbf{Z}^{\mathrm{T}}\gamma_1 + \text{Normal}(0, \sigma_x^2)$, and if $V_c \sim \text{Normal}(0, \sigma_v^2)$, then, with $\lambda = \sigma_x^2/(\sigma_x^2 + \sigma_v^2)$,

$$
\begin{aligned}
X_* &= (\gamma_0 + \mathbf{Z}^{\mathrm{T}}\gamma_1)(1 - \lambda) + \lambda W + \text{Normal}(0, \sigma_v^2\lambda) \\
&= E(X_*|W, \mathbf{Z}) + \text{Normal}(0, \sigma_v^2\lambda).
\end{aligned}
$$

If we define $\alpha_* = \alpha + \sigma_v^2\lambda/2$, and if we make the exponential approximation, then by using moment generating calculations,

$$
\begin{aligned}
P(D = 1|W, \mathbf{Z}) &\approx \exp[\alpha_* + E(X_*|W, \mathbf{Z})\beta_1 + \mathbf{Z}^{\mathrm{T}}\boldsymbol{\beta}_2] \\
&\approx \text{expit}[\alpha_* + E(X_*|W, \mathbf{Z})\beta_1 + \mathbf{Z}^{\mathrm{T}}\boldsymbol{\beta}_2].
\end{aligned}
$$

Hence, to obtain consistent (asymptotically unbiased) estimates of the risk parameters $\boldsymbol{\beta} = (\beta_1, \boldsymbol{\beta}_2)$, we should run logistic regression by replacing X_* by $E(X_*|W, \mathbf{Z})$.

Of course, how to get the regression calibration function requires additional data. We will focus later on its use in the case-control context.

10.2 An example of case-control studies with measurement error

As an illustration, Carroll *et al.* (1993) describe a data set (cf. Table 10.1) where X_* and W are binary on exposure to herpes simplex virus type 2, while D is invasive cervical cancer: there are no error-free covariates $\mathbf{Z}$. Carroll *et al.* (1993) discuss that the misclassification appears to be differential, i.e., it depends on disease status D. The log odds ratio when using the smaller data set where X_* is observed is estimated as 0.68, with standard error 0.40. The odds ratio using the error-prone covariates W is 0.45 with standard error 0.09. The corresponding odds ratios are 1.98 and 1.55. The effect of using only the error-prone data is immediate: underestimation of relative risk. The pseudo-likelihood method of Carroll *et al.* (1993) (see Section 10.5.2.1) under differential misclassification has a log odds ratio estimated as 0.62 with standard error 0.36.

10.3   Introduction to case-control studies

10.3.1   Background

Case-control studies have important differences with prospective cohort studies, and these differences are especially important for a measurement error analysis.

Once again, the true exposure is X_*, the exposure measured with error is W, the co-variates/confounders measured without error is $\mathbf{Z}$, and the predictors in the model are $\mathbf{X} = (X_*, \mathbf{Z})$. Almost without exception in case-control studies, the outcome D is binary, with $D = 1$ meaning the subject has a disease and $D = 0$ meaning that the subject is without disease. Much, but not all, of the literature is based on the idea of a *prospective* logistic risk model of the form

$$P(D = 1|\mathbf{X}) = \text{expit}(\alpha + \mathbf{X}^{\mathrm{T}}\boldsymbol{\beta}) = \text{expit}(\alpha + X_*\beta_1 + \mathbf{Z}^{\mathrm{T}}\boldsymbol{\beta}_2). \tag{10.5}$$

We focus here on (population-based) case-control studies, which we will simply call a case-control study, and at the end we will mention some work on matched case-control studies. In a case-control study, the sampling distribution is that of $(W, X_*, \mathbf{Z})$ given $D = d$, and is thus inherently retrospective. This differs from the case of simple random sampling, where the sampling distribution is typically thought of as that of D given $(W, X_*, \mathbf{Z})$.

It is well known (Cornfield, 1956; Anderson, 1972; Prentice and Pyke, 1979) that if (a) general logistic model (10.5); and (b) the true exposure X_* were observable, then $\boldsymbol{\beta}$ can be estimated and inference can be made about it by a simple logistic regression of D on $\mathbf{X}$. Indeed, doing an ordinary logistic regression analysis even gives correct standard errors for the components of $\boldsymbol{\beta}$. This profound result means, of course, that if the true exposure X_* is observed, then to estimate $\boldsymbol{\beta}$, the case-control sampling scheme can be ignored. Unfortunately, when the true exposure is not observed, then the case-control sampling scheme generally must be taken fully into account, as we show below.

As an aside, it is perhaps less well recognized that the parameter α in (10.5) actually cannot be identified from case-control data, no matter what the sample size is. Indeed, if $\pi_d = P(D = d)$ in the source population, and if n_d is the number of case-control study participants with $D = d$, the intercept estimated from ordinary logistic regression is $\alpha_* = \alpha + \log(n_1/n_0) - \log(\pi_1/\pi_0)$. The special nature of the logistic function, however, makes this fact irrelevant for estimating $\boldsymbol{\beta}$; see below.

10.3.2   Bootstrapping

The bootstrap for case-control studies is different from the ordinary bootstrap for prospective studies. What one does is to resample the data, with replacement, separately among the cases and the controls. Thus, each bootstrap data set has the same number of cases and controls; see Wang *et al.* (1997).

10.4 The binary and categorical cases

10.4.1 Background

Almost all expositions of case-control sampling with mismeasured exposure start with the case that the true exposure X_* and its observed version W are binary. In addition, such treatments generally start out by ignoring the possibility of covariates $\mathbf{Z}$. Here we briefly review those developments.

10.4.2 Odds ratios with binary X_* observed without error

The literature generally starts with the case that there are no covariates $\mathbf{Z}$, and that X_* is binary as well. The logistic model is (10.5).

If X_* is binary, this means that

$$P(D = 1|X_* = 0) = \text{expit}(\alpha)$$

and

$$P(D = 1|X_* = 1) = \text{expit}(\alpha + \beta).$$

In this case, it is known (Cornfield, 1956; Anderson, 1972; Prentice and Pyke, 1979) that the odds ratio for the case-control study is the same as in a simple random sample, so that

$$
\begin{aligned}
\exp(\beta) &= \frac{P(X_* = 1|D = 1)/P(X_* = 0|D = 1)}{P(X_* = 1|D = 0)/P(X_* = 0|D = 0)} \\
&= \frac{P(D = 1|X_* = 1)/P(D = 0|X_* = 1)}{P(D = 1|X_* = 0)/P(D = 0|X_* = 0)}.
\end{aligned}
\tag{10.6}
$$

More generally, if X_* is not binary, and for any (x_0, x_1),

$$\exp\{(x_1 - x_0)\beta\} = \frac{P(X_* = x_1|D = 1)/P(X_* = x_0|D = 1)}{P(X_* = x_1|D = 0)/P(X_* = x_0|D = 0)}.$$

10.4.3 Odds ratios with binary X_* observed with error

We can see from (10.6) that we can estimate β if we can obtain information about $P(X_* = x|D = d)$. Suppose now that we observe a binary W instead of the binary X_*. Then the likelihood of the observed retrospective data is

$$P(W = w|D = d) = \sum_{x=0}^{1} P(W = w|X_* = x, D = d)P(X_* = x|D = d). \tag{10.7}$$

In the case of nondifferential measurement error,

$$P(W = w|X_* = x, D = d) = P(W = w|X_* = x),$$

and (10.7) simplifies accordingly.

Equation (10.7) reveals that the *critical* piece of information needed to correct for the effect of misclassification is the misclassification matrix $P(W = 1|X_* = x, D = d)$. For the moment, let us pretend that we know this information.

Define

$$p_{xy} = P(W = 1 | X_* = x, D = d),$$
$$\pi_{Wwy} = P(W = w | D = d),$$
$$\tilde{\pi}_W = (\pi_{W00}, \pi_{W01}, \pi_{W10}, \pi_{W11})^{\mathrm{T}},$$
$$\pi_{Xxy} = P(X_* = x | D = d),$$
$$\tilde{\pi}_X = (\pi_{X00}, \pi_{X01}, \pi_{X10}, \pi_{X11})^{\mathrm{T}}.$$

Numerous authors (Greenland and Kleinbaum, 1983; Greenland, 1988a,b; Morrissey and Spiegelman, 1999) have noticed that

$$\tilde{\pi}_W = \begin{bmatrix} 1 - p_{00} & 0 & 1 - p_{10} & 0 \\ 0 & 1 - p_{01} & 0 & 1 - p_{11} \\ p_{00} & 0 & p_{10} & 0 \\ 0 & p_{01} & 0 & p_{11} \end{bmatrix} \tilde{\pi}_X = A\tilde{\pi}_X.$$

This has led to the *matrix method*, wherein $\tilde{\pi}_W$ is estimated from the observed data, and then a matrix inversion is done to recover $\tilde{\pi}_X$, i.e., $\tilde{\pi}_X = A^{-1}\tilde{\pi}_W$.

An alternative calculation is given in Marshall (1990) (see also Morrissey and Spiegelman, 1999), resulting in what is called the *inverse matrix method*, which is based not on the misclassification matrix, but instead on the positive and negative predicted values $PPV_y = P(X_* = 1 | W = 1, D = d)$ and $PNV_y = P(X_* = 0 | W = 0, D = d)$, respectively, noting that $P(X_* = x | W = w, D = d) = P(W = w | X_* = x, D = d)/\pi_{Xxy}$, in which case there is a matrix B, given in formula (3) of Morrissey and Spiegelman (1999), so that $\tilde{\pi}_X = B\tilde{\pi}_W$.

Carrying on the fiction that the misclassification matrix or the positive and negative predicted values are known, both the matrix method and the inverse matrix method are simple to compute, yielding estimates of $\tilde{\pi}_X$, which can then be plugged into (10.6) to estimate β.

10.4.4   Estimating the misclassification matrix

10.4.4.1   Validation data

Of course, the fiction that the misclassification matrix is known, or that the positive and negative predicted values are known, is generally just that: a fiction. Thus, consideration has been given to a number of possible alternatives.

A commonly discussed case is when, in addition to the main study, there is a *validation* study in which X_* is also observed. Suppose that for the first $i = 1, ..., n_1$ observations, the main study, we only observe (W_i, D_i), while for the last $i = n_1 + 1, ..., n$ observations, the validation study, we observe (W_i, D_i, X_{*i}). Then the loglikelihood of the case-control data is

$$\sum_{i=1}^{n_1} \log\{P(W_i | D_i)\} + \sum_{i=n_1+1}^{N} \log\{P(W_i | X_{*i}, D_i)P(X_{*i} | D_i)\}; \tag{10.8}$$

see equation (7) of Morrissey and Spiegelman (1999). That paper recognizes that the unknown parameters are β, $\theta = P(X_* = 1 | D = 0)$, and for $y = 0, 1$,

$$P_y = P(W = 1 | X_* = 1, D = d)$$

and

$$R_y = P(W = 0 | X_* = 0, D = d),$$

and that, based on (10.6),

$$P(X_* = 1|D = 0) = \theta;$$

$$P(X_* = 1|D = 1) = \frac{\theta \exp(\beta)}{1 - \theta + \theta \exp(\beta)};$$

$$P(W = 1|D = 0) = P_0\theta + (1 - R_0)(1 - \theta);$$

$$P(W = 1|D = 1) = \frac{P_1\theta \exp(\beta) + (1 - R_1)(1 - \theta)}{1 - \theta + \theta \exp(\beta)}.$$

From this, the loglikelihood can be maximized. Morrissey and Spiegelman (1999) show that this likelihood-based method is more efficient than either of the two matrix methods. In the nondifferential error case, $P_0 = P_1$ and $R_0 = R_1$, and this can be exploited for further gains in efficiency.

A complete asymptotic theory for case-control studies when there is measurement error, a validation study, and either nondifferential or differential error is given in Carroll *et al.* (1993).

10.4.4.2   Replication or multiple instruments data

More difficult is the case that there are no validation data. Suppose that the measurement error is nondifferential. Chapter 5 of Gustafson (2004) describes what can be done; see the earlier work of Hui and Walter (1980) and Drews *et al.* (1993). This work considers the case that there are sub-samples among the case and controls that have two binary, nondifferentially mismeasured variables on the same subject, say (W_1, W_2): they could be replicates or not. If they are not replicates, these papers show that there are six parameters in the model: $r_1 = P(X_* = 1|D = 1)$, $r_0 = P(X_* = 0|D = 0)$, $p_1 = P(W_1 = 1|X_* = 1)$, $q_1 = P(W_1 = 1|X_* = 0)$, $p_2 = P(W_2 = 1|X_* = 1)$ and $q_2 = P(W_2 = 0|X_* = 0)$. Also, via the 2×2 tables separately for cases and controls, there are six sufficient statistics, so that β is technically identified, in the sense that as the sub-sample sizes increase, β can be estimated consistently. See equations (5.9)-(5.10) of Gustafson (2004) for the likelihood function. In the case of replicates, there are only four parameters, and in the aforementioned equation (5.10), $p_1 = p_2$ and $q_1 = q_2$. As is emphasized by Gustafson (2004), however, unless $r_1 = P(X_* = 1|D = 1)$ and $r_0 = P(X_* = 1|D = 0)$ are well separated, estimation of β will have large variation.

10.4.5   Categorical covariates

The developments in Sections 10.4.3-10.4.4 also equally apply to problems where X_* is categorical rather than binary. A nice example of this is given in Rice and Holmans (2003), wherein X_* can be the values of a single nucleotide polymorphism (SNP), which takes on the values 0, 1 and 2 depending on the number of minor alleles. Then the risk model might be

$$P(D = 1|X_*) = \text{expit}\{\alpha + I(X_* = 1)\beta_1 + I(X_* = 2)\beta_2\}.$$

Just as in (10.6), we can identify $\boldsymbol{\beta} = (\beta_1, \beta_2)^{\mathrm{T}}$ from odds ratios in the case-control study, e.g., for $x = 1, 2$,

$$\exp(\beta_x) = \frac{P(X_* = x|D = 1)P(X_* = 0|D = 0)}{P(X_* = 0|D = 1)P(X_* = x|D = 0)},$$

and the crucial step is to identify the misclassification matrix $P(W = w|X_* = x, D = d)$, or the positive and negative predicted values.

10.4.6   When there are additional predictors **Z**

The simple methods described above have all been introduced in the context that there are no additional covariates **Z**, and when X_* and W are binary (or categorical, see Section 10.4.5). In practice, though, it is more the rule than the exception that case-control studies also include covariates/confounders, sometimes of rather high dimension.

For binary X_* and W, nondifferential measurement error, and rare disease, and with reference to Section 10.4.4.2, Gustafson (2004) suggests replacing r_0 and r_1 in Section 10.4.4.2 by $r_y(\mathbf{Z}) = \operatorname{expit}(\lambda_0 + \lambda_1 y + \mathbf{Z}^{\mathrm{T}} \lambda_2)$ and interpreting λ_1 as if it were the log odds ratio for X_*; see that paper's equation (5.18). As described there, λ_1 is a reasonable approximation for the log odds ratio as long as the disease is rare and the effects of the covariates **Z** are not large.

Another approach to incorporating **Z** (Satten and Kupper, 1993b) is described in Section 10.5.2.2.

10.5   Case-control studies with continuous exposure

10.5.1   Background

As in the binary X_* case, to correct for the biases induced by measurement error, generally one needs either a validation study, in which X_* is observed for a subset of study participants, or one needs either replicate measures of W or multiple instruments that are proxies for W. We discuss the former in Section 10.5.2 and the latter in Section 10.5.3.

10.5.2   Validation data

10.5.2.1   Pseudo-likelihood: Modeling only the error distribution

For the case of validation data, Section 3 of Carroll *et al.* (1993) develops a method based on the idea of pseudo-likelihood (Gong and Samaniego, 1981). Their method assumes that selection into the validation study depends only on disease status D. They allow for differential measurement error, and they only model the distribution of the measurement error process W given $(X_*, \mathbf{Z}, D)$.

Carroll *et al.* (1993) do not explicitly allow for covariates **Z** measured without error. Sticking to the desire to model only the distribution of W given $(X_*, \mathbf{Z}, D)$, one can handle covariates measured without error by defining their W exactly the same as our $(W, \mathbf{Z})$, and their X as our $\mathbf{X} = (X_*, \mathbf{Z})$. What this means though is that, in implementing Carroll *et al.* (1993), one must pretend that not only is X_* not observed, but also that **Z** is not observed.

Carroll *et al.* (1993) thus present a pseudo-likelihood, which can be maximized to obtain parameter estimates. They provide formulae for asymptotic standard errors, and of course as a simple alternative the bootstrap as described in Section 10.3.2 can be used.

10.5.2.2   Likelihood when modeling the distribution of the true exposure

Carroll *et al.* (2006) state that Satten and Kupper (1993b) *is an important paper with major implications for the analysis of retrospective studies in the presence of missing data*, and is of course applicable to the measurement error problem. The methodology assumes nondifferential measurement error, allows for covariates **Z** measured without error, includes various scenarios including cases where X_* is partially observed through validation data, and allows the selection of such validation data to be a complex process. It is based on estimating

$P(X_* = x|W, \mathbf{Z}, D = 0)$ among the controls, either via validation data or from external data, although one has to be careful with external data, because often the distributions of the exposure X_* will differ between data sets. This latter issue is called the *transportability* issue in Section 2.2 of Carroll *et al.* (2006).

The methodology in Satten and Kupper (1993b) is written for the case that all of $(X_*, W, \mathbf{Z})$ take on a finite number of values, although the number of those values may be large, and indeed in their Example 2 in their Section 2.4, $\mathbf{Z}$ is total cholesterol measured at the integer level. The seemingly discrete nature of $(X_*, W, \mathbf{Z})$, although motivated by genetics, along with the many seemingly endless summations in the paper, has masked a stunning piece of research, because the work is far more general.

For the general case, in the situation where selection into the validation study is random, Carroll *et al.* (1995) translated the so-called unconditional method of Satten and Kupper (1993b) into a notation closer to what we have been using. For $i = 1, ..., n$, let $\delta_i = 1$ mean that X_{*i} is observed in the validation study, and $\delta_i = 0$ otherwise. Referring to (10.5), let the density or mass function of X_* given $(W, \mathbf{Z}, D = 0)$ be denoted as $f_{X|W,Z,D}(X_*, W, \mathbf{Z}, D = 0, \boldsymbol{\gamma}, \beta_1)$. Define $R(W, \mathbf{Z}, \beta_1, \boldsymbol{\gamma}) = \log[E\{\exp(X_*\beta_1)|W, \mathbf{Z}, D = 0\}]$. Then

$$\frac{f_{X|W,Z,D}(X_*, W, \mathbf{Z}, D = 1, \boldsymbol{\gamma}, \beta_1)}{f_{X|W,Z,D}(X_*, W, \mathbf{Z}, D = 0, \boldsymbol{\gamma})} = \exp\{X_*\beta_1 + R(W, \mathbf{Z}, \beta_1, \boldsymbol{\gamma})\}.$$

Satten and Kupper (1993b) also showed that

$$P(D = 1|W, \mathbf{Z}) = \text{expit}\{\alpha + \mathbf{Z}^{\mathrm{T}}\boldsymbol{\beta}_2 + R(W, \mathbf{Z}, \beta_1, \boldsymbol{\gamma})\}.$$

Then the translation in Carroll *et al.* (1995) shows that the loglikelihood function is

$$\sum_{i=1}^{n} \left[\delta_i \log\{f_{X|W,Z,D}(X_{*i}, W_i, \mathbf{Z}_i, D_i, \boldsymbol{\gamma}, \beta_1)\} \right.$$
$$\left. + D_i \log\{P(D_i = 1|W_i, \mathbf{Z}_i)\} + (1 - D_i)\log\{1 - P(D_i = 1|W_i, \mathbf{Z}_i)\} \right].$$

The loglikelihood can then be maximized to estimate the parameters $(\alpha, \beta_1, \boldsymbol{\beta}_2, \boldsymbol{\gamma})$. The appendix in Carroll *et al.* (1995) shows that the usual Fisher information standard errors are also correct. Of course, the bootstrap as described in Section 10.3.2 can also be used.

10.5.3   Regression calibration, validation, replicates, multiple proxies

Often, obtaining validation data in a case-control study is impossible. Instead, in these cases, it is sometimes possible to obtain replicate versions, as in Section 10.4.4.2, and, since here X_* is a continuous variable, to use regression calibration. This is discussed in Section 4.3 of Carroll *et al.* (1993), who also mention the normal discriminant analysis method which assumes a distribution for (X_*, W) given $(D, \mathbf{Z})$; see Michalek and Tripathi (1980); Armstrong *et al.* (1989); Buonaccorsi (1990). In prospective studies, regression calibration involves the replacement of X_* by an estimate of its calibration function $E(X_*|W, \mathbf{Z})$. The discussion in Carroll *et al.* (1993) includes situations where the replicates occur in both the cases and the controls. However, a simple analysis can be done when the disease is rare, typical for a case-control study, and replicates are done only among the controls. Then, by methods described in Carroll *et al.* (1993), one simply replaces X_* by the estimate of $E(X_*|W, \mathbf{Z})$ and runs an ordinary logistic regression. Standard errors can be obtained as in Carroll *et al.* (1993), or, far more simply, by the bootstrap as described in Section 10.3.2.

In some cases, the proxy/surrogate, W, is not unbiased for X_*, so that the classical measurement error model (10.3) does not hold. However, there may be another variable, W_* say, that is measured for some of the controls and for which (10.3) holds. Then one replaces X_* by the regression of W_* on $(W, \mathbf{Z})$.

10.6 Bayesian methods for case-control studies

There is a small literature on Bayesian analysis of case-control studies with measurement error in covariates: the papers we know of are Müller and Roeder (1997); Gustafson *et al.* (2002); Gustafson (2004); Richardson *et al.* (2002). Müller and Roeder (1997) is extremely general, allowing the distribution of X_* to be a Dirichlet mixture of normal distributions, part of the trend to nonparametric Bayes methodology. Gustafson *et al.* (2002) takes a much simpler approach, but it assumes that X_* is univariate and independent of, or at least only weakly related to, any covariates $\mathbf{Z}$ measured without error. The book by Gustafson (2004), especially its Chapter 5, is a sophisticated discussion of issues that arise in the case that X_* is binary: readers will appreciate the directness of its interpretations as it pertains to extant methods. The paper by Richardson *et al.* (2002) is a semiparametric approach to the problem allowing a flexible distribution for the true exposure when there are validation data.

One of the issues with the discussion of Bayesian analysis of case-control studies is that even without measurement error, it is complex. Reconciling prospective and retrospective analysis of case-control data is trivial for frequentist statisticians and epidemiologists, since in the logistic context, as we have already mentioned, Prentice and Pyke (1979) showed that the case-control sampling design can be ignored for the estimation of $\boldsymbol{\beta}$. In the Bayesian context, finding prior distributions that do this is not easy (see Seaman and Richardson, 2004), and extensions of that work to account for measurement error will be harder still.

10.7 Matched case-control studies

In a 1-1 matched case-control study, which we consider here, a case and a control are matched on variables such as age, gender, etc. Then an exposure is measured for each matched case and control. For the ith matched pair, we observe the unordered case and control (D_{i1}, D_{i2}), and, ideally, the corresponding true exposures (X_{i1*}, X_{i2*}). In survival analysis, such matching on time yields a nested case-control study.

There is a substantial literature on matched case-control studies when the exposure is binary or categorical, but instead of the true exposures (X_{i1*}, X_{i2*}), what is observed is measured exposures (W_{i1}, W_{i2}). These papers make different assumptions about whether the measurement error is or is not differential, and different assumptions about what is being assumed about the misclassification probabilities. For this literature, see Greenland (1982); Greenland and Kleinbaum (1983); Greenland (1989); Satten and Kupper (1993a,b); Rice (2003).

For example, Satten and Kupper (1993a) work with categorical data, but in the case of binary data, they assume nondifferential misclassification, and that, in our notation, $P(X_* = x | D = 0, W = w)$ is known. Like the other papers cited above, they develop clever ways of working with the discrete data to estimate the odds ratio $\exp(\beta)$ in the population, and to make inference about it. Other papers, see for example Greenland (1989), work with the misclassification matrix (see Section 10.4.3), assuming that it is either known or estimable in the source population. Rice (2003) provides interesting generalizations.

There are some problems though that this literature may not address directly. The first is the case that the true exposure X_* is continuous and univariate. None of the aforementioned papers address this directly, although it might be reasonable to discretize X_* to make it a discrete variable to which these papers may be applicable. In addition, none of them allow the addition of complex, multivariate variables $\mathbf{Z}$ observed without error. Again, in some cases it might be possible to reduce $\mathbf{Z}$ to strata, use the methods to estimate the odds ratios in each strata, and then somehow combine them to estimate the overall odds ratio for true exposure. Another issue is that the matching variables might affect the distribution of X_* given (D, W).

To handle more complex cases, such as continuous exposures and variables measured without error, the literature is quite small: we know of McShane *et al.* (2001), Guolo and Brazzale (2008) and Espino-Hernandez *et al.* (2011). The former describes version of the *conditional scores* approach (Stefanski and Carroll, 1987) and regression calibration, what they call Regression Calibration 2, which applies regression calibration to the cases and controls and then does a conditional logistic regression on the calibrated estimates. The latter includes SIMEX (Cook and Stefanski, 1994; Stefanski and Cook, 1995; Carroll *et al.*, 2006) and a prospective likelihood analysis, and does a large simulation study. The overall conclusion of Guolo and Brazzale (2008) is that the prospective likelihood analysis is the overall winner, but computationally difficult, while Regression Calibration 2 is a reasonable and computationally simpler alternative.

Finally, we once again mention Satten and Kupper (1993b), which is also applicable to matched case-control studies; see Example 1 in its Section 4. As mentioned previously in the unmatched case, the methodology assumes nondifferential measurement error, allows for covariates $\mathbf{Z}$ measured without error, includes various scenarios including cases where X_* is partially observed through validation data, and allows the selection of such validation data to be a complex process. It is based on estimating $P(X_* = x | W, \mathbf{Z}, D = 0)$. The methodology is written for the case that all of $(X_*, W, \mathbf{Z})$ take on a finite number of values, and a translation of that work to the continuous case would be useful to have.

A fully Bayesian treatment is given in Espino-Hernandez *et al.* (2011), developing a method that has WinBUGS software. Here, they treat each matched pair as a stratum, and they allow that, within the matched pair, (X_{i1*}, X_{i2*}) are normally distributed with a covariance matrix independent of the stratum and with a mean that is normally distributed as well. They also assume that the measurement error structure is normally distributed with a common covariance matrix. It would be interesting to see whether these assumptions of normality can be relaxed in a way that allows practical (as opposed to theoretical) implementation.

10.8 Open problems

In summary, with respect to case-control studies, there is a substantial body of work available for users to deal with the issue of measurement errors, as we have outlined here. The real practical issue is to get investigators to understand that if they ignore measurement error, then the relative risks they report are in error, sometimes grossly so, and the inferences they make may be in error as well.

There are numerous other papers that describe different approaches to the problem of measurement error in case-control studies (Thürigen *et al.*, 2000; Keogh and White, 2014).

An examination of the reference list in this chapter shows that essentially almost every paper that has to do with case-control studies and measurement error was written at least a decade ago, and the seminal work was done in the 1980s and 1990s. There are exceptions: in the author's experience see Lobach *et al.* (2008) for gene-environment interactions and Gail *et al.* (2016) for matched studies involving calibrating Vitamin D levels to a central laboratory. There is obviously far more work needed in the Bayesian analysis of case-control studies. Also far more work is needed in matched case-control studies. For example, even at a prosaic level, it would be useful to translate the work in Satten and Kupper (1993b) to matched case-control studies to allow for continuous $(X_*, W, \mathbf{Z})$, as was done in Carroll *et al.* (1995) for unmatched studies.

In contrast, for considerations of measurement error in prospective studies there are a host of new concepts, and much new work (time-varying X_*, longitudinal and functional data, multivariate $\mathbf{X}_*$, deconvolution in new directions, multivariate excess zeros and measurement error, semiparametric advances, etc.). In prospective studies there are many new data types that have complex forms of measurement error, and the data for handling the issues are readily available, e.g., for prospective studies in nutrition, and the myriad ways of measuring physical activity (two fields of current interest to the author) and also many other fields. Hopefully, these new ideas and concepts will translate to case-control studies. A possible caveat is that case-control studies allow us to estimate odds ratios, but not the full range of exposure effect measures that are possible with cohort data, unless the case-control data are supplemented by knowing $P(D = 1)$.

Bibliography

Anderson, J. A. (1972). Separate sample logistic discrimination. *Biometrika*, **59**, 19–35.

Armstrong, B. G., Whittemore, A. S., and Howe, G. R. (1989). Analysis of case-control data with covariate measurement error: Application to diet and colon cancer. *Statistics in Medicine*, **8**, 1151–1163.

Buonaccorsi, J. P. (1990). Double sampling for exact values in the normal discriminant model with application to binary regression. *Communications in Statistics-Theory and Methods*, **19**, 4569–4586.

Buonaccorsi, J. P. (2010). *Measurement Error: Models, Methods and Applications*. Chapman & Hall.

Carroll, R. J., Gail, M. H., and Lubin, J. H. (1993). Case-control studies with errors in covariates. *Journal of the American Statistical Association*, **88**, 185–199.

Carroll, R. J., Wang, S., and Wang, C. Y. (1995). Prospective analysis of logistic case-control studies. *Journal of the American Statistical Association*, **90**, 157–169.

Carroll, R. J., Ruppert, D., Stefanski, L. A., and Crainiceanu, C. M. (2006). *Measurement Error in Nonlinear Models: A Modern Perspective, Second Edition*. Chapman and Hall.

Cook, J. R. and Stefanski, L. (1994). Simulation-Extrapolation estimation in parametric measurement error models. *Journal of the American Statistical Association*, **89**, 1314–1328.

Cornfield, J. (1956). A statistical problem arising from retrospective studies. In *Proceedings of the Third Berkeley Symposium on Mathematical Statistics and Probability*, volume 4, pages 135–148. University of California Press, Berkeley.

Drews, C. D., Flanders, W. D., and Kosinski, A. S. (1993). Use of two data sources to estimate odds ratios in case-control studies. *Epidemiology*, **4**, 327–335.

Espino-Hernandez, G., Gustafson, P., and Burstyn, I. (2011). Bayesian adjustment for measurement error in continuous exposures in an individually matched case-control study. *BMC Medical Research Methodology*, **11**, 67.

Gail, M. H., Wu, J., Wang, M., Yaun, S.-S., Cook, N. R., Eliassen, A. H., McCullough, M. L., Yu, K., Zeleniuch, A., Smith-Warner, S. A., Ziegler, R. G., and Carroll, R. J. (2016). Calibration and seasonal adjustment for matched case-control studies of vitamin D and cancer. *Statistics in Medicine*, **35**, 2133–2148.

Gong, G. and Samaniego, F. J. (1981). Pseudo maximum likelihood estimation: Theory and applications. *The Annals of Statistics*, **9**, 861–869.

Greenland, S. (1982). The effect of misclassification in matched-pair case-control studies. *American Journal of Epidemiology*, **116**, 402–406.

Greenland, S. (1988a). Statistical uncertainty due to misclassification: Implications for validation substudies. *Journal of Clinical Epidemiology*, **41**, 1167–1174.

Greenland, S. (1988b). Variance estimation for epidemiologic effect estimates under misclassification. *Statistics in Medicine*, **7**, 745–757.

Greenland, S. (1989). On correcting for misclassification in twin studies and other matched-pair studies. *Statistics in Medicine*, **8**, 825–829.

Greenland, S. and Kleinbaum, D. G. (1983). Correcting for misclassification in two-way tables and matched-pair studies. *International Journal of Epidemiology*, **12**, 93–97.

Guolo, A. and Brazzale, A. R. (2008). A simulation-based comparison of techniques to correct for measurement error in matched case-control studies. *Statistics in Medicine*, **27**, 3755–3775.

Gustafson, P. (2004). *Measurement Error and Misclassification in Statistics and Epidemiology*. Chapman and Hall/CRC.

Gustafson, P., Le, N., and Vallée, M. (2002). A Bayesian approach to case-control studies with errors in covariables. *Biostatistics*, **3**, 229–243.

Hui, S. L. and Walter, S. D. (1980). Estimating the error rates of diagnostic tests. *Biometrics*, **36**, 167–171.

Keogh, R. H. and Cox, D. R. (2014). *Case-Control Studies*. Cambridge University Press.

Keogh, R. H. and White, I. R. (2014). A toolkit for measurement error correction, with a focus on nutritional epidemiology. *Statistics in Medicine*, **33**, 2137–2155.

Li, Y., Guolo, A., Hoffman, F. O., and Carroll, R. J. (2007). Shared uncertainty in measurement error problems, with application to Nevada Test Site fallout data. *Biometrics*, **63**, 1226–1236.

Lobach, I., Carroll, R. J., Spinka, C., Gail, M. H., and Chatterjee, N. (2008). Haplotype-based regression analysis and inference of case-control studies with unphased genotypes and measurement errors in environmental exposures. *Biometrics*, **64**, 673–684.

Mallick, B., Hoffman, F. O., and Carroll, R. J. (2002). Semiparametric regression modeling with mixtures of Berkson and classical error, with application to fallout from the Nevada Test Site. *Biometrics*, **58**, 13–20.

Marshall, R. J. (1990). Validation study methods for estimating exposure proportions and odds ratios with misclassified data. *Journal of Clinical Epidemiology*, **43**, 941–947.

McShane, L., Midthune, D. N., Dorgan, J. F., Freedman, L. S., and Carroll, R. J. (2001). Covariate measurement error adjustment for matched case-control studies. *Biometrics*, **57**, 62–73.

Michalek, J. E. and Tripathi, R. C. (1980). The effect of errors in diagnosis and measurement on the estimation of the probability of an event. *Journal of the American Statistical Association*, **75**, 713–721.

Morrissey, M. J. and Spiegelman, D. (1999). Matrix methods for estimating odds ratios with misclassified exposure data: Extensions and comparisons. *Biometrics*, **55**, 338–344.

Müller, P. and Roeder, K. (1997). A Bayesian semiparametric model for case-control studies with errors in variables. *Biometrika*, **84**, 523–537.

Prentice, R. L. and Pyke, R. (1979). Logistic disease incidence models and case-control studies. *Biometrika*, **66**, 403–411.

Reeves, G. K., Cox, D. R., Darby, S. C., and Whitley, E. (1998). Some aspects of measurement error in explanatory variables for continuous and binary regression models. *Statistics in Medicine*, **17**, 2157–2177.

Rice, K. (2003). Full-likelihood approaches to misclassification of a binary exposure in matched case-control studies. *Statistics in Medicine*, **22**, 3177–3194.

Rice, K. and Holmans, P. (2003). Allowing for genotyping error in analysis of unmatched case-control studies. *Annals of Human Genetics*, **67**, 165–174.

Richardson, S., Leblond, L., Jaussent, I., and Green, P. J. (2002). Mixture models in measurement error problems, with reference to epidemiological studies. *Journal of the Royal Statistical Society: Series A*, **165**, 549–566.

Satten, G. A. and Kupper, L. L. (1993a). Conditional regression analysis of the exposure-disease odds ratio using known probability of exposure values. *Biometrics*, **49**, 429–440.

Satten, G. A. and Kupper, L. L. (1993b). Inferences about exposure-disease associations using probability-of-exposure information. *Journal of the American Statistical Association*, **88**, 200–208.

Seaman, S. R. and Richardson, S. (2004). Equivalence of prospective and retrospective models in the Bayesian analysis of case-control studies. *Biometrika*, **91**, 15–25.

Stefanski, L. A. and Carroll, R. J. (1987). Conditional scores and optimal scores in generalized linear measurement error models. *Biometrika*, **74**, 703–716.

Stefanski, L. A. and Cook, J. R. (1995). Simulation-Extrapolation: The measurement error jackknife. *Journal of the American Statistical Association*, **90**, 1247–1256.

Thürigen, D., Spiegelman, D., Blettner, M., Heuer, C., and Brenner, H. (2000). Measurement error correction using validation data: A review of methods and their applicability in case-control studies. *Statistical Methods in Medical Research*, **9**, 447–474.

Wang, C. Y., Wang, S., and Carroll, R. J. (1997). Estimation in choice-based sampling with measurement error and bootstrap analysis. *Journal of Econometrics*, **77**, 65–86.

Part III

Case-control Studies that Use Full-Cohort Information

11

Alternative Formulation of Models in Case-Control Studies

William E. Barlow

University of Washington

John B. Cologne

Radiation Effects Research Foundation, Hiroshima

11.1 Introduction

Most models for the odds ratio typically assume an additive model on the log scale so that effects of covariates are multiplicative on the odds ratio. Standard models for the hazard ratio, rate ratio, or odds ratio are typically of the form $e^{\mathbf{x}^{\mathrm{T}}\boldsymbol{\beta}}$ that implies a multiplicative effect among risk factors denoted by the vector included in the model. Multiplicative models are simple to interpret and behave well in model fitting when data are not sparse. However, epidemiologists argue that such models do not reflect public health impact or underlying biology (i.e., they might lack biological plausibility) and may not adequately describe the interactions of two risk factors on outcome (Walker and Rothman, 1982; Greenland, 1983; Figueroa *et al.*, 2014; Moonesinghe *et al.*, 2011; Han *et al.*, 2012). Consequently, alternative models for risk, risk ratios, or odds ratios have been suggested to represent more realistic models for excess risk associated with risk factors or their interaction. The simplest alternative model is the linear model for risk of the form $1 + \mathbf{x}^{\mathrm{T}}\boldsymbol{\beta}$ so that each risk factor acts additively on the risk. However, such models have constraints on estimability as well as poor statistical properties. In this chapter, we consider alternative models for the odds ratio, rate ratio, hazard ratio, or probability of an event. We explore linear models as well as hybrid mixture models that address some of the concerns. Estimation of absolute risk is possible from stratified case-control studies when the sampling fraction is known. As an example we consider results from a full cohort estimation of breast cancer risk following a screening mammogram. We show that sampling controls with known sampling fraction can produce comparable absolute risk predictions, risk differences, or odds ratios depending on the model form chosen.

11.2   Case-control studies with unknown sampling fractions

In many case-control studies all cases are identified and selected controls are chosen from the larger population. It is assumed that these controls are representative of all potential controls even though the entire population of controls may not be able to be enumerated. The controls may be individually matched to cases or frequency matched on the basis of age or other stratification variables. Such studies incur constraints when the sampling fractions for controls are unknown. While the odds ratios may be estimated, the actual underlying absolute risks cannot be. Both unconditional and conditional models for estimation of the odds ratio remain possible even though estimation of absolute risk is not.

11.3   Conditional logistic regression models for stratified designs

For conditional models with a stratification factor, it will be assumed that the parameter associated with the stratum s operates multiplicatively on the remaining risk function:

$$\gamma_s r(\mathbf{x}; \boldsymbol{\beta})$$

so that the stratum effect γ_s will be factored out in the odds ratio, which is presumed constant over strata. Of course, this assumption of homogeneity of the odds ratio across strata can be tested. This then leads to the odds ratio risk function $\psi(\mathbf{x}; \boldsymbol{\beta})$, which can be either linear

$$\psi = 1 + \mathbf{x}^{\mathrm{T}} \boldsymbol{\beta} = 1 + x_1\beta_1 + x_2\beta_2 + \ldots + x_p\beta_p$$

or log-linear

$$\log\psi = x_1\beta_1 + x_2\beta_2 + \ldots + x_p\beta_p$$

with the intercept and the stratum effect γ_s conditioned out of the likelihood by stratification. Storer *et al.* (1983) describe procedures for model fitting of the linear model that were subsequently included in PECAN – a conditional logistic regression program. Departure from pure additive effects can be tested on either scale by adding interaction terms (see for example Stevens *et al.* (2011)). Unfortunately, the linear model suffers from boundary issues requiring the covariates to be coded in a constrained way. It was also shown by Storer *et al.* (1983) and Barlow (1985) that the Wald test for the linear model is unreliable as are the Wald derived confidence intervals on the estimated parameters. The score test using the expected information matrix is preferable to the score test using the observed information matrix (Storer *et al.*, 1983), though the likelihood ratio test may be best.

To overcome some of the statistical difficulties with the linear additive model, Barlow (1985) proposed a reparametrization called an exponential additive model:

$$\psi = 1 + \sum_{k=1}^{p} x_k \left(e^{\beta_k} - 1\right).$$

This model has better Wald standard errors than the standard linear model, but has the same likelihood and therefore the same overall likelihood ratio test of model fit. Another potential model is the following:

$$\psi = 1 + p^{-1} \sum_{k=1}^{p} (e^{x_k \beta_k} - 1) = p^{-1} \sum_{k=1}^{p} e^{x_k \beta_k}.$$

This model includes only positive additive terms that are monotonic with each x_k. However, neither model has found its way into contemporary practice.

11.4   Mixed linear and multiplicative models

If one assumes that all risk factors either act collectively as multiplicative or additive, then one can embed the linear additive and the log-linear multiplicative model into a generalized framework where a single parameter can index the model form. Thomas (1981) suggested the model

$$\psi = \left(e^{\mathbf{x}^{\mathrm{T}} \boldsymbol{\beta}} \right)^{1-\alpha} \left(1 + \mathbf{x}^{\mathrm{T}} \boldsymbol{\beta} \right)^{\alpha}$$

with $\alpha = 0$ the multiplicative form and $\alpha = 1$ the additive form. One illustration of this model as fit using the Epicure software (Preston *et al.*, 2017) is provided by Cologne *et al.* (2004). Breslow and Storer (1985) also proposed a general model with risk function

$$\log \psi = \begin{cases} \frac{(1 + \mathbf{x}^{\mathrm{T}} \boldsymbol{\beta})^{\lambda} - 1}{\lambda} & \text{if} \quad \lambda \neq 0 \\ \log \left(1 + \mathbf{x}^{\mathrm{T}} \boldsymbol{\beta} \right) & \text{if} \quad \lambda = 0 \end{cases}$$

with $\lambda = 0$ the additive form and $\lambda = 1$ the multiplicative form. In most cases values of 0 or 1 for the index parameter will be of greatest interest. One can test α or λ against these alternatives using a likelihood ratio test. However, Barlow (1985) suggests a simple approach for testing departure from the multiplicative form, which is to fit the standard multiplicative model (estimating $\boldsymbol{\beta}$) and then conduct a score test of the additional covariate

$$z = \begin{cases} \left(1 + \mathbf{x}^{\mathrm{T}} \hat{\boldsymbol{\beta}} \right) \cdot \log \left(1 + \mathbf{x}^{\mathrm{T}} \hat{\boldsymbol{\beta}} \right) & \text{if using the Breslow-Storer model} \\ \log \left(1 + \mathbf{x}^{\mathrm{T}} \hat{\boldsymbol{\beta}} \right) & \text{if using the Thomas model.} \end{cases}$$

If the covariate z adds to the multiplicative model, then it indicates that the multiplicative model is not appropriate for that collection of covariates.

These generalized risk models suggest that all covariates must enter either multiplicatively or additively. However, there have been proposed models that allow both multiplicative and additive factors. Barlow (1985) had a general model that allowed each covariate to have either a multiplicative or additive effect on the odds ratio that generalizes the approach of Thomas (1981):

$$\psi = \left(e^{\sum_{k=1}^{p} (1 - \alpha_k) x_k \beta_k} \right) \left(p^{-1} \sum_{k=1}^{p} e^{\alpha_k x_k \beta_k} \right).$$

Each individual term's effect is determined by α_k, which is estimated from the data. One drawback of mixture type models is that the same risk parameter $\boldsymbol{\beta}$ occurs in both the additive (excess relative odds) and multiplicative (log odds) terms. Estimating distinct risk parameters for these two terms in the case that the index parameter is neither 0 nor 1 can be difficult (Little *et al.*, 1999).

However, rather than determining empirically which model is more appropriate, it may be better to postulate a scientific model for the variable of interest. In many cases this may suggest an excess risk (or additive) model for the exposure variable while the potential confounders are included as multiplicative factors in order to control for them in the background. Such types of models are frequently used in radiation risk assessment; see for example Cologne *et al.* (2010) and Ohishi *et al.* (2014).

11.5   Cohort models

In case-control studies with unknown fractions, one is limited to modeling the odds ratio. However, in cohort studies one can model either the relative or absolute risk of an event. Survival time models (e.g., Cox model) may be appropriate for modeling the hazard ratio or relative risk ratio. The linear risk form for hazard ratio in the Cox model still suffers from poor statistical properties (Barlow and Sun, 1989). For the moment we will consider classical rate models that depend on person-time at risk. Consider a simple situation where we are interested in the risk of disease for high versus low exposure adjusted for potential confounders. Muirhead and Darby (1987) describe a general model for the rate parameter that allows one to choose between modeling absolute risk versus modeling the relative risk. Assume that an exposed individual has risk $\lambda_i(1)$ and an unexposed individual risk $\lambda_i(0)$; then the general model is as follows:

$$\lambda_i(1) = \left[\lambda_i{}^{\gamma}(0) + \left\{ 1 + \exp(\mathbf{x}_i^{\mathrm{T}}\boldsymbol{\beta}) \right\}^{\gamma} - 1 \right]^{1/\gamma} \tag{11.1}$$

where the absolute risk model applies if $\gamma = 1$ and the relative risk model applies as $\gamma \to 0$. The absolute risk model implies that the difference between exposed and unexposed $\lambda_i(1) - \lambda_i(0)$ is constant across all covariate combinations while the relative risk model implies the ratio $\lambda_i(1)/\lambda_i(0)$ is constant. One can then use a likelihood ratio test or score test to identify the appropriate model empirically.

In many situations one prefers to model the risk directly. We will assume a common follow-up time for each individual so that a binomial probability can be used to model the event rate as a function of the covariate vector $\mathbf{x}$. Typically, a logit link is preferred but a log link can be used if one prefers a relative risk interpretation instead of odds ratios. However, an identity link yields a standard additive model for the risk:

$$P(D = 1|\mathbf{x}) = \mathbf{x}^{\mathrm{T}}\boldsymbol{\beta}. \tag{11.2}$$

These models can have difficulty in model fitting due to constraints on the parameter space. However, a recent paper by Kovalchik and Varadhan (2013) describes a constrained maximization procedure developed as the R package `blm`. A robust variance is constructed using the influence function. This allows the excess risk to be expressed as a direct difference between the exposed and unexposed probabilities. This model was generalized into a model that has both linear and multiplicative components called the lexpit model (Kovalchik *et al.*, 2013a)

$$P(D = 1|\mathbf{x}, \mathbf{z}) = \mathbf{x}^{\mathrm{T}}\boldsymbol{\beta} + \mathrm{expit}\left(\mathbf{z}^{\mathrm{T}}\boldsymbol{\gamma}\right), \tag{11.3}$$

where $\mathrm{expit}(x) = \exp(x)/(1 + \exp(x))$ is the inverse-logit function. The covariates included in $\mathbf{x}$ and $\mathbf{z}$ in the model need not be distinct. Typically, the intercept term is included in the multiplicative part only. The model allows one to model excess risk due to exposure as a linear effect, but with adjustment for potential confounders in a multiplicative framework. This model is also included in the R package `blm` and also uses constrained maximization. The authors illustrate this approach in a case-control examination of lung cancer considering smoking amount interacting with gender as additive effects and the remainder of the covariates as multiplicative effects (Kovalchik *et al.*, 2013b).

11.6   Case-control samples with known sampling fractions

Large cohort studies often lend themselves to case-control studies when specific additional covariates need to be collected, but it is not plausible or efficient to collect those covariates on all members of the cohort. In these embedded case-control studies all cases may be selected, but controls are sampled using known sampling fractions that may depend on well-established risk factors. In this latter case, one can ignore the sampling fractions and model the odds ratio or the relative risk. Alternatively, one can accommodate the sampling fractions and estimate the absolute risk of the event using a multiplicative, additive, or lexpit model described above. Inverse sampling weights are used to adjust the predicted risk back to the distribution in the original case-control population.

11.7   Breast cancer incidence example

Using a population-based cohort study, Barlow *et al.* (2006) predicted the risk of a breast cancer diagnosis within one year of a screening mammogram. Separate models were constructed for premenopausal and postmenopausal women. The intent was to produce a model that would be simple to use in practice, but have stronger predictive ability than the widely used Gail model (Gail *et al.*, 1989). We focus on the premenopausal model as an example since it had only four significant covariates in the model: (1) age group (35-39; 40-44; 45-49; 50-54); number of first degree relatives with breast cancer (0; 1; 2 or more; unknown); previous breast procedure such as a biopsy (no; yes; unknown); and breast density on the BI-RADS scale (1: Almost entirely fat; 2: Scattered fibroglandular densities; 3: Heterogeneously dense; 4: Extremely dense; 9: Unknown). Because of the large sample size we required that a risk factor be significant at $p < 0.0001$ to be included and we did not attempt to fit interaction terms. This was because we wanted to keep the model simple and interest was in predicting breast cancer, rather than identifying specific risk factors. The original model treated unknown as a separate category for number of biopsies and previous breast procedure, but as both risk factors have low frequency and the beta coefficient for Unknown did not differ from the No category we fold the unknowns into "no" here for those two variables. However, unknown breast density was common so we continue to model it as a separate category. It has been suggested that a complete record analysis (or complete case analysis excluding subjects with missing data) may be less biased than an analysis using a missing or unknown category (Greenland and Finkle, 1995). Excluding subjects with unknown density would result in loss of about 23% of the sample, and in practice breast density may be an unknown risk factor for many women so we include missing density as a separate category. Table 11.1 shows the frequencies for the four risk factors and the crude incidence rate per 1,000 women. For the purpose of this illustration we will assume that our primary interest is in breast density as the "novel" risk factor and that age, family history of breast cancer, and previous breast procedures are potential confounders of that association with outcome.

11.8   Full cohort analysis

We first explore a standard logistic regression model to obtain estimated probabilities of breast cancer within one year. We will then model it as a linear model in the probability. Standard programs in SAS and Stata have difficulty with this estimation, but the constrained optimization in the R package `blm` converges. Table 11.2 shows the results of different modeling approaches for the full cohort analysis. Four main effects are fitted in each model as categorical covariates: age group, prior breast procedure, number of first degree relatives with breast cancer, and breast density. The multiplicative model represents the usual cohort approach for a binary outcome and is most often interpreted through the odds ratios. Since breast cancer is rare, one would expect the odds ratio to be close to the relative risk ratio as well. The linear additive model represents risk differences and has been scaled to be per 1,000 observations to be more interpretable. For example, women with breast density 3: Heterogeneously dense have an increased absolute risk of breast cancer of 1.93 per 1,000 compared to breast density 1: Almost entirely fat. The mixture model treats breast density as an additive effect, but the other risk factors as multiplicative adjustment factors. Thus, one can interpret the odds ratio as the residual risk for breast density category 1. The breast density coefficients represent the excess risk per 1,000 as breast density increases. For the three models, the estimated number of breast cancer cases per 1,000 is given for each breast density category adjusted to the overall combination of all other risk factors. While comparable at higher levels of breast density, the multiplicative model shows a low risk for the baseline density value of 1. In fact, multiplicative models may produce more extreme estimates of risk than additive models when the joint effects are assessed so that interaction terms with negative coefficients are needed to mitigate multiplicative joint effects. Those interactions can then be misinterpreted as scientific interactions.

11.9   Stratified case-control analysis

We now demonstrate a stratified case-control approach to estimation if we choose all cases in the population, but only an age-stratified set of controls for comparison. Suppose that we can enumerate case status and age on everyone in the population but had to collect breast density and other risk factors from medical record abstraction. For each case we want approximately 5 age-matched controls. Thus, we choose sampling fractions of 1.0%, 1.1%, 1.8%, and 2.2% for the four age groups. This constitutes our age-stratified case-control study with known sampling fractions. We can then estimate odds ratios, risk ratios, and absolute risk estimates by inversely weighting the controls by the reciprocal sampling fraction. In a standard case-control design we may be able to enumerate the cases, but not all members of the control population. Thus, we could still choose 5 controls per case, but the sampling fraction would be unknown and we would be restricted to estimation of the odds ratio.

   Table 11.1 shows one randomly chosen sample of controls according to the sampling fractions above. We now illustrate estimation using the sampling fractions showing the

TABLE 11.1

Description of the cohort and sample. Premenopausal women undergoing screening mammography and breast cancer diagnosed within one year of the mammogram.

Risk factor	Population	Women with breast cancer	Cancer rate per 1,000	Age-stratified controls
Age group (sampling fraction)				
35-39 (1.0%)	37043	75	2.02	375
40-44 (1.1%)	239273	539	2.25	2594
45-49 (1.8%)	194584	693	3.56	3501
50-54 (2.2%)	97315	419	4.31	2213
Prior breast procedure				
No (or unknown)	486831	1348	2.77	7332
Yes	81384	378	4.62	1351
First-degree relatives with BC				
0 or unknown	490286	1376	2.81	7522
1	75106	332	4.42	1112
2+	2823	18	6.38	49
Breast density				
1: Almost entirely fat	18183	19	1.04	277
2: Scattered fibroglandular densities	146721	306	2.09	2332
3: Heterogeneously dense	200896	704	3.50	3070
4: Extremely dense	61413	251	4.09	942
9: Unknown	141002	446	3.16	2062
Total	568215	1726	3.04	8683

analytic results in Table 11.3. If the control frequencies are inversely weighted, then the sample produces estimates very close to those of the full cohort (first columns of Table 11.3 versus first columns of Table 11.2). The model based SEs are close to those of Table 11.2 as well, but in fact are underestimates. The sandwich variance (empirical) SEs correctly reflect the sampling and the expected increase in error. For comparison we show the results of the case-control analysis ignoring the sampling weights. The correct age odds ratio cannot be estimated due to the sampling and cannot show the true variation by age. Nonetheless, the remaining odds ratios for the other risk factors are relevant and can be estimated with standard errors similar to the weighted approach.

Table 11.3 also shows the linear model based on the weighted sample and the mixture model allowing density to have additive effects, but adjusted for other risk factors using multiplicative effects. Results are similar to the full model when the weighting is accounted for.

11.10   Summary

While multiplicative models are well behaved statistically they make strong assumptions about joint effects of risk factors. In many cases there may be a significant interaction between two covariates that mutes the joint effects when both factors are present. That is, the joint effects may be subadditive on the log scale. However, on the linear risk scale an interaction may not be necessary. The additive models can be interpreted as risk differences, often may better reflect biological interactions, and may be more directly relevant to public

TABLE 11.2
Three models of the full cohort predicting breast cancer incidence

Effect	Multiplicative Model Odds Ratio Model					Additive Model Risk difference (per 1,000)				Mixed Model OR (multiplicative)/Risk difference (additive)					
	Parameter estimate	Model SE	OR	Coef 95% CI Lower limit	Upper limit	Parameter estimate	SE	Wald 95% CI Lower limit	Upper limit	Parameter estimate	Modeled as	SE	OR	Wald 95% CI Lower limit	Upper limit
Intercept	−7.525	0.257				2.27E−06	1.80E−04			−7.327	Mult	0.118			
Age															
40-44 vs. 35-39	0.204	0.124	1.23	−0.032	0.455	0.393	0.167	0.067	0.720	0.328	Mult	0.124	1.39	0.085	0.571
45-49 vs. 35-39	0.655	0.122	1.93	0.423	0.902	1.523	0.197	1.137	1.909	1.038	Mult	0.122	2.82	0.798	1.277
50-54 vs. 35-39	0.872	0.126	2.39	0.631	1.127	2.324	0.251	1.832	2.815	1.312	Mult	0.126	3.72	1.065	1.560
Prior breast procedure	0.396	0.059	1.49	0.279	0.510	1.433	0.240	0.963	1.902	0.583	Mult	0.059	1.79	0.468	0.698
First-degree relatives with BC															
One	0.444	0.062	1.56	0.322	0.564	1.499	0.241	1.027	1.971	0.637	Mult	0.062	1.89	0.516	0.758
Two or more	0.759	0.238	2.14	0.254	1.194	3.706	1.518	0.730	6.682	1.017	Mult	0.238	2.77	0.550	1.484
Breast density															
2 vs 1	0.690	0.237	1.99	0.256	1.189	0.646	0.179	0.295	0.998	0.247	Add	0.268	NA	−0.277	0.772
3 vs 1	1.204	0.233	3.34	0.779	1.696	1.934	0.196	1.550	2.319	1.574	Add	0.273	NA	1.038	2.110
4 vs 1	1.368	0.238	3.93	0.929	1.869	2.425	0.287	1.862	2.988	2.114	Add	0.352	NA	1.425	2.803
Unknown vs 1	1.183	0.235	3.27	0.753	1.678	1.677	0.201	1.283	2.071	1.301	Add	0.282	NA	0.748	1.855
	Expected cases per 1,000					Expected cases per 1,000				Expected cases per 1,000					
Breast density															
1	1.03					1.51				1.87					
2	2.05					2.15				2.11					
3	3.42					3.44				3.44					
4	4.03					3.93				3.98					
9 (unknown)	3.35					3.18				3.17					

TABLE 11.3
Models based on the stratified case-control sample

Effect	Multiplicative Model Weighted Sample				Multiplicative Model Unweighted Sample				Additive Model Weighted Sample (per 1,000)		Mixed Model OR (multi)/Risk difference per 1,000 (add)		
	Parameter estimate	Model SE	Empirical SE	OR	Parameter estimate	Model SE	Empirical SE	OR	Parameter estimate	Empirical SE	Parameter estimate	Modeled as	SE
Intercept	−7.461	0.258	0.270		−2.861	0.271	0.270		0.000	0.000	−7.216	Mult	0.053
40-44 vs. 35-39	0.222	0.124	0.137	1.25	0.130	0.137	0.136	1.14	0.449	0.061	0.292	Mult	0.055
45-49 vs. 35-39	0.664	0.122	0.135	1.94	0.084	0.135	0.134	1.09	1.562	0.076	0.967	Mult	0.055
50-54 vs. 35-39	0.839	0.126	0.140	2.31	0.062	0.139	0.139	1.06	2.216	0.099	1.193	Mult	0.057
Prior breast procedure	0.350	0.059	0.068	1.42	0.354	0.067	0.067	1.43	1.240	0.174	0.505	Mult	0.045
One first-degree relative with BC	0.447	0.062	0.070	1.56	0.453	0.070	0.070	1.57	1.571	0.195	0.638	Mult	0.048
Two or more first-degree relatives with BC	0.574	0.239	0.284	1.78	0.615	0.281	0.290	1.85	3.316	1.425	0.722	Mult	0.218
Breast density 2 vs 1	0.624	0.237	0.245	1.87	0.618	0.245	0.246	1.86	0.607	0.071	0.180	Add	0.123
Breast density 3 vs 1	1.159	0.233	0.241	3.19	1.156	0.241	0.242	3.18	1.955	0.101	1.565	Add	0.140
Breast density 4 vs 1	1.259	0.239	0.248	3.52	1.260	0.249	0.249	3.53	2.262	0.181	1.905	Add	0.217
Unknown density vs 1	1.108	0.235	0.243	3.03	1.102	0.244	0.244	3.01	1.637	0.100	1.227	Add	0.145

health concerns. While case-control models have limitations when the sampling fraction is unknown, these limitations are removed by knowledge about the size of the population that can be incorporated into the model. Weighted analyses can return absolute risk estimates as well as risk ratios and odds ratios. The underlying model can be multiplicative, additive, or a mixture of the two. All of these may be appropriate depending on biological and scientific insights.

Bibliography

Barlow, W. E. (1985). General relative risk models in stratified epidemiologic studies. *Journal of the Royal Statistical Society, Series C*, **34**, 246–257.

Barlow, W. E. and Sun, W. H. (1989). Bootstrapped confidence intervals for the Cox model using a linear relative risk form. *Statistics in Medicine*, **8**, 927–935.

Barlow, W. E., White, E., Ballard-Barbash, R., Vacek, P. M., Titus-Ernstoff, L., Carney, P. A., Tice, J. A., Buist, D. S., Geller, B. M., Rosenberg, R., Yankaskas, B. C., and Kerlikowske, K. (2006). Prospective breast cancer risk prediction model for women undergoing screening mammography. *Journal of the National Cancer Institute*, **98**, 1204–1214.

Breslow, N. E. and Storer, B. E. (1985). General relative risk functions for case-control studies. *American Journal of Epidemiology*, **122**, 149–162.

Cologne, J., Cullings, H., Furukawa, K., and Ross, P. (2010). Attributable risk for radiation in the presence of other risk factors. *Health Physics*, **99**, 603–612.

Cologne, J. B., Pawel, D. J., Sharp, G. B., and Fujiwara, S. (2004). Uncertainty in estimating probability of causation in a cross-sectional study: Joint effects of radiation and hepatitis-C virus on chronic liver disease. *Journal of Radiological Protection*, **24**, 131–145.

Figueroa, J. D., Han, S. S., Garcia-Closas, M., Baris, D., Jacobs, E. J., Kogevinas, M., Schwenn, M., Malats, N., Johnson, A., Purdue, M. P., Caporaso, N., Landi, M. T., Prokunina-Olsson, L., Wang, Z., Hutchinson, A., Burdette, L., Wheeler, W., Vineis, P., Siddiq, A., Cortessis, V. K., Kooperberg, C., Cussenot, O., Benhamou, S., Prescott, J., Porru, S., Bueno-de Mesquita, H. B., Trichopoulos, D., Ljungberg, B., Clavel-Chapelon, F., Weiderpass, E., Krogh, V., Dorronsoro, M., Travis, R., Tjønneland, A., Brenan, P., Chang-Claude, J., Riboli, E., Conti, D., Gago-Dominguez, M., Stern, M. C., Pike, M. C., Van Den Berg, D., Yuan, J. M., Hohensee, C., Rodabough, R., Cancel-Tassin, G., Roupret, M., Comperat, E., Chen, C., De Vivo, I., Giovannucci, E., Hunter, D. J., Kraft, P., Lindstrom, S., Carta, A., Pavanello, S., Arici, C., Mastrangelo, G., Karagas, M. R., Schned, A., Armenti, K. R., Hosain, G. M., Haiman, C. A., Fraumeni, J. F. J., Chanock, S. J., Chatterjee, N., Rothman, N., and Silverman, D. T. (2014). Genome-wide interaction study of smoking and bladder cancer risk. *Carcinogenesis*, **35**, 1737–1744.

Gail, M. H., Brinton, L. A., Byar, D. P., Corle, D. K., Green, S. B., Schairer, C., and Mulvihill, J. J. (1989). Projecting individualized probabilities of developing breast cancer for white females who are being examined annually. *Journal of the National Cancer Institute*, **81**, 1879–1886.

Greenland, S. (1983). Tests for interaction in epidemiologic studies: A review and a study of power. *Statistics in Medicine*, **2**, 243–251.

Greenland, S. and Finkle, W. D. (1995). A critical look at methods for handling missing covariates in epidemiologic regression analysis. *American Journal of Epidemiology*, **142**, 1255–1264.

Han, S. S., Rosenberg, P. S., Garcia-Closas, M., Figueroa, J. D., Silverman, D., Chanock, S. J., Rothman, N., and Chatterjee, N. (2012). Likelihood ratio test for detecting gene (G)-environment (E) interactions under an additive risk model exploiting G-E independence for case-control data. *American Journal of Epidemiology*, **176**, 1060–1067.

Kovalchik, S. and Varadhan, R. (2013). Fitting additive binomial regression models with the R package blm. *Journal of Statistical Software*, **54**, 1–18.

Kovalchik, S. A., Varadhan, R., Fetterman, B., Poitras, N. E., Wacholder, S., and Katki, H. A. (2013a). A general binomial regression model to estimate standardized risk differences from binary response data. *Statistics in Medicine*, **32**, 808–821.

Kovalchik, S. A., De Matteis, S., Landi, M. T., Caporaso, N. E., Varadhan, R., Consonni, D., Bergen, A. W., Katki, H. A., and Wacholder, S. (2013b). A regression model for risk difference estimation in population-based case-control studies clarifies gender differences in lung cancer risk of smokers and never smokers. *BMC Medical Research Methodology*, **13**, 143.

Little, M. P., Muirhead, C. R., and Charles, M. W. (1999). Describing time and age variations in the risk of radiation-induced solid tumour incidence in the Japanese atomic bomb survivors using generalized relative and absolute risk models. *Statistics in Medicine*, **18**, 17–33.

Moonesinghe, R., Khoury, M. J., Liu, T., and Janssens, A. C. (2011). Discriminative accuracy of genomic profiling comparing multiplicative and additive risk models. *European Journal of Human Genetics*, **19**, 180–185.

Muirhead, C. R. and Darby, S. C. (1987). Modelling the relative and absolute risks of radiation-induced cancers. *Journal of the Royal Statistical Society, Series A*, **150**, 83–118.

Ohishi, W., Cologne, J. B., Fujiwara, S., Suzuki, G., Hayashi, T., Niwa, Y., Akahoshi, M., Ueda, K., Tsuge, M., and Chayama, K. (2014). Serum interleukin-6 associated with hepatocellular carcinoma risk: A nested case-control study. *International Journal of Cancer*, **134**, 154–163.

Preston, D. L., Lubin, J. H., Pierce, D. A., McConney, M. E., and Shilnikova, N. S. (2017). *Epicure: Risk Regression Model Software*. Risk Sciences International, Ottawa, Canada. https://www.risksciences.com/project/epicure/.

Stevens, R. G., Cologne, J. B., Nakachi, K., Grant, E. F., and Neriishi, K. (2011). Body iron stores and breast cancer risk in female atomic bomb survivors. *Cancer Science*, **102**, 2236–2240.

Storer, B. E., Wacholder, S., and Breslow, N. E. (1983). Maximum likelihood fitting of general risk models to stratified data. *Journal of the Royal Statistical Society, Series C*, **32**, 172–181.

Thomas, D. C. (1981). General relative-risk models for survival time and matched case-control analysis. *Biometrics*, **37**, 673–686.

Walker, A. M. and Rothman, K. J. (1982). Models of varying parametric form in case-referent studies. *American Journal of Epidemiology*, **115**, 129–137.

12

Multi-Phase Sampling

Gustavo Amorim, Alastair J. Scott, and Chris J. Wild

University of Auckland

12.1   Introduction

12.1.1   Two-phase and multi-phase sampling

In a two-phase study, some variables are measured on all the units in a large initial sample of units drawn from a cohort. Then, based on the values of these variables, a subsample of units is drawn and the values of additional variables are obtained for members of the subsample. The idea was first introduced in survey sampling by Neyman (1938) – he called it "double sampling" – and in epidemiology by White (1982) – she called it "two-stage sampling." Such designs are particularly useful when the additional variables are expensive, invasive, or difficult to measure, and can result in considerable savings. Xu and Zhou (2012), Chatterjee and Chen (2007) and others point to the increasing importance of such sampling designs in genetic epidemiology, where they can reduce the cost of studies by limiting expensive ascertainments of genetic and environmental exposure to an efficiently selected subsample of the main study. They also have other uses besides reducing the cost of obtaining expensive covariates. For example, adding an extra phase of sampling can provide an efficient way of making an after-the-fact adjustment for a confounder that was overlooked and not measured in the original study – in fact this was the motivation for White (1982) – or even an exposure that was not recorded in the original study but has later become of particular interest.

The process of subsampling can be continued indefinitely. In a three-phase study, some of the extra covariates are not measured on all the units sampled at the second phase, but only on a subsample drawn from them. Whittemore and Halpern (1997) discuss several studies with three or more phases of sampling. For example, in a study to investigate the relationship of prostate cancer risk to diet and other lifestyle characteristics, cases (men with a history of prostate cancer) and controls (men without such a history) were identified in the initial phase. Then, at the second phase, all the cases and a sample of controls were asked whether or not they had a family history of the disease (father or brother). This information was then used to draw the third-phase sample in which more detailed information on family size and structure, age at prostate cancer occurrence or censoring, and place and date of prostate cancer diagnosis was collected. Subjects who had three or more family members with prostate cancer were asked to participate in phase four, in which family members provided blood and/or tissue samples for DNA analysis.

The class includes some studies that are not normally thought of as multi-phase designs. For example, if we have administrative or other population information available on some variables for all individuals in the cohort from which the study data has been sampled, then efficiency can often be increased by considering this whole-cohort data as the first phase and the study data as coming from one or more subsequent phases. Case-control studies, where case status and perhaps the values of other variables are ascertained for the whole cohort, are a special case of this. Breslow *et al.* (2013) illustrate how efficiency can be improved by using any such whole-cohort data. The methods of this chapter may also be useful in some missing-data situations when, under missing-at-random assumptions, the observed/missing mechanism can be thought of as corresponding to an additional phase of sampling. The missing data example of Arbogast *et al.* (2002), for example, has exactly the same structure as a three-phase case-control sample. In concluding this paragraph, we must note that there are real dangers in supplementing study data using data sources external to the study that need careful consideration and handling (see Chatterjee *et al.*, 2016).

Note that what we are calling multi-*phase* studies have been more commonly called multi-*stage* studies in the biostatistics literature, following White (1982) (see Whittemore and Halpern, 1997, for example). Multi-phase sampling is the term used in the survey sampling literature where multi-stage sampling already has another well-established meaning (Cochran, 1977). We follow Breslow and Holubkov (1997) in using the survey terminology. We note the following in passing. Our interest is in fitting regression models, rather than population totals, which has been the main emphasis in the survey sampling literature. Additionally, the "two-phase" designs of Breslow and Holubkov (1997), in which the initial phase is a case-control sample, are actually three-phase designs in our terminology with the first phase being the selection of cases and controls.

12.1.2   Women's Health Initiative Example

Throughout the chapter we will use a set of data from the Women's Health Initiative (WHI) study (https://www.nhlbi.nih.gov/whi/). Study details that are not pertinent to use of the data to exemplify the methods in the chapter will be suppressed. A fuller discussion is given by Breslow *et al.* (2013) (see also Rossouw *et al.*, 2002, 2008).

We have used a cohort consisting of postmenopausal women aged between 50 and 79 years old from WHI who were part of two trials of hormone therapy (HT) to reduce coronary heart disease (CHD). The women with an intact uterus were randomized to a combination of estrogen plus progestin (E+P) versus placebo, while the remaining women (who had a prior hysterectomy) were randomized to estrogen alone (E) versus placebo. These trials were stopped early because of adverse outcomes and lack of CHD benefit.

A followup case-control study was conducted using subjects from this cohort to investigate the mechanisms through which HT might increase the risk of CHD (Rossouw *et al.*, 2008). This involved the CHD cases and nearly three times as many controls selected on a variety of factors including trial (E versus E+P) and age. For those in the case-control study, blood samples that had been stored at baseline were assayed giving additional data.

12.1.3 Subsampling strategies

In this chapter we will particularly highlight the two simplest strategies for taking subsamples (Lawless *et al.*, 1999):

1. **Basic stratified sampling (BSS)**: Here the set of individuals in the current phase is divided into K strata, and a pre-specified number of subjects, or a pre-specified fraction of subjects, is selected from each stratum for the next phase.

2. **Variable probability sampling (VPS)**: Here units are inspected sequentially as they arise and are selected for the next phase independently with some probability π which would typically depend on what was observed at the current and any previous phases. For the special case of a stratified VPS, each unit has its stratum identified and if the ith unit belongs to stratum S_j, it is selected for the next phase with probability π_j.

Note that, for BSS the sample size n_j selected from stratum S_j is considered fixed given N_j, the total number of Phase-1 individuals in stratum S_j, while for stratified VPS the n_j's are random for strata that are not fully sampled.

12.1.4 Chapter organization

This chapter is organized as follows. Section 12.2 describes the form of likelihoods, and conditional likelihoods, for fitting regression models to two-phase data. Section 12.3 develops the resulting methods for two-phase case-control data, while Section 12.4 generalises this beyond case-control sampling. Section 12.5 describes survey-weighted (Horvitz-Thompson, or inverse-probability weighted) alternatives to the likelihood-based methods. Section 12.6 applies all of the methods covered thus far to the Women's Health Initiative example introduced in Section 12.1.2. Section 12.7 extends the methodological discussion to allow for the design variables that are not included in the regression model of interest. Section 12.8 then generalizes the methods to three and more phases of sampling. All analyses were performed using an R package implementing the methods described in the chapter that is available from the Handbook website.

12.2 Likelihood methods for two-phase sampling

Before starting we pause for a notational aside. Throughout this handbook the standard notation for case-control status is $D = 1$ for cases and $D = 0$ for controls. This chapter uses a notation which lets us deal with general response (outcome) variables Y with a binary case-control indicator variable being a possible special case. So even with a case-control response we will use Y rather than D.

The context for this chapter is that we want to fit some parametric regression model

$$f(\boldsymbol{y}|\boldsymbol{x};\boldsymbol{\beta})$$

whereby the conditional density of the response variable(s) $\boldsymbol{Y}$ are a function of explanatory variables (covariates) $\boldsymbol{X}$ depending on a vector of parameters $\boldsymbol{\beta}$.

At the first phase, we have a sample (often the whole cohort) of N subjects having values $\{(\boldsymbol{x}_i, \boldsymbol{y}_i), i = 1, \ldots, N\}$. If we had complete data on $\{\boldsymbol{x}_i, \boldsymbol{y}_i\}$ for all Phase-1 units, the likelihood would be of the form

$$L_{complete}(\boldsymbol{\beta}, g) = \prod_{i=1}^{N} P(\boldsymbol{Y} = \boldsymbol{y}_i, \boldsymbol{x}_i) = \prod_{i=1}^{N} f(\boldsymbol{y}_i \mid \boldsymbol{x}_i; \boldsymbol{\beta}) g(\boldsymbol{x}_i), \qquad (12.1)$$

where $g()$ is the marginal distribution of the covariates. Since, in (12.1), information on the covariate distribution is orthogonal to information on the parameters of interest $\boldsymbol{\beta}$, we would then be able to ignore it and base our inferences about $\boldsymbol{\beta}$ on

$$L_{complete}(\boldsymbol{\beta}) = \prod_{i=1}^{N} f(\boldsymbol{y}_i \mid \boldsymbol{x}_i; \boldsymbol{\beta}). \qquad (12.2)$$

For a two-phase study, however, we have whole-cohort information only on a subset $\boldsymbol{Y}^{(1)}$ of $\boldsymbol{Y}$ (often all of $\boldsymbol{Y}$) and a subset $\boldsymbol{X}^{(1)}$ of $\boldsymbol{X}$, with the remainder of $\boldsymbol{Y}$ and $\boldsymbol{X}$ being observed only on a subsample. Define the selection indicator R_i by setting $R_i = 1$ if the ith unit is in the subsample and $R_i = 0$ otherwise, $i = 1, \ldots, N$. We will assume that the probability that $R_i = 1$ depends only on the variables observed at Phase 1 (in a designed study, this can be accomplished purposefully), so that

$$P(R_i = 1 \mid \boldsymbol{y}_i, \boldsymbol{x}_i) = P(R_i = 1 \mid \boldsymbol{y}_i^{(1)}, \boldsymbol{x}_i^{(1)}) = \pi(\boldsymbol{y}_i^{(1)}, \boldsymbol{x}_i^{(1)}).$$

Thus the unsampled components of $\boldsymbol{Y}$ and $\boldsymbol{X}$ are missing at random (MAR) in the terminology of Rubin (1976). We also need to assume that $\pi(\boldsymbol{y}_i^{(1)}, \boldsymbol{x}_i^{(1)}) > 0$ for all Phase-1 units. We cannot, in general, just ignore the sampling design and use a standard prospective analysis based on applying (12.2) to the fully observed (i.e., subsampled) individuals unless the conditional inclusion probabilities, $\pi(\boldsymbol{y}_i, \boldsymbol{x}_i)$, depend only on the value of $\boldsymbol{x}_i^{(1)}$ and not on $\boldsymbol{y}_i$; in other words, unless the sample is not response-biased.

12.2.1 Ascertainment-corrected likelihood

One way forward is to use only the units that have been fully observed ($R_i = 1$) together with a likelihood that conditions on this fact (i.e., is "ascertainment corrected"). Under variable probability sampling (VPS), because individuals are subsampled independently, the ascertainment-corrected likelihood is

$$L_C(\boldsymbol{\beta}; \pi()) = \prod_{R_i=1} f_C(\boldsymbol{y}_i \mid \boldsymbol{x}_i; \boldsymbol{\beta}, \pi()), \qquad (12.3)$$

where

$$f_C(\boldsymbol{y}_i \mid \boldsymbol{x}_i; \boldsymbol{\beta}, \pi()) = f(\boldsymbol{y}_i \mid \boldsymbol{x}_i, R_i = 1) = \frac{f(\boldsymbol{y}_i|\boldsymbol{x}_i; \boldsymbol{\beta})\pi(\boldsymbol{y}_i^{(1)}, \boldsymbol{x}_i^{(1)})}{\int f(\boldsymbol{y}|\boldsymbol{x}_i; \boldsymbol{\beta})\pi(\boldsymbol{y}^{(1)}, \boldsymbol{x}_i^{(1)}) d\mu(\boldsymbol{y})}. \qquad (12.4)$$

The $d\mu(\boldsymbol{y})$ notation in the denominator is a shorthand for saying that we integrate over the possible values of $\boldsymbol{y}$ for continuous $\boldsymbol{Y}$s but sum over the possible values of $\boldsymbol{y}$ for discrete $\boldsymbol{Y}$s.

Expression (12.4) underpins the "conditional maximum likelihood" (CML) method developed by Breslow and Cain (1988) for fitting logistic regression models to data from case-control studies (see also Hausman and Wise, 1981). Under VPS, (12.3) is an ordinary likelihood with the usual properties. Under basic stratified sampling (BSS) the resulting score function, treated in the working-independence-model sense of Liang and Zeger (1986), can be used to obtain consistent estimating equations for $\boldsymbol{\beta}$ and we will find that it plays an important part in maximum-likelihood estimation based on the full set of data.

Logistic regression for binary data

Here we specialize to the case of a *logistic regression* model for a univariate binary response Y (taking values $1, 0$), e.g., case or control status, whereby

$$f(1 \mid \boldsymbol{x}) = P(Y = 1 \mid \boldsymbol{x}) = \frac{e^{\boldsymbol{x}^T \boldsymbol{\beta}}}{1 + e^{\boldsymbol{x}^T \boldsymbol{\beta}}} = \text{expit}(\boldsymbol{x}^T \boldsymbol{\beta}), \qquad (12.5)$$

where Y is observed at Phase 1. By applying Bayes' Theorem, the conditional distribution of Y conditional on $\boldsymbol{x}$ and being subsampled has the same logistic-regression form but with an added offset:

$$P_C(Y = 1 \mid \boldsymbol{x}) = P(Y = 1 \mid \boldsymbol{x}, R = 1) = \text{expit}(o_{\boldsymbol{x}} + \boldsymbol{x}^T \boldsymbol{\beta}), \qquad (12.6)$$

where $o_{\boldsymbol{x}} = \log\{\pi(1, \boldsymbol{x}^{(1)})/\pi(0, \boldsymbol{x}^{(1)})\}$ is the log of the relative-sampling-rates of cases to controls at $\boldsymbol{X}^{(1)} = \boldsymbol{x}^{(1)}$. So under VPS with $\pi()$ known, maximum ascertainment-corrected, or "conditional," likelihood estimation can be implemented by running a standard (prospective) logistic regression program with the appropriate set of offset values. For BSS this also gives the right estimates but standard errors need to be adjusted (see Lee *et al.*, 2010, p. 367). Note that (12.3) with (12.4) makes no use of the partially observed units. We will find that, even where we know $\pi(y_i, \boldsymbol{x}_i^{(1)}) = P(R_i = 1 \mid y_i, \boldsymbol{x}_i^{(1)})$, it is more efficient to estimate it from the data than to apply the known function.

12.2.2 Full likelihood

We now turn our attention to the likelihood based upon all of the data. Under either VPS or the more common BSS, following the arguments of Scott and Wild (2001, Appendix B) the likelihood is given by

$$
\begin{aligned}
L_{full}(\boldsymbol{\beta}, g) &= \prod_{R_i=1} P(\boldsymbol{y}_i, \boldsymbol{x}_i) \prod_{R_i=0} P(\boldsymbol{y}_i^{(1)}, \boldsymbol{x}_i^{(1)}) \qquad (12.7) \\
&= \prod_{R_i=1} f(\boldsymbol{y}_i \mid \boldsymbol{x}_i; \boldsymbol{\beta}) g(\boldsymbol{x}_i) \prod_{R_i=0} \int_{\boldsymbol{y}:\boldsymbol{y}_i^{(1)}} \int_{\boldsymbol{x}:\boldsymbol{x}_i^{(1)}} f(\boldsymbol{y} \mid \boldsymbol{x}; \boldsymbol{\beta}) dG(\boldsymbol{x}) d\mu(\boldsymbol{y}),
\end{aligned}
$$

where $g()$ is the marginal density of $\boldsymbol{X}$ and $G()$ is its distribution function. The notation "$\boldsymbol{x} : \boldsymbol{x}_i^{(1)}$" is used to signify that the integration is over all $\boldsymbol{x}$ consistent with $\boldsymbol{x}_i^{(1)}$ and similarly for $\boldsymbol{y}$. We can no longer ignore $g()$ in (12.7). We could model it parametrically, but $g(\boldsymbol{x})$ is of no interest in its own right, and modelling it can be difficult and essentially impossible when $\boldsymbol{x}$ contains a large number of variables. Thus, when we have a response-biased sample, we are driven to consider *semi-parametric* methods that require no modelling of the covariate distribution $g()$, making it a potentially infinite-dimensional nuisance parameter.

Empirical-likelihood/semiparametric-maximum-likelihood approaches replace $g()$ in (12.7) by a discrete distribution which places an atom of probability, δ_k say, at every distinct observed value of $\boldsymbol{x}$ and maximizes $L_{full}(\boldsymbol{\beta}, \boldsymbol{\delta})$. If $\boldsymbol{X}$ contains any continuous variable measured exactly, the number of free $\boldsymbol{\delta}$ parameters equals one less than the entire size of the subsampled data set. The famous result of Prentice and Pyke (1979), which tells us to estimate covariate effects in ordinary case-control studies (cf. Section 8.1.3 in Chapter 8) by using prospective logistic regression, can be deduced from applying semiparametric-maximum likelihood in this sense. [For an empirical likelihood development, see Wang and Zhou (2006); Wang *et al.* (2009) and a comparison, Amorim (2014, p. 20-22).]

Semiparametric maximum likelihood solutions are possible with brute force methods such as the EM algorithm (cf. Chen, 2004; Jiang, 2004; Scott and Wild, 2006). However, there is a set of important special cases which allow the problem to be simplified, resulting in analytic dimension reduction to a finite (and often small) dimensional nuisance parameter.

12.3 Two-phase case-control sampling

In this section, we specialize to two-phase case-control sampling. The response variable Y is binary, taking values of $Y = 1$ for the cases and $Y = 0$ for the controls. We are interested in fitting the logistic regression model (12.5).

At Phase 1, we observe the case-control status Y and the values of some explanatory variables, say $\boldsymbol{X}^{(1)}$, for all the units in the cohort (or Phase-1 sample). We start by assuming that the components of $\boldsymbol{X}^{(1)}$ have finite support, with $\boldsymbol{X}^{(1)}$ having possible values $\boldsymbol{v}_1, \dots, \boldsymbol{v}_J$ say. Let N_{hj} be the number of Phase-1 units with $Y = h$ and $\boldsymbol{X}^{(1)} = \boldsymbol{v}_j$. The cohort is stratified by case-control status (Y) alone or by the cross-product of Y and some subset of the $\boldsymbol{X}^{(1)}$ variables (cf. Section 11.9 in Chapter 11 on stratified case-control analysis). A random sample is drawn from each of these strata, and the values of the remaining variables in $\boldsymbol{X}$, say $\boldsymbol{X}^{(2)}$, are measured at Phase 2. Let $\{\boldsymbol{x}_{hjk}; k = 1, \dots, n_{hj}\}$ be the $\boldsymbol{X}$ values measured for the n_{hj} Phase-2 units sampled from the stratum defined by $Y = h$ and $\boldsymbol{X}^{(1)} = \boldsymbol{v}_j$ ($h = 0, 1; j = 1, \dots, J$). For $Y = h$ and $\boldsymbol{X}^{(1)} = \boldsymbol{v}_j$, write $\pi(y, \boldsymbol{x}^{(1)}) = \pi_{hj}$, and let $\boldsymbol{\pi}$ denote the vector of π_{hj} values.

Estimating $\boldsymbol{\beta}$ by semiparametric maximum likelihood (maximizing $L_{full}(\boldsymbol{\beta}, \boldsymbol{\delta})$) has been shown by Scott and Wild (2011) to be equivalent to solving the score equations from

$$\ell^*(\boldsymbol{\beta}, \boldsymbol{\pi}) = \ell_C(\boldsymbol{\beta}, \boldsymbol{\pi}) - \widetilde{\ell}(\boldsymbol{\pi}), \qquad (12.8)$$

jointly for $\boldsymbol{\phi} = (\boldsymbol{\beta}, \boldsymbol{\pi})$, where $\ell_C(\boldsymbol{\beta}, \boldsymbol{\pi})$ is the log of the conditional-likelihood (12.3) and

$$\widetilde{\ell}(\boldsymbol{\pi}) = \sum_{h,j} \left[n_{hj} \log \pi_{hj} + (N_{hj} - n_{hj}) \log(1 - \pi_{hj}) \right]. \qquad (12.9)$$

Thus we can get the semiparametric maximum-likelihood estimate, $\widehat{\boldsymbol{\beta}}$, of $\boldsymbol{\beta}$ by setting

$$\frac{\partial \ell^*(\boldsymbol{\phi})}{\partial \boldsymbol{\phi}} = \begin{pmatrix} \frac{\partial \ell^*(\boldsymbol{\beta}, \boldsymbol{\pi})}{\partial \boldsymbol{\beta}} \\ \frac{\partial \ell^*(\boldsymbol{\beta}, \boldsymbol{\pi})}{\partial \boldsymbol{\pi}} \end{pmatrix} = \begin{pmatrix} \frac{\partial \ell_C(\boldsymbol{\beta}, \boldsymbol{\pi})}{\partial \boldsymbol{\beta}} \\ \frac{\partial \ell_C(\boldsymbol{\beta}, \boldsymbol{\pi})}{\partial \boldsymbol{\pi}} - \frac{\partial \widetilde{\ell}(\boldsymbol{\pi})}{\partial \boldsymbol{\pi}} \end{pmatrix} = \boldsymbol{0}. \qquad (12.10)$$

Moreover, Scott and Wild (2011) have shown that we can estimate the variance-covariance matrix of $\widehat{\boldsymbol{\beta}}$ using the upper left-hand ($\boldsymbol{\beta}$-) block of

$$\boldsymbol{\mathcal{J}}(\widehat{\boldsymbol{\phi}})^{-1} = -\frac{\partial^2 \ell^*(\boldsymbol{\phi})}{\partial \boldsymbol{\phi} \partial \boldsymbol{\phi}^T}\bigg|_{\boldsymbol{\phi} = \widehat{\boldsymbol{\phi}}}^{-1}. \qquad (12.11)$$

The resulting estimation is semiparametric efficient (Breslow *et al.*, 2003; Lee and Hirose,

2010). While it looks as though ℓ^* is behaving like a likelihood, the solution does not occur at a maximum of ℓ^* but at a saddle point (Scott and Wild, 2001). We note that the original semiparametric maximum-likelihood problem of maximizing $L_{full}(\boldsymbol{\beta}, \boldsymbol{\delta})$, where the potential number of nuisance parameters δ_k is just one less than the entire size of the Phase-2 sample, has been reduced to a problem involving only $\boldsymbol{\pi}$ whose dimension is only the number of strata.

Inspection of the $\widetilde{\ell}$ term, (12.9), reveals that it is the log-likelihood you would get from modelling the binary sampling indicator R in terms of the stratum sampling-probabililities π_{hj}. Use of $\widetilde{\ell}$ alone results in the maximum likelihood estimator of the true sampling rate π_{hj} in the $(Y = h, \boldsymbol{x}^{(1)} = \boldsymbol{v}_j)$ stratum being the observed sampling rate $\widetilde{\pi}_{hj} = n_{hj}/N_{hj}$.

While semiparametric maximum likelihood solves the score equations from (12.8), (12.9) for $\boldsymbol{\beta}$ and $\boldsymbol{\pi}$ jointly, the conditional maximum-likelihood (CML) approach developed by Breslow and Cain (1988) is equivalent to a two-step plug-in method whereby we first use $\widetilde{\ell}(\boldsymbol{\pi})$ to obtain $\widetilde{\boldsymbol{\pi}}$, an estimate of the parameters of the sampling-rates model, and then "plug that in" to ℓ_C and estimate $\boldsymbol{\beta}$ by maximizing $\ell_C(\boldsymbol{\beta}, \widetilde{\boldsymbol{\pi}})$. We will find that this idea of coupling the "ascertainment corrected" log-likelihood ℓ_C with a model for the sampling-rate probabilities in either of the ways we discussed above [joint estimation via (12.8) or the two-step plug-in method] is useful much more generally than just for the current setting.

For logistic regression, we saw in equation (12.6) that $P_C(Y = 1 \mid \boldsymbol{x})$ is an offset-adjusted version of the original model. Specializing (12.6) to the current stratified-sampling situation gives, when $\boldsymbol{x}^{(1)} = \boldsymbol{v}_j$,

$$P_C(Y = 1 \mid \boldsymbol{x}) = \text{expit}(o_j(\boldsymbol{\pi}) + \boldsymbol{x}^T \boldsymbol{\beta})$$

with $o_j(\boldsymbol{\pi}) = \log(\pi_{1j}/\pi_{0j})$. The corresponding expression for ℓ_C is

$$\ell_C(\boldsymbol{\beta}, \boldsymbol{\pi}) = \sum_{h,j,k} \left[\{o_j(\boldsymbol{\pi}) + \boldsymbol{x}_{hjk}^T \boldsymbol{\beta}\}h - \log(1 + e^{o_j(\boldsymbol{\pi}) + \boldsymbol{x}_{hjk}^T \boldsymbol{\beta}}) \right].$$

Recall $\{\boldsymbol{v}_j\}$ contains all the distinct values $\boldsymbol{X}^{(1)}$ can take. In the standard case-control analysis we use a completely saturated model for the dependence of Y on the set of Phase-1-variables, say with coefficient $\beta_j^{(1)}$ for a dummy variable indicating whether or not $\boldsymbol{x}^{(1)} = \boldsymbol{v}_j$ $(j = 1 \ldots, J)$. (Other equivalent formulations could be used.) When we have a completely saturated model for the Phase-1 variables, the joint and two-step plug-in estimation methods coincide and the variance-covariance matrix from (12.11) has a very simple form (see Lee *et al.*, 2010, Section 2.4). If we are only interested in the parameters corresponding to the Phase-2 variables $\boldsymbol{X}^{(2)}$ and run the logistic regression model through a standard logistic regression program, the program output gives the semi-parametric-efficient estimate of $\boldsymbol{\beta}^{(2)}$ and its appropriate variance estimates. The $\beta_j^{(1)}$'s are also correctly estimated if we include the offsets; otherwise we end up estimating $\beta_j^{(1)*} = \beta_j^{(1)} + o_j(\boldsymbol{\pi})$ rather than $\beta_j^{(1)}$ (we also need to make a small reduction to the estimate of the variance of $\widehat{\beta}_j^{(1)}$ that the program supplies). For related discussion on how these models arise, see Sections 3.2.6, 8.1.2, and 8.1.3 in Chapters 3 and 8.

In many two-phase studies we may well want to fit more sophisticated regression models for at least some of the variables measured at Phase 1. This can be managed exactly as in standard case-control fitting. The only difference is that we no longer get the simplifications that allow us to use prospective logistic regression programs and so need special-purpose programs that use (12.10) and (12.11) directly, or equivalent formulations and parameterizations (see Wild, 1991; Qin, 1993; Scott and Wild, 1991, 1997, 2001, 2006; Lawless *et al.*, 1999; Amorim, 2014, pp. 20-21).

The joint method (12.8) is the semi-parametric efficient method if the Phase-1 variables, $\boldsymbol{X}^{(1)}$, are all discrete (Breslow *et al.*, 2003; Lee and Hirose, 2010) so that it is more efficient than the two-step plug-in method (CML). The difference in efficiency is often small but there are situations when it is appreciable (see Lawless *et al.*, 1999 and the extensive simulations of Amorim, 2014). As pointed out by Lumley *et al.* (2011), however, this extra efficiency depends on the validity of the assumed regression model so the two-step plug-in method may still be a better choice if we are worried about further exposure to model misspecification.

12.4 Two-phase studies more generally

Let us now go back to the general case of an arbitrary regression model $f(\boldsymbol{y}|\boldsymbol{x};\boldsymbol{\beta})$ where both $\boldsymbol{y}$ and $\boldsymbol{x}$ may be vectors. The Phase-1 variables that selection is based on must be in the regression model; we will relax this later. Let $\boldsymbol{V}$ contain all variables recorded at Phase 1 that we want to feed into the analysis. It must include those on which selection into Phase 2 is based but may include more. (Variables used in a sampling plan are termed *design variables* in the survey literature.)

For both VPS and BSS, for a fully observed unit

$$E_{R=1,\boldsymbol{x}}\left\{\frac{\partial}{\partial\boldsymbol{\beta}}\log f_C(\boldsymbol{y}\mid\boldsymbol{x};\boldsymbol{\beta},\pi())\right\}=\boldsymbol{0}\qquad(12.12)$$

under regularity conditions that allow the interchange of integration over $\boldsymbol{y}$ and differentiation. Thus, for known $\pi(\boldsymbol{y}^{(1)},\boldsymbol{x}^{(1)})$, setting the score vector from $\ell_C(\boldsymbol{\beta},\pi())$ to zero provides unbiased estimating equations for $\boldsymbol{\beta}$.

We can embed $\pi(\boldsymbol{y}^{(1)},\boldsymbol{x}^{(1)})$ in a larger function, $\pi(\boldsymbol{v};\boldsymbol{\alpha})$, which depends on a vector of parameters $\boldsymbol{\alpha}$ and contains the true selection probabilities, so that $\pi(\boldsymbol{y}^{(1)},\boldsymbol{x}^{(1)})=\pi(\boldsymbol{v};\boldsymbol{\alpha}_0)$ for some $\boldsymbol{\alpha}_0$. For example, in the context of the previous section, the α's are the stratum selection-probabilities thought of as unknowns. We will call $\pi(\boldsymbol{v};\boldsymbol{\alpha})$ a *selection model*. In the $\pi()$ known case, we set the score equations for $\boldsymbol{\beta}$ from ℓ_C (12.3) to zero. More precisely, we set $\boldsymbol{S}_{0,\boldsymbol{\beta}}(\boldsymbol{\beta},\boldsymbol{\alpha}_0)$ to zero, where

$$\boldsymbol{S}_{0,\boldsymbol{\beta}}(\boldsymbol{\beta},\boldsymbol{\alpha})=\sum_{i=1}^{N}R_i\frac{\partial}{\partial\boldsymbol{\beta}}\log f_C(\boldsymbol{y}_i\mid\boldsymbol{x}_i;\boldsymbol{\beta},\boldsymbol{\alpha}).$$

This still provides consistent estimates for $\boldsymbol{\beta}$ if $\boldsymbol{\alpha}_0$ is replaced by a consistent estimator $\widetilde{\boldsymbol{\alpha}}$ and we can obtain such an $\widetilde{\boldsymbol{\alpha}}$ using just the Phase-1 information. Under VPS the log likelihood for $\boldsymbol{\alpha}$ based on the Phase-1 information alone is

$$\widetilde{\ell}(\boldsymbol{\alpha})=\sum_{i=1}^{N}\left[R_i\log\pi(\boldsymbol{v}_i;\boldsymbol{\alpha})+(1-R_i)\log\left\{1-\pi(\boldsymbol{v}_i;\boldsymbol{\alpha})\right\}\right],$$

for which the corresponding score equations set the following to $\boldsymbol{0}$:

$$\boldsymbol{S}_1(\boldsymbol{\alpha})=\sum_{i=1}^{N}\left[\frac{R_i}{\pi_i}-\frac{1-R_i}{1-\pi_i}\right]\frac{\partial\pi_i}{\partial\boldsymbol{\alpha}}=\sum_{i=1}^{N}\frac{(R_i-\pi_i)}{\pi_i(1-\pi_i)}\frac{\partial\pi_i}{\partial\boldsymbol{\alpha}}=\sum_{i=1}^{N}\boldsymbol{S}_{1i},\qquad(12.13)$$

where $\pi_i=\pi(\boldsymbol{v}_i;\boldsymbol{\alpha})$. For basic stratified sampling we can think of (12.13) as coming from a working independence model in the sense of Liang and Zeger (1986). We generally use a logistic regression model for $P(R=1\mid\boldsymbol{v})$ so that $\boldsymbol{S}_1$ is just the components of the logistic-regression score-vector.

Let us consider the three likelihood-based estimation methods to follow. In each case the resulting estimators are consistent and asymptotically normal under mild regularity conditions (Scott and Wild, 2011). We reiterate that the methods discussed are implemented in a R package available from the Handbook website.

12.4.1 Known $\pi()$ or equivalently known $\boldsymbol{\alpha}_0$

Solve $\boldsymbol{S}_{0,\boldsymbol{\beta}}(\boldsymbol{\beta}, \boldsymbol{\alpha}_0) = \boldsymbol{0}$ for $\boldsymbol{\beta}$. When the R_i's are independent, the asymptotic variance-covariance matrix of $\widehat{\boldsymbol{\beta}}$ is given by

$$\text{AVar}\{\widehat{\boldsymbol{\beta}}\} = \boldsymbol{\mathcal{I}}_{00}^{-1}\boldsymbol{\mathcal{C}}_{00}\boldsymbol{\mathcal{I}}_{00}^{-1},$$

where $\boldsymbol{\mathcal{I}}_{00} = E\{-\partial \boldsymbol{S}_0/\partial \boldsymbol{\beta}^T\}$ and $\boldsymbol{\mathcal{C}}_{00} = \text{Var}(\boldsymbol{S}_0) = \text{Cov}(\boldsymbol{S}_0, \boldsymbol{S}_0)$.

12.4.2 Two-step plug-in

Solve $\boldsymbol{S}_1(\boldsymbol{\alpha}) = \boldsymbol{0}$ to obtain $\widetilde{\boldsymbol{\alpha}}$ and then $\boldsymbol{S}_{0,\boldsymbol{\beta}}(\boldsymbol{\beta}, \widetilde{\boldsymbol{\alpha}}) = \boldsymbol{0}$ for $\boldsymbol{\beta}$, or equivalently, solve for $\boldsymbol{\phi} = (\boldsymbol{\beta}, \boldsymbol{\alpha})$:

$$\boldsymbol{S}(\boldsymbol{\phi}) = \boldsymbol{S}(\boldsymbol{\beta}, \boldsymbol{\alpha}) = \begin{pmatrix} \boldsymbol{S}_{0,\boldsymbol{\beta}}(\boldsymbol{\beta}, \boldsymbol{\alpha}) \\ \boldsymbol{S}_1(\boldsymbol{\alpha}) \end{pmatrix} = \sum_{i=1}^{N} \boldsymbol{S}_i = \boldsymbol{0}. \tag{12.14}$$

We then have asymptotic variance-covariance matrix $\text{AVar}\{\widehat{\boldsymbol{\phi}}\} = \boldsymbol{\mathcal{I}}^{-1}\boldsymbol{\mathcal{C}}(\boldsymbol{\mathcal{I}}^T)^{-1}$ where $\boldsymbol{\mathcal{C}} = \text{Var}\{\boldsymbol{S}\}$ and $\boldsymbol{\mathcal{I}} = \boldsymbol{\mathcal{I}}(\boldsymbol{\phi}) = E\{-\partial \boldsymbol{S}/\partial \boldsymbol{\phi}^T\}$. When the R_i's are independent,

$$\text{AVar}\{\widehat{\boldsymbol{\beta}}\} = \boldsymbol{\mathcal{I}}_{00}^{-1}\boldsymbol{\mathcal{C}}_{00}\boldsymbol{\mathcal{I}}_{00}^{-1} - \boldsymbol{\mathcal{I}}_{00}^{-1}\boldsymbol{\mathcal{C}}_{01}\boldsymbol{\mathcal{C}}_{11}^{-1}\boldsymbol{\mathcal{C}}_{01}^T\boldsymbol{\mathcal{I}}_{00}^{-1} \tag{12.15a}$$

$$= \boldsymbol{\mathcal{I}}_{00}^{-1}\boldsymbol{\mathcal{C}}_R\boldsymbol{\mathcal{I}}_{00}^{-1}, \tag{12.15b}$$

where $\boldsymbol{\mathcal{C}}_R = \boldsymbol{\mathcal{C}}_{00} - \boldsymbol{\mathcal{C}}_{01}\boldsymbol{\mathcal{C}}_{11}^{-1}\boldsymbol{\mathcal{C}}_{01}^T$. Here $\boldsymbol{\mathcal{C}}_{rs} = \text{Cov}(\boldsymbol{S}_r, \boldsymbol{S}_s)$ for $r = 0, 1; s = 0, 1$.

This tells us two things. First, the initial term in (12.15a) is the value of $\text{AVar}\{\widehat{\boldsymbol{\beta}}\}$ when known values of the π_i's are used, so that the second term represents the effect of estimating π_i's, or equivalently $\boldsymbol{\alpha}$. Note that the last term is nonnegative definite. This means that $\text{AVar}\{\widehat{\boldsymbol{\beta}}\}$ is always smaller when we use estimated values for the inclusion probabilities than when we use the true values. In other words, even if we know the π_is exactly, as we usually will in designed studies since they are determined by us, we are still better off estimating them! This type of "estimated better than known" result has been noted in similar contexts by a number of authors, in particular by Robins *et al.* (1994) (see also Carroll *et al.*, 1995 and the general treatment of Henmi and Eguchi, 2004), and is not quite as paradoxical as it might seem at first glance. $\boldsymbol{S}_{0,\boldsymbol{\beta}}(\boldsymbol{\beta}, \boldsymbol{\alpha}_0)$ on its own makes no use of the partially observed (Phase-1 only) units. In the process of estimating the inclusion probabilities, we bring in information on $\boldsymbol{y}$ and $\boldsymbol{x}^{(1)}$ from the unsampled units, just as we do when we use post-stratification or calibration in survey sampling (Deville and Särndal, 1992). Thus the estimators based on estimated inclusion probabilities make use of additional information that is not used with known inclusion probabilities, which makes the consequent variance reduction much less surprising.

Second, (12.15b) tells us something about how this works. We note that $\boldsymbol{\mathcal{C}}_R$ is the variance-covariance matrix of the residual vector when $\boldsymbol{S}_0(\boldsymbol{\phi})$ is regressed on $\boldsymbol{S}_1(\boldsymbol{\phi})$, i.e., $\boldsymbol{\mathcal{C}}_R = \inf_{\boldsymbol{B}} \text{AVar}\{\boldsymbol{S}_0 - \boldsymbol{B}\boldsymbol{S}_1\}$. Clearly, adding any extra variables on which we have the required information to the inclusion model can never increase, and may decrease, $\boldsymbol{\mathcal{C}}_R$, even if the inclusion probabilities do not actually depend on these variables. In fact, we can see immediately from the form of $\boldsymbol{\mathcal{C}}_R$ that the size of reduction depends on the relationship between the score for the added variable and $\boldsymbol{S}_0(\boldsymbol{\phi}_0)$ and not at all on the strength of its effect on the inclusion probabilities. If $\boldsymbol{v}$ has finite support then, asymptotically, the most efficient strategy will be to fit a saturated model for $\boldsymbol{\pi}$. The resulting reduction in $\mathrm{AVar}\{\widehat{\boldsymbol{\beta}}\}$ can be substantial, as illustrated in the simulation results in Scott and Wild (2011); Amorim (2014, Chapters 2-4). Of course, this is an asymptotic result and there is a lower-order penalty to pay for estimating extra parameters. Thus throwing in a large number of variables may not be optimal in small samples. More work is required in this area.

12.4.3   Joint Estimation

Solve for $\boldsymbol{\phi} = (\boldsymbol{\beta}, \boldsymbol{\alpha})$:

$$\widetilde{\boldsymbol{S}}(\boldsymbol{\phi}) = \widetilde{\boldsymbol{S}}(\boldsymbol{\beta}, \boldsymbol{\alpha}) = \begin{pmatrix} \boldsymbol{S}_{0,\beta}(\boldsymbol{\beta}, \boldsymbol{\alpha}) \\ \boldsymbol{S}_{0,\alpha}(\boldsymbol{\beta}, \boldsymbol{\alpha}) - \boldsymbol{S}_1(\boldsymbol{\alpha}) \end{pmatrix} = \sum_{i=1}^{N} \widetilde{\boldsymbol{S}}_i = \boldsymbol{0}. \qquad (12.16)$$

This differs from (12.14) by the inclusion of

$$S_{0,\alpha}(\boldsymbol{\beta}, \boldsymbol{\alpha}) = \sum_{i=1}^{N} R_i \frac{\partial}{\partial \boldsymbol{\alpha}} \log f_C(\boldsymbol{y}_i \mid \boldsymbol{x}_i; \boldsymbol{\beta}, \boldsymbol{\alpha}).$$

If all of the Phase-1 variables are discrete and $\pi(\boldsymbol{v}; \boldsymbol{\alpha})$ is a completely saturated model for all combinations of values of the Phase-1 variables then use of (12.16) is the empirical-likelihood/semiparametric-maximum-likelihood solution, is semiparametric efficient, and we can estimate the variance-covariance matrix of $\widehat{\boldsymbol{\beta}}$ with the upper left-hand corner of

$$\boldsymbol{\mathcal{J}}(\widehat{\boldsymbol{\phi}})^{-1} = -\left. \frac{\partial \widetilde{\boldsymbol{S}}(\boldsymbol{\phi})}{\partial \boldsymbol{\phi}^T} \right|_{\boldsymbol{\phi}=\widehat{\boldsymbol{\phi}}}^{-1}.$$

The beauty of both (12.14) and (12.16) is that they allow us to gain efficiency by bringing in Phase-1 variables not used for sampling and this may include continuous Phase-1 variables. It is done very simply – by including them as additional variables in the selection model. While use of (12.16) can no longer be shown to be semiparametric efficient once we introduce continuous Phase-1 variables, Amorim (2014, pp. 40-43) has shown that (12.16) is the most efficient linear combination of $\boldsymbol{S}_0(\boldsymbol{\phi})$ and $\boldsymbol{S}_1(\boldsymbol{\alpha})$.

   While simulations in Amorim (2014) show substantial efficiency gains from richer selection models (i.e., including more Phase-1 variables) optimal strategies for doing this have not yet been found.

   If we have continuous Phase-1 variables there is no theory that says that use of (12.16) behaves essentially like likelihood estimation. At some small cost in efficiency, however, we can use discrete coarsenings of continuous $\boldsymbol{X}^{(1)}$ variables together with (12.10) and (12.11). This avoids the need to worry about different stratified-sampling structures in computing the variance of the score equations. Otherwise, (12.10) has to be treated in the working-independence-model sense of Liang and Zeger (1986) with variance estimates computed using sandwich estimators of the form, $\mathrm{AVar}\{\widehat{\boldsymbol{\phi}}\} = \boldsymbol{\mathcal{I}}^{-1}\boldsymbol{\mathcal{C}}(\boldsymbol{\mathcal{I}}^{\mathrm{T}})^{-1}$. Here $\boldsymbol{\mathcal{C}} = \mathrm{Var}\{\widetilde{\boldsymbol{S}}\}$ should take the sampling scheme into account, although ignoring stratified sampling and assuming independence of the R_i's is conservative.

12.5   Survey-weighted approach

We will very briefly discuss the survey-weighted (Horvitz-Thompson, or inverse-probability weighted) approach whereby the contribution from each fully observed unit to the complete-data likelihood score (12.2) is weighted inversely to its probability of selection rather than allowed for by conditioning (cf. Binder, 1983; Pfeffermann, 1993). Where the π_i's are known, naive application of this idea results in solving for $\boldsymbol{\beta}$

$$\boldsymbol{S}_W(\boldsymbol{\beta}) = \sum_{i=1}^N \frac{R_i}{\pi_i} \frac{\partial}{\partial \boldsymbol{\beta}} \log f(\boldsymbol{y}_i \mid \boldsymbol{x}_i; \boldsymbol{\beta}, \boldsymbol{\alpha}) = \boldsymbol{0}.$$

This includes no information on Phase-1 individuals who were not selected into Phase 2 (for whom $R_i = 0$). There are various ways of bringing in Phase-1 information. The method which directly parallels the two-step plug-in method of the previous subsection is to model $P(R_i = 1)$ in terms of all desired Phase-1 variables $\boldsymbol{v}_i$ with parameters $\boldsymbol{\alpha}$ (e.g., with a logistic regression model) which gives us an estimate $\widetilde{\boldsymbol{\alpha}}$ of $\boldsymbol{\alpha}$. We then estimate $\boldsymbol{\beta}$ by solving

$$\boldsymbol{S}_W(\boldsymbol{\beta}; \widetilde{\boldsymbol{\alpha}}) = \sum_{i=1}^N \frac{R_i}{\pi(\boldsymbol{v}_i; \widetilde{\boldsymbol{\alpha}})} \frac{\partial}{\partial \boldsymbol{\beta}} \log f(\boldsymbol{y}_i \mid \boldsymbol{x}_i; \boldsymbol{\beta}) = \boldsymbol{0}.$$

Variance estimation uses sandwich estimators (12.15a) with $\boldsymbol{S}_W$ replacing $\boldsymbol{S}_0$ in (12.14).

In the survey-weighted approach we can straightforwardly use any Phase-1 variables in the fitted selection model, whether or not they are present in the regression model, something which is much more problematic with the methods based on conditioning (see Section 12.7).

An alternative to modelling the inclusion probabilities as above is *calibrating the weights*; see Chapter 13. In the special case where $\boldsymbol{V}$ has finite support and inclusion probabilities are fitted using a saturated model, then the results produced by modelling the inclusion probabilities as above are identical to those from poststratification (which is available in many major statistical packages) and to calibrating the weights to the Phase-1 cell totals. Calibration has been explored more generally for two-phase sampling by Breslow *et al.* (2009) and Lumley *et al.* (2011) and they found that it was better to calibrate on population totals of functions that are highly correlated with the scores in $\boldsymbol{S}_W$ rather than on variables that are correlated with $\boldsymbol{y}$, a very similar conclusion to the one that we have reached in the previous section. Their method, which is the subject of Chapter 8 of Lumley (2010), is implemented in Thomas Lumley's R package `survey`.

Although typically less efficient than the conditional methods, and sometimes considerably so for the effects of Phase-2 variables, survey-weighted estimation is attractive for three main reasons. One is the wide availability of software to implement it – most major statistical packages can handle linear and logistic models with poststratification, and both *Stata* and the `survey` package in R can handle arbitrary Generalized Linear Models. The second is that it has the property of estimating the same quantity that we would estimate if we had data from the full cohort, even if the model $f(\boldsymbol{y}|\boldsymbol{x}; \boldsymbol{\beta})$ is misspecified. The third is that it is much easier to deal with sampling designs based on design variables that are not present in the regression model. These issues are explored in detail by Amorim (2014). More details of the survey-weighting approach are given in Chapter 13 in this Handbook.

12.6   Two-phase analyses for the WHI Example

Recall from Section 12.1.2 that at Phase 1 we have data on postmenopausal women aged between 50 and 79 years old from WHI trials of hormone therapy (HT) intended to reduce coronary heart disease (CHD). The women with an intact uterus had been part of a trial in which they were randomized to a combination of estrogen plus progestin (E+P) versus placebo, while the remaining women (who had a prior hysterectomy) were part of a trial randomized to estrogen alone (E) versus placebo.

Phase 2 corresponds to a followup case-control study. For those subjects selected into the case-control study, blood samples that had been stored at baseline were assayed giving additional data for inflammatory, lipid, thrombotic, and genetic markers. The controls were selected matched to cases by date of randomization, trial, age, and prevalence of the particular cardiovascular disease (CVD) at baseline. After exclusions for missing data as explained in Breslow *et al.* (2013, p. 234), the size of the Phase-1 cohort size was 23,301, and at Phase 2 there were 248 cases and 617 controls.

Rossouw *et al.* (2008) analyzed the original case-control data by ordinary logistic regression, with CHD case-control status as the outcome and HT treatment as the primary risk factor. All analyzes were adjusted for baseline age, trial, body mass index, waist-hip ratio, smoking, alcohol, physical activity, diabetes, history of high cholesterol, prevalent CVD, left ventricular hypertrophy, systolic blood pressure (SBP), use of anti-hypertensive medications, aspirin, and statins. Among the more interesting findings was a positive interaction between HT and the LDL/HDL ratio (on a log scale). Presence of the GpIIIa leu33pro polymorphism was also associated with increased risk.

Breslow *et al.* (2013) used a model for CHD with log(LDL/HDL) ratio (centred at log 3), HT, their interaction and the GpIIIa leu33pro polymorphism as variables of primary interest. Seven of the fifteen variables mentioned above were used for adjustment. The other eight variables were retained for use as design or auxiliary variables.

Recall that the actual case-control sampling was performed matched on case-control status (cc), Trial, prevalent CVD and AgeG consisting of the 3 age-groups: 49-59, 60-69, and 70-79. To properly account for that, selection models need to include a saturated model for the full set of interactions between these four variables (`cc*Trial*CVD*AgeG`). The analysis that produced Table 12.1 used more Phase-1 information. The selection models used also included `cc*HT + cc*(SBP/100) + cc*Statins + cc*Smoking + cc*Diabetes + cc*AgeG3` where `AgeG3` contains the five age groups 49-54, 55-60, 61-66, 67-72, and 73-79. Very similar results are obtained using continuous age.

All three two-phase methods corrected for the bias in the control sample that was serious with respect to the design variables age and prevalent CVD. The regression coefficients for these variables were considerably higher, and the standard errors somewhat lower (as expected because of additional Phase-1 information). The weighted method estimated a noticeably smaller interaction between HT and the log(LDL/HDL) ratio than the conditional methods. As expected, the weighted method produced standard errors that were generally larger than those for the conditional methods, including even the standard method, but the differences were generally small except for the design variable SBP. Despite quite large efficiency differences between methods being evident for some scenarios in simulations, the results from the four types of analysis were remarkably similar for these data.

TABLE 12.1
Comparing results for the model for CHD from the two-phase analysis methods (exception is Std which refers to ordinary logistic regression).

	Std		Weighted		Plug-in		Joint	
	Est	SE	Est	SE	Est	SE	Est	SE
log(LDL/HDL)	0.83	0.35	0.99	0.39	0.81	0.35	0.82	0.35
HT	0.16	0.17	0.14	0.16	0.24	0.15	0.23	0.15
HT*log(LDL/HDL)	0.97	0.49	0.60	0.51	0.99	0.48	0.99	0.48
GpIIIa	0.43	0.18	0.45	0.20	0.46	0.18	0.45	0.18
Age/10	0.07	0.14	0.64	0.13	0.67	0.12	0.67	0.12
Current smoker	1.45	0.24	1.49	0.20	1.41	0.18	1.41	0.18
Diabetes	1.30	0.28	1.26	0.20	1.15	0.19	1.13	0.19
Prevalent CVD	0.64	0.21	1.21	0.19	1.19	0.18	1.19	0.18
SBP/100	2.30	0.49	1.97	0.50	1.88	0.42	1.91	0.42
Statins	0.67	0.25	0.67	0.22	0.67	0.21	0.68	0.21
Trial E+P	0.24	0.17	0.12	0.17	0.15	0.15	0.16	0.15

12.7 Design variables outside the regression model

Recall the *design variables* are variables used in a sampling plan. The theory above assumes that the true selection probabilities depend only on design variables that are obtained at Phase 1 and are present in the regression model. The selection model being fitted can use other Phase-1 variables, including variables external to the regression model, provided they are redundant as far as predicting selection is concerned (auxiliary variables). This is done to add efficiency to the estimation of regression-model parameters (for the reasons described above). But these external Phase-1 variables cannot themselves be determinants of selection. The reason for this is that estimating equations (12.12) are asymptotically unbiased using f_C defined in (12.4) with a consistent estimator of $\pi(\boldsymbol{x}^{(1)}, \boldsymbol{y}^{(1)})$, but may not be otherwise.

What happens if there are other design variables known for the whole population and used in selecting the sample but not included in the model? One very simple solution is to include them as extra $\boldsymbol{x}$ variables in the model. This often works well, but there are situations where it makes no scientific sense and it may change the natural interpretation of the other regression coefficients. For example, Lee *et al.* (1997) used data from a case-control study on Sudden Infant Death Syndrome (SIDS) to model the chance that a child will receive the standard childhood inoculations. The main design variable was an indicator of whether or not a child was a SIDS victim and it makes no sense to include this as a predictor of inoculation status.

Let $\boldsymbol{Z}$ contain the design variables not present in the regression model. There are a couple of alternative approaches, both of which require us to build a model for $f(\boldsymbol{z} \mid \boldsymbol{x}^{(1)}, \boldsymbol{y}^{(1)})$, say $f(\boldsymbol{z} \mid \boldsymbol{x}^{(1)}, \boldsymbol{y}^{(1)}; \boldsymbol{\gamma})$. The first is to add the extra variables to the response, forming a modified response $\boldsymbol{y}^* = (\boldsymbol{y}, \boldsymbol{z})$, and then apply the methods discussed above to

$$f(\boldsymbol{y}^* \mid \boldsymbol{x}; \boldsymbol{\beta}, \boldsymbol{\gamma}) = f(\boldsymbol{z} \mid \boldsymbol{y}, \boldsymbol{x}; \boldsymbol{\gamma}) f(\boldsymbol{y} \mid \boldsymbol{x}; \boldsymbol{\beta}).$$

This is the approach used, by example in Jiang *et al.* (2006) for secondary analysis of case-control data and Neuhaus *et al.* (2014) for longitudinal data from outcome-dependent sampling designs. The other approach is to build a model for the selection probability, π_i, as a function of $\boldsymbol{z}, \boldsymbol{x}^{(1)}, \boldsymbol{y}^{(1)}$ and then set

$$\pi\left(\boldsymbol{x}^{(1)}, \boldsymbol{y}^{(1)}\right) = \int \pi\left(\boldsymbol{z}, \boldsymbol{x}^{(1)}, \boldsymbol{y}^{(1)}\right) dF\left(\boldsymbol{z} \mid \boldsymbol{x}^{(1)}, \boldsymbol{y}^{(1)}; \boldsymbol{\gamma}\right). \tag{12.17}$$

A great deal more work is needed before we can say much about the relative merits of these two approaches. They can be very difficult to implement adequately, particularly if we have large numbers of extra design variables. They tend also to expose us to additional modelling assumptions.

The additional level of modelling described above is not, however, necessary in the survey-weighted approach. We do not actually need to take the additional, often difffcult, step of modelling design variables external to the regression model, $\boldsymbol{Z}$, in terms of $(\boldsymbol{X}, \boldsymbol{Y})$ and then using $\pi(\boldsymbol{x}_i^{(1)}, \boldsymbol{y}_i^{(1)})$ via (12.17), though it may be more efficient to do so (cf. Kim and Skinner, 2013). We can just use $\pi\left(\boldsymbol{z}, \boldsymbol{x}^{(1)}, \boldsymbol{y}^{(1)}\right)$ directly.

12.8   Three and more phases of sampling

We will now add more phases of sampling to our two-phase structure. Certain components of the outcome and the covariate vector, say $\boldsymbol{y}^{(1)}$ and $\boldsymbol{x}^{(1)}$, are observed for all subjects at Phase 1 and these data are used to construct strata or sampling probabilities for a random sample of Phase-2 subjects ($R_1 = 1$), and additional components $\boldsymbol{y}^{(2)}$ and $\boldsymbol{x}^{(2)}$ are measured for those who are sampled. Now a further stratified sample of Phase-2 subjects is selected for Phase 3 ($R_2 = 1$) based on $(\boldsymbol{y}^{(1)}, \boldsymbol{y}^{(2)}, \boldsymbol{x}^{(1)}, \boldsymbol{x}^{(2)})$ information available after Phase 2, and the entire and remaining $\boldsymbol{y}$ and $\boldsymbol{x}$ variables are observed for those selected ($R_2 = 1$; these also have $R_1 = 1$).

We now need two selection models:

$$\pi_1(\boldsymbol{y}^{(1)}, \boldsymbol{x}^{(1)}; \boldsymbol{\alpha}_1) = P(R_1 = 1 \mid \boldsymbol{y}^{(1)}, \boldsymbol{x}^{(1)}; \boldsymbol{\alpha}_1)$$

into Phase 2, and

$$\pi_2(\boldsymbol{y}^{(1)}, \boldsymbol{y}^{(2)}, \boldsymbol{x}^{(1)}, \boldsymbol{x}^{(2)}; \boldsymbol{\alpha}_2) = P(R_2 = 1 \mid R_1 = 1, \boldsymbol{y}^{(1)}, \boldsymbol{y}^{(2)}, \boldsymbol{x}^{(1)}, \boldsymbol{x}^{(2)}; \boldsymbol{\alpha}_2)$$

from Phase 2 into Phase 3. The observational conditioning event in $f_C(\boldsymbol{y} \mid \boldsymbol{x}; \boldsymbol{\beta}, \boldsymbol{\alpha})$ is that $R = R_1 R_2 = 1$ which has probability

$$\pi(\boldsymbol{\alpha}) = \pi_1(\boldsymbol{y}^{(1)}, \boldsymbol{x}^{(1)}; \boldsymbol{\alpha}_1)\pi_2(\boldsymbol{y}^{(1)}, \boldsymbol{y}^{(2)}, \boldsymbol{x}^{(1)}, \boldsymbol{x}^{(2)}; \boldsymbol{\alpha}_2).$$

The working-independence-model estimating equations for the α_j's from the selection models are, into Phase 2:

$$\boldsymbol{S}_1(\boldsymbol{\alpha}_1) = \sum_{i=1}^{N} \left[\frac{R_{1i}}{\pi_{1i}} - \frac{1 - R_{1i}}{1 - \pi_{1i}} \right] \frac{\partial \pi_{1i}}{\partial \boldsymbol{\alpha}_1} = \boldsymbol{0},$$

where $\pi_{1i} = \pi_1(\boldsymbol{y}_i^{(1)}, \boldsymbol{x}_i^{(1)}; \boldsymbol{\alpha}_1)$, and from Phase 2 into Phase 3 (observed only if $R_1 = 1$):

$$\boldsymbol{S}_2(\boldsymbol{\alpha}_2) = \sum_{i=1}^{N} R_{1i} \left[\frac{R_{2i}}{\pi_{2i}} - \frac{1 - R_{2i}}{1 - \pi_{2i}} \right] \frac{\partial \pi_{2i}}{\partial \boldsymbol{\alpha}_2} = \boldsymbol{0}, \tag{12.18}$$

where $\pi_{2i} = \pi_2(\boldsymbol{y}_i^{(1)}, \boldsymbol{y}_i^{(2)}, \boldsymbol{x}_i^{(1)}, \boldsymbol{x}_i^{(2)}; \boldsymbol{\alpha}_2)$. The joint-estimation estimating equations for $\boldsymbol{\phi} = (\boldsymbol{\beta}, \boldsymbol{\alpha})$ are

$$\widetilde{\boldsymbol{S}}(\boldsymbol{\phi}) = \widetilde{\boldsymbol{S}}(\boldsymbol{\beta}, \boldsymbol{\alpha}) = \begin{pmatrix} \boldsymbol{S}_{0,\boldsymbol{\beta}}(\boldsymbol{\beta}, \boldsymbol{\alpha}) \\ \boldsymbol{S}_{0,\boldsymbol{\alpha}_1}(\boldsymbol{\beta}, \boldsymbol{\alpha}_1) - \boldsymbol{S}_1(\boldsymbol{\alpha}_1) \\ \boldsymbol{S}_{0,\boldsymbol{\alpha}_2}(\boldsymbol{\beta}, \boldsymbol{\alpha}_2) - \boldsymbol{S}_2(\boldsymbol{\alpha}_2) \end{pmatrix} = \boldsymbol{0} \tag{12.19}$$

where $\boldsymbol{S}_{0,\boldsymbol{\alpha}_j}(\boldsymbol{\beta},\boldsymbol{\alpha}_j) = \sum_{i=1}^N R_i \partial \log f_C(\boldsymbol{y}_i \mid \boldsymbol{x}_i; \boldsymbol{\beta},\boldsymbol{\alpha})/\partial \boldsymbol{\alpha}_j$.

Extending to four or more phases simply involves adding more terms following the same pattern (one for each phase). At the kth phase, R_k records selection or not of those who were selected at Phase $(k-1)$ (and thus all previous phases) in to Phase k, and the equivalent of (12.18) requires a leading $R_{1i} \cdots R_{(k-1)i}$. Again, this gives the semiparametric maximum likelihood solution in the case where all variable information used in all phases but the last is discrete and fully-saturated selection models are used. The plug-in method is equivalent to omitting the $\boldsymbol{S}_{0,\boldsymbol{\alpha}_j}$ terms in (12.19).

We note that Lee *et al.* (2010) gives a different approach to solving this problem that is equivalent to the above for the special case, which was the subject of that paper, in which subsampling depends only on discrete variables.

12.8.1 The WHI Example continued

The data we have discussed to date have been viewed as a *two-phase* sample, where the main cohort is the Phase-1 sample, assumed to have been drawn by simple random sampling from a "superpopulation" and the Phase-2 sample is the case-control sample, drawn by outcome-dependent, stratified sampling from the phase-1 sample.

A particular feature of the WHI study, however, invites consideration of a more complex design. In order to assess adherence to treatment, the investigators selected a 8.6% cohort random sample, stratified on trial and ethnicity, for assay of baseline and subsequent blood samples for selected biomarkers (Anderson *et al.*, 2003). The baseline LDL and HDL levels were thus also available for an additional 2,158 controls who were not sampled for the case-control study. Putting this together, the resulting data may be regarded as having arisen from a *three-phase* design, with the main cohort as Phase 1, all subjects with known LDL and HDL levels as Phase 2 and the case-control sample, for which genotype is also known, as Phase 3.

As the additional individuals were selected into Phase 2 on the basis of ethnicity and trial, we added the term `cc*Trial*Ethnicity` to the terms used in the selection model used in the two-phase analyses to form the first selection model (Phase 1 into Phase 2). The second selection model (Phase 2 into Phase 3) used the same set of variables and added a `cc*HT*log.ratio` term to bring in the new cholesterol information now available at Phase 2. The model of interest is unchanged. The results of the various forms of analysis are given in Table 12.2.

Incorporation of the additional information on LDL and HDL from the 8.6 % sample had a noticeable effect on precision for three of the variables of prime interest, namely, log(LDL/HDL), HT and their interaction. In comparison with results from Table 12.1, standard errors for these variables were reduced for all three methods (Weighted, Plug-in, Joint). There was stronger evidence from the conditional methods (Plug-in and Joint) for an interaction between HT and log(LDL/HDL); the results from the Weighted method were still inconclusive. The standard errors for the adjustment variables decreased for the Weighted method whereas several increased slightly for the conditional methods in comparison with the two-phase results. Consequently, the loss of precision from using weighted method relative to the conditional methods was reduced.

TABLE 12.2
Comparing results for the model for CHD from the three-phase analysis methods (exception is Std which refers to ordinary logistic regression).

	Std		Weighted		Plug-in		Joint	
	Est	SE	Est	SE	Est	SE	Est	SE
log(LDL/HDL)	0.83	0.35	1.16	0.35	0.99	0.31	1.00	0.31
HT	0.16	0.17	0.09	0.16	0.19	0.15	0.15	0.15
HT*log(LDL/HDL)	0.97	0.49	0.69	0.46	1.05	0.43	1.05	0.43
GpIIIa	0.43	0.18	0.45	0.20	0.46	0.18	0.45	0.18
Age/10	0.07	0.14	0.66	0.13	0.61	0.12	0.64	0.12
Current smoker	1.45	0.24	1.40	0.21	1.25	0.19	1.28	0.19
Diabetes	1.30	0.28	1.24	0.22	1.15	0.21	1.11	0.20
Prevalent CVD	0.64	0.21	1.13	0.19	1.15	0.18	1.13	0.18
SBP/100	2.30	0.49	1.84	0.50	1.72	0.43	1.82	0.43
Statins	0.67	0.25	0.61	0.23	0.64	0.21	0.67	0.21
Trial E+P	0.24	0.17	0.10	0.17	0.10	0.15	0.14	0.15

12.9 Summary

In a two-phase study, some variables are measured on all the units in a large initial sample of units drawn from a cohort or finite population (Phase 1). Then, based on the values of these variables, a subsample of units is drawn and the values of additional variables are obtained for members of the subsample (Phase 2). For simplicity of exposition we refer to any variable that we have data on for the full cohort a full-cohort variable.

Our main focus has been on likelihood-based methods (Section 12.2), and on a particular formulation of the semiparametric maximum-likelihood methods that have been developed and are semiparametric-efficient when all the full-cohort variables used are discrete (Section 12.3). This formulation permits easy incorporation of continuous variables for the whole cohort and also makes other generalisations possible (Sections 12.4 and 12.7). The formulation is based upon fitting the conditional, ascertainment-corrected model

$$f_C(\boldsymbol{y}_i \mid \boldsymbol{x}_i; \boldsymbol{\beta}) = \mathrm{P}(\boldsymbol{y}_i \mid \boldsymbol{x}_i, R_i = 1)$$

to just those units with $R_i = 1$ (signifying selection into Phase 2.) For logistic models this simply involves an offset adjustment to the model of interest. Full-cohort information enters into the analysis through a model for selection into Phase 2,

$$\pi(\boldsymbol{v}_i; \boldsymbol{\alpha}) = \mathrm{P}(R_i = 1 \mid \text{full-cohort data}).$$

Additional information from variables that are unnecessary for modelling selection but are correlated with elements of the scores for the model of interest adds efficiency (see the discussion following equation (12.15b)). We have discussed joint and two-step plug-in variations. We have also discussed survey-weighted (inverse-probability weighted) methods based on solving

$$\sum_{i=1}^N \frac{R_i}{\pi(\boldsymbol{v}_i; \boldsymbol{\alpha})} \frac{\partial}{\partial \boldsymbol{\beta}} \log f(\boldsymbol{y}_i \mid \boldsymbol{x}_i; \boldsymbol{\beta}) = \boldsymbol{0}$$

(see Section 12.5). These methods are generally less efficient. An alternative way of including such full-cohort information is through "calibrating the weights" (see Chapter 13).

There are restrictions on how full-cohort information is treated for these conditional methods that are unnecessary for the inverse-probability weighted methods (see Section 12.7).

There is a live issue about the trade-off between increased efficiency of the conditional methods when models are true versus biases when models are misspecified. For some discussion see Chapter 14 and Lumley (2017). This is an area that needs more research.

Section 12.8 generalised the above discussion to three or more phases of sampling.

Bibliography

Amorim, G. (2014). *Semiparametric Methods for Outcome-Dependent Samples with Discrete and Continuous Outcomes*. Ph.D. thesis, Department of Statistics, University of Auckland.

Anderson, G. L., Manson, J., Wallace, R., Lund, B., Halla, D., Davis, S., Shumaker, S., Wan, C. Y., Stein, E., and Prentice, R. L. (2003). Implementation of the Women's Health Initiative study design. *Annals of Epidemiology*, **14**, S5–S17.

Arbogast, P. D., Lin, D. Y., Siscovick, D. S., and Schwartz, S. M. (2002). Estimating incidence rates from population-based case-control studies in the presence of nonrespondents. *Biometrical Journal*, **44**, 227–240.

Binder, D. A. (1983). On the variances of asymptotically normal estimators from complex surveys. *International Statistical Review*, **51**, 279–292.

Breslow, N. E. and Cain, K. C. (1988). Logistic regression for two-stage case-control data. *Biometrika*, **75**, 11–20.

Breslow, N. E. and Holubkov, R. (1997). Maximum likelihood estimation of logistic regression parameters under two-phase, outcome-dependent sampling. *Journal of the Royal Statistical Society, Series B (Statistical Methodology)*, **59**, 447–461.

Breslow, N. E., McNeney, B., and Wellner, J. A. (2003). Large sample theory for semi-parametric regression models with two-phase, outcome dependent sampling. *Annals of Statistics*, **31**, 1110–1139.

Breslow, N. E., Lumley, T., Ballantyne, C. M., Chambless, L. E., and Kulich, M. (2009). Improved Horvitz-Thompson estimation of model parameters from two-phase stratified samples: Applications in epidemiology. *Statistics in Biosciences*, **1**, 32–49.

Breslow, N. E., Amorim, G., Pettinger, M. B., and Rossouw, J. (2013). Using the whole cohort in the analysis of case-control data: Application to the Women's Health Initiative. *Statistics in Biosciences*, **5**, 232–249.

Carroll, R. J., Ruppert, D., and Stefanski, L. A. (1995). *Measurement Error in Nonlinear Models*. Chapman and Hall, New York.

Chatterjee, N. and Chen, Y.-H. (2007). Maximum likelihood inference on a mixed conditionally and marginally specified regression model for genetic epidemiologic studies with two-phase sampling. *Journal of the Royal Statistical Society: Series B (Statistical Methodology)*, **69**, 123–142.

Chatterjee, N., Chen, Y.-H., Maas, P., and Carroll, R. J. (2016). Constrained maximum likelihood estimation for model calibration using summary-level information from external big data sources (with discussion). *Journal of the American Statistical Association*, **111**, 107–131.

Chen, H. Y. (2004). Nonparametric and semiparametric models for missing covariates in parametric regression. *Journal of the American Statistical Association*, **99**, 1176–1189.

Cochran, W. G. (1977). *Sampling Techniques*. John Wiley & Sons, Hoboken, New Jersey.

Deville, J.-C. and Särndal, C.-E. (1992). Calibration estimators in survey sampling. *Journal of the American Statistical Association*, **87**, 377–382.

Hausman, J. A. and Wise, D. A. (1981). Stratification on endogenous variables and estimation: The Gary income maintenance experiment. In C. F. Manski and D. L. McFadden, editors, *Structural Analysis of Discrete Data with Econometric Applications*, chapter 10, pages 365–391. MIT Press, Cambridge, Massachusetts.

Henmi, M. and Eguchi, S. (2004). A paradox concerning nuisance parameters and projected estimating functions. *Biometrika*, **91**, 929–941.

Jiang, Y. (2004). *Semiparametric Maximum Likelihood for Multi-phase Response-Selective Sampling and Missing Data Problems*. Ph.D. thesis, Department of Statistics, University of Auckland.

Jiang, Y., Scott, A. J., and Wild, C. J. (2006). Secondary analysis of case-control data. *Statistics in Medicine*, **25**, 1323–1339.

Kim, J. K. and Skinner, C. J. (2013). Weighting in survey analysis under informative sampling. *Biometrika*, **100**, 385–398.

Lawless, J. F., Kalbfleisch, J. D., and Wild, C. J. (1999). Semiparametric methods for response-selective and missing data problems in regression. *Journal of the Royal Statistical Society: Series B (Statistical Methodology)*, **61**, 413–438.

Lee, A. and Hirose, Y. (2010). Semi-parametric efficiency bounds for regression models under response-selective sampling: The profile likelihood approach. *Annals of the Institute of Statistical Mathematics*, **62**, 1023–1052.

Lee, A. J., Scott, A. J., and McMurchy, A. L. (1997). Re-using data from case-control studies. *Statistics in Medicine*, **16**, 1377–1389.

Lee, A. J., Scott, A. J., and Wild, C. J. (2010). Efficient estimation in multi-phase case-control studies. *Biometrika*, **97**, 361–374.

Liang, K.-Y. and Zeger, S. L. (1986). Longitudinal data analysis using generalized linear models. *Biometrika*, **73**, 13–22.

Lumley, T. (2010). *Complex Surveys: A Guide to Analysis Using R*. John Wiley & Sons Inc., Hoboken, New Jersey.

Lumley, T. (2017). Robustness of semiparametric efficiency in nearly-true models for two-phase samples. ArXiv e-print: 1707.05924.

Lumley, T., Shaw, P. A., and Dai, J. Y. (2011). Connections between survey calibration estimators and semiparametric models for incomplete data. *International Statistical Review*, **79**, 200–220.

Neuhaus, J. M., Scott, A. J., Wild, C. J., Jiang, Y., McCulloch, C. E., and Boylan, R. (2014). Likelihood-based analysis of longitudinal data from outcome-related sampling designs. *Biometrics*, **70**, 44–52.

Neyman, J. (1938). Contribution to the theory of sampling human populations. *Journal of the American Statistical Association*, **33**, 101–116.

Pfeffermann, D. (1993). The role of sampling weights when modeling survey data. *International Statistical Review*, **61**, 317–337.

Prentice, R. L. and Pyke, R. (1979). Logistic disease incidence models with case-control studies. *Biometrika*, **66**, 403–411.

Qin, J. (1993). Empirical likelihood in biased sample problems. *Annals of Statistics*, **21**, 1182–1196.

Robins, J. M., Rotnitzky, A., and Zhao, L. P. (1994). Estimation of regression coefficients when some regressors are not always observed. *Journal of the American Statistical Association*, **89**, 846–867.

Rossouw, J. E., Anderson, G. L., Prentice, R. L., LaCroix, A. Z., Kooperberg, C., Stefanick, M. L., Jackson, R. D., Beresford, S. A. A., Howard, B. V., Johnson, K. C., Kotchen, M., and Ockene, J. (2002). Risks and benefits of estrogen plus progestin in healthy postmenopausal women. Principal results from the Women's Health Initiative randomized controlled trial. *Journal of the American Medical Association*, **288**, 321–333.

Rossouw, J. E., Cushman, M., Greenland, P., Lloyd-Jones, D. M., Bray, P., Kooperberg, C., Pettinger, M., Robinson, J., Hendrix, S., and Hsia, J. (2008). Inflammatory, lipid, thrombotic, and genetic markers of coronary heart disease risk in the Women's Health Initiative trials of hormone therapy. *Archives of Internal Medicine*, **168**, 2245–2253.

Rubin, D. B. (1976). Inference and missing data. *Biometrika*, **63**, 581–592.

Scott, A. J. and Wild, C. J. (1991). Fitting logistic regression models in stratified case-control studies. *Biometrics*, **47**, 497–510.

Scott, A. J. and Wild, C. J. (1997). Fitting regression models to case-control data by maximum likelihood. *Biometrika*, **84**, 57–71.

Scott, A. J. and Wild, C. J. (2001). Maximum likelihood for generalised case-control studies. *Journal of Statistical Planning and Inference*, **96**, 3–27.

Scott, A. J. and Wild, C. J. (2006). Calculating efficient semiparametric estimators for a broad class of missing-data problems. In E. P. Liski, J. Isotalo, J. Niemelä, S. Puntanen, and G. P. H. Styan, editors, *Festschrift for Tarmo Pukkila on his 60th Birthday*, pages 301–314. University of Tampere, Tampere, Finland.

Scott, A. J. and Wild, C. J. (2011). Fitting regression models with response-biased samples. *Canadian Journal of Statistics*, **39**, 519–536.

Wang, X. and Zhou, H. (2006). A semiparametric empirical likelihood method for biased sampling schemes with auxiliary covariates. *Biometrics*, **62**, 1149–1160.

Wang, X., Wu, Y., and Zhou, H. (2009). Outcome- and auxiliary-dependent subsampling and its statistical inference. *Journal of Biopharmaceutical Statistics*, **19**, 1132–1150.

White, J. E. (1982). A two stage design for the study of the relationship between a rare exposure and a rare disease. *American Journal of Epidemiology*, **115**, 119–128.

Whittemore, A. S. and Halpern, J. (1997). Multi-stage sampling in genetic epidemiology. *Statistics in Medicine*, **16**, 153–167.

Wild, C. J. (1991). Fitting logistic regression models in stratified case-control studies. *Biometrics*, **47**, 497–510.

Xu, W. and Zhou, H. (2012). Mixed effect regression analysis for a cluster-based two-stage outcome-auxiliary-dependent sampling design with a continuous outcome. *Biostatistics*, **13**, 650–664.

13

Calibration in Case-Control Studies

Thomas Lumley

University of Auckland

13.1 Introduction

Calibration of weights (Deville and Särndal, 1992; Deville *et al.*, 1993) is a technique for using the whole cohort in analysis of a subsample. In common with many other techniques from survey sampling, it is simple and requires no assumptions for valid inference, but may be less efficient than approaches relying more heavily on models. In this chapter I will explain how calibration works; how it is related to other, possibly more familiar, techniques; and how to do it in R. The name 'calibration' is unfortunate, since it is used for so many unrelated techniques across statistics (and science). It is often better to use the less ambiguous, if more obscure, term *generalised raking*, a name that comes from one of the computational algorithms used for an early version of the method. Not many people will know what it means, but search engines will find the right results.

We are interested in fitting a logistic regression model

$$\text{logit } P(D = 1) = \mathbf{X}^T \boldsymbol{\beta} \tag{13.1}$$

relating a binary outcome D to predictors $\mathbf{X}$. In a perfect world, we would measure D and $\mathbf{X}$ on everyone in the cohort and simply fit the model. In practice, though, some components of $\mathbf{X}$ may not be available on the whole cohort; we may only be able to afford to measure them on a subsample. In this chapter I will consider case-control subsamples; Chapter 17 considers case-cohort subsamples and the Cox model.

Because calibration relates the case-control sample to the whole cohort from which it is taken, we need notation that describes both the sample and the cohort. I will write $R_i = 1$ if individual i is in the sample, $R_i = 0$ if individual i is not in the sample. The sampling probability for individual i is $\pi_i = P(R_i = 1) = E(R_i)$; it will typically be 1 for cases and a small value for controls. I will write N for the size of the cohort and n for the size of the sample. I will assume that the case-control outcome D is known for everyone in the cohort, and so are some other variables $\mathbf{Z}$. Variables $\mathbf{X}$ in our regression model will include variables $\mathbf{X}_\star$ measured only on the case-control sample, and may also include some components of $\mathbf{Z}$ available for the whole cohort. I will refer to the cohort as the *phase 1 sample* and the variables available for the whole cohort as the phase-1 variables. The individuals in the subsample will be referred to as the *phase 2 sample*, and the variables $\mathbf{X}_\star$ as phase-2 variables. The use of 'phase' rather than 'stage' is a technical distinction in survey sampling: in two-phase sampling the probabilities π_i are allowed to depend on the phase-1 variables.

Sections 13.2 and 13.3 describe where calibration estimators come from and how they work, starting with the simpler problem of estimating a population mean and then extending the procedure to logistic regression models; they can be skipped by readers who only want to use the estimators. Section 13.4 gives a strategy based on imputation for using the estimators in practice, with an example in Section 13.5. Section 13.6 discusses when calibration is likely to be effective.

13.2   Constructing the calibration estimator

13.2.1   Using the whole cohort to estimate a mean

In order to understand how calibration uses information from the whole cohort, it is useful to step back from regression models and consider simply estimating the mean of a continuous variable X. Since we know the sampling probabilities π_i for each individual in the subsample, we could use the Horvitz-Thompson estimator (Horvitz and Thompson, 1952) of the cohort total and divide by the cohort size N

$$\hat{\mu}_{HT} = \frac{1}{N} \sum_{i=1}^{N} \frac{R_i}{\pi_i} X_i. \tag{13.2}$$

The Horvitz–Thompson estimator is unbiased, and easy to compute, but it does not make use of the information we have for everyone in the cohort. The full-cohort variables $\mathbf{Z}$ are potentially informative: they may be correlated with X.

13.2.2   Estimating a mean by regression

Suppose we fit a linear regression model to predict X from phase-1 variables $\mathbf{Z}$ (including a column of 1s for an intercept)

$$X = \mathbf{Z}^T \boldsymbol{\gamma} + \epsilon.$$

Since X is available only in the sample, we should fit this model using the sampling weights and choosing $\hat{\boldsymbol{\gamma}}$ to minimise

$$\sum_{i=1}^{N} \frac{R_i}{\pi_i} \left(X_i - \mathbf{Z}_i \boldsymbol{\alpha} \right)^2.$$

There's no assumption here that the model is a good one: it might be, but it might also be horribly misspecified. We will see later where that matters. Let's write $\hat{X}_i$ for the fitted value of X_i, available now for everyone in the cohort.

Based on this fit, we have the classical regression estimator of μ

$$\hat{\mu}_R = \frac{1}{N} \sum_{i=1}^{N} \frac{R_i}{\pi_i} (X_i - \hat{X}_i) + \frac{1}{N} \sum_{i=1}^{N} \hat{X}_i. \tag{13.3}$$

The second term looks like a pure imputation estimator. The first term looks like a bias correction: it estimates the mean residual $X_i - \hat{X}_i$ using just the sample. However, as the model was fitted by design-weighted least squares and the first term is just the weighted mean of the residuals, the term is exactly zero by construction.

A useful next step in analysing the estimator is to think about an unrealistic prediction that would be obtained from the full cohort. If we had X on everyone in the cohort we could still (pointlessly) predict X from $\mathbf{Z}$ by unweighted least-squares regression, to get a prediction $\tilde{X} = \mathbf{Z}^T \hat{\gamma}$. Regardless of the goodness of fit of the model, as long as it has an intercept parameter, we have

$$\sum_{i=1}^{N} \tilde{X}_i = \sum_{i=1}^{N} X_i.$$

We can now expand the estimator from equation (13.3) in terms of $\hat{X}$ and $\tilde{X}$

$$\hat{\mu}_R = \frac{1}{N} \sum_{i=1}^{N} \frac{R_i}{\pi_i} (X_i - \tilde{X}_i) + \frac{1}{N} \sum_{i=1}^{N} \tilde{X}_i + \left(\frac{1}{N} \sum_{i=1}^{N} \left(1 - \frac{R_i}{\pi_i} \right) (\hat{X}_i - \tilde{X}_i) \right).$$

The first term has zero mean because it is the Horvitz–Thompson estimator of a quantity that is exactly zero for the cohort. It has smaller variance than the Horvitz–Thompson estimator from equation (13.2) because it only deals with the residuals $X - \tilde{X}$. The second term is the cohort mean of X and so is an unbiased estimator of the population μ. The third term will be negligibly small if the sample size is large: under typical survey asymptotics it will be $o_p(n^{-1/2})$ when the first term is $O_p(n^{-1/2})$. Again, we have *made no assumption about the accuracy of the model* here.

The regression estimator $\hat{\mu}_R$ will be more accurate than $\hat{\mu}_{HT}$ to the extent that $X - \hat{X}$ has smaller variance than $\hat{X}$. If the model for predicting X from $\mathbf{Z}$ has a high R^2, the reduction in variance will be large; if it has a low R^2, the reduction in variance will be small. But, in contrast to more familiar imputation approaches, the regression estimator cannot be worse (in large enough sample sizes) than the Horvitz–Thompson estimator. A poor choice of model will be ineffective, but cannot be harmful.

13.2.3 Estimating a mean by calibration

Somewhat surprisingly, the classical regression estimator $\hat{\mu}_R$ can be written as a weighted sum with the auxiliary variables $\mathbf{Z}$ only appearing as small ($o_p(1)$) adjustments to the weights. We saw that

$$\hat{\mu}_R = \frac{1}{N} \sum_{i=1}^{N} \hat{X}_i.$$

Now, $\hat{X}_i$ is a linear combination of $\mathbf{Z}_i$ and $\hat{\gamma}$, and the standard matrix formula for linear regression estimators shows that $\hat{\gamma}$ is a linear combination of X_i with coefficients depending on the matrix of $\mathbf{Z}$ values and the weights. So there is *some* set of weights ω_i such that

$$\hat{\mu}_R = \frac{1}{N} \sum_{i=1}^{N} R_i \omega_i X_i.$$

These weights can be worked out explicitly (e.g., equations 1.3–1.7 of Deville and Särndal 1992), but the result is not very illuminating. At the moment, it is enough to know that suitable ω_i *exist* and that they depend *only* on $\mathbf{Z}$, R, and the sampling probabilities, not on X.

That is, we can calibrate the sampling weights from π_i^{-1} to $\omega_i = g_i \pi_i^{-1}$ to increase the accuracy of estimation of a mean. The improvement depends on how well we can predict the variable whose mean we want from variables we know for everyone, and misspecifying this prediction model will give small improvements in accuracy but will not introduce bias.

One reason for not looking too closely at the form of ω implied by the regression estimator is that we also want to consider other forms of ω. In deriving these, it is useful to consider the artificial problem of predicting the mean of a variable $\mathbf{Z}$ that we actually have measured for the whole cohort. Since the calibration adjustments g do not depend on X, we could estimate the mean of $\mathbf{Z}$ with the same weights ω, and since $\mathbf{Z}$ is a perfect predictor of itself, the regression estimator would have zero error

$$\sum_{i=1}^{N} R_i \omega_i \mathbf{Z}_i = \sum_{i=1}^{N} \mathbf{Z}_i. \tag{13.4}$$

Equation (13.4) is called the *calibration constraint*. Calibration on auxiliary variables $\mathbf{Z}$ has the effect of constraining the estimated sample mean of $\mathbf{Z}$ to exactly match the cohort mean. In effect, we are forcing the sample to be more representative of the cohort for the variable $\mathbf{Z}$. If $\mathbf{Z}$ were a set of indicator variables for demographic strata such as age by sex by race, calibration of weights would be exactly equivalent to direct standardisation of the sample to the whole-cohort age-sex-race distribution; like direct standardisation, calibration can also be used to correct bias when the sample is not representative of the whole cohort.

The calibration constraint is not enough on its own to determine ω. We also choose a distance function $G(\cdot, \cdot)$ and define ω as the values that minimise the total distance between ω and the sampling weights

$$\sum_{i:R_i=1} G(\omega_i, \pi_i^{-1})$$

subject to the calibration constraint. With $G(a, b) = (a - b)^2/2b$, defining ω in this way produces the classical regression estimator $\hat{\mu}_R$.

Other choices of $G(\cdot, \cdot)$ are available, leading to estimators that are asymptotically equivalent (Deville and Särndal, 1992), but with different small sample properties. In particular, using

$$G(a, b) = a\log(a/b) - a + b$$

forces ω to be nonnegative and leads to another classical survey estimator, the *raking estimator*. There is no *theoretical* difficulty presented by a small number of negative weights, but the practical difficulties can be substantial: software may refuse to accept them or may handle them incorrectly. Using raking is convenient, and since the two estimators are asymptotically equivalent, we can still use the classical regression estimator to develop heuristics for choosing auxiliary variables.

13.3 Calibration for logistic regression

In case-control studies we are actually interested in estimating regression coefficients in some logistic model, not in estimating a mean. That is, we want to estimate $\boldsymbol{\beta}$ in the model

$$\operatorname{logit} P(D = 1) = \mathbf{X}^T \boldsymbol{\beta}, \tag{13.5}$$

where some of the $\mathbf{X}$ variables may be elements of $\mathbf{Z}$, available for the whole cohort, and even the others may be predictable from $\mathbf{Z}$. We will call this the *outcome model*.

An obvious idea is to calibrate using $\mathbf{X}$ (where available), or predictions of $\mathbf{X}$, as auxiliary variables. This does not work; there is no gain in precision. One explanation of why it doesn't work is that that outcome model already adjusts for $\mathbf{X}$, so that differences in the distribution of $\mathbf{X}$ between sample and cohort will have little or no influence on $\hat{\boldsymbol{\beta}}$. To understand the choice of good auxiliary variables it's useful to approximate $\hat{\boldsymbol{\beta}}$ by a whole-cohort mean or total, since we do understand the precision gain for means and totals.

Normally distributed parameter estimates in statistics are typically asymptotically linear, meaning that they are well approximated by simple sums. For logistic regression, we can construct the approximation from the score equations used to fit the model. If $\mathbf{X}$ were available for everyone in the cohort, we would solve (writing expit( ) for the inverse of the logit function)

$$\sum_{i=1}^{N} \mathbf{x}_i \{d_i - \text{expit}(\mathbf{x}_i^T \boldsymbol{\beta})\} = 0.$$

The estimator $\hat{\boldsymbol{\beta}}_{\text{cohort}}$ would satisfy

$$\sqrt{N}(\hat{\boldsymbol{\beta}}_{\text{cohort}} - \boldsymbol{\beta}) = -\mathcal{I}^{-1} \sum_{i=1}^{N} \mathbf{x}_i \{d_i - \text{expit}(\mathbf{x}_i^T \boldsymbol{\beta})\} + o_p(N^{-1/2}), \qquad (13.6)$$

where $\mathcal{I}$ is the whole-cohort Fisher information for $\boldsymbol{\beta}$. The terms

$$\mathcal{I}^{-1} \mathbf{x}_i \{d_i - \text{expit}(\mathbf{x}_i^T \boldsymbol{\beta})\}$$

are called *influence functions*. They are approximately the same as the delta-betas, the changes in $\hat{\boldsymbol{\beta}}$ when a single observation is removed from the data.

Since $\hat{\boldsymbol{\beta}}_{\text{cohort}}$ is approximately a sum, a weighted survey estimator $\hat{\boldsymbol{\beta}}_w$ can be constructed by solving

$$\sum_{i=1}^{N} \frac{R_i}{\pi_i} \mathbf{x}_i \{d_i - \text{expit}(\mathbf{x}_i^T \boldsymbol{\beta})\} = 0$$

and will satisfy

$$\sqrt{n}(\hat{\boldsymbol{\beta}}_w - \boldsymbol{\beta}) = -\mathcal{I}^{-1} \sum_{i=1}^{N} \frac{R_i}{\pi_i} \mathbf{x}_i \{d_i - \text{expit}(\mathbf{x}_i^T \boldsymbol{\beta})\} + o_p(n^{-1/2}). \qquad (13.7)$$

The use of n rather than N in scaling equation (13.7) is to emphasize that the available information about $\boldsymbol{\beta}$ depends only on the sample here. This weighted estimator can be computed using survey logistic regression procedures in standard software; using weights in software for ordinary logistic regression will give correct point estimates but incorrect standard errors.

The simple weighted estimator does not use any information from the unsampled observations, but the weights can now be calibrated. Equation (13.7) also tells us what auxiliary variables will be helpful: they should be variables that we can compute for the whole cohort and that are linearly correlated with the influence functions, that is, with the entries of $\mathbf{x}_i \{d_i - \text{expit}(\mathbf{x}_i^T \boldsymbol{\beta})\}$.

The most straightforward way to come up with variables correlated with the influence functions for $\boldsymbol{\beta}$ is to construct another model, using only phase-1 data, which estimates $\boldsymbol{\beta}$ (or something close to it) and use the influence functions from that model (which we will call the *phase-1 model*). One generally applicable way to construct the phase-1 model is to impute the unavailable variables $\mathbf{X}_\star$ for everyone in the cohort and then fit the intended phase-2 model with the imputed data (Breslow *et al.*, 2009a; Lumley *et al.*, 2011; Han, 2015). The next section describes this process in detail.

13.4 Imputation for calibration

The first step is to fit an imputation model using only phase-1 data to impute $\mathbf{X}_\star$, using any convenient predictive modelling technique. Initially, we will assume a single-imputation approach, where a single predicted $\hat{\mathbf{X}}_\star$ is produced for everyone in the cohort (including those for whom $\mathbf{X}_\star$ is actually known).

Next, we fit the intended phase-2 model to the whole cohort, but using $\hat{\mathbf{X}}_\star$ in place of $\mathbf{X}_\star$ even when $\mathbf{X}_\star$ is known. Since this model includes every individual in the cohort, no sampling weights are needed. The result is a model that uses only phase-1 data, but is trying to estimate the same parameters as the target model. We'll call this the auxiliary model.

The influence functions from the phase-1 model are then extracted and used as auxiliary variables in calibration, to produce calibrated sampling weights $\omega_i = g_i \pi_i^{-1}$ for each individual i in the phase 2 sample. Finally, the phase-2 model is fitted with the calibrated weights to obtain the final estimates of $\boldsymbol{\beta}$.

Algorithm 1 Basic calibration by imputation

1: Fit imputation model to impute $\mathbf{X}_\star$ by $\hat{\mathbf{X}}_\star$
2: Fit target model with $\hat{\mathbf{X}}_\star$ instead of $\mathbf{X}$ to obtain auxiliary model
3: Compute influence functions for auxiliary model
4: Calibrate subsample to cohort using influence functions
5: Fit target model to calibrated subsample to get final estimates $\hat{\boldsymbol{\beta}}$

There are two straightforward modifications that can be made, which will be improvements in sufficiently large sample sizes. First, in the original algorithm the influence functions from auxiliary model are evaluated at the parameter estimates from the auxiliary model. These parameter estimates may not be very good. We can iterate the process, creating new auxiliary variables by evaluating the influence functions of the auxiliary model at the parameter estimates from the target model and re-calibrating.

Algorithm 2 Iterated calibration by imputation

1: Fit imputation model to impute $\mathbf{X}_\star$ by $\hat{\mathbf{X}}_\star$
2: Fit target model with $\hat{\mathbf{X}}_\star$ instead of $\mathbf{X}$ to obtain auxiliary model
3: Compute influence functions for auxiliary model
4: Calibrate subsample to cohort using influence functions
5: Fit target model to calibrated subsample to get interim estimates $\hat{\boldsymbol{\beta}}^{(i)}$
6: Compute influence functions for auxiliary model at $\boldsymbol{\beta} = \hat{\boldsymbol{\beta}}^{(i)}$
7: Calibrate subsample to cohort using influence functions
8: Fit target model to calibrated subsample to get final estimates $\hat{\boldsymbol{\beta}}$

Second, we can use multiple imputation instead of single imputation. The ideal auxiliary variable for estimating $\boldsymbol{\beta}$ is the expected value of the influence functions in the target model given the phase-1 data and the model parameters. Multiple imputation lets us approximate the analytical expected value by a straightforward average of samples.

With multiple imputation, rather than estimating the expected value of an unavailable $\mathbf{X}_\star$ with the imputation model we sample M possible values $\tilde{\mathbf{X}}_\star^{(m)}$ from the predictive distribution of the imputation model, to get M complete data sets. The target model is then fitted to each of the M data sets to give M auxiliary models and M sets of influence functions. These influence functions are then averaged to give a single set of auxiliary variables.

One way to think about the difference between single and multiple imputation is that single imputation averages over the uncertainty in $\hat{\mathbf{X}}_\star$ before fitting the auxiliary model (to save computational effort), and multiple impuation averages after fitting the auxiliary model. Han (2015) has shown that multiple imputation for calibration gives the most efficient doubly-robust estimator, which in this setting means the most efficient estimator that relies only on the sampling probabilities being correct.

Algorithm 3 Calibration by multiple imputation

1: Fit imputation model to impute $X_\star$ by $m = 1, \ldots, M$ possible $\tilde{\mathbf{X}}_\star^{(m)}$
2: Fit target model with each set $\tilde{\mathbf{X}}_\star^{(m)}$ instead of $\mathbf{X}$ to obtain auxiliary models
3: Compute influence functions for each auxiliary model and average them
4: Calibrate subsample to cohort using averaged influence functions
5: Fit target model to calibrated subsample to get final estimates $\hat{\boldsymbol{\beta}}$

13.5   Example: Predicting relapse of Wilms' Tumour

Data from the National Wilms' Tumour Group trials (Gren *et al.*, 1998; D'Angio *et al.*, 1989) have been a popular example for illustrating incomplete-data estimators (Breslow and Chatterjee, 1999; Kulich and Lin, 2004; Breslow *et al.*, 2009b). Wilms' Tumour is a rare childhood kidney cancer, which is successfully treated in the majority of cases. There is interest in predicting recurrence risk because of the potential for using less damaging treatments. The strongest predictor of relapse is the histological classification of the original tumour, and the histology assessment by the NWTSG central lab is more predictive than that from institutional labs. In this analysis we follow previous analyses by pretending that the central-lab histology variable is available only for a subsample of study participants, and so is our phase-two variable $X_\star$. Specifically, we take a case-control subsample with all the cases of relapse ($D = 1$) and an equal number of controls ($D = 0$).

We are interested in fitting a model with predictors ($\mathbf{X}$) histology (favourable or unfavourable), tumour diameter, disease stage (1 or 2 versus 3 or 4), a linear spline in age with a knot at 1 year, and age by histology and diameter by stage interactions. We have one variable Z available for the whole cohort but not in the model of interest: the histological classification from the local institution. We compare the basic weighted and unweighted (maximum likelihood) logistic regression estimates for a case-control sample with three calibrated estimators. Code and data are available on the website for the book and also at github.com/tslumley/calib-chapter.

Table 13.1 shows log odds ratios from the basic weighted and unweighted estimators and from a model fitted to the full cohort (i.e., $\hat{\boldsymbol{\beta}}_{\text{cohort}}$, as if all of $\mathbf{X}$ was available for everyone). In this example the weighted and unweighted estimators are very similar, which is fairly common when the most important predictors are discrete.

The first calibration estimator we consider simply imputes the histology $\hat{X}_\star$ as the value from the institutional lab. We then follow Algorithm 1: fitting the model of interest using the imputed variable, extracting the influence functions, calibrating the weights, and finally fitting the model of interest to the subsample.

The second calibration estimator imputes the histology using all the available data. Our

TABLE 13.1
Comparison to full-cohort regression: weighted and unweighted estimators give
similar results for prediction of relapse.

	Full cohort		Unweighted		Weighted	
	$\hat{\beta}_{\text{cohort}}$	Std Err	$\hat{\beta}$	Std Err	$\hat{\beta}$	Std Err
Intercept	-2.61	0.34	-2.19	0.44	-2.58	0.35
Histology (at age=0)	5.66	0.98	4.46	1.12	5.09	1.24
age (/yr) ($<$ 1yr)	-0.73	0.35	-1.13	0.46	-0.71	0.34
age (/yr) ($>$ 1yr)	0.12	0.02	0.22	0.03	0.12	0.02
Histol: age ($<$ 1yr)	-4.20	1.10	-2.08	1.31	-3.83	1.32
Histol: age ($>$ 1yr)	-0.03	0.05	-0.10	0.08	0.01	0.06
stage $>$ 2	1.51	0.30	2.25	0.43	1.45	0.31
tumour diameter (/cm)	0.07	0.02	0.09	0.02	0.07	0.02
stage $>$ 2 : diameter	-0.09	0.02	-0.13	0.03	-0.08	0.02

TABLE 13.2
Differences from full-cohort regression coefficients: calibration based on direct use of a
surrogate, single regression imputation, and multiple imputation.

	$\hat{\beta}_{\text{cohort}}$	Uncalibrated $\hat{\beta} - \hat{\beta}_{\text{cohort}}$	Using `instit` $\hat{\beta} - \hat{\beta}_{\text{cohort}}$	Imputation $\hat{\beta} - \hat{\beta}_{\text{cohort}}$	MI $\hat{\beta} - \hat{\beta}_{\text{cohort}}$
Intercept	-2.61	0.09	0.03	0.04	0.04
Histology (at age=0)	5.66	-2.17	-0.57	-0.61	-0.89
age (/yr) ($<$ 1yr)	-0.73	-0.16	0.02	-0.02	0.01
age (/yr) ($>$ 1yr)	0.12	0.03	-0.01	-0.00	-0.01
Histol: age ($<$ 1yr)	-4.20	2.31	0.36	0.38	0.73
Histol: age ($>$ 1yr)	-0.03	-0.02	0.04	0.06	0.04
stage $>$ 2	1.51	0.07	-0.06	-0.01	-0.07
tumour diameter (/cm)	0.07	0.01	0.01	0.00	0.01
stage $>$ 2 : diameter	-0.09	0.01	0.01	0.00	0.01

model, following Kulich and Lin (2004), uses local institution histology, case status, age,
and stage to impute central-lab histology. Again, the details are as in Algorithm 1.

Finally, we consider a multiple imputation estimator using Algorithm 3. Our $X_\star$, central-
lab histology, is imputed and influence functions computed $M = 50$ times and the resulting
influence functions are averaged to give the auxiliary variables for calibration.

Table 13.2 shows $\hat{\beta} - \hat{\beta}_{\text{cohort}}$ for the three calibration estimators. They give comparable
results. All three move the regression estimator closer to the true value that would be obtained with complete data. The benefit is greater for variables that are actually available for
everyone, but even for the phase-2 variables, central-lab histology and its interactions, there
is a benefit. Ordinarily, one would expect better performance from the second estimators
than for the first, but in this case local-institution histology predicts so strongly that the
benefits of the other variables are marginal.

These values are for a single data set – anecdote, rather than data. Table 13.3 summarises
500 replicates of the analysis, where a different case-control sample is taken each time. The
standard errors in Table 13.3 are for $\hat{\beta} - \hat{\beta}_{\text{cohort}}$ for each estimator: they compare the phase-
two component of the uncertainty, the additional uncertainty due to not measuring $X_\star$ on
the whole cohort. The variance of $\hat{\beta}$ for each estimator would be the sum of the variance of
$\hat{\beta}_{\text{cohort}}$ and the square of the standard errors in the table.

This simulation gives the same message: there are gains in precision; they are greater
when the variable is available for the whole cohort or is an interaction; they do not differ
greatly depending on how calibration is done.

TABLE 13.3

Impact of calibration on phase-two sampling errors: the median absolute deviation of $\hat{\beta} - \hat{\beta}_{\text{cohort}}$ for the maximum likelihood estimator, the simple weighted estimator, and the three calibration estimators.

	SE	Uncalibrated SE	Using `instit` SE	Imputation SE	MI SE
Intercept	0.23	0.23	0.03	0.04	0.04
Histology (at age=0)	1.43	1.53	0.78	0.86	1.24
age (/yr) (< 1yr)	0.27	0.28	0.03	0.04	0.04
age (/yr) (> 1yr)	0.02	0.02	0.01	0.01	0.01
Histol: age (< 1yr)	1.51	1.59	0.91	0.92	1.25
Histol: age (> 1yr)	0.06	0.07	0.06	0.06	0.06
stage > 2	0.25	0.27	0.08	0.09	0.07
tumour diameter (/cm) $\times 10$	0.11	0.13	0.03	0.04	0.03
stage > 2 : diameter $\times 10$	0.19	0.21	0.06	0.07	0.06

13.6 When is calibration useful?

Calibration is always worth trying, except in very small samples: it does not change the target of inference, does not introduce bias, and can sometimes increase precision usefully. Often, though, it has little impact because the phase-1 data are not sufficiently predictive of $\mathbf{X}_\star$.

Calibration is likely to result in a worthwhile precision gain for coefficients of:

1. variables that are actually in the phase-1 data (i.e., in $\mathbf{X}$ but not $\mathbf{X}_\star$)
2. variables in $\mathbf{X}_\star$ that can be predicted well from the phase-1 data

In a case-control study, these criteria are likely to be met for the parameters of interest when $\mathbf{X}_\star$ are confounders rather than exposures, when there is a good surrogate for $\mathbf{X}_\star$ measured at phase 1, or when the primary research question is about interactions between exposure and a phase-1 variable.

A particularly promising area of future application is where $\mathbf{Z}$ is administratively collected data and $\mathbf{X}_\star$ is the validated version of these data on a subsample. Calibration allows the (often very large) administrative database to contribute information, but does not allow it to bias the results. In more-traditional epidemiology, calibration is also likely to be valuable when self-reported exposures are available for the whole cohort, with biomarker-validated exposures for a subsample. Calibration will also generally decrease the standard errors of all coefficients to the extent that D is predictable from $\mathbf{Z}$, but it is relatively unusual for this to have a large impact.

The 'free lunch' aspect of calibration is reminiscent of the gains from adjusting for baseline in linear regression analyses of randomised trials. Lumley *et al.* (2011) shows there is a formal connection, thinking of randomisation as sampling from potential outcomes. Tsiatis *et al.* (2008) show how to construct similar estimators for other randomised-trial analyses (though they do not describe the connection to sampling).

13.6.1 Other ways to use the information

The other question, when there is sufficient phase-1 information to make calibration useful, is whether there are other techniques that can use the information more effectively.

When a good surrogate for $\mathbf{X}_\star$ or a strong predictor of D is available at phase 1 it may also be possible to use a different sampling design, such as balanced two-phase sampling or countermatching. Using phase-1 information in the design will always be preferable to using the same information only at analysis, but design variables typically have to be discrete, and only a small number of sampling strata may be feasible. Calibration is still likely to be useful as a way to use all the phase-1 data.

In the usual setting where the complete cohort is treated as an independent and identically distributed sample from some probability model, calibration estimators are Augmented Inverse-Probability-Weighted estimators in the sense of Robins *et al.* (1994) and share their advantages and disadvantages. In particular, estimators that make stronger assumptions about the relationships between D and $\mathbf{X}$, D and $\mathbf{Z}$, or $\mathbf{X}$ and $\mathbf{Z}$ can be more precise.

Bibliography

Breslow, N. E. and Chatterjee, N. (1999). Design and analysis of two-phase studies with binary outcome applied to Wilms tumour prognosis. *Journal of the Royal Statistical Society, Series C: Applied Statistics*, **48**, 457–468.

Breslow, N. E., Lumley, T., Ballantyne, C. M., Chambless, L. E., and Kulich, M. (2009a). Using the whole cohort in the analysis of case-cohort data. *American Journal of Epidemiology*, **169**, 1398–405.

Breslow, N. E., Lumley, T., Ballantyne, C. M., Chambless, L. E., and Kulich, M. (2009b). Using the whole cohort in the analysis of case-cohort data. *American Journal of Epidemiology*, **169**, 1398–1405.

D'Angio, G., Breslow, N., Beckwith, J., Evans, A., Baum, H., de Lorimer, A., Ferbach, D., Hrabovsky, E., Jones, G., Kelalis, P., *et al.* (1989). Treatment of Wilms' tumor. Results of the Third National Wilms Tumor Study. *Cancer*, **64**, 349–60.

Deville, J.-C. and Särndal, C.-E. (1992). Calibration estimators in survey sampling. *Journal of the American Statistical Association*, **87**, 376–382.

Deville, J.-C., Särndal, C.-E., and Sautory, O. (1993). Generalized raking procedures in survey sampling. *Journal of the American Statistical Association*, **88**, 1013–1020.

Gren, D., Breslow, N., Beckwith, J., Finkelstein, F., Grundy, P., Thomas, P., Kim, T., Shochat, S., Haase, G., Ritchey, M., Kelalis, P., and D'Angio, G. (1998). Comparison between single-dose and divided-dose administration of dactinomycin and doxorubicin for patients with Wilms' tumor: A report from the National Wilms' Tumor Study Group. *Journal of Clinical Oncology*, **16**, 237–245.

Han, P. (2015). Combining inverse probability weighting and multiple imputation to improve robustness of estimation. *Scandinavian Journal of Statistics*, **43**, 246–260.

Horvitz, D. G. and Thompson, D. J. (1952). A generalization of sampling without replacement from a finite universe. *Journal of the American Statistical Association*, **47**, 663–685.

Kulich, M. and Lin, D. (2004). Improving the efficiency of relative-risk estimation in case-cohort studies. *Journal of the American Statistical Association*, **99**, 832–844.

Lumley, T., Shaw, P. A., and Dai, J. Y. (2011). Connections between survey calibration estimators and semiparametric models for incomplete data. *International Statistical Review*, **79**, 200–220.

Robins, J. M., Rotnitzky, A., and Zhao, L.-P. (1994). Estimation of regression coefficients when some regressors are not always observed. *Journal of American Statistical Association*, **89**, 846–866.

Tsiatis, A. A., Davidian, M., Zhang, M., and Lu, X. (2008). Covariate adjustment for two-sample treatment comparisons in randomized clinical trials: A principled yet flexible approach. *Statistics in Medicine*, **27**, 4658–4677.

14

Secondary Analysis of Case-Control Data

Chris J. Wild

University of Auckland

14.1 Introduction

Case-control studies often collect data on large numbers of variables. This can make their data a treasure trove to mine subsequently for inexpensive additional research (secondary research studies) involving *secondary outcomes*; outcomes other than the disease outcome that defined case-control status in the original (primary) study. The analyses done are called *secondary analyses*.

There are several areas in which secondary research using already-available case-control data have become quite common. According to Tchetgen Tchetgen (2014), "secondary outcomes analyses are now routine in genetic epidemiology, with several recent papers on genetic variants influencing human quantitative traits such as height, body mass index, and lipid levels, using data mostly from case-control studies of complex diseases (diabetes, cancer, and hypertension)." He also gives recent examples in environmental epidemiology, such as a study that uses data taken, in part, from a case-control study nested within the Nurses Health Study (NHS). "In the NHS Lead Study, Boston-area NHS participants had extensive lead exposure assessment (bone and blood measures). Associations of lead measures with hypertension, bone mineral density/metabolism, and cognition were then assessed ... the Lead Study selected women on the basis of their blood pressure status."

Disproportionate-growth example

The following example, from Jiang *et al.* (2006), will be used as a running example through this chapter. The data comes from the Auckland Birthweight Collaborative (ABC) Study described in Thompson *et al.* (2001) which was conducted to investigate risk factors for the condition of 'low birthweight' in newborn babies. The study group was of full-term babies, defined as those with a gestational age of 37 weeks or greater. It was designed as a case-control study in which the cases were those SGA (small for gestational age) babies defined

TABLE 14.1
Cross-tabulation of SGA- and
DG-status.

	DG=1	DG=0	Total
SGA=1	257	521	778
SGA=0	88	729	817
Total	345	1250	1595

as being at or below the sex-specific 10th percentile for gestational age in the New Zealand population. The remaining babies were classified as AGA (appropriate for gestational age).

The response variable of interest for a secondary analysis was DG, an indicator variable for 'disproportionate growth' defined as having a ponderal index below the 10th percentile. The *ponderal index*, due to Rohrer (1921), is defined as weight in grams divided by the cube of height in centimetres. Ponderal indices below the 10th percentile are considered to be indicators of poor nutritional status at birth.

A priori, an association between birthweight and ponderal index would be expected. Table 14.1 cross-classifies SGA-status and DG-status. There is clearly a very strong association between these two variables. The unadjusted odds ratio is 4.1 with a 95% confidence interval extending from 3.1 to 5.3.

A variety of types of analysis make sense here using either DG (binary), or ponderal index (continuous), as the response of interest. Model fitting is complicated by the fact the sampling is biased by including far too many SGA babies which will in turn also bring in too many DG babies. But, since the data is not sampled conditional on DG status, standard results underlying case-control analyses do not apply and standard logistic regression analyses are not valid.

We use the following notation consistently with the notation in Chapter 12 on multiphase sampling which this chapter draws on heavily. Y_1 is the binary variable that was the outcome of interest for the original, or primary, case-control study. Y_2 is the outcome variable for the secondary analyses (the theory also applies to a vector of outcome variables). X denotes the other available variables that we want to use. The usual reason for having data available on Y_2 is that this variable was collected for use as an explanatory variable for the primary study. We thus have data on Y_1, Y_2 and X for a sample of n_1 Y_1-cases (individuals with $Y_1 = 1$) and a sample of n_0 Y_1-controls (individuals with $Y_1 = 0$). The models used for the secondary analysis are of the form

$$f(y_2 \mid x; \boldsymbol{\beta}). \tag{14.1}$$

Most work in this area has emphasized logistic regression models for binary Y_2 or linear regression models for continuous Y_2. Depending on the scientific questions being asked, an entry for y_1 may or may not be included in x. Whether or not y_1 is included has consequences for the analysis.

This chapter is organised as follows. Section 14.2 discusses ad hoc methods that have historically been used for secondary analyses of case-control data but are not fit for purpose. Section 14.3 discusses the (inverse probability) weighted method, which is a special case of the weighted method in Section 12.5 (in Chapter 12). Section 14.4 introduces the semi-parametric maximum-likelihood (SPML) methods of Lee *et al.* (1997) and Jiang *et al.* (2006). These are also special cases of the methods in Chapter 12. In addition to fitting the model of interest, the SPML methods involve fitting additional (nuisance) models that enable us to correct biases arising from the sampling design. Section 14.5 applies all of these methods to the disproportionate-growth example, and also discusses conclusions from simulations based on the data looking at bias, relative efficiencies and confidence-interval coverage. Deficiencies in the ad hoc methods are demonstrated as are increased efficiencies of estimation that can occur for the SPML methods compared with the weighted method. These can sometimes be quite substantial.

Section 14.6 discusses simulations looking at the effects of misspecifying the nuisance models that SPML methods use to correct for biases due to the sampling design. Such mis-specifications can sometimes cause important biases in estimates of coefficients of the model of interest even when the nuisance-model deficiencies are small enough that they can seldom be detected. Section 14.7 discusses recent developments growing out of both the semipara-metric maximum-likelihood tradition and out of the augmented inverse-probability-weighted (AIPW) tradition that aim to weaken assumptions to point where only the crucially im-portant components of the model of interest need to be correctly specified and the effect of additional modelling is just to increase efficiency when posited additional models are true or nearly true, but without risk of biases when they are misspecified.

14.2   Ad hoc approaches

Studies of secondary outcomes using existing data from a case-control study generally need special methods of analysis. We should be highly suspicious of any analysis that ignores the way the data was assembled (case-control sampling) and applies standard techniques. Most case-control studies are conducted because their primary outcome of interest is relatively rare so a combined data set of cases and controls vastly overrepresents a small group of very unusual individuals. It is thus not at all representative in general and may well not be representative with respect to the data features of interest either. This does not stop the results of such analyses being reported. The background idea that if we use logistic regression to obtain information about odds ratios we can ignore case-control sampling (because of the result of Prentice and Pyke, 1979), may be a contributing factor. The Prentice-Pyke result, however, applies only to logistic models for a case-control study's primary outcome. It does not apply to models for any secondary outcome.

Recall that the data was sampled conditionally on the value of Y_1 (the primary case-control study's outcome variable) but Y_2 is the (secondary) outcome of interest for a new research question. The model of interest is $f(y_2 \mid \boldsymbol{x}; \boldsymbol{\beta})$ [equation (14.1)]. Jiang *et al.* (2006, Section 2) outlined a number of ad hoc approaches that have been used for estimating elements of $\boldsymbol{\beta}$ using standard methods: (i) fit (14.1) by standard methods ignoring the sampling scheme; (ii) fit (14.1) using only the controls ($Y_1 = 0$); and (iii) include Y_1 as an additional covariate, i.e. fit $f(y_2 \mid \boldsymbol{x}, y_1; \boldsymbol{\beta}, \boldsymbol{\gamma})$ using standard methods. Each of these can work in special circumstances, often under conditions that are hard to verify, but they are in general flawed. Empirical investigations demonstrating this have been conducted by, among others, Jiang (2004), Jiang *et al.* (2006), Lin and Zeng (2009), Ghosh *et al.* (2013), and Tchetgen Tchetgen (2014).

Ignoring case-control, sampling, (i), is justified if Y_2 and Y_1 are independent given $\boldsymbol{x}$. Typically, however, they are associated, and often strongly associated. This can result in severe biases. Using only the controls, (ii), works when the cases are sufficiently rare in the parent population (e.g., $< 1\%$, Lin and Zeng, 2009). But because it does not use any information from the cases we can expect some efficiency losses. Re (iii), if we condition on Y_1 then standard methods can legitimately be applied. In some cases Y_1 may be a legitimate covariate for inclusion in the model of interest (14.1) on substantive scientific grounds. But if it is not, and conditioning is applied simply to adjust for the sampling design, then we are fitting an incorrect regression model, $f(y_2 \mid \boldsymbol{x}, y_1; \boldsymbol{\beta}, \boldsymbol{\gamma})$, in the hope of getting a good approximation to what we would have obtained from a valid fit of the model of interest, $f(y_2 \mid \boldsymbol{x}; \boldsymbol{\beta})$. Unless you also have a valid fitting method it is basically impossible to tell.

What about analysing the Y_1-case and Y_1-control groups separately? This is a form of conditioning on Y_1 so the comments under (iii) in the previous paragraph apply. We have to be able to answer the following question in the affirmative, "Are these scientifically meaningful subgroups for which we want separate models for $f(y_2 \mid \boldsymbol{x}; \boldsymbol{\beta})$?" Of course if Y_1-cases are rare, analysis of Y_1-controls only is justified as discussed under (ii) in the previous paragraph.

14.3   Weighted approach

Let π_{case} be the probability that any given Y_1-case is sampled and similarly π_{con} for Y_1-controls. If these values are known exactly (e.g., by design under variable probability sampling; see Section 12.1.3) we can use the survey-weighted approach (cf. Section 12.5) in which the contribution of individuals to the usual score function for the model of interest is inversely weighted by their probabilities of selection. Here that reduces to solving

$$\frac{1}{\pi_{\text{case}}} \sum_{Y_1\text{-cases}} \frac{\partial}{\partial \boldsymbol{\beta}} \log f(y_{2i} \mid \boldsymbol{x}_i; \boldsymbol{\beta}) + \frac{1}{\pi_{\text{con}}} \sum_{Y_1\text{-controls}} \frac{\partial}{\partial \boldsymbol{\beta}} \log f(y_{2i} \mid \boldsymbol{x}_i; \boldsymbol{\beta}) = \mathbf{0}.$$

(We note that the relative sampling rate $\pi_{\text{case}}/\pi_{\text{con}}$ is all that is actually needed here, not the individual values.) The selection rates π_{case} and π_{con} can also easily be deduced from the Y_1-case and control sample sizes and a known Y_1-case rate in the population.

In reality the true rates are seldom known exactly and we use estimates. The weighted method gives consistent estimates of the parameters $\boldsymbol{\beta}$ for a true model of interest if the weights use consistent estimates of the selection probabilities. However, the weights are then no longer constant so uncertainty in the weights should also be accounted for in the analysis.

If the cases and controls are selected from a well-defined cohort or finite population we have a very simple special case of the two-phase designs discussed in Chapter 12. At Phase 1 we observe Y_1-case-control status for all N people in the cohort. At Phase 2 we have just two strata (Y_1-cases and Y_1-controls) and observe both Y_2 and $\boldsymbol{x}$ for a sample of n_1 of the N_1 individuals in the Y_1-case stratum and of n_0 of the N_0 individuals in the Y_1-control stratum. Further details of the weighted approach can be found in Section 12.5. Analyses can be performed using the two-phase capabilities of the **survey** package in R with Y_1 specified as a stratification variable.

If we do not have a well-defined cohort with known N_1 and N_0 but do have an estimate $\widehat{p}_1$ of $p_1 = P(Y_1 = 1)$, we can incorporate that estimate and a level of uncertainty about it, represented by $v_p = \text{Var}(\widehat{p}_1)$, by solving $v_p = \widehat{p}_1(1 - \widehat{p}_1)/N$ for N and using $N_1 = N\widehat{p}_1$ and $N_0 = N(1 - \widehat{p}_1)$. The argument for this comes from the binomial form of the contribution that N_1 and N_0 make to the two-phase likelihood. We can do this for both the weighted method and for semiparametric maximum likelihood methods. A sensitivity analysis allows exploration of the sensitivity of the results to the choices of N and $\widehat{p}_1$.

14.4 Semiparametric maximum likelihood

We will continue to use the two-phase formulation of the secondary analysis problem at the end of the previous section and will now discuss the semiparametric maximum-likelihood methods of Jiang *et al.* (2006, Section 2.3). Denote $\mathbf{y} = (y_1, y_2)$ and consider a model for the joint response,

$$f(\mathbf{y} \mid \boldsymbol{x}; \boldsymbol{\theta}), \tag{14.2}$$

that satisfies the property that the marginal distribution of Y_2 given $\boldsymbol{x}$ is the model of interest, $f(y_2 \mid \boldsymbol{x}; \boldsymbol{\beta})$. This enables us to apply the two-phase methodology of Section 12.4 directly, no matter whether Y_2 is categorical, discrete, continuous or even multivariate. But in what sense are the resulting methods semiparametric? They deal with the conditional distributions of Y_1 and Y_2 given $\boldsymbol{x}$ parametrically and the marginal distribution of $\boldsymbol{x}$ non-parametrically. (We will discuss methods that make even fewer parametric assumptions in Section 14.7.)

Jiang *et al.* (2006, Section 2.3) constructed the joint model (14.2) in two different ways. The most straightforward and easily generalisable approach is a conditional break up

$$f(\mathbf{y} \mid \boldsymbol{x}; \boldsymbol{\theta}) = f_2(y_2 \mid \boldsymbol{x}; \boldsymbol{\beta}) f_{1|2}(y_1 \mid y_2, \boldsymbol{x}; \boldsymbol{\gamma}). \tag{14.3}$$

This approach, which they labelled SPML2, requires building a nuisance binary regression model $f_{1|2}(y_1 \mid y_2, \boldsymbol{x}; \boldsymbol{\gamma})$; they used a logistic regression model. This is the form of modelling that the original case-control study was designed for. In the main example of Jiang *et al.* (2006), Y_2 was also binary so they also used a logistic regression model for f_2 as well as for $f_{1|2}$.

Their other approach, which they labelled SPML3, was to use joint models for $\mathbf{Y} = (Y_1, Y_2)$ constructed from individual marginal models for Y_1 and Y_2 given $\boldsymbol{x}$ and combine them using some other model to deal with any association. The simplest model in the binary case is the Palmgren model (see Lee *et al.*, 1997; Neuhaus *et al.*, 2002) which combines separate marginal logistic regression models for Y_1 and Y_2 with a model for the log odds ratio between Y_1 and Y_2 that is assumed to be linear in $\boldsymbol{x}$. A more general strategy, also used in Jiang *et al.* (2006), is to combine individual marginal models by using a copula to model the (conditional on $\boldsymbol{x}$) association between them.

Subsequently Lin and Zeng (2009) developed an SPML2 solution for continuous Y_2 that does not involve N_1 and N_0 but does involve either knowledge of the true Y_1-case rate, $P(Y_1 = 1)$, or a "rare disease" assumption $P(Y_1 = 1) < 0.01$. They use a standard linear-regression model to provide $f(y_2 \mid \boldsymbol{x})$, i.e., they assume that $Y_2 = \boldsymbol{\beta}^T \boldsymbol{x} + \sigma \epsilon$ with $\epsilon \sim N(0, 1)$. No allowance is made for uncertainty of estimation of $P(Y_1 = 1)$ when a "known" value is used, so sensitivity analyses around the user-specified estimate are desirable to address that. Calculations involve numeric integrals over the normal error-density. Software implementing the approach is available from Lin's website at http://dlin.web.unc.edu/software/spreg-2/. Their software also deals with the binary Y_2 case.

Ghosh *et al.* (2013) developed an SPML3 solution for continuous Y_2 which also used a standard linear-regression model for Y_2. Their motivation was to force the analysis to preserve the marginal model for Y_1 obtained in the original case-control study. It is arguable whether this is important for what is just a nuisance model being used to try to get a good fit to the joint distribution of Y_1 and Y_2. There was no mention of software but Sofer *et al.* (2017) speak of using software obtained from the authors of Ghosh *et al.* (2013).

14.5   Disproportionate growth example continued

Recall that our outcome of interest for our secondary analysis is the binary variable disproportionate growth (DG). Selection into the case-control study was stratified on SGA (small for gestational age). All eligible SGA-cases were taken and SGA-controls were sampled at a rate of approximately 1 in 9.

Our main interest in this section is in comparing the results of the different forms of analysis. After some exploration, Jiang *et al.* (2006) decided to model DG-status in terms of mother's marital status, ethnicity, marijuana smoking and age using a logistic regression model.

The fitted regression coefficients and standard errors from each of the methods are given in Table 14.2. The first column relates to a Palmgren model fitted by semiparametric maximum likelihood (SPML3). To do this they had also to build two additional models, a logistic regression for SGA-status in terms of covariates and a linear model for the log odds ratio between DG and SGA in terms of covariates. The model for SGA-status contained occupational class, ethnicity, smoking, hypertension, primiparity, a quadratic in mother's weight and mother's height (almost the same as the model in Thompson *et al.*, 2001). The log odds ratio model contained marital status, ethnicity and marijuana smoking.

The second column of Table 14.2 relates to a (SPML2) semiparametric maximum likelihood analysis in which a joint model for $Y_1 = \text{SGA}$ and $Y_2 = \text{DG}$ is constructed using a logistic model $f(y_2 \mid \boldsymbol{x}; \boldsymbol{\beta})$ for Y_2 in terms of covariates and a logistic model $f_{1|2}(y_1 \mid y_2, \boldsymbol{x}; \boldsymbol{\gamma})$ for Y_1 given Y_2 and covariates. This second model used the same explanatory variables as the SGA component of the Palmgren model, as well as DG and its interactions with marital status, occupational status, ethnicity and marijuana smoking.

The first two columns of Table 14.2 use different modelling frameworks to deal with the nuisance terms in the likelihood. In both cases the modelling strategy used was just a crude "put in all of the 'significant' variables" in a manual stepwise fashion. Given all the background modelling that went into producing the first two columns of Table 14.2, the results for the model of interest are reassuringly similar. We note, however, that if we did not include the nominally "significant" interactions with $Y_2 = \text{DG}$ in the $(Y_1 \mid Y_2, \boldsymbol{X})$-model, then the two methods produced quite different answers. The weighted method also produced fairly similar answers, although the standard errors from the weighted approach are usually slightly bigger than those from the semiparametric maximum likelihood approaches. The biggest difference is in the standard error for the "Agepreg" variable which is 38% larger for the weighted method than for the SPML methods. Simulations to follow show more extreme differences.

The results from the three ad hoc methods are very different, however, from those for the theoretically justified methods. The ad hoc methods are, in that sense, quite misleading. Because the proportion of cases in the population is nearly 10% for this data, ordinary logistic regression analysis with only the SGA-controls involves using a seriously biased sample from the population. We also note that the variables whose effects are badly estimated in the "Ignore" (simply logistic, ignoring the sampling scheme) and "Cond Y_1" (add Y_1 as another explanatory variable to the Y_2 model) methods are those variables which, in the SPML3 method, are significant in the logOR-model (log-linear model for the conditional odds ratio of Y_1 and Y_2 given $\boldsymbol{X}$). These results are not shown here. Similar effects appear in the simulation studies that follow.

TABLE 14.2
Coefficients (std errors) for fitted logistic model for $P(DG = 1 \mid \boldsymbol{x})$.

Theoretically Justified Methods			
Parameters	*SPML3*	*SPML2*	*Wtd*
Intercept	-0.675 (0.426)	-0.665 (0.434)	-0.793 (0.611)
Marital status *(baseline is "Married")*			
defacto	-0.482 (0.253)	-0.513 (0.257)	-0.683 (0.290)
single	-0.731 (0.329)	-0.870 (0.334)	-0.931 (0.335)
singoth	-0.262 (0.647)	-0.197 (0.669)	-0.232 (0.659)
Ethnicity *(baseline is "European")*			
maori	0.473 (0.320)	0.548 (0.320)	0.358 (0.358)
pacific	-0.101 (0.264)	-0.167 (0.262)	-0.034 (0.260)
indian	0.847 (0.334)	0.833 (0.330)	0.795 (0.345)
chinese	0.191 (0.362)	0.196 (0.367)	0.156 (0.376)
asian	0.284 (0.460)	0.284 (0.465)	0.349 (0.461)
others	1.337 (0.507)	1.361 (0.512)	1.307 (0.510)
Smokemar	0.735 (0.356)	0.774 (0.355)	0.917 (0.377)
Agepreg	-0.042 (0.013)	-0.043 (0.013)	-0.038 (0.019)
Ad hoc Methods			
Parameters	*Ignore*	*Controls*	*Cond* Y_1
Intercept	0.019 (0.421)	-1.182 (0.858)	-0.918 (0.441)
Marital status *(baseline is "Married")*			
defacto	0.025 (0.185)	-1.132 (0.436)	-0.082 (0.192)
single	-0.091 (0.242)	-1.536 (0.622)	-0.202 (0.247)
singoth	0.026 (0.482)	-0.373 (0.844)	-0.038 (0.495)
Ethnicity *(baseline is "European")*			
maori	0.207 (0.231)	0.354 (0.494)	0.108 (0.239)
pacific	-0.174 (0.191)	0.091 (0.329)	-0.009 (0.198)
indian	0.715 (0.221)	0.640 (0.527)	0.313 (0.230)
chinese	0.120 (0.252)	0.156 (0.470)	-0.083 (0.260)
asian	0.100 (0.316)	0.422 (0.568)	-0.129 (0.325)
others	0.522 (0.394)	1.563 (0.590)	0.368 (0.410)
Smokemar	-0.045 (0.263)	1.399 (0.462)	-0.107 (0.269)
Agepreg	-0.047 (0.013)	-0.030 (0.026)	-0.039 (0.013)
SGA			1.343 (0.143)

14.5.1   Simulations

Jiang *et al.* (2006, Section 4.1) investigated the comparative performances of the various methods under conditions in which the true models were known by using data generated from the fitted Palmgren model for $f(y_1, y_2 \mid \boldsymbol{x})$ for the DG example. Their simulations used the same sample and population sizes as in the real data. They looked at relative efficiencies and confidence-interval coverage for coefficients in the model of interest.

For the ad hoc "Ignore" and "Condition on Y_1" methods, they found serious biases in estimates and undercoverage of confidence intervals for all variables that were "significant" in the model for the Y_1-Y_2 odds-ratio, i.e., for the variables linked to the form of the association between Y_1 and Y_2. The ad hoc methods often had better efficiency and quite good coverage for variables not implicated in the Y_1-Y_2 association but this is of little relevance in practice because the appeal of the ad hoc methods is not having to do the additional modelling of the form of the association. For this simulation the "Y_1-controls only" method had good coverage but showed serious inefficiencies even compared with the weighted method. Relative efficiencies of coefficient estimates for SPML compared to the weighted method ranged from a little over 1 to 2.

In some simulations, generating from simpler Palmgren models, relative-efficiency advantages of SPML over the weighted method were at best modest when the Y_1-case-rate was smaller (5%) but could be substantial when the Y_1-cases were less rare (10%). In the latter situation the relative efficiency advantages became large when the association between Y_1 and Y_2 was strongly related to a continuous variable.

We do not want to read too much into the results of a small number of simulations and all this was happening, of course, under conditions in which not only was the model of interest correctly specified but so were the nuisance models.

14.6   Model misspecification and robustness

The robustness issues of concern here are a lack of robustness against model misspecification, and particularly lack of robustness against the misspecification of any nuisance model whose only purpose in an analysis is to help correct for the effects of a sampling design, e.g., a model for $f_{1|2}(y_1 \mid y_2, \boldsymbol{x})$ in (14.3). The weighted method, of course, incurs no risks of nuisance-model misspecification because it does not use any nuisance models! The weighted method, on the other hand, can be quite inefficient.

It is not good enough that model assumptions be testable. Lack of robustness against model misspecification is an important problem in practice whenever model *deficiencies smaller than those that can be detected reasonably reliably* result in practically important distortions to inferences about parameters of interest. (If a model was detectably inadequate we would try to find a better model.)

Jiang *et al.* (2006, Section 5) performed some limited investigations of the effects of nuisance-model misspecification when Y_2 is binary. Simulating from the model fitted to the ABC study data above, they found that when the true joint model was Palmgren (SPML3) but a SPML2 analysis was used employing a logistic regression model for $f_{1|2}(y_1 \mid y_2, \boldsymbol{x}; \boldsymbol{\gamma})$, then there were some severe biases in model-of-interest coefficients and problems with confidence interval coverage when the $f_{1|2}(y_1 \mid y_2, \boldsymbol{x})$ model contained no $y_2 \times \boldsymbol{x}$ interaction terms but the method performed well when the "significant" $y_2 \times x_k$ interactions were included. It seems that these interactions had permitted the fitted misspecified model to get close enough to the true model that the results were not affected.

Within the Palmgren model, Jiang *et al.* (2006, Section 5) also did simulations investigating the effects of mistakenly omitting an x-variable from the nuisance models. In some simulations they investigated the effects of a crude nuisance-model building approach in which the term was included when it was "significant" and omitted otherwise. With coefficient-value settings in which the term was "detectable" about 40% of the time there were some instances of nominally 95% confidence intervals for coefficients of interest falling to as low as 72%. For the range of values they considered, the missing term in the log odds ratio models caused worse problems than one in the marginal model for Y_1.

Methods that are more efficient than the weighted method but have lower risks from nuisance-model misspecification than the SPML methods described above have an obvious practical appeal. We will describe some of the work in this area in the next section.

While guarding against misspecification of nuisance models is one direction that work in this area has taken, another is robustness against misspecification of the model of interest. To motivate this, consider the example of maximum likelihood estimation for the usual normal-errors regression model. In the case of independent sampling, this leads to least-squares estimation of the regression coefficients, a method that still works well under a number of departures from the assumptions that gave rise to it. However, when coupled with response-biased sampling, maximum likelihood estimation for the usual normal-errors regression model is much less robust in this regard. So research has taken place on using models that are not fully specified (Wei *et al.*, 2013; Tchetgen Tchetgen, 2014; Ma and Carroll, 2016; Sofer *et al.*, 2017). There is a basic philosophy behind this that says "formulate parametric models for just those elements that are of primary scientific interest and make everything else as nonparametric as possible." If this can be done successfully then we have much reduced any exposure to errors from *nonessential model* misspecifications.

14.7   Model-misspecification robust methods

This brief section concentrates on linear regression models for a continuous Y_2.

Wei *et al.* (2013) dispensed with the assumption of normal errors in the regression model for Y_2 as a function of x but still assumed heteroscedastic errors and made a rare disease approximation. This method also uses a logistic model for $f_{1|2}(y_1 \mid y_2, x)$ so does not address the problem of misspecification of this nuisance model.

Ma and Carroll (2016) went further and developed an approach which does not require a known true case-rate $P(Y_1 = 1)$ or a rare-disease assumption, and does not assume either normality or homoscedasticity of the regression error. They only require a model for the mean function $E(Y_2 \mid x)$ that is correctly specified and a correctly specified (nuisance) model for $f_{1|2}(y_1 \mid y_2, x)$. Their semiparametric estimator involves positing density functions for $P(x)$ and $P(Y_2 \mid x)$ that may or may not be true, as a means of gaining efficiency. The resulting estimators are consistent and asymptotically normal if the posited functions are incorrectly specified, but become efficient if the posited functions are correctly specified. Internally several additional conditional distributions arise in the likelihood formulation, including quantities conditional on the covariates. This leads to the need to perform several nonparametric regressions on the covariates in their estimator which cause problems as the covariate dimension increases. There is ongoing work on methods for reducing these problems. Software and test data for the approach is available at `http://www.stat.tamu.edu/~carroll/matlab_programs/software.php` (see "Programs for the method of secondary linear regression analysis of case-control studies").

Another approach by Sofer *et al.* (2017), building on work by Tchetgen Tchetgen (2014), is based upon augmenting the estimating equations from the (inverse probability) weighted method, using a so-called control function, in a way that leads to efficiency gains when posited models are true but gives consistent estimates regardless of this. (Control functions are an idea arising from econometrics to control for certain types of selection bias.) Sofer *et al.* (2017) require a model for the mean function $E(Y_2 \mid x)$ that is correctly specified, that the true case rate $P(Y_1 = 1)$ be known, and a correctly specified model for the marginal density of X. However, parametric or semiparametric models for the marginal density of X can be specified. Features of a posited model for $f_{1|2}(y_1 \mid y_2, x)$ are used to gain efficiency when they are correct but can be misspecified. At the time of writing the R package mentioned at the end of Sofer *et al.* (2017) is no longer on CRAN but a 2013 version is available from `https://cran.r-project.org/src/contrib/Archive/RECSO/`.

Virtually all models used in statistical practice are misspecified to some degree. The secondary analysis of data from case-control studies is much more vulnerable to the effects of model misspecification than are primary analyses. Excellent progress is being made on methods which have the robustness of the (inverse probability) weighted method but can recoup much of the efficiency gains of the earlier semiparametric maximum likelihood methods. Their use will never be entirely routine to apply, however, because the efficiency gains are reliant on a lot of modelling of aspects of the data above and beyond building and fitting the model of interest.

Bibliography

Ghosh, A., Wright, F. A., and Zou, F. (2013). Unified analysis of secondary traits in case–control association studies. *Journal of the American Statistical Association*, **108**, 566–576.

Jiang, Y. (2004). *Semiparametric Maximum Likelihood for Multi-phase Response-Selective Sampling and Missing Data Problems*. Ph.D. thesis, Department of Statistics, University of Auckland.

Jiang, Y., Scott, A. J., and Wild, C. J. (2006). Secondary analysis of case-control data. *Statistics in Medicine*, **25**, 1323–1339.

Lee, A. J., Scott, A. J., and McMurchy, A. L. (1997). Re-using data from case-control studies. *Statistics in Medicine*, **16**, 1377–1389.

Lin, D. Y. and Zeng, D. (2009). Proper analysis of secondary phenotype data in case-control association studies. *Genetic Epidemiology*, **33**, 256–265.

Ma, Y. and Carroll, R. J. (2016). Semiparametric estimation in the secondary analysis of case–control studies. *Journal of the Royal Statistical Society: Series B (Statistical Methodology)*, **78**, 127–151.

Neuhaus, J., Scott, A., and Wild, C. (2002). The analysis of retrospective family studies. *Biometrika*, **89**, 23–37.

Prentice, R. L. and Pyke, R. (1979). Logistic disease incidence models with case-control studies. *Biometrika*, **66**, 403–411.

Rohrer, R. (1921). Der Index der Köperfulle als Maß des Ernährungszustandes. *Münchener Medizinische Wochenschrift*, **68**, 580–582.

Sofer, T., Cornelis, M. C., Kraft, P., and Tchetgen Tchetgen, E. J. (2017). Control function assisted IPW estimation with a secondary outcome in case-control studies. *Statistica Sinica*, **27**, 785–804.

Tchetgen Tchetgen, E. J. (2014). A general regression framework for a secondary outcome in case-control studies. *Biostatistics*, **15**, 117–128.

Thompson, J. M. D., Clark, P. M., Robinson, E., Becroft, D. M. O., Pattison, N. S., Glavish, N., Pryor, J. E., Rees, K., and Mitchell, E. A. (2001). Risk factors for small-for-gestational-age babies: The Auckland Birthweight Collaborative Study. *Journal of Paediatrics and Child Health*, **37**, 369–375.

Wei, J., Carroll, R. J., Müller, U. U., Keilegom, I. V., and Chatterjee, N. (2013). Robust estimation for homoscedastic regression in the secondary analysis of case–control data. *Journal of the Royal Statistical Society: Series B (Statistical Methodology)*, **75**, 185–206.

15

Response Selective Study Designs Using Existing Longitudinal Cohorts

Paul J. Rathouz

University of Wisconsin School of Medicine & Public Health

Jonathan S. Schildcrout

Vanderbilt University Medical Center

Leila R. Zelnick and Patrick J. Heagerty

University of Washington

15.1 Introduction

Over the past thirty-five years, longitudinal data collection has become a ubiquitous design element in epidemiology, clinical trials, program evaluation, natural history studies, and related areas of biomedical and public health investigation (Diggle *et al.*, 2002). Longitudinal data are powerful because with them, we can model individual trajectories of growth or can compare trajectories of, say, disease progression or remission between treated (or exposed) versus untreated (unexposed) groups of individuals. Such designs and accompanying methods of analysis are well described in several key texts (Diggle *et al.*, 2002; Fitzmaurice *et al.*, 2012). In addition, longitudinal designs permit the study of within-subject covariation of disease response and time-varying predictors, and this feature allows study participants to "serve as their own control" when examining time-varying treatments or exposures, thereby opening potential to control confounders that may not be measured or even known (Neuhaus and Kalbfleisch, 1998; Begg and Parides, 2003). In many designs, longitudinal data yield increases in statistical efficiency relative to cross-sectional data, owing to beneficial effects of within-subject correlation of responses over time.

With the regular exploitation of such study designs have come a host of well-characterized statistical models and methods for data analysis. Linear mixed models (Laird and Ware, 1982) is one anchoring method for continuous data, providing a highly flexible modeling framework that allows for various correlation structures and/or randomly varying slopes and intercepts from subject to subject to capture between-individual variability in trajectories. Analysis is typically likelihood-based and as such applies equally well to both small and large samples.

When data are binary or counts, the go-to approach has been marginal models with analysis based on generalized estimating equations (GEE) (Zeger and Liang, 1986; Liang and Zeger, 1986). GEE is based on the premise of a correctly specified regression model for the mean response over time, while allowing for various association structures linking the repeated measures. Importantly, however, GEE inferences about the mean regression model are robust to misspecification or poor estimation of the association model, so long as sample sizes are large enough to drive the empirical estimator of the sampling variance-covariance matrix of the regression parameter estimates (Royall, 1986). It is worth noting that if interest lies in likelihood-based approaches to estimating marginal model parameters, marginalized models are available (Azzalini, 1994; Heagerty, 1999; Heagerty and Zeger, 2000).

Despite these remarkable advances in methods of analysis, longitudinal studies can be very expensive to implement. In addition, their efficiency can be threatened by domains within the data that lack covariability between response and predictors of interest. Many longitudinal designs are based on a model of simple random sampling (SRS) of individuals from a population, wherein those sampled individuals are then followed up prospectively over time. We have found, however, that, per unit of data collected, the SRS plan can lead to underpowered hypothesis tests, and to unnecessarily uncertain estimates relative to designs that are more carefully tailored to the inferential targets of the study. Non-SRS sampling plans may lead to greater statistical efficiency, and a commensurate more efficient use of research resources.

In the past several decades, there have been substantial advances in enhanced, non-SRS, sampling plans in other areas of epidemiology. The case-control study (Cornfield, 1951; Anderson, 1972; Prentice and Pyke, 1979; Breslow and Day, 1980) dramatically oversamples affected individuals versus unaffected controls in order to generate efficient inferences about the association of disease and various exposures of interest. Extending that idea to disease events arising over time, the nested case-control (Borgan and Langholz, 1993; Borgan *et al.*, 1995; Langholz and Goldstein, 1996) and case-cohort (Prentice, 1986) designs are based on over-sampling cases (or, equivalently, undersampling controls) as those cases arise in a population or cohort over time. In parallel to developments in epidemiology and biostatistics, survey samplers have long designed studies that oversample important subpopulations. Extending these ideas into the domain of epidemiology, then, two-phase designs, pioneered by Prof. Breslow (e.g. Breslow and Day, 1980; Breslow and Cain, 1988; Breslow and Holubkov, 1997; Breslow and Chatterjee, 1999; Breslow, 1996), have been developed and exploited to bring the benefits of the case-control concept into more complex domains where affected versus unaffected status may not be so crisp, where multiple diseases may be studied simultaneously, and/or where expensive exposure measures can only be afforded on a restricted sample of individuals.

Whereas longitudinal designs have largely been excluded from these developments in the area of enhanced sampling, there are exceptions. Crossover trials for treatment interventions expose subjects longitudinally to both treatment and control conditions, thereby allowing subjects to act as their own control and eliminating between-subject variance in resulting inferences. Similarly, the case-crossover design (Maclure, 1991; Navidi, 1998) for observational data contrasts acute exposure at event times to that at "nearby" nonevent times on the same subject; in this design, allowing subjects to act as their own control over longitudinal arcs of time eliminates both between-subject variance and confounding in estimation of exposure effects. Both of these designs can be formally characterized as based on sampling individual time points for analysis, within a population or cohort that is being followed in structured longitudinal way.

Aside from these leading examples, it is only recently that sampling plans for longitudinal designs have been deeply and formally considered more generally. Whereas the foregoing two examples sample both individuals and, for each individual, time points, we and others have made substantial inroads into designs that sample individuals in ways that depart considerably from SRS, and then follow those individuals over time in typical structured longitudinal fashion. We see these newer designs as leading cases in a broad effort to expand the two-phase sampling paradigm advanced by Prof. Breslow into the rich and important domain of longitudinal data. The purpose of this chapter is to describe and illustrate some of these leading cases, accompanied by appropriate data analysis models and methods for estimating treatment effects while accounting for enhanced sampling designs.

We begin in the next section with an important illustration of how case-control sampling works. Then, in Section 15.3, we describe a design for continuous response data wherein the entire longitudinal vector is observed in Phase I of sampling, and Phase II is devoted to subsampling individuals for enriched exposure assessment, perhaps, for example, based on assays applied to stored tissue samples. Anticipating interest in either baseline levels of mean response, and/or the time-slope of the mean response in the context of a linear mixed model, sampling plans will be based on a combination of the linear regression intercept and slope for each individual. Full closed-form likelihood analysis, corrected for enhanced ascertainment (sampling), obtains and yields valid inferences, and contrasts with SRS.

In Section 15.4, we describe a design for longitudinal binary responses which for shorthand can be labeled "longitudinal follow up after case-control sampling." In these designs, Phase I sampling will typically yield a baseline (time zero) measure of binary response Y or a binary surrogate measure Z closely related to baseline Y. Phase II is then, essentially, case-control sampling based on baseline Y or Z; cases and controls are then followed over time in typical longitudinal fashion. Analysis is based on a marginal modeling approach with an extension of GEE to account for enhanced sampling.

15.2 Leading case: Retrospective sampling for binary data

The overriding motivation behind two-phase, response-selective designs is to increase statistical efficiency while controlling sample size in Phase II. The heuristic notion is to sample in such a way to increase the variability in some aspect of the response variable, with the hope of a commensurate increase in the statistical information in the sample about key parameters of interest; such information is often directly related to response variation and/or the response-predictor covariation. For example, in Section 15.3, we study sampling designs based on oversampling extreme values of the longitudinal response vector, where extreme is defined in terms of either absolute level or the slope over time. Before turning to that case, however, we examine the classic setting of case-control sampling.

As is well known, the statistical information in binary response data is directly related

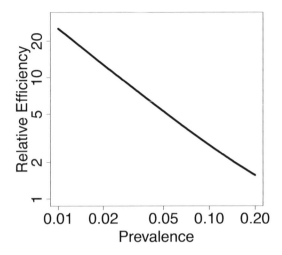

FIGURE 15.1
Relative statistical efficiency of 1:1 case-control sampling versus simple random sampling, as a function of population disease prevalence.

(and exactly proportional in logistic regression) to the response variance, which in turn is equal to $\mu(1-\mu)$ where μ is the expected positive proportion in the sample. When the response is a disease indicator and the disease is rare in the population, therefore, information about the exposure-disease relationship can be considerably enhanced by over-sampling cases relative to controls, either directly from the reference population, or in Phase II of a two-phase study. This is exactly what case-control sampling does.

To illustrate, consider a case-control study wherein cases are sampled in a 1:1 ratio relative to controls, and interest is on the exposure disease log odds ratio for some exposure of interest. The asymptotic relative efficiency of the case-control design, versus a SRS design, is plotted in Figure 15.1. As can be seen, the rarer the disease, the greater the efficiency gain in using the case-control design. For prevalence less than 2%, gains can be substantial.

With this basic heuristic in mind, our goal has been to extend the general case-control paradigm into the domain of longitudinal data. In this vein, we have explored a variety of longitudinal epidemiologic study designs, including those for continuous, count, and binary data; and those that oversample either entire subjects or specific longitudinal timepoints within subjects. In this chapter, we focus on two key designs for the former: One for continuous data wherein the emphasis might be on either time-invariant or time-varying exposure variables. And a second design wherein "case" and "control" subjects, defined as such at baseline, are sampled and followed up over time longitudinally.

Of course, in any setting, there are two main statistical issues to be considered. First, as indicated, we need to consider sampling plans to enhance inferences about key parameters of interest. Second, we need to craft methods of inference that account for the chosen biased sampling design. The following two sections consider both of these factors in two key classes of design.

15.3 Two-phase retrospective designs for quantitative longitudinal outcomes

Because primary data are very expensive to collect and curate, increasingly researchers are expected to address new scientific questions with existing data contained in resources such as electronic health records and cohort studies. Often these resources have, readily available, nearly all data necessary to address scientific questions, except for a key exposure or confounder variable that must be collected retrospectively. Perhaps the most common examples include genetic or biomarker research where the biomarker data are not readily available, but can be ascertained retrospectively by analyzing stored biospecimen. Assuming the original Phase I cohort is large, then exposure ascertainment costs limit sample size. In what follows, we describe retrospective study designs for quantitative longitudinal data when most data are readily available, with the one exception that an expensive to ascertain, time-fixed, exposure variable must be collected, but in Phase II can only be collected on a fraction of the cohort.

15.3.1 Model

In Phase I, assume a cohort of N subjects with longitudinal outcome vector $\boldsymbol{Y}_i$, $i \in \{1, 2 \ldots N\}$, covariate data $\boldsymbol{X}_{o,i}$ available on all N subjects, and a key exposure $\boldsymbol{X}_{e,i}$ that must be ascertained retrospectively for analyses. Exposure variable $\boldsymbol{X}_{e,i}$ is often a biomarker that can only be collected when stored biospecimen are analyzed. Further, assume interest is in the mixed-effect Laird and Ware model (Laird and Ware, 1982): $\boldsymbol{Y}_i = \boldsymbol{X}_i \boldsymbol{\beta} + \boldsymbol{Z}_i \boldsymbol{b}_i + \boldsymbol{\epsilon}_i$, where $\boldsymbol{\beta}$ is a p-vector of fixed-effect coefficients, $\boldsymbol{X}_i = (\boldsymbol{1}, \boldsymbol{T}_i, \boldsymbol{X}_{e,i}, \boldsymbol{X}_{e,i} \cdot \boldsymbol{T}_i, \boldsymbol{X}_{o,i})$, $\boldsymbol{T}_i = \{T_{ij}\}_{j \in 1,2,\ldots n_i}$ is the vector of times, $\boldsymbol{Z}_i = (\boldsymbol{1}, \boldsymbol{T}_i)$ is a $n_i \times 2$ design matrix for the random effects, $\boldsymbol{b}_i = (b_{0i}, b_{1i})^{\mathrm{T}} \sim N(\boldsymbol{0}, \boldsymbol{D})$, and $\boldsymbol{\epsilon}_i \sim N(\boldsymbol{0}, \boldsymbol{\Sigma})$. Here, $\boldsymbol{D}_i$ is the 2×2 covariance matrix that contains the variance components $(\sigma_0^2, \sigma_1^2, \rho)$, where ρ is the correlation between b_{0i} and b_{1i}. Assume $\boldsymbol{\Sigma} = \sigma_e^2 \boldsymbol{I}_{n_i}$ where $\boldsymbol{I}_{n_i}$ is a diagonal identity matrix. The multivariate density for this model is given by:

$$f(\boldsymbol{Y}_i \mid \boldsymbol{X}_i; \boldsymbol{\theta}) = (2\pi)^{-n_i/2} |\boldsymbol{V}_i|^{-1/2} \exp\left\{ -\frac{1}{2}(\boldsymbol{Y}_i - \boldsymbol{\mu}_i)^{\mathrm{T}} \boldsymbol{V}_i^{-1}(\boldsymbol{Y}_i - \boldsymbol{\mu}_i) \right\} ,$$

where $\boldsymbol{\theta} = (\boldsymbol{\beta}, \sigma_0, \sigma_1, \rho)$, $\boldsymbol{\mu}_i = \boldsymbol{X}_i \boldsymbol{\beta}$, $\boldsymbol{V}_i = \boldsymbol{Z}_i \boldsymbol{D}_i \boldsymbol{Z}_i^{\mathrm{T}} + \sigma_e^2 \boldsymbol{I}$. If a random sample of N_s subjects was drawn, inferences could be made by maximizing the log-likelihood:

$$l(\boldsymbol{\theta}; \boldsymbol{Y}, \boldsymbol{X}) = \sum_{i=1}^{N_s} l_i(\boldsymbol{\theta}; \boldsymbol{Y}_i, \boldsymbol{X}_i) = \sum_{i=1}^{N_s} \log f(\boldsymbol{Y}_i \mid \boldsymbol{X}_i; \boldsymbol{\theta}).$$

See Laird and Ware (1982); Lindstrom and Bates (1988); McCulloch and Searle (2001) for details regarding maximization.

15.3.2 Outcome dependent sampling (ODS) study designs

We consider Phase II sampling based on strata defined by low-dimensional summaries of the outcome vector $\boldsymbol{Y}_i$. These summaries represent key features of the outcome distribution that are used to identify informative individuals for estimating target parameters. Specifically, let $Q_i = g(\boldsymbol{Y}_i, \boldsymbol{X}_{oi})$ define a function of the response and observed covariates that summarizes key features of the response vectors. For example, let $Q_i = \boldsymbol{W}_i \boldsymbol{Y}_i$ where $\boldsymbol{W}_i = (\boldsymbol{X}_{Ti}^{\mathrm{T}} \boldsymbol{X}_{Ti})^{-1} \boldsymbol{X}_{Ti}^{\mathrm{T}}$, and $\boldsymbol{X}_{Ti} = (\boldsymbol{1}, \boldsymbol{T}_i)$, then $\boldsymbol{W}_i \boldsymbol{Y}_i$ contains the intercept and slope of

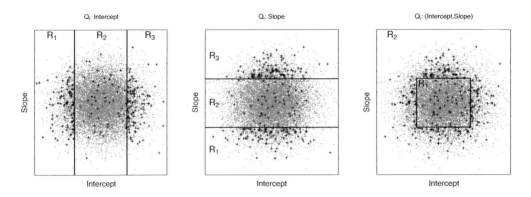

FIGURE 15.2
Study designs based on strata defined by subject-specific regressions of quantitative responses on time. In all panels, the central stratum pertains to the 'less informative' individuals whose Q_i values are in the center of the respective distributions. In contrast, the outer strata pertain to the 'more informative' individuals. Here central strata contain the central 80 percent of all data points. Black pluses denote sampled subjects and grey dots denote unsampled subjects.

subject i's regression of Y_i on T_i. While more general Q_i exist, we focus on Q_i that is linear in Y_i. Further, even though one could sample directly based on Q_i itself, we define strata based on coarsened summaries of Q_i that are easy to implement, and that do not lead to an over-conditioning when conducting analysis of the resulting biased sample.

Figure 15.2, adapted from Schildcrout *et al.* (2015), shows designs based on sampling strata defined by subject-specific simple linear regressions of the response vector on a time variable. In all panels, black pluses correspond to sampled subjects and grey dots correspond to unsampled subjects. In a) and b), we show three sampling strata that are based on the intercept and slope, respectively. In c), we show a design that samples on the subject-specific, bivariate intercept and slope. Common to all designs, there is a central region, R_2 in a) and b), and R_1 in c), that captures the relatively "typical" individuals. Outside this region, R_1 and R_3 in a) and b), and R_2 in c), are those subjects who are less "typical" in that their Q_i value tends towards the extremes of the distributions. In general, the goal of these designs is to overrepresent these subjects in the ODS because they are likely to be relatively informative for particular regression parameters. We highlight this over-representation of the less typical subjects by showing the sampled subjects with black pluses. We are able to further overrepresent informative subjects by broadening the central strata and/or increasing within-stratum sampling probabilities in the outlying strata.

Intuitively, efficiency gains from ODS are obtained by improving response and exposure (co)-variation, and the choice of Q_i should target the appropriate source of variation. We have shown in Schildcrout *et al.* (2013, 2015) that sampling based on the intercept leads to efficiency improvements in time-invariant covariate coefficients because it leads to over-representation of those with low and high average response values, associated with time-fixed traits. Such average values often are approximations to a subject-specific predisposition or tendency to have especially high or low Y_{ij} values. In contrast, sampling based on the slope leads to improvements in time-varying covariate coefficient estimates since it results in increased within-subject variability over time. Further, sampling based jointly on the subject-specific intercept and slope has been shown to improve efficiency for a larger range of coefficients than sampling based on either one individually.

15.3.3 Estimation

15.3.3.1 Ascertainment corrected maximum likelihood

Because these ODS designs lead to nonrepresentative samples, naive likelihood analyses will usually result in invalid inferences. We discuss an ascertainment corrected likelihoood that conditions on having $\boldsymbol{X}_{e,i}$ (or its scalar version) ascertained. Because $f(\boldsymbol{Y}_i \mid \boldsymbol{X}_i; \boldsymbol{\theta})$ is the multivariate density for subject i under random sampling, the corresponding density for someone included in the ODS is given by

$$f(\boldsymbol{Y}_i \mid \boldsymbol{X}_i, S_i = 1; \boldsymbol{\theta}) = \pi(q_i) f(\boldsymbol{Y}_i \mid \boldsymbol{X}_i; \boldsymbol{\theta}) \left\{ P(S_i = 1 \mid \boldsymbol{X}_i; \boldsymbol{\theta}) \right\}^{-1} ,$$

where the indicator S_i is 1 if individual i is included in the sample, q_i is the observed value of Q_i and $\pi(q_i)$ is the sampling probability given $Q_i = q_i$. Letting $\pi(R_k)$ be the sampling probability for all of region R_k, then if N_s subjects are selected into the ODS, the ascertainment corrected log-likelihood is given by

$$l^C(\boldsymbol{\theta}; \boldsymbol{Y}, \boldsymbol{X}) = \sum_{i=1}^{N_s} \left[l_i(\boldsymbol{\theta}; \boldsymbol{Y}_i, \boldsymbol{X}_i) - \log \left\{ \underbrace{\sum_{k=1}^{K} \pi(R_k) \int_{R_k} f(q_i \mid \boldsymbol{X}_i; \boldsymbol{\theta}) dq_i}_{\text{AC}_i} \right\} \right] ,$$

where $l_i(\boldsymbol{\theta}; \boldsymbol{Y}_i, \boldsymbol{X}_i) = \log f(\boldsymbol{Y}_i \mid \boldsymbol{X}_i; \boldsymbol{\theta})$. Thus, AC_i is a correction to the original likelihood contribution that is due to the study design. This ascertainment corrected log-likelihood (ACL) is a "complete data" likelihood (Carroll *et al.*, 2006; Lawless *et al.*, 1999) because it only includes subjects with complete data in the analysis. Since $Q_i = \boldsymbol{W}_i \boldsymbol{Y}_i$ is a linear function of the response profile, and $\boldsymbol{Y}_i \mid \boldsymbol{X}_i \sim N(\boldsymbol{\mu}_i, \boldsymbol{V}_i)$, then $Q_i \mid \boldsymbol{X}_i \sim N(\boldsymbol{\mu}_{qi}, \boldsymbol{\Sigma}_{qi})$ where $\boldsymbol{\mu}_{qi} = \boldsymbol{W}_i \boldsymbol{\mu}_i$ and $\boldsymbol{\Sigma}_{qi} = \boldsymbol{W}_i \boldsymbol{V}_i \boldsymbol{W}_i^{\mathrm{T}}$. If Q_i is univariate, $\boldsymbol{\mu}_{qi} = \mu_{qi}$ and $\boldsymbol{\Sigma}_{qi} = \sigma_{qi}^2$, and we can write

$$\text{AC}_i = \sum_{l=1}^{K} \pi(R_k) \left\{ \Phi \left(\frac{l_k - \mu_{qi}}{\sigma_{qi}} \right) - \Phi \left(\frac{l_{k-1} - \mu_{qi}}{\sigma_{qi}} \right) \right\} ,$$

where $l_0 < l_1 < \cdots < l_K$ is a partition of the real line that defines the sampling regions R_k, and $\Phi(c)$ is the standard normal cumulative distribution function.

15.3.3.2 Weighted likelihood

Weighted likelihood (WL) (Horvitz and Thompson, 1952; Manski and Lerman, 1977; Robins *et al.*, 1994; Breslow and Holubkov, 1997; Scott and Wild, 2001, 2002) is a popular approach for addressing planned nonrepresentative sampling in survey sampling and unplanned non-representative sampling in missing data scenarios. In order to generalize results from a biased sample to the target population represented by the original cohort, we can augment the standard score equation (i.e., the derivative of the log-likelihood) with a weight representing the inverse probability $\pi(Q_i)$ of each subject being sampled in Phase II. In the setting discussed here, the weighted likelihood score equation is given by

$$\sum_{i=1}^{N_s} \frac{1}{\pi(Q_i)} \frac{\partial l_i(\boldsymbol{\theta}; \boldsymbol{Y}_i, \boldsymbol{X}_i)}{\partial \boldsymbol{\theta}} = \boldsymbol{0} .$$

To estimate uncertainty, standard sandwich-based (Horvitz and Thompson, 1952) approaches are usually used. Weighted likelihood is, however, known to be inefficient (Robins *et al.*, 1994) due to weight variability and inefficient use of available data.

15.3.3.3 Full likelihood

The ACL and WL approaches described in the last two subsections use only those subjects with complete data (i.e., those for whom $S_i = 1$) in order to estimate regression parameters and perform inference. However, the outcome Y and available exposures X_o may be available for all, and additional information about the parameters of interest may be gleaned by including unsubsampled individuals in the analysis. While unsubsampled subjects do not have the exposure of interest measured, and cannot directly provide information on the relationship of the expensive covariate to the outcome, the observed outcomes of unsubsampled individuals provide information on the population-level mixture of covariate-specific mean outcomes. Thus, including these individuals in inference (at an added computational but no additional logistical cost) could improve inference on some parameters or combinations of parameters.

Writing the full likelihood that includes data from both sampled and unsampled individuals shows all potential sources of information that may be used to estimate target parameters. In the following representation, we focus on the simple situation where $X_i = X_{e,i}$ or where no additional observed covariates are explicitly denoted. Any observed covariates $X_{o,i}$ would be conditioned on for each component of the full likelihood. The parameter vector $\boldsymbol{\theta}$ would now need to be expanded to include parameters that also describe the marginal of the covariates. Here we decompose the full likelihood into key components, and connect to the more focused ACL:

$$
\begin{aligned}
L(\boldsymbol{\theta}; \boldsymbol{Y}, \boldsymbol{X}, \boldsymbol{S}) &= \prod_{i=1}^{N} f(\boldsymbol{Y}_i, \boldsymbol{X}_i, S_i; \boldsymbol{\theta}) \\
&= \prod_{S_i=1} P(S_i = 1; \boldsymbol{\theta}) \cdot f(\boldsymbol{Y}_i, \boldsymbol{X}_i | S_i = 1; \boldsymbol{\theta}) \cdot \prod_{S_i=0} f(\boldsymbol{Y}_i | S_i = 0; \boldsymbol{\theta}) \cdot P(S_i = 0; \boldsymbol{\theta}) \\
&= \prod_{S_i=1} P(S_i = 1; \boldsymbol{\theta}) \cdot f(\boldsymbol{X}_i | S_i = 1; \boldsymbol{\theta}) \cdot f(\boldsymbol{Y}_i | \boldsymbol{X}_i, S_i = 1; \boldsymbol{\theta}) \cdot \prod_{S_i=0} f(\boldsymbol{Y}_i | S_i = 0; \boldsymbol{\theta}) \cdot P(S_i = 0; \boldsymbol{\theta})
\end{aligned}
$$

subsampled + unsubsampled, joint

subsampled + unsubsampled, conditional

$$
= \prod_{S_i=1} f(\boldsymbol{X}_i | S_i = 1; \boldsymbol{\theta}) \cdot \underbrace{f(\boldsymbol{Y}_i | \boldsymbol{X}_i, S_i = 1; \boldsymbol{\theta})}_{\text{subsampled only, conditional}} \cdot \prod_{S_i=0} f(\boldsymbol{Y}_i | S_i = 0; \boldsymbol{\theta}) \cdot \prod_{i=1}^{N} P(S_i; \boldsymbol{\theta}).
$$

subsampled only, joint

The unconditional observed data likelihood can be factored into a number of terms that could be utilized to yield valid estimators of $\boldsymbol{\theta}$. The ACL discussed in Section 15.3.3.1 corresponds to a component of the full likelihood obtained by analyzing only those individuals in whom the exposure has been ascertained, and by conditioning on that exposure (denoted "subsampled only, conditional" in the equation above). Other approaches (Neuhaus *et al.*, 2014, 2006) have likewise analyzed information from subsampled individuals, but included information from exposures via a joint, as opposed to conditional, likelihood (denoted "subsampled only, joint" above).

The inclusion of unsubsampled subjects, either conditional on $[f(\boldsymbol{Y}_i \mid \boldsymbol{X}_i, S_i = 1; \boldsymbol{\theta})]$ or considered jointly with $[f(\boldsymbol{Y}_i, \boldsymbol{X}_i, \mid S_i = 1; \boldsymbol{\theta})]$ exposures, may provide additional information. While unsubsampled subjects do not have the marker measured, and cannot directly

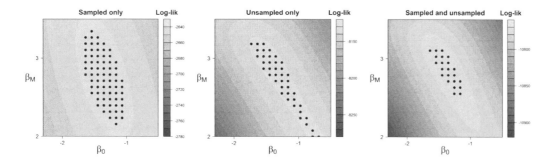

FIGURE 15.3
Profile log-likelihood contours and 95% confidence region obtained by inversion, showing the contribution of unsubsampled subjects under random sampling and true regression parameter $\beta^T = (\beta_0, \beta_T, \beta_M, \beta_{M \times T}) = (-1.5, -0.15, 3, -0.15)$. Marker prevalence for the cohort of 1000 was 25%, and 250 subjects were subsampled. The characteristic "ridge" in the middle panel reflects the fact that only the estimated population-level mean outcome is observed in these subjects. While many different combinations of regression parameters could give rise to the observed data, adding this information to an analysis based on subsampled subjects alone (left panel) may potentially improve inference for some parameters. The inclusion of unsubsampled individuals both changes the precision and orientation of the confidence region (right panel).

provide information on the relationship of the expensive covariate to the outcome, the observed outcomes of unsubsampled individuals provide information on the population-level mixture of marker-specific mean outcomes. For example, for a binary biomarker $X_{e,i} = 0/1$, at baseline, the mean outcomes for subjects with $X = 0$ and $X = 1$ under the usual linear mixed model are β_0 and $\beta_0 + \beta_X$, respectively. If p is the prevalence of the marker, observing the mean of Y among all cohort members at baseline would then give an estimate of $E(Y|T = 0) = \beta_0 + \beta_X p$; the variance of Y is likewise related to a combination of regression parameters.

In order to demonstrate the potential information that is available from components of the full likelihood we use simulated data and plots of profile likelihoods. Specifically, we generated simulated data with a single binary covariate, X_e, or biomarker denoted as M, under regression parameters $\beta^T = (\beta_0, \beta_T, \beta_M, \beta_{M \times T}) = (-1.5, -0.15, 3, -0.15)$ for $N = 1000$ cohort members each with $n_i = 6$ observations per member, of whom $N_S = 250$ were randomly subsampled; the marker population prevalence was 25%. Figure 15.3 shows representative contours from subsampled and unsubsampled subjects' contributions to the profile log-likelihood for these parameters under random sampling, and illustrates the possible impact of including these individuals in the analysis. Notably, the log-likelihood contribution of unsubsampled subjects (middle panel of Figure 15.3) describes a ridge of linear combinations of the parameters related to the baseline mean of Y among all subjects, subject to constraints imposed by the observed variance. Adding information from the unsubsampled subjects to the usual log-concave likelihood contributions from subsampled subjects (left panel of Figure 15.3) has the potential to affect both estimation (i.e, orientation) and precision (the area of a 95% confidence region obtained by inversion), as seen in the right panel of Figure 15.3.

Ultimately full-likelihood analysis may provide additional information but requires additional computational burden to program all elements of the likelihood. One pragmatic alternative is to simply use multiple imputation as a strategy that does use all available information yet is frequently straightforward to implement.

15.3.3.4   Multiple imputation

Because the ACL and WL approaches only use data from those in whom the expensive exposure, $\boldsymbol{X}_{e,i}$, was ascertained (i.e., with $S_i = 1$), one might consider a multiple imputation strategy (MI) (Rubin, 1976) that imputes $\boldsymbol{X}_{e,i}$ in those with $S_i = 0$ so that data available on such subjects are used in analysis. MI recovers some but not much information about the coefficient for $\boldsymbol{X}_{e,i}$, but it can recover far more information about coefficients associated with $\boldsymbol{X}_{o,i}$. Recall that $\boldsymbol{X}_{o,i}$ is available in subjects with $S_i = 0$, but it is not used in complete data analyses such as ACL and WL. The key to MI analysis is to build imputation data sets from the conditional exposure distribution, $[\boldsymbol{X}_{e,i} \mid \boldsymbol{Y}_i, \boldsymbol{X}_{o,i}, S_i = 0]$. Because our design sampled based on observed response and covariate data $(\boldsymbol{Y}_i, \boldsymbol{X}_{o,i})$, the missing data mechanism for the imputation model is at random (MAR). Specifically, the assumption ensuring model identification is that

$$P(\boldsymbol{X}_{e,i} \mid \boldsymbol{X}_{o,i}, \boldsymbol{Y}_i, S_i = 0) = P(\boldsymbol{X}_{e,i} \mid \boldsymbol{X}_{o,i}, \boldsymbol{Y}_i) = P(\boldsymbol{X}_{e,i} \mid \boldsymbol{X}_{o,i}, \boldsymbol{Y}_i, S_i = 1) \;,$$

so that we may build imputation models for $\boldsymbol{X}_{e,i}$ in unsampled participants directly from an analysis from the sampled subjects without adjusting for nonrepresentative sampling. Two approaches towards building this model, described in Schildcrout *et al.* (2015), produced similar results in simulations under proper model specification. Once the exposure model is constructed, M multiple imputation data sets can be estimated. Standard imputation approaches for analysis of the complete data sets and for combining results from the data sets can then be implemented, e.g., Rubin (1976); Little and Rubin (2014); Schafer and Graham (2002) .

15.3.4   Childhood Asthma Management Program (CAMP)

We now briefly summarize results published in Schildcrout *et al.* (2015) which depict several take-home points regarding the utility of the design and analysis procedures discussed here. This is done via plasmode simulation (Franklin *et al.*, 2014) wherein we simulate the conduct of a longitudinal genetic association substudy from the CAMP study (CAMP Research Group, 1999, 2000). We conceive of a circumstance where 555 children with sufficient data were available in the original cohort for inclusion into the substudy; however, only approximately 250 blood samples can be analyzed for retrospective ascertainment of a genetic biomarker IL-10 due to costs. At each of 30 replications of the plasmode simulation, we sampled subjects either with a RS design or with one of three ODS designs described in Section 15.3.2. We then conducted the analysis using maximum likelihood (under RS), ACL (under ODS designs), and MI (under all designs). We summarize the results via average parameter and standard error estimates.

Our interest is the Laird and Ware (1982) random effects model given by

$$E[Y_{ij} \mid \boldsymbol{X}_i, \boldsymbol{b}_i] = (\beta_0 + b_{0i}) + (\beta_t + b_{1i}) \cdot t_{ij} + \beta_s \cdot \mathrm{IL10}_i + \beta_{st} \cdot t_{ij} \cdot \mathrm{IL10}_i + \boldsymbol{\beta}_C^{\mathrm{T}} \cdot \mathrm{covariates}_{ij} \;,$$

where Y_{ij} is the observed post-bronchodilator percent of predicted forced vital capacity (FVC%) for child i at visit j, t_{ij} is the number of years since baseline, $\mathrm{IL10}_i$ is an indicator variable that child i had at least one variant allele at the IL10 cytokine, and $\boldsymbol{b}_i = (b_{0i}, b_{1i})^{\mathrm{T}}$ contains subject i's random intercept and slope. Other covariates are also included (including randomized treatment assignment) but will not be discussed here. Table 15.1, excerpted

TABLE 15.1

Characteristics of children participating in the CAMP study with genotype and covariate data available representing the original cohort. Continuous variables are summarized with the 10th, 50th, and 90th percentiles, and categorical variables are summarized with proportions.

Variable	
Cohort size (N)	555
Age at randomization (years)	6.23, 8.81, 11.71
Male gender	0.65
Black race	0.10
Other (non-Caucasian) race	0.26
IL10 Variant Allele	0.50
Observations per subject	9, 10, 10
Follow-up time (years)	3.85, 3.99, 4.1
Post-Bronchodilator Percent Predicted	92, 105, 116

from Schildcrout *et al.* (2015), shows that 50% of the children possessed the variant allele, that the majority of children were observed for the scheduled 10 follow-up visits, and that most children were followed for the entire 4 years of planned follow-up.

To generate ODS designs, we computed all estimated intercepts and slopes from subject-specific simple linear regressions of FVC% on time since randomization. Sampling was then based on: the estimated intercept (ods.i), the estimated slope (ods.s), or the estimated intercept and slope jointly (ods.b). In order to obtain 250 subjects, the cutoff points that define strata in the ods.i and ods.s designs are given by the 16th and 84th percentiles of the original cohort. We sampled all subjects below (above) the 16th (84th) percentile and with probability 0.19 all subjects falling in the central 68% stratum. For ods.b, we sampled with probability 0.19 all subjects who fell in the central 68% region of the joint intercept and slope distribution in the original cohort and with probability 1 all of those falling outside this region. Random sampling (RS) of 250 subjects is also simulated as a comparator.

Results from 30 replications of the plasmode simulation are shown in Table 15.2. We highlight several key points: 1) All design by analysis procedure combinations largely reproduced the point estimates from the original cohort across replications; 2) The ods.s design is most efficient for time trends and for the difference between the time trends (i.e., the interaction) but was inefficient for time-fixed covariate coefficients; 3) The ods.i design was most efficient for the time-fixed IL10 coefficient at all timepoints, but was inefficient for time-varying covariate effects; 4) MI led to fully efficient estimates of baseline covariate coefficients irrespective of the design; 5) The extent to which MI (versus complete data, CD) led to efficiency gains for coefficients linked to the imputed IL-10 depended upon the design (i.e., if the design was already efficient for a coefficient, MI did not improve efficiency); on the other hand, MI did not degrade the efficiency relative to CD; 6) While not shown, the efficiency of the ods.b design was reasonably high for all parameters, but not optimal for any of them.

Our conclusion is that outcome dependent sampling designs can deliver efficiency performance nearly paralleling analysis of the much larger full cohort. To realize this efficiency, we recommend ACL complemented with MI, which is not hard to implement.

TABLE 15.2

CAMP Results: Average estimates (average standard error estimates) based on 30 replications of each study design. At each replication, twenty imputation samples were used. Although other covariate effects are not shown, they were included in analyses. See Schildcrout et al. (2015). The Original Cohort column displays results from the analysis of the full cohort of 555 participants. Analysis methods are: CD=Complete data analysis using ACL; MI="Direct" multiple imputation as described in Schildcrout et al. (2015)

Variable	Original Cohort	RS		ods.s		ods.i	
		CD	MI	CD	MI	CD	MI
Time trend (per year) irrespective of treatment							
No VAs	0.14 (0.16)	0.11 (0.23)	0.09 (0.19)	0.14 (0.17)	0.10 (0.16)	-0.04 (0.22)	0.09 (0.18)
With VAs	-0.25 (0.15)	-0.19 (0.23)	-0.19 (0.19)	-0.19 (0.17)	-0.21 (0.16)	-0.38 (0.22)	-0.21 (0.18)
Difference	-0.39 (0.22)	-0.30 (0.33)	-0.27 (0.31)	-0.33 (0.24)	-0.31 (0.24)	-0.35 (0.31)	-0.30 (0.29)
IL10 (VA vs no VA) in the placebo arm at baseline and year 4							
$t_{ij}=0$	-1.65 (1.15)	-1.67 (1.70)	-1.78 (1.69)	-2.20 (1.65)	-2.13 (1.67)	-1.72 (1.30)	-1.90 (1.32)
$t_{ij}=4$	-3.20 (1.17)	-2.87 (1.73)	-2.88 (1.71)	-3.51 (1.68)	-3.35 (1.68)	-3.11 (1.5)	-3.12 (1.52)
Other baseline variable coefficients							
Male (vs female)	-1.14 (0.72)	-1.47 (1.08)	-1.22 (0.73)	-1.47 (1.07)	-1.13 (0.72)	-0.71 (0.86)	-1.16 (0.72)
Black (vs white)	0.51 (1.21)	0.52 (1.87)	0.53 (1.25)	1.22 (1.85)	0.76 (1.23)	1.19 (1.56)	0.47 (1.24)
Other (vs white)	-0.81 (0.98)	-0.95 (1.44)	-0.74 (0.99)	-1.31 (1.44)	-0.59 (1.00)	-0.01 (1.15)	-0.71 (0.99)
Age ($t_{ij}=0$)	-0.21 (0.17)	-0.23 (0.26)	-0.22 (0.17)	-0.40 (0.26)	-0.23 (0.17)	-0.50 (0.21)	-0.22 (0.17)

15.4   Auxiliary variable, outcome related, sampling designs for longitudinal binary data

We now discuss a class of designs that, in Phase II, samples from an existing cohort or directly from a reference population based on an outcome-related, auxiliary variable. Subjects are then followed longitudinally in time. The sampling scheme is intended to enrich the sample with response and exposure (co)variation. The auxiliary variable is related to the longitudinal outcome and is used for building a sample that can estimate exposure-outcome associations more efficiently than can SRS designs. The design may be described as "longitudinal follow-up after case-control sampling." We describe marginal model parameter estimation using extensions of the semiparametric generalized estimating equations (GEE) method (Liang and Zeger, 1986; Zeger and Liang, 1986). Other authors, including Neuhaus *et al.* (2014), have developed likelihood based approaches to estimate subject-specific, generalized mixed effect model (Stiratelli *et al.*, 1984; Breslow and Clayton, 1993) parameters in such designs. Whereas the modeling and estimation issues differ, the study design considerations are very similar regardless of marginal versus subject-specific modeling approach.

15.4.1   Model under random sampling

In addition to the notation introduced in the foregoing section, let $\boldsymbol{X}_i^{\mathrm{T}} = (\mathbf{x}_{i1}, \ldots, \mathbf{x}_{in_i})$. Assume interest lies in the marginal probability that $Y_{ij} = 1$ (i.e., the prevalence) given $\boldsymbol{X}_i$,

$$\mu_{ij}^p = P(Y_{ij} = 1 | \boldsymbol{X}_i) = g^{-1}(\beta_0 + \boldsymbol{x}_{ij}^{\mathrm{T}}\boldsymbol{\beta}_1) \tag{15.1}$$

(superscript p for population), where $g(\cdot)$ is a link function and $\boldsymbol{\beta}_1$ is the parameter of interest. Note that (15.1) implicitly assumes the full covariate conditional mean assumption that

$$P(Y_{ij} = 1 | \boldsymbol{X}_i) = P(Y_{ij} = 1 | \boldsymbol{x}_{ij}) \ ,$$

i.e., that predictors available in $\boldsymbol{X}_i$ provide no additional predictive value for Y_{ij} over and above the information available in $\boldsymbol{x}_{ij}$. Let S_i be an indicator variable for the ith subject in the Phase I cohort or the population being selected into the sample, and assume that the sampling indicators, S_i, are independent. Then, under simple random sampling, or exposure ($\boldsymbol{X}_i$) dependent sampling, we may directly estimate $\boldsymbol{\beta} = (\beta_0, \boldsymbol{\beta}_1^{\mathrm{T}})^{\mathrm{T}}$, say with GEE with a working correlation model appropriate to the longitudinal design (Liang and Zeger, 1986; Zeger and Liang, 1986).

15.4.2   Auxiliary variable sampling design

Under rare outcome scenarios, however, simple random sampling may yield very few observed events, thereby limiting power to detect outcome-exposure associations. To enrich the sample with events, consider a univariate auxiliary sampling variable Z_i related to response vector $\boldsymbol{Y}_i$. We consider the case wherein Z_i is binary, although other cases are possible. Although Z_i is not used for analytical purposes (that is, we are interested in $\boldsymbol{\mu}_i^p$), it is intended to enrich the sample with events in order to improve precision of $\boldsymbol{\beta}$ estimates. We refer to designs that sample exclusively on Z_i as *auxiliary variable sampling* (AVS). Further, if one is interested in the relationship between $\boldsymbol{Y}_i$ and a relatively rare baseline covariate $X_{1i} \subset \boldsymbol{X}_i$, one may also stratify the sampling scheme jointly on (Z_i, X_{1i}). Designs of this sort are termed *exposure and auxiliary variable sampling* (EAVS). We consider the case where X_{1i} is a binary indicator, but other, including multidimensional, forms of X_1 are possible.

Broadly, the goals of AVS and EAVS designs are to improve observed variability in outcome and covariability between outcome and exposure. Under these designs, we sample subjects *independently* with *investigator specified* probability

$$\pi(z) \equiv P(S_i = 1 \mid \boldsymbol{Y}_i, \boldsymbol{X}_i, Z_i = z) = P(S_i = 1 \mid Z_i = z) \tag{15.2}$$

under AVS, and

$$\pi(z, X_{1i}) \equiv P(S_i = 1 \mid \boldsymbol{Y}_i, \boldsymbol{X}_i, Z_i = z) = P(S_i = 1 \mid X_{1i}, Z_i = z) \tag{15.3}$$

under EAVS. Assuming the marginal prevalences of Z_i and X_{1i} are low, we would anticipate that $\pi(1)$ would be large compared to $\pi(0)$ under AVS, and that $\pi(1, 1)$ would be large compared to $\pi(0, 0)$, while $\pi(0, 1)$ and $\pi(1, 0)$ would fall somewhere in between under EAVS.

15.4.3   Estimation with GEE using sequential offsetted regressions

Because sampling under the proposed design class is based on a Z_i that is related to reponse vector $\boldsymbol{Y}_i$, the sample is not representative of the target population. To address this issue, we have developed an estimation strategy that conducts GEE analyses based on a sequence of two offsetted logistic regressions. To describe the program, define the sampling probability as a function of the entire design matrix and as a function of the jth response value with $\rho_{ij}(y, \boldsymbol{X}_i) \equiv P(S_i = 1 | Y_{ij} = y, \boldsymbol{X}_i)$. Note that $\rho_{ij}(y, \boldsymbol{X}_i)$ can vary within i over timepoints j due to variability in y_{ij} and the time-varying components of $\boldsymbol{X}_i$. Now, when (15.1) is a logistic regression model, i.e., when $g(u) = \log\{u/(1 - u)\}$, then we show in an appendix that

$$\mu_{ij}^s = P(Y_{ij} = 1 | \boldsymbol{X}_i) = g^{-1}\left[\beta_0 + \boldsymbol{x}_{ij}^{\mathrm{T}} \boldsymbol{\beta}_1 + \underbrace{\log\{\rho_{ij}(1, \boldsymbol{X}_i)/\rho_{ij}(0, \boldsymbol{X}_i)\}}_{\text{offset}} \right] \tag{15.4}$$

(superscript s indicating the pseudo-population represented by the enriched sample). Thus, if $\rho_{ij}(y, \boldsymbol{X}_i)$ were known, we would be able to conduct offsetted logistic regression using GEE with a working correlation model for $\mathrm{corr}(Y_{ij}, Y_{ik} | \boldsymbol{X}_i, S_i = 1)$ in the sample.

The ratio $\rho_{ij}(1, \boldsymbol{X}_i)/\rho_{ij}(0, \boldsymbol{X}_i)$ is, however, generally not known and must be estimated. In fact, sampling depends upon $(\boldsymbol{Y}_i, \boldsymbol{X}_i)$ through Z_i with AVS, and upon (Z_i, X_{1i}) with EAVS. By (15.2)-(15.3), we may use the known $\pi(1, X_{1i})/\pi(0, X_{1i})$ to estimate $\rho_{ij}(1, \boldsymbol{X}_i)/\rho_{ij}(0, \boldsymbol{X}_i)$, which is then used to make inferences about $\boldsymbol{\beta}$ in (15.1) via the off-setted model (15.4). To proceed, define the intermediate, auxiliary model,

$$\lambda_{ij}^p(y, \boldsymbol{X}_i) = P(Z_i = 1 | Y_{ij} = y, \boldsymbol{X}_i), \quad y = 0, 1.$$

Similar to $\rho_{ij}(y, \boldsymbol{X}_i)$, $\lambda_{ij}^p(y, \boldsymbol{X}_i)$ is conditional on the entire design matrix $\boldsymbol{X}_i$, but only on the jth response Y_{ij}. When $\lambda_{ij}^p(y, \boldsymbol{X}_i)$ is a logistic regression model, we show in an appendix that

$$\mathrm{logit}\{\lambda_{ij}^s(y, \boldsymbol{X}_i)\} = \mathrm{logit}\{\lambda_{ij}^p(y, \boldsymbol{X}_i)\} + \underbrace{\log\{\pi(1, X_{1i})/\pi(0, X_{1i})\}}_{\text{offset}}, \tag{15.5}$$

so that $\lambda_{ij}^p(y, \boldsymbol{X}_i)$ is estimable by performing logistic regression for Z_i in the sample with a known offset $\log\{\pi(1, X_{1i})/\pi(0, X_{1i})\}$. In addition, with estimated $\lambda_{ij}^p(y, \boldsymbol{X}_i)$, the ratio

$$\frac{\rho_{ij}(1, \boldsymbol{X}_i)}{\rho_{ij}(0, \boldsymbol{X}_i)} = \frac{1 - \lambda_{ij}^p(1, \boldsymbol{X}_i) + \{\pi(1, X_{1i})/\pi(0, X_{1i})\}\lambda_{ij}^p(1, \boldsymbol{X}_i)}{1 - \lambda_{ij}^p(0, \boldsymbol{X}_i) + \{\pi(1, X_{1i})/\pi(0, X_{1i})\}\lambda_{ij}^p(0, \boldsymbol{X}_i)}, \tag{15.6}$$

can be estimated which in turn leads to estimation of μ_{ij}^p.

To summarize this "sequential offsetted regression" (SOR) approach, we first estimate λ_{ij}^p using offsetted logistic regression of Z_i on $\boldsymbol{X}_i$ and Y_{ij}. We then combine, for all i and j, the estimated $\widehat{\lambda}_{ij}^p$ with the known sampling ratio $\pi(1, X_{1i})/\pi(0, X_{1i})$ to estimate ratio (15.6). This ratio is then used in another offsetted logistic regression to estimate marginal mean model parameters $\boldsymbol{\beta}$ in (15.1) by using relationship (15.4). Because (15.6) is estimated, standard errors are a bit more complicated than standard robust standard errors, and calculations are described in Schildcrout and Rathouz (2010) and Schildcrout *et al.* (2012).

15.4.4   Practical considerations for estimating the auxiliary model

Proper specification of the auxiliary model λ_{ij}^p is required for the analysis approach to be valid. In most circumstances, the strongest predictor in this model will (hopefully) be Y_{ij}. One must then carefully consider which covariates in $\boldsymbol{X}_i$ and which interactions with Y_{ij} should be included. One would expect that, with longitudinal data, the $Y_{ij} \times t_{ij}$ interaction will be required if a serial component to the longitudinal structure exists. While one might be conservative and include all pairwise interaction with Y_{ij}, we have observed (unpublished work) that including a large number of unimportant $\boldsymbol{X}_i \times Y_{ij}$ interactions can result in efficiency losses for $\boldsymbol{\beta}$ estimates. Scientific knowledge, exploratory data analysis, and variable selections should be considered to balance the bias-variance tradeoff associated a rich – versus parsimonious – model for λ_{ij}^p; further research is warranted.

15.4.5   Extensions and alternatives

15.4.5.1   Observation-level sampling

Thus far, we have described an estimation approach for marginal model parameters when we subsample *subjects* from a larger cohort for inclusion into a substudy. Conveniently, the estimation program we described translates, with little modification, to observation-level sampling designs, in which we sample specific *time points* j within subjects at which response Y_{ij} is observed. Similar to subject-level sampling, we may consider AVS or EAVS designs, replacing Z_i with Z_{ij}, X_{1i} with $\boldsymbol{x}_{1,ij}$, and S_i with S_{ij} in the foregoing description (Schildcrout *et al.*, 2012). One important consideration with observation-level sampling is that the full covariate conditional mean assumption (Pepe and Anderson, 1994; Whittemore, 1995; Diggle *et al.*, 2002; Schildcrout and Heagerty, 2005) is likely to be violated because, even if $P(Y_{ij} = 1 \mid \boldsymbol{X}_i) = P(Y_{ij} = 1 \mid \boldsymbol{x}_{ij})$, $P(Y_{ij} = 1 \mid \boldsymbol{X}_i, S_{ij} = 1)$ may not equal $P(Y_{ij} = 1 \mid \boldsymbol{x}_{ij}, S_{ij} = 1)$ due to the (possibly indirect) relationship between $\boldsymbol{S}_i$ and $\boldsymbol{X}_i$ through $\boldsymbol{Z}_i = (Z_{i1}, \ldots, Z_{in_i})^{\mathrm{T}}$. Thus, when conducting analyses of observation-level sampling designs using GEE, we recommend using a working independence covariance structure.

15.4.5.2   Other exponential family members

We are also able to extend the SOR analysis procedure to other exponential family members in a relatively straightforward manner. Let $F_P(y|\boldsymbol{x}_{ij})$ be the marginal distribution function of $Y_{ij} \mid \boldsymbol{x}_i$ in the target population, where Y_{ij} may be binary, continuous, or count-valued, and assume the density $dF_P(y \mid \boldsymbol{x}_{ij})$ is an exponential family member,

$$dF_P(y|\boldsymbol{x}_{ij}) \equiv f(y|\boldsymbol{x}_{ij}) = \exp\left\{ [\theta_{ij}y - b(\theta_{ij})]/\phi + c(y; \phi) \right\} .$$

Specifying $\mathrm{E}(Y_{ij}|\boldsymbol{x}_{ij}) = b'(\theta_{ij}) = g^{-1}(\eta_{ij})$ and $\eta_{ij} = \beta_0 + \boldsymbol{x}_{ij}^{\mathrm{T}}\boldsymbol{\beta}_1$, this is a generalized linear model with canonical parameter θ_{ij}, cumulant function $b(\theta_{ij})$, and dispersion parameter ϕ.

We note that we can write $dF_p(\cdot)$ in terms of the population odds

$$\text{odds}_P(y|\boldsymbol{x}_{ij}) \equiv \frac{dF_P(y|\boldsymbol{x}_{ij})}{dF_P(y_0|\boldsymbol{x}_{ij})} = \exp\{\theta_{ij}(y-y_0)/\phi + c(y;\phi) - c(y_0;\phi)\} \,,$$

where y_0 is an appropriate reference value of the response distribution (e.g., the population median). Even though the odds ratio representation is natural in the binary data case ($y_0 = 0$), as shown in Rathouz and Gao (2009), it can also be applied to other exponential family members.

Just as with the binary case, wherein the logistic form of the model in the population is retained in the sample, as in (15.4), in this more general setting, the induced model in the sample is still in the exponential family, with the same support and same canonical parameter θ_{ij}, so long as the sampling ratio (15.6) does not depend on $\boldsymbol{\beta}$. Much of the same theoretical development applies. Similar to the case with binary logistic regression, we obtain an estimate of the ratio (15.6). The mean model analyses for $\boldsymbol{\beta}$ then involve a generalization of the GEE approach outlined above.

Importantly, even though analysis considerations for other members of the exponential family are similar to those for the binary logistic model, design considerations differ. These results and indications for ongoing research are given in McDaniel *et al.* (2016).

15.4.5.3 Weighting

As discussed in Section 15.3.3.2, for analyses of samples that are biased by design or are nonrepresentative due to missing data, augmenting score equations or estimating equations with appropriate weights can permit valid inferences from the sample to the population. Two obvious approaches to inverse probability weighting include: 1) weighting subjects by the inverse of the known sampling probability, $\pi(Z_i)$ or $\pi(Z_i, X_{1i})$, to approximate the original population, and 2) weighting individual observations by the inverse of the estimated $\hat{\rho}_{ij}(Y_{ij}, \boldsymbol{X}_i)$ described in Section 15.4.3. To our investigation thus far, approach 1) does not appear to be as statistically efficient – and is often less efficient – than the SOR approach advanced here, although 2) may be more competitive from an efficiency standpoint.

15.4.6 ADHD natural history study

The Attention Deficit Hyperactivity Disorder (ADHD) Study (Lahey *et al.*, 1998; Hartung *et al.*, 2002) studied 255 children to examine the natural history of ADHD symptoms in boys and girls over time over 8 waves (years). The study enrolled 138 children referred to a participating clinic and a demographically similar group of 117 nonreferred children. At each visit, ADHD symptom expression was assessed using the Diagnostic and Statistical Manual of Mental Disorders (4th ed.; DSM-IV; American Psychatric Association, 1994) criteria. Participant referral, our auxiliary variable, Z_i, was a very strong predictor of the binary ADHD symptoms at the first visit (Y_{i1}) in that 92% (2%) of referred (nonreferred) children met the criteria for expressing at least some ADHD symptoms. The study was matched on gender, G_i; it can be considered an EAVS design since the probability of being sampled depended upon (Z_i, G_i).

Referred ($Z_i = 1$) and nonreferred ($Z_i = 0$) children possessed similar demographic characteristics. They were approximately 82% male, 64% white, 31% African-American; 6% were classified as "other" ethnicity; and the median age at baseline was 5 years. Similar to Schildcrout and Rathouz (2010), we show the impact of assumptions about $\pi(1,g)/\pi(0,g)$ and those in auxiliary model (15.5). We operate under the assumption that five percent of girls in the population would qualify for referral and, as a sensitivity analysis, 5 or 15 percent of boys would qualify. That is $P(Z_i = 1 \mid G_i = 1) = 0.05$ and $P(Z_i = 1 \mid G_i =$

TABLE 15.3

ADHD Study results: Linear t_{ij} columns correspond to estimates where the functional form of t_{ij} in the auxiliary model (15.5) was assumed linear. With flexible t_{ij}, time-specific indicator variables were used. Results are given for two different assumptions about sampling probabilities. We display logistic regression parameter estimates and 95% confidence intervals.

| Variable | $P(Z_i = 1 \mid G_i = 1) = 0.05$ | | $P(Z_i = 1 \mid G_i = 1) = 0.15$ | | Naive |
	Flexible t_{ij}	Linear t_{ij}	Flexible t_{ij}	Linear t_{ij}	
Time (years)	0.13	0.10	0.06	0.06	-0.04
	(0.06, 0.19)	(0.05, 0.16)	(0.02, 0.11)	(0.01, 0.10)	(-0.07, -0.01)
Age (years) -5	-0.25	-0.18	-0.17	-0.14	-0.09
	(-0.59, 0.09)	(-0.51, 0.14)	(-0.45, 0.12)	(-0.42, 0.13)	(-0.34, 0.15)
Female	-0.41	-0.50	-1.05	-1.05	0.00
	(-1.12, 0.30)	(-1.18, 0.17)	(-1.72, -0.37)	(-1.71, -0.39)	(-0.66, 0.66)
Female $\times$ Time	-0.12	-0.10	-0.06	-0.06	-0.09
	(-0.23, -0.01)	(-0.20, -0.01)	(-0.16, 0.05)	(-0.16, 0.04)	(-0.19, 0.01)
Afr Am Ethnicity	1.29	0.96	0.94	0.82	0.54
	(0.73, 1.85)	(0.43, 1.48)	(0.48, 1.41)	(0.37, 1.27)	(0.13, 0.95)
Other Ethnicity	0.11	0.00	0.22	0.17	0.38
	(-0.97, 1.18)	(-1.05, 1.06)	(-0.74, 1.17)	(-0.77, 1.12)	(-0.51, 1.27)
Intercept	-2.21	-2.05	-1.55	-1.49	-0.05
	(-2.66, -1.77)	(-2.48, -1.63)	(-1.89, -1.20)	(-1.83, -1.16)	(-0.36, 0.25)

$0) \in \{0.05, 0.15\}$. In the sample, 25 of 46 girls and 113 of 209 boys were cases. Thus, $\pi(1,1)/\pi(0,1) = (25 \cdot 0.95)/(21 \cdot 0.05) = 22.6$ and $\pi(1,0)/\pi(0,0) \in \{22.4, 6.7\}$. We also specify predictors in auxiliary model (15.5) in two distinct functional forms. In the first, the linear predictor includes Y_{ij}, t_{ij}, age at baseline, gender, African American ethnicity, "other" ethnicity, and all pairwise interactions with Y_{ij}. In the second, all terms were the same as in the first, except that the main effect of t_{ij} and its interaction with Y_{ij} were replaced with time-specific indicator variables.

Results from these analyses are displayed in Table 15.3. A naive analysis that ignored the design yielded quite different conclusions than analyses that acknowledge the biased study design for the time trend in boys (i.e., the main effect of time). Study wave, t_{ij}, was positively associated with ADHD prevalence in boys ($G_i = 0$) in the bias corrected analyses and negatively associated with ADHD in the naive analysis. The association of gender at baseline appeared unassociated with ADHD prevalence in the naive analysis. Though it was estimated to be negatively associated with ADHD prevalence in both SOR-based analyses, it was only statistically significantly associated under the higher prevalence assumption for boys. In this analysis, the assumption regarding the linear predictor in auxiliary model (15.5) did not have a substantial impact on estimates from regression parameters. Interestingly, in the four SOR-based analyses, the time trend among females agreed quite closely. That is, they were all quite close to 0, as can be seen by the fact that the coefficients for t_{ij} and $t_{ij} \cdot G_i$ were similar in magnitude and in the opposite directions.

15.5 Conclusion

In this chapter, we have elaborated study designs for longitudinal data which aim to enhance outcome variability and outcome-exposure covariability through nonrepresentative sampling. We have presented two leading examples: One with a continuous response in which sampling is based on subject-specific intercept, time-slope, or both; and, one with a binary response in which sampling is based on an auxiliary variable related to positive responses through the longitudinal trajectory. In each case, we have also presented previously developed and well-characterized methods of analysis. Whereas these analysis methods are of strong statistical interest, other designs may require variations on these approaches. More important is the message about exploiting the concepts herein to increase statistical precision for model parameters and tests in the context of epidemiologic designs. Biostatisticians play a critical role in conveying the strength of these ideas to their epidemiologist colleagues.

Appendix

Details on Equation (15.4):

By Bayes' Theorem, we may relate the marginal odds in the pseudo-population that is represented by the sample ($S_i = 1$) to the marginal odds in the target population model (15.1) with

$$\frac{P(Y_{ij} = 1|\boldsymbol{X}_i, S_i = 1)}{P(Y_{ij} = 0|\boldsymbol{X}_i, S_i = 1)} = \frac{\mu_{ij}^S}{1 - \mu_{ij}^S} = \frac{\mu_{ij}^p}{1 - \mu_{ij}^p} \frac{\rho_{ij}(1, \boldsymbol{X}_i)}{\rho_{ij}(0, \boldsymbol{X}_i)} .$$

Details on Equations (15.5)-(15.6):

Again, via Bayes' Theorem, calculations yield an odds model for Z_i in the pseudo-population represented by the sample,

$$\frac{P(Z_i = 1|Y_{ij} = y, \boldsymbol{X}_i, S_i = 1)}{P(Z_i = 0|Y_{ij} = y, \boldsymbol{X}_i, S_i = 1)} = \frac{\lambda_{ij}^S(y, \boldsymbol{X}_i)}{1 - \lambda_{ij}^S(y, \boldsymbol{X}_i)} = \frac{\lambda_{ij}^P(y, \boldsymbol{X}_i)}{1 - \lambda_{ij}^P(y, \boldsymbol{X}_i)} \frac{\pi(1, X_{1i})}{\pi(0, X_{1i})} ,$$

$y = 0, 1$, where $\lambda_{ij}^S(y, \boldsymbol{X}_i) = P(Z_i = 1|Y_{ij} = y, \boldsymbol{X}_i, S_i = 1)$, yielding (15.5). Additionally, due to (15.2)-(15.3),

$$\rho_{ij}(y, \boldsymbol{X}_i) = \pi(0, X_{1i})\{1 - \lambda_{ij}^P(y, \boldsymbol{X}_i)\} + \pi(1, X_{1i})\lambda_{ij}^P(y, \boldsymbol{X}_i) , \quad y = 0, 1 ,$$

from which we can write ratio (15.6).

Bibliography

Anderson, J. A. (1972). Separate sample logistic discrimination. *Biometrika*, **59**, 19–35.

Azzalini, A. (1994). Logistic regression for autocorrelated data with application to repeated measures. *Biometrika*, **81**, 767–775. Correction **84**, 989.

Begg, M. D. and Parides, M. K. (2003). Separation of individual-level and cluster-level covariate effects in regression analysis of correlated data. *Statistics in Medicine*, **22**, 2591–2602.

Borgan, Ø. and Langholz, B. (1993). Nonparametric estimation of relative mortality from nested case-control studies. *Biometrics*, **49**, 593–602.

Borgan, Ø., Goldstein, L., and Langholz, B. (1995). Methods for the analysis of sampled cohort data in the Cox proportional hazards model. *The Annals of Statistics*, **23**, 1749–1778.

Breslow, N. E. (1996). Statistics in epidemiology: The case-control study. *Journal of the American Statistical Association*, **91**, 14–28.

Breslow, N. E. and Cain, K. C. (1988). Logistic regression for two-stage case-control data. *Biometrika*, **75**, 11–20.

Breslow, N. E. and Chatterjee, N. (1999). Design and analysis of two-phase studies with binary outcome applied to Wilms tumour prognosis. *Journal of the Royal Statistical Society, Series C: Applied Statistics*, **48**, 457–468.

Breslow, N. E. and Clayton, D. G. (1993). Approximate inference in generalized linear mixed models. *Journal of the American Statistical Association*, **88**, 9–25.

Breslow, N. E. and Day, N. E. (1980). *Statistical Methods in Cancer Research. Vol. 1: The Analysis of Case-control Studies*. IARC, Lyon.

Breslow, N. E. and Holubkov, R. (1997). Maximum likelihood estimation of logistic regression parameters under two-phase, outcome-dependent sampling. *Journal of the Royal Statistical Society: Series B (Statistical Methodology)*, **59**, 447–461.

CAMP Research Group (1999). The Childhood Asthma Management Program (CAMP): Design, rationale, and methods. *Controlled Clinical Trials*, **20**, 91–120.

CAMP Research Group (2000). Long-term effects of budesonide or nedocrimil in children with asthma. *New England Journal of Medicine*, **343**, 1054–1063.

Carroll, R., Ruppert, D., Stefanski, D. R., and Crainiceanu, C. M. (2006). *Measurement Error in Nonlinear Models: A Modern Perspective. 2nd ed.* Chapman & Hall/CRC, Boca Raton.

Cornfield, J. (1951). A method of estimating comparative rates from clinical data; applications to cancer of the lung, breast, and cervix. *Journal of the National Cancer Institute*, **11**, 1269–1275.

Diggle, P., Heagerty, P. J., Liang, K.-Y., and Zeger, S. L. (2002). *Analysis of Longitudinal Data*. Oxford University Press, Oxford.

Fitzmaurice, G. M., Laird, N. M., and Ware, J. H. (2012). *Applied Longitudinal Analysis. 2nd ed.* John Wiley & Sons, New York.

Franklin, J. M., Schneeweiss, S., Polinski, J. M., and Rassen, J. A. (2014). Plasmode simulation for the evaluation of pharmacoepidemiologic methods in complex healthcare databases. *Computational Statistics & Data Analysis*, **72**, 219–226.

Hartung, C., Willcutt, E., Lahey, B., Pelham, W., Loney, J., Stein, M., and Keenan, K. (2002). Sex differences in young children who meet criteria for attention deficit hyperactivity disorder. *Journal of Clinical Child & Adolescent Psychology*, **31**, 453–464.

Heagerty, P. J. (1999). Marginally specified logistic-normal models for longitudinal binary data. *Biometrics*, **55**, 688–698.

Heagerty, P. J. and Zeger, S. L. (2000). Multivariate continuation ratio models: Connections and caveats. *Biometrics*, **56**, 719–732.

Horvitz, D. G. and Thompson, D. J. (1952). A generalization of sampling without replacement from a finite universe. *Journal of the American Statistical Association*, **47**, 663–685.

Lahey, B., Pelham, W., Stein, M., Loney, J., Trapani, C., Nugent, K., Kipp, H., Schmidt, E., Lee, S., Cale, M., Gold, E., Hartung, C., Willcutt, E., and Baumann, B. (1998). Validity of DSM-IV attention-deficit/hyperactivity disorder for younger children. *Journal of the American Academy of Child and Adolescent Psychiatry*, **37**, 695–702.

Laird, N. M. and Ware, J. H. (1982). Random-effects models for longitudinal data. *Biometrics*, **38**, 963–974.

Langholz, B. and Goldstein, L. (1996). Risk set sampling in epidemiologic cohort studies. *Statistical Science*, **11**, 35–53.

Lawless, J. F., Kalbfleisch, J., and Wild, C. J. (1999). Semiparametric methods for response-selective and missing data problems in regression. *Journal of the Royal Statistical Society Series B-Statistical Methodology*, **61**, 413–438.

Liang, K.-Y. and Zeger, S. L. (1986). Longitudinal data analysis using generalized linear models. *Biometrika*, **73**, 13–22.

Lindstrom, M. and Bates, D. (1988). Newton-Raphson and EM algorithms for linear mixed-effects models for repeated-measures data. *Journal of the American Statistical Association*, **83**, 1014–1022.

Little, R. J. and Rubin, D. B. (2014). *Statistical Analysis with Missing Data*. John Wiley & Sons, New York.

Maclure, M. (1991). The case-crossover design: A method for studying transient effects on the risk of acute events. *American Journal of Epidemiology*, **133**, 144–153.

Manski, C. F. and Lerman, S. R. (1977). The estimation of choice probabilities from choice based samples. *Econometrica*, **45**, 1977–1988.

McCulloch, C. E. and Searle, S. R. (2001). *Generalized, Linear and Mixed Models*. Wiley, New York.

McDaniel, L. S., Schildcrout, J. S., Schisterman, E. F., and Rathouz, P. J. (2016). Generalized linear models for longitudinal data with biased sampling designs: A sequential offsetted regressions approach. Technical report, University of Wisconsin.

Navidi, W. (1998). Bidirectional case-crossover designs for exposures with time trends. *Biometrics*, **54**, 596–605.

Neuhaus, J., Scott, A., and Wild, C. (2006). Family-specific approaches to the analysis of case-control family data. *Biometrics*, **62**, 488–494.

Neuhaus, J. M. and Kalbfleisch, J. D. (1998). Between- and within-cluster covariate effects in the analysis of clustered data. *Biometrics*, **54**, 638–645.

Neuhaus, J. M., Scott, A. J., Wild, C. J., Jiang, Y., McCulloch, C. E., and Boylan, R. (2014). Likelihood-based analysis of longitudinal data from outcome-related sampling designs. *Biometrics*, **70**, 44–52.

Pepe, M. S. and Anderson, G. L. (1994). A cautionary note on inference for marginal regression models with longitudinal data and general correlated response data. *Communications in Statistics: Simulation and Computation*, **23**, 939–951.

Prentice, R. L. (1986). A case-cohort design for epidemiologic cohort studies and disease prevention trials. *Biometrika*, **73**, 1–11.

Prentice, R. L. and Pyke, R. (1979). Logistic disease incidence models and case-control studies. *Biometrika*, **66**, 403–412.

Rathouz, P. J. and Gao, L. (2009). Generalized linear models with unspecified reference distribution. *Biostatistics*, **10**, 205–218.

Robins, J. M., Rotnitzky, A., and Zhao, L. P. (1994). Estimation of regression coefficients when some regressors are not always observed. *Journal of the American Statistical Association*, **89**, 846–866.

Royall, R. M. (1986). Model robust confidence intervals using maximum likelihood estimators. *International Statistical Review*, **54**, 221–226.

Rubin, D. B. (1976). Inference and missing data. *Biometrika*, **63**, 581–592.

Schafer, J. L. and Graham, J. W. (2002). Missing data: Our view of the state of the art. *Psychological Methods*, **7**, 147–177.

Schildcrout, J. S. and Heagerty, P. J. (2005). Regression analysis of longitudinal binary data with time-dependent environmental covariates: Bias and efficiency. *Biostatistics*, **6**, 633–652.

Schildcrout, J. S. and Rathouz, P. J. (2010). Longitudinal studies of binary response data following case–control and stratified case–control sampling: Design and analysis. *Biometrics*, **66**, 365–373.

Schildcrout, J. S., Mumford, S. L., Chen, Z., Heagerty, P. J., and Rathouz, P. J. (2012). Outcome-dependent sampling for longitudinal binary response data based on a time-varying auxiliary variable. *Statistics in Medicine*, **31**, 2441–2456.

Schildcrout, J. S., Garbett, S. P., and Heagerty, P. J. (2013). Outcome vector dependent sampling with longitudinal continuous response data: Stratified sampling based on summary statistics. *Biometrics*, **69**, 405–416.

Schildcrout, J. S., Rathouz, P. J., Zelnick, L. R., Garbett, S. P., and Heagerty, P. J. (2015). Biased sampling designs to improve research efficiency: Factors influencing pulmonary function over time in children with asthma. *The Annals of Applied Statistics*, **9**, 731–753.

Scott, A. and Wild, C. (2001). Case–control studies with complex sampling. *Journal of the Royal Statistical Society: Series C (Applied Statistics)*, **50**, 389–401.

Scott, A. and Wild, C. (2002). On the robustness of weighted methods for fitting models to case–control data. *Journal of the Royal Statistical Society: Series B (Statistical Methodology)*, **64**, 207–219.

Stiratelli, R., Laird, N., and Ware, J. H. (1984). Random-effects models for serial observations with binary response. *Biometrics*, **40**, 961–971.

Whittemore, A. S. (1995). Logistic regression of family data from case-control studies. *Biometrika*, **82**, 57–67. Correction. **84**, 989–990.

Zeger, S. L. and Liang, K.-Y. (1986). Longitudinal data analysis for discrete and continuous outcomes. *Biometrics*, **42**, 121–130.

Part IV

Case-Control Studies for Time-to-Event Data

16

Cohort Sampling for Time-to-Event Data: An Overview

Ørnulf Borgan and Sven Ove Samuelsen

University of Oslo

16.1   Introduction

Cohort studies are considered to be the most reliable study design in epidemiology, while case-control studies are easier and quicker to implement. The logistic regression model, which is typically used in traditional case-control studies (cf. Chapters 3 and 4), does not explicitly consider the time aspect of the development of a disease. In contrast, in cohort studies of the time to death of a particular cause or the time to onset of a specific disease (generically denoted "failure"), it is common to use Cox's regression model to assess the influence of risk factors and other covariates on mortality or morbidity. In this chapter, we will assume that failures (i.e., deaths or disease occurrences) in the cohort are modelled by Cox's regression model, and we discuss how various cohort sampling designs make it possible to adopt Cox regression also for certain types of case-control data. The purpose of the chapter is both to give an overview of case-control methods for failure time data and to provide a background for the succeeding chapters in Part IV of the handbook.

There are two main types of cohort sampling designs: nested case-control studies and case-cohort studies. For both types of designs, covariate information has to be recorded for all failing individuals ("cases"), but only for a sample of the individuals who do not fail ("controls"). This may drastically reduce the workload of data collection and error checking compared to a full cohort study. Further when covariate measurements are based on stored biological material, it may save valuable material for future studies.

The two types of cohort sampling designs differ in the way controls are selected. For nested case-control sampling, one selects for each case a small number of controls from those at risk at the case's failure time, and a new sample of controls is selected for each case. For the case-cohort design, a subcohort is selected from the full cohort, and the individuals in the subcohort are used as controls at all failure times when they are at risk. In their original forms, the designs use simple random sampling without replacement for the selection of controls and subcohort (Thomas, 1977; Prentice, 1986). Later the designs have been modified to allow for stratified random sampling (Langholz and Borgan, 1995; Borgan *et al.*, 2000).

In this chapter we present nested case-control and case-cohort designs with simple or stratified random sampling of the controls/subcohort, and we review basic results on statistical inference for Cox regression for these cohort sampling designs. Later chapters in Part IV of the handbook give more detailed treatments of cohort sampling methods and also discuss how other regression models for time-to-event data may be used for sampled cohort data. Case-cohort studies and nested case-control studies are discussed further in Chapters 17 and 18, respectively, while in Chapter 19 it is described how one may treat nested case-control data as if they were case-cohort data with a nonstandard sampling scheme for the subcohort. The commonly used inference methods for case-cohort and nested case-control data only use information for individuals in the case-control sample (i.e., the cases and controls/subcohort). Chapters 20 and 21 discuss methods that use all available information for the full cohort; multiple imputation is considered in Chapter 20 while maximum likelihood estimation is discussed in Chapter 21. The topic of Chapter 22 differs somewhat from the other chapters in Part IV. In this chapter it is shown how the self-controlled case series method may be used to evaluate the association between an adverse event and a time-varying exposure. The method only uses information from the cases, and it has been applied most frequently in pharmacoepidemiology, notably in the study of vaccine safety.

No data examples are provided in this chapter. But the later chapters in Part IV give a number of practical data illustrations.

16.2   Cox regression for cohort data

We first review Cox regression for cohort data. Consider a cohort $\mathcal{C} = \{1, \ldots, N\}$ of N independent individuals, and let $\lambda_i(t)$ be the hazard rate for the ith individual with vector of covariates $\mathbf{x}_i$. The time variable t may be age, time since the onset of a disease, or some other time scale relevant to the problem at hand. The covariates may be time-fixed or time-dependent, but we have suppressed the time-dependency from the notation. We assume that the covariates of individual i are related to its hazard rate by Cox's regression model:

$$\lambda_i(t) = \lambda(t \mid \mathbf{x}_i) = \lambda_0(t) \exp(\boldsymbol{\beta}^{\mathrm{T}} \mathbf{x}_i). \tag{16.1}$$

Here $\boldsymbol{\beta}$ is a vector of regression coefficients describing the effects of the covariates, while the baseline hazard rate $\lambda_0(t)$ corresponds to the hazard rate of an individual with all covariates equal to zero. In particular we may interpret e^{β_j} as the hazard ratio (or more loosely speaking, relative risk) per unit change in the jth covariate, when all other covariates are kept the same.

The individuals in the cohort may be followed over different periods of time, from an entry time to an exit time corresponding to failure or censoring. The risk set $\mathcal{R}(t)$ is the collection of all individuals who are under observation just before time t, and $n(t) = |\mathcal{R}(t)|$ is the number at risk at that time. We denote by $t_1 < t_2 < \cdots < t_{n_d}$ the times when failures are observed and, assuming no tied failure times, we let i_j denote the individual who fails at t_j.

We assume throughout that late entries and censorings are independent in the sense that the additional knowledge of which individuals have entered the study or have been censored before time t does not carry information on the risks of failure at t, cf. Kalbfleisch and Prentice (2002, Sections 1.3 and 6.2). Then the vector of regression coefficients in (16.1) is estimated by $\widehat{\boldsymbol{\beta}}$, the value of $\boldsymbol{\beta}$ maximizing Cox's partial likelihood

$$L_{\mathrm{full}}(\boldsymbol{\beta}) = \prod_{j=1}^{n_d} \frac{\exp(\boldsymbol{\beta}^{\mathrm{T}} \mathbf{x}_{i_j})}{\sum_{k \in \mathcal{R}(t_j)} \exp(\boldsymbol{\beta}^{\mathrm{T}} \mathbf{x}_k)}. \tag{16.2}$$

It is well known that $\widehat{\boldsymbol{\beta}}$ can be treated as an ordinary maximum likelihood estimator (Andersen and Gill, 1982). In particular, $\widehat{\boldsymbol{\beta}}$ is approximately multivariate normally distributed around the true value of $\boldsymbol{\beta}$ with a covariance matrix that may be estimated by the inverse information matrix, and nested models may be compared by likelihood ratio tests.

16.3 Nested case-control studies

In this section we consider nested case-control studies. We start out by a general description of how the controls are sampled. Then we consider the classical nested case-control design where the controls are selected by simple random sampling and the situation where the controls are selected by stratified random sampling ("counter-matching"). Other sampling schemes for the controls are discussed in Chapter 18. Finally we discuss nested case-control designs where the controls are matched on one or more confounding variables.

16.3.1 Selection of controls

The controls in a nested case-control study are selected as follows. If a case occurs at time t (in the study time scale), one selects a small number of controls among the nonfailing individuals in the risk set $\mathcal{R}(t)$. (In Sections 16.3.2 and 16.3.3 we describe two sampling schemes for the controls.) The set consisting of the case and the selected controls is called a sampled risk set and denoted $\widetilde{\mathcal{R}}(t)$. Covariate values are ascertained for the individuals in the sampled risk sets, but are not needed for the remaining individuals in the cohort.

Figure 16.1 illustrates the basic features of a nested case-control study for a hypothetical cohort of ten individuals when one control is selected per case. Each individual in the cohort

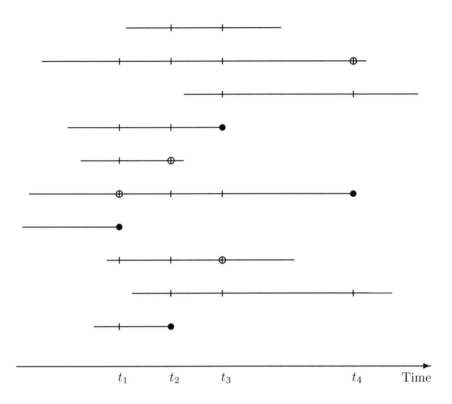

FIGURE 16.1
Illustration of nested case-control sampling, with one control per case, from a hypothetical cohort of ten individuals. Each individual is represented by a line starting at an entry time and ending at an exit time corresponding to failure or censoring. Failure times are indicated by dots (•), potential controls are indicated by bars (|), and the sampled controls are indicated by circles (○).

is represented by a horizontal line starting at some entry time and ending at some exit time. If the exit time corresponds to a failure, this is represented by a "•" in the figure. In the hypothetical cohort considered, four individuals are observed to fail. The potential controls for the four cases are indicated by a "|" in the figure, and are given as all individuals at risk at the times of the failures, cases excluded. Among the potential controls one is selected as indicated by a "○" in the figure. The four sampled risk sets are then represented by the four •, ○ pairs in Figure 16.1. Note that the selection of controls is done independently at the different failure times. Thus subjects may serve as controls for multiple cases, and a case may serve as control for other cases that failed when the case was at risk. For example, the case at time t_4 in the figure had been selected as control at the earlier time t_1.

A basic assumption for valid inference in nested case-control studies is that not only delayed entries and censorings, but also the sampling of controls, are independent in the sense that the additional knowledge of which individuals have entered the study have been censored or have been selected as controls before time t does not carry information on the risks of failure at t. This assumption will be violated if, e.g., in a prevention trial, individuals selected as controls change their behavior in such a way that their risk of failure is different from similar individuals who have not been selected as controls.

16.3.2   Simple random sampling

In the classical form of the nested case-control design (Thomas, 1977), the controls are selected by simple random sampling. More specifically, if a case occurs at time t, one selects at random m controls from the $n(t) - 1$ nonfailing individuals in the risk set $\mathcal{R}(t)$. So the sampled risk set $\widetilde{\mathcal{R}}(t)$ contains $m + 1$ individuals, the case and its m controls.

For classical nested case-control data, the vector of regression coefficients in (16.1) may be estimated by $\widehat{\boldsymbol{\beta}}_{\mathrm{ncc}}$, the value of $\boldsymbol{\beta}$ that maximizes the partial likelihood

$$L_{\mathrm{ncc}}(\boldsymbol{\beta}) = \prod_{j=1}^{n_d} \frac{\exp(\boldsymbol{\beta}^{\mathrm{T}} \mathbf{x}_{i_j})}{\sum_{k \in \widetilde{\mathcal{R}}(t_j)} \exp(\boldsymbol{\beta}^{\mathrm{T}} \mathbf{x}_k)}, \tag{16.3}$$

cf. Chapter 18. Note that (16.3) is similar to the full cohort partial likelihood (16.2), except that the sum in the denominator is only over subjects in the sampled risk set. Also note that (16.3) coincides with a conditional likelihood for matched case-control data under a logistic regression model (Chapter 4).

Inference concerning the regression coefficients, using usual large sample likelihood methods, can be based on the partial likelihood (16.3). In particular, $\widehat{\boldsymbol{\beta}}_{\mathrm{ncc}}$ is approximately multivariate normally distributed around the true value of $\boldsymbol{\beta}$ with a covariance matrix that may be estimated by the inverse information matrix (Goldstein and Langholz, 1992; Borgan *et al.*, 1995). Furthermore nested models may be compared by likelihood ratio tests. For computing one may use standard software for Cox regression (like `coxph` in the `survival` library in R), formally treating the label of the sampled risk sets as a stratification variable in the Cox regression, or software for conditional logistic regression.

The relative efficiency of a simple nested case-control study compared to a full cohort study is the ratio of the variance of the estimator for full cohort data to the variance of the estimator based on nested case-control data. If there is only one covariate in the model, and its regression coefficient equals zero, the relative efficiency of the nested case-control design compared to a full cohort study is $m/(m+1)$, independent of censoring and covariate distributions (Goldstein and Langholz, 1992). When the regression coefficient differs from zero, and when two or more regression coefficients are estimated, the efficiency may be lower (Borgan and Olsen, 1999).

16.3.3   Counter-matching

To select a simple random sample of controls, we only need to know the at risk status for the individuals in the cohort. Often, however, some additional information is available for all cohort members, e.g., a surrogate measure of an exposure of interest may be available for everyone. Langholz and Borgan (1995) have developed a stratified version of the nested case-control design, which makes it possible to incorporate such information into the sampling process in order to obtain a more informative sample of controls. For this design, which is called *counter-matching*, one applies the information available for all cohort members to classify each individual at risk into one of, say, S strata. We denote by $\mathcal{R}_s(t)$ the subset of the risk set $\mathcal{R}(t)$ that belongs to stratum s, and let $n_s(t) = |\mathcal{R}_s(t)|$ be the number at risk in this stratum just before time t. If a failure occurs at time t, we want to sample our controls such that the sampled risk set will contain a specified number m_s of individuals from each stratum $s = 1, \ldots, S$. This is achieved as follows. Assume that an individual i who belongs to stratum $s(i)$ fails at t. Then for each $s \neq s(i)$ one samples randomly without replacement

m_s controls from $\mathcal{R}_s(t)$. From the case's stratum $s(i)$ only $m_{s(i)} - 1$ controls are sampled. The failing individual is, however, included in the sampled risk set $\widetilde{\mathcal{R}}(t)$, so this contains a total of m_s from each stratum. Even though it is not made explicit in the notation, we note that the classification into strata may be time-dependent; e.g., one may stratify according to the quartiles of a time-dependent surrogate measure of an exposure of main interest. A crucial assumption, however, is that the information on which the stratification is based has to be known just before time t.

Inference for counter-matched nested case-control data may be based on a partial likelihood similar to (16.3). However, as shown in Chapter 18, weights have to be inserted in the partial likelihood in order to reflect the different sampling probabilities. Specifically, using the weights $w_k(t) = n_{s(k)}(t)/m_{s(k)}$ the partial likelihood takes the form

$$L_{\text{cm}}(\boldsymbol{\beta}) = \prod_{j=1}^{n_d} \frac{\exp(\boldsymbol{\beta}^{\mathrm{T}}\mathbf{x}_{i_j})w_{i_j}(t_j)}{\sum_{k\in\widetilde{\mathcal{R}}(t_j)} \exp(\boldsymbol{\beta}^{\mathrm{T}}\mathbf{x}_k)w_k(t_j)}. \tag{16.4}$$

Inference concerning the regression coefficients, using usual large sample maximum likelihood methods, can be based on this weighted partial likelihood (Borgan *et al.*, 1995; Langholz and Borgan, 1995). Moreover, software for Cox regression can be used to fit the model provided the software allows us to specify the logarithm of the weights as "offsets."

16.3.4 A note on additional matching

In order to keep the presentation simple, we have above considered the proportional hazards model (16.1), where the baseline hazard rate is the same for all individuals. Often this will not be reasonable. To control for the effect of one or more confounding variables, one may adopt a stratified version of (16.1), where the baseline hazard differs between population strata generated by the confounders. The regression coefficients are, however, assumed to be the same across population strata. Thus the hazard rate of an individual i from population stratum c is assumed to take the form

$$\lambda_i(t) = \lambda_{0c}(t)\exp(\boldsymbol{\beta}^{\mathrm{T}}\mathbf{x}_i). \tag{16.5}$$

When the stratified proportional hazards model (16.5) applies, the sampling of controls in a nested case-control study should be restricted to the nonfailing individuals at risk in the same population stratum as the case. We say that the controls are matched on the stratification variable(s).

In particular for simple random sampling, if an individual in population stratum c fails at time t, one selects at random m controls from the $n_c(t) - 1$ nonfailing individuals at risk in this population stratum. Then the partial likelihood (16.3) still applies, and the estimation of the vector of regression coefficients is carried out as described in Section 16.3.2. One may also combine matching and counter-matching by selecting the controls among those in the sampling strata used for counter-matching who belong to the population stratum of the case. Then the partial likelihood (16.4) still applies if we use the weights $w_k(t) = n_{s(k),c}(t)/m_{s(k)}$, where $n_{s,c}(t)$ is the number of individuals at risk in sampling stratum s who belong to population stratum c (cf. Chapter 18).

16.4 Case-cohort studies

Case-cohort studies are considered in this section. We start out with the original version of the design, where the subcohort is selected by simple random sampling, and discuss two ways of analysing the case-cohort data. Then the modification with stratified sampling of the subcohort is considered, and finally some comments on post-stratification are given.

16.4.1 Sampling of the subcohort

The case-cohort design was first suggested by Prentice (1986), although related designs without taking a time-perspective into consideration had previously been considered (Kupper *et al.*, 1975; Miettinen, 1982). For the original version of the case-cohort design, one selects a subcohort $\widetilde{C}$ of size $\widetilde{m}$ from the full cohort by simple random sampling. The individuals in the subcohort are used as controls at all failure times when they are at risk. Covariate values are ascertained for the individuals in $\widetilde{C}$ as well as for the cases occurring outside the subcohort, but they are not needed for the nonfailures outside the subcohort. Similarly to nested case-control sampling, an assumption for valid inference is that individuals sampled to the subcohort do not change their behavior in such a way that their risk of failure is different from (similar) individuals who have not been selected to the subcohort. Figure 16.2 illustrates a case-cohort study for the hypothetical cohort of Figure 16.1 with subcohort size $\widetilde{m} = 4$.

16.4.2 Prentice's estimator

Different methods have been suggested for estimating the regression coefficients in (16.1) from case-cohort data. The original suggestion of Prentice (1986) consists of maximizing what is referred to as a pseudo-likelihood:

$$L_\mathrm{P}(\boldsymbol{\beta}) = \prod_{j=1}^{n_d} \frac{\exp(\boldsymbol{\beta}^\mathrm{T}\mathbf{x}_{i_j})}{\sum_{k \in \mathcal{S}(t_j)} \exp(\boldsymbol{\beta}^\mathrm{T}\mathbf{x}_k)}. \tag{16.6}$$

Here the sum in the denominator is over the set $\mathcal{S}(t_j)$ consisting of the subcohort individuals at risk with the case i_j added when it occurs outside the subcohort.

Each factor of the product in (16.6) is of the same form as a factor of the product in the partial likelihood (16.3). In (16.6), however, controls from the subcohort are used over again for each case and thus the factors are dependent. This has the consequence that (16.6) is not a partial likelihood (Langholz and Thomas, 1991). Thus standard errors can not be computed directly from the information matrix derived from (16.6) and likelihood ratio statistics will not follow chi-square distributions. But (16.6) provides unbiased estimating equations (Prentice, 1986), and one may show that the maximum pseudo-likelihood estimator $\widehat{\boldsymbol{\beta}}_\mathrm{P}$ is approximately normally distributed (Self and Prentice, 1988).

More specifically, for the information matrix $\mathbf{I}_\mathrm{P}(\boldsymbol{\beta}) = -\partial^2 \log L_\mathrm{P}(\boldsymbol{\beta})/\partial\boldsymbol{\beta}^\mathrm{T}\partial\boldsymbol{\beta}$ we have under standard assumptions that $N^{-1}\mathbf{I}_\mathrm{P}(\widehat{\boldsymbol{\beta}}_\mathrm{P}) \to \boldsymbol{\Sigma}$ in probability, where $\boldsymbol{\Sigma}$ is the same limit as for the cohort information matrix. For the case-cohort estimator we then have that

$$\sqrt{N}(\widehat{\boldsymbol{\beta}}_\mathrm{P} - \boldsymbol{\beta}) \xrightarrow{d} \mathrm{N}\left(\mathbf{0}, \boldsymbol{\Sigma}^{-1} + \frac{1-p}{p}\boldsymbol{\Sigma}^{-1}\boldsymbol{\Xi}\boldsymbol{\Sigma}^{-1}\right), \tag{16.7}$$

where p is the (limiting) proportion of the cohort that is sampled to the subcohort, and $\boldsymbol{\Xi}$ is the limit in probability of the covariance matrix of the individual score-contributions

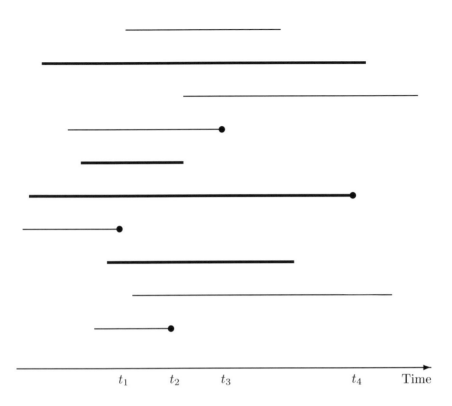

FIGURE 16.2
Illustration of case-cohort sampling, with subcohort size $\widetilde{m} = 4$, from the hypothetical cohort of Figure 16.1. Failure times are indicated by dots ($\bullet$), and the individuals in the subcohort are indicated by thick lines.

(Self and Prentice, 1988; Borgan *et al.*, 2000). An interpretation of the covariance matrix for $\widehat{\beta}_P$ is that it is the sum of the covariance matrix for the cohort estimator and a term that accounts for additional variation due to sampling of the subcohort.

For testing simple associations in Cox's model (16.1), the relative efficiency of a simple nested case-control study with m controls per case is $m/(m+1)$ when compared to a full cohort study (cf. Section 16.3.2). It does not seem possible to derive a similar simple result for the case-cohort design (Self and Prentice, 1988). But although published results are somewhat conflicting (Langholz and Thomas, 1991; Barlow *et al.*, 1999), the relative efficiencies of nested case-control and case-cohort studies seem to be about the same when they involve the same number of individuals for whom covariate information has to be collected. However, case-cohort studies may be more sensitive to large amounts of right censoring and left truncation (Langholz and Thomas, 1991).

The covariance matrix of the case-cohort estimator can be estimated by a straightforward plug-in procedure using (16.7). The estimate of $\boldsymbol{\Sigma}$ is obtained from $\mathbf{I}_P(\widehat{\boldsymbol{\beta}}_P)$ and in programs that allow for calculation of score-contributions and *dfbetas*, the covariance matrix $\boldsymbol{\Xi}$ is just replaced by the empirical counterpart; see Therneau and Li (1999) for details. An alternative to this model based estimator is to use a robust sandwich type estimator (Lin and Ying, 1993; Barlow, 1994).

16.4.3 IPW estimators

Prentice's pseudo-likelihood (16.6) can be calculated for time-dependent covariates also when covariate information for cases outside the subcohort are ascertained only at their failure times. This may be useful in some situations. However, with fixed covariates (or when the full covariate paths of time-dependent covariates are easily retrieved) it would seem that information may be lost by this estimating procedure. Another proposal for case-cohort studies, first suggested by Kalbfleisch and Lawless (1988), is to maximize the weighted likelihood (or, more precisely, weighted pseudo-likelihood)

$$L_{\mathrm{W}}(\boldsymbol{\beta}) = \prod_{j=1}^{n_d} \frac{\exp(\boldsymbol{\beta}^{\mathrm{T}} \mathbf{x}_{i_j})}{\sum_{k \in \widetilde{\mathcal{S}}(t_j)} \exp(\boldsymbol{\beta}^{\mathrm{T}} \mathbf{x}_k) w_k}, \tag{16.8}$$

where $\widetilde{\mathcal{S}}(t_j)$ is the set consisting of the subcohort individuals at risk at time t_j together with all cases that are at risk at that time. The weights are $w_k = 1$ for cases (whether in the subcohort or not) and $w_k = 1/p_k$ for nonfailures in the subcohort, where the p_k's are appropriate inclusion probabilities. Note that we have assumed that cases are sampled with probability one, so inverse probability weighting (IPW) is used. The estimator is thus an application of the Horvitz-Thompson method (Horvitz and Thompson, 1952). IPW estimation for case-cohort studies is further discussed in Chapter 17.

Kalbfleisch and Lawless (1988) assumed that the inclusion probabilities p_k were known. Later Borgan *et al.* (2000), in the context of stratified case-cohort studies (Section 16.4.4), suggested to set p_k equal to the proportion of nonfailures in the subcohort compared to all nonfailures. We denote the estimator thus obtained by $\widehat{\boldsymbol{\beta}}_{\mathrm{W}}$. For a standard case-cohort study with simple random sampling of the subcohort, this estimator coincides with a suggestion by Chen and Lo (1999). We may show that

$$\sqrt{N}(\widehat{\boldsymbol{\beta}}_{\mathrm{W}} - \boldsymbol{\beta}) \xrightarrow{d} \mathrm{N}(\mathbf{0}, \boldsymbol{\Sigma}^{-1} + \frac{q(1-p)}{p} \boldsymbol{\Sigma}^{-1} \boldsymbol{\Xi}_0 \boldsymbol{\Sigma}^{-1}), \tag{16.9}$$

where $\boldsymbol{\Sigma}$ and p are defined in connection with (16.7), q is the (limiting) proportion of nonfailures in the cohort, and $\boldsymbol{\Xi}_0$ is the limit in probability of the covariance matrix of the individual score-contributions among nonfailures. The result is a special case of (16.10) below. Since $q < 1$ and the variance of score-contributions over nonfailures is smaller than over the full cohort, we find, by comparing (16.7) and (16.9), that the variance of $\widehat{\boldsymbol{\beta}}_{\mathrm{W}}$ is smaller than the variance of the original Prentice estimator $\widehat{\boldsymbol{\beta}}_{\mathrm{P}}$. However, in practice this matters little unless there is a fairly large proportion of cases, and in such situations the case-cohort design will typically not be used.

Estimation of the covariance matrix of the IPW estimator may be performed by a slight modification of the plug-in procedure described at the end of Section 16.4.2; see, e.g., Langholz and Jiao (2007). We may also use the robust estimator, although now this estimator is theoretically conservative.

16.4.4 Stratified sampling of the subcohort

In Section 16.3.3 we discuss stratified sampling of the controls for the nested case-control design. In a similar manner one may adopt a stratified version of the case-cohort design (Samuelsen, 1989; Borgan *et al.*, 2000). One then applies information that is available for all cohort subjects to classify the cohort individuals into S distinct strata. With n_s individuals in stratum s, one selects a random sample of $\widetilde{m}_s$ individuals to the subcohort $\widetilde{\mathcal{C}}$ from each stratum s; $s = 1, 2, \ldots, S$. By selecting the subcohort by stratified sampling, one may increase the variation in the subcohort of a covariate of main interst, and thereby achieve a more efficient estimation of the effect of this covariate (Samuelsen, 1989; Borgan *et al.*, 2000).

As for the simple case-cohort design, there are different options for analysing stratified case-cohort data. Borgan *et al.* (2000) discussed three estimators. We will here restrict attention to their Estimator II, denoted $\widehat{\boldsymbol{\beta}}_{\mathrm{II}}$, which is a generalization of the IPW estimator of Section 16.4.3. The estimator is further discussed in Chapter 17. For this estimator we use the weighted likelihood (16.8) with weights $w_k = 1$ for cases and $w_k = n_s^0/\widetilde{m}_s^0$ for nonfailing subcohort members from stratum s. Here n_s^0 and $\widetilde{m}_s^0$ are the number of nonfailures in the cohort and subcohort, respectively, who belong to stratum s.

For Estimator II we have (Borgan *et al.*, 2000; Samuelsen *et al.*, 2007)

$$\sqrt{N}(\widehat{\boldsymbol{\beta}}_{\mathrm{II}} - \boldsymbol{\beta}) \xrightarrow{d} \mathrm{N}(\mathbf{0}, \boldsymbol{\Sigma}^{-1} + \sum_{s=1}^{S} \frac{q_s(1 - p_s)}{p_s} \boldsymbol{\Sigma}^{-1} \boldsymbol{\Xi}_{0s} \boldsymbol{\Sigma}^{-1}). \tag{16.10}$$

Here q_s is the (limiting) proportion of nonfailures who belong to stratum s and p_s is the (limiting) proportion of nonfailures in this stratum who are sampled to the subcohort. Furthermore $\boldsymbol{\Xi}_{0s}$ is the limit in probability of the covariance matrix of the individual score-contributions among nonfailures in stratum s. We may estimate the covariance matrix of Estimator II by a plug-in procedure using (16.10); details are provided in Langholz and Jiao (2007) and Samuelsen *et al.* (2007). For stratified case-cohort data, one should avoid using the robust covariance estimator as this tends to give variance estimates that can be quite a bit too large.

16.4.5   Post-stratification and calibration

When describing the stratified case-cohort design in Section 16.4.4 we assume, for the ease of presentation, that the cohort is stratified according to some background information (like a surrogate measure for exposure) that is available for everyone. However, all information that is recorded for every cohort member may be used for stratification, including information on entry and follow-up times and whether an individual is a case or not. When such additional information is used to stratify the cohort, it is common to say that the cohort is post-stratified.

Note that we may use stratified sampling to select the subcohort at the outset of the study, and later redefine the strata by post-stratification. In fact, this is what we do in Section 16.4.4 when we define the cases as a separate stratum. Another possibility is to post-stratify on follow-up time (appropriately partitioned). As shown by Samuelsen *et al.* (2007), this corresponds to the "local averaging" estimator of Chen (2001).

The idea of post-stratification can also be applied to background variables known for the entire cohort. Suppose a simple or stratified case-cohort sample has been selected at the outset of a study. At the analysis stage, one may then post-stratify according to known background variables, thereby modifying the sampling fractions. Such an approach may lead to improved efficiency when the background variables are strongly related to the covariates of the Cox model. In particular, if the background variables are included as covariates in (16.1), the efficiency of the corresponding regression coefficients will improve greatly. But such an approach will break down with very fine post-stratification. Then one option is to modify the weights using the calibration technique discussed in Chapter 17 so that they better reflect the full cohort information.

16.5   Comparison of the cohort sampling designs

If one wants to apply a cohort sampling design, a choice between a nested case-control and a case-cohort study has to be made. The choice between the two designs depends on a number of issues, and it has to be made on a case to case basis. We here discuss some issues that should be considered to arrive at a useful design for a particular study.

16.5.1   Statistical efficiency and analysis

As mentioned in Section 16.4.2, the statistical efficiencies of the nested case-control and case-cohort designs seem to be about the same when they involve comparable numbers of individuals for whom covariate information has to be ascertained. Thus efficiency considerations are usually not important for design decisions when studying a single disease endpoint. If multiple endpoints are of interest, the situation may be different; cf. Section 16.5.2.

The statistical analysis of nested case-control data by Cox's regression model (16.1) parallels the analysis of cohort data, and it may be performed by means of the usual partial likelihood based methods and standard Cox regression software (or by software for conditional logistic regression). For case-cohort data, likelihood methods do not apply, and even though standard Cox regression software may be "tricked" to do the analysis (Therneau and Li, 1999; Langholz and Jiao, 2007), this has made inference for case-cohort data more cumbersome. But with the development of specialized computer software for case-cohort data (like cch in the survival library in R), this drawback has become less important.

In a nested case-control study, the controls are sampled from those at risk at the cases' failure times. Therefore one has to decide the time scale to be used in the analysis (e.g., age or time since the onset of a disease) before the controls are selected. This does not apply to a case-cohort study, where the subcohort is selected without consideration of at risk status. Moreover, while other failure time models than (16.1) may be used to analyze case-cohort data (cf. Chapter 17), the analysis options for nested case-control data are more restricted. Thus case-cohort data allow for more flexibility in model choice at the analysis stage (see, however, Section 16.6 and Chapter 19).

16.5.2   Study workflow and multiple endpoints

Cohort sampling is useful both for prospective studies, like disease prevention trials, and for retrospective studies, where the events have already happened, but covariate information is costly to retrieve (e.g., from paper files or biological samples). For the former case, the workflow can be made more predictable with a case-cohort design. Since the subcohort is sampled at the outset of the study, more efforts can be used in early phases on processing subcohort information, while the information on the cases may be processed later. For a nested case-control study, however, control selection and ascertainment of covariate values for the controls have to wait until the cases occur.

In a nested case-control study, the controls are matched to their cases. So if one wants to study more than one type of endpoint (e.g., more than one disease), new controls have to be selected for each endpoint. Here a case-cohort design may give large savings by allowing the subcohort individuals to be used as controls for multiple endpoints. See, however, Section 16.6.

Cohort sampling designs are much used in studies of biomarkers from cohorts with stored biological samples. For such studies one should be aware of possible effects of analytic batch and long-term storage. If these effects are substantial, a case-cohort study may give biased results, and it is advisable to use a nested case-control design with matching on storage time with the cases and their controls analyzed in the same batch. Otherwise a case-cohort design may be the preferred approach, since it allows us to reuse the biomarkers for other endpoints (Rundle *et al.*, 2005).

16.5.3 Simple or stratified sampling

In Sections 16.3.3 and 16.4.4 we discuss the possibility of selecting the controls and the subcohort by stratified random sampling. Stratified sampling may be a useful option when stratification can be based on a surrogate measure of an exposure of main interest. One should be aware, however, that the efficiency gain for the exposure of main interest will often be accompanied by a loss in efficiency for other covariates. Thus stratified sampling may be a useful option for studies with a focused research question, but less so for a subcohort that is assembled to serve as controls for multiple endpoints.

16.6 Reuse of controls in nested case-control studies

In the partial likelihood (16.3), a case and its controls are included only at the failure time of the case. When the covariate information obtained for cases and controls is time-fixed (or the full trajectories of time-dependent covariates can be obtained), one may consider to break the matching between a case and its controls and analyse the nested case-control data as if they were case-cohort data (with a nonstandard sampling scheme for the subcohort); cf. Chapter 19. In this way the covariate information for cases and controls may be used whenever the individuals are at risk. Such reuse of controls may lead to more efficient estimators and counter some of the limitations of nested case-control studies discussed in Section 16.5. One should be aware, however, that in some situations the matching is needed to avoid bias (Section 16.5.2), and then one should avoid breaking the matching between a case and its controls.

As described in Chapter 19, one way to reuse the controls is by estimating the probability that an individual is ever sampled as control, and then apply the weighted likelihood (16.8). For instance Samuelsen (1997) suggested using the weights $w_k = 1/\pi_k$, where $\pi_k = 1$ for cases and

$$\pi_k = 1 - \prod \left(1 - \frac{m}{n(t_j) - 1} \right) \tag{16.11}$$

for control individual k. The product in (16.11) is over failure times t_j when individual k is at risk. As further discussed in Chapter 19, one may alternatively estimate the inclusion probabilities by logistic regression using the indicator of being sampled among noncases as response and the entry and exit times as covariates. As for case-cohort data, the weighted likelihood does not possess likelihood properties, so variance estimation requires special attention; see Chapter 19 for details.

16.7   Using the full cohort

Nested case-control and case-cohort studies take place within a well-defined cohort $\mathcal{C}$, and it is assumed that the at-risk status is known for all individuals in $\mathcal{C}$. Often some cheaply measured covariates are also available for all individuals in the cohort, while expensive covariate measurements are only available for the case-control sample $\mathcal{S}$, i.e., for the cases and controls/subcohort. We have discussed how the information available for the full cohort may be used to obtain a counter-matched nested case-control sample (Section 16.3.3) or a stratified sample of the subcohort (Section 16.4.4), and we have also mentioned the possibility of post-stratification and calibration of case-cohort data (Section 16.4.5). But in any case, the partial likelihoods (16.3) and (16.4) and the pseudo-likelihoods (16.6) and (16.8) only use data for the case-control sample. In this section we briefly describe two methods that use all the available information for the full cohort. For ease of presentation we will assume that there is a single expensive covariate, and restrict attention right-censored survival data; see Chapters 20 and 21 for a full account.

Let X denote the covariate that is expensive to measure, and let $\mathbf{Z}$ denote the vector of cheaply measured covariates. Conditional on $X = x$ and $\mathbf{Z} = \mathbf{z}$, we assume that failures in the cohort occur according to the Cox regression model

$$\lambda(t) = \lambda_0(t) \exp(\beta x + \boldsymbol{\gamma}^{\mathsf{T}} \mathbf{x}), \tag{16.12}$$

where we assume that all the covariates are time-fixed. We consider a cohort $\mathcal{C} = \{1, \ldots, N\}$ of N independent individuals, and denote the values of X_i, $\mathbf{Z}_i$ for individual i by x_i, $\mathbf{z}_i$. Then $\mathbf{z}_i$ is observed for all individuals in the cohort ($i \in \mathcal{C}$), while x_i is only observed for the case-control sample ($i \in \mathcal{S}$). Each individual in the cohort is observed until failure or censoring. For individual i we let T_i be the time of failure or censoring, and let Δ_i be an indicator taking the value 1 if the individual fails at T_i and the value 0 if the individual is censored. The values of T_i and Δ_i are observed for all $i \in \mathcal{C}$ and are denoted t_i and δ_i. (Note that t_i has a different meaning here than in Sections 16.2, 16.3, 16.4, and 16.6, where the t_j's are the ordered failure times.)

16.7.1   Maximum likelihood estimation

Data from a nested case-control or case-cohort study may be viewed as full cohort data where observation of the covariate X is missing by design for the cohort members who are not in the case-control sample (i.e., for $i \in \mathcal{C} \backslash \mathcal{S}$). Therefore, under certain assumptions given in Chapter 21 (see also Saarela *et al.*, 2008), the likelihood will have the same form regardless if the case-control sample $\mathcal{S}$ is a (possibly counter-matched) nested case-control sample or a (possibly stratified) case-cohort sample. In any case an individual $i \in \mathcal{S}$ contributes a factor

$$P(t_i, \delta_i, x_i \mid \mathbf{z}_i) = P(t_i, \delta_i \mid x_i, \mathbf{z}_i) P(x_i \mid \mathbf{z}_i)$$

to the likelihood, while the contribution from an individual $i \in \mathcal{C} \setminus \mathcal{S}$ is given by

$$P(t_i, \delta_i \mid \mathbf{z}_i) = \int P(t_i, \delta_i \mid x, \mathbf{z}_i) \, dP(x \mid \mathbf{z}_i).$$

Thus the likelihood becomes (conditional on the covariates $\mathbf{z}_i$):

$$L = \prod_{i \in \mathcal{S}} P(t_i, \delta_i \mid x_i, \mathbf{z}_i) P(x_i \mid \mathbf{z}_i) \times \prod_{i \in \mathcal{C} \setminus \mathcal{S}} \int P(t_i, \delta_i \mid x, \mathbf{z}_i) \, dP(x \mid \mathbf{z}_i). \tag{16.13}$$

To achieve a full maximum likelihood solution, we need to specify the conditional distributions in (16.13). We assume the Cox model (16.12) for the hazard of the ith individual. Then the conditional density of (T_i, Δ_i) given $(X_i, \mathbf{Z}_i) = (x_i, \mathbf{z}_i)$ takes the form

$$P(t_i, \delta_i \mid x_i, \mathbf{z}_i) = \{\lambda_0(t_i) \exp(\beta x_i + \boldsymbol{\gamma}^{\mathrm{T}} \mathbf{z}_i)\}^{\delta_i} \tag{16.14}$$

$$\times \exp\left\{-\exp(\beta x_i + \boldsymbol{\gamma}^{\mathrm{T}} \mathbf{z}_i) \int_0^{t_i} \lambda_0(u) du\right\}.$$

For a full likelihood solution, we also need to specify $P(x_i \mid \mathbf{z}_i)$; the conditional distribution of X_i given $\mathbf{Z}_i = \mathbf{z}_i$.

A number of authors have considered maximum likelihood estimation for the full cohort using the likelihood (16.13); see, e.g., Scheike and Martinussen (2004); Scheike and Juul (2004); Zeng *et al.* (2006); Zeng and Lin (2014). An up-to-date review based on Zeng and Lin (2014) is given in Chapter 21.

16.7.2 Multiple imputation

An alternative to maximum likelihood estimation for the full cohort is to use multiple imputation (e.g. Carpenter and Kenward, 2013). For this method, the missing values of X are imputed for all individuals who are not in the case-control sample. In Chapter 20 it is described in detail how multiple imputation is performed for nested case-control and case-cohort data. Here we will just give a brief review.

The multiple imputation procedure involves following three steps:

1. The missing values of X (i.e., x_i for $i \in \mathcal{C} \setminus \mathcal{S}$) are imputed from the distribution of the missing data given all the observed data (i.e., x_i for $i \in \mathcal{S}$ and $\mathbf{z}_i$, t_i and δ_i for $i \in \mathcal{C}$). This is done K times and gives us K "complete" data sets for the full cohort.

2. Cox's regression model (16.12) is fitted to each of the K imputed data sets using the full cohort partial likelihood (cf. Section 16.2). This gives K estimates $\widehat{\beta}_1, \ldots, \widehat{\beta}_K$ of β with corresponding estimated variances $\widehat{\mathrm{Var}}(\widehat{\beta}_1), \ldots, \widehat{\mathrm{Var}}(\widehat{\beta}_K)$.

3. The estimates $\widehat{\beta}_k$ and their variance estimates $\widehat{\mathrm{Var}}(\widehat{\beta}_k)$ are combined using "Rubin's rules" (Rubin, 1987) to obtain the multiple imputation estimate

$$\widehat{\beta}_{\mathrm{MI}} = \frac{1}{K} \sum_{k=1}^{K} \widehat{\beta}_k$$

and its variance estimate

$$\widehat{\mathrm{Var}}(\widehat{\beta}_{\mathrm{MI}}) = \widehat{W} + \left(1 + \frac{1}{K}\right) \widehat{B}.$$

Here

$$\widehat{W} = \frac{1}{K} \sum_{k=1}^{K} \widehat{\mathrm{Var}}(\widehat{\beta}_k) \qquad \text{and} \qquad \widehat{B} = \frac{1}{K-1} \sum_{k=1}^{K} (\widehat{\beta}_k - \widehat{\beta}_{\mathrm{MI}})^2$$

are the average within imputation variance and the between imputation variance.

In Chapter 20 it is described in detail how the imputations in step 1 are performed.

16.7.3 Efficiency gains

When the number of controls per case in a nested case-control study is fairly large (say five or more) or when a case-cohort study has a fairly large subcohort, the traditional analysis methods based on partial likelihoods and weighted pseudo-likelihoods give very good efficiencies compared to a full cohort analysis. So in these situations there is not much to gain by using multiple imputation or a full maximum likelihood approach. But with a small number of controls (say one or two) or a small subcohort, multiple imputation or a full maximum likelihood approach may give important efficiency gains compared to the traditional analysis methods. The gain may be substantial for estimation of the effects of the covariates $\mathbf{Z}$ that are observed for everyone, but is typically smaller for the covariate X that is only observed for the case-control sample; Chapters 20 and 21 provide numerical illustrations.

16.8 Closing remarks

Nested case-control and case-cohort designs are increasingly being used in epidemiology and biomarker studies. In this chapter we have given an overview of methods for analysing nested case-control and case-cohort data using Cox's regression model. The focus has been on the estimation of regression coefficients (and hence hazard ratios) for Cox's regression model using partial likelihood and weighted pseudo-likelihood methods. But we have also discussed the possibility of considering the covariates that are only measured for the case-control sample as missing by design for the other cohort members, and performing the estimation by means of multiple imputation or maximum likelihood estimation.

The other chapters in Part IV of the handbook give an in-depth treatment of the topics discussed in this chapter, and also include a number of topics that are not discussed here. Chapter 17 considers case-cohort data and discusses in detail how estimation for Cox's model may be performed by inverse probability weighted (IPW) likelihood methods. Estimation of the baseline hazard and absolute risks for Cox regression, and estimation for the Lin-Ying (1994) additive hazards model, are also considered in this chapter. Chapter 18 presents a general framework for nested case-control sampling and discusses partial likelihood methods, baseline hazard estimation and model checking for Cox's regression model for quite general control sampling schemes (that include simple random sampling and counter-matched sampling of the controls as special cases). Chapter 19 is also concerned with nested case-controls studies. But here it is shown how one may consider nested case-control data as case-cohort data with a nonstandard sampling scheme for the subcohort, and use IPW likelihood methods for estimation in Cox regression and other regression models. Nested case-control and case-cohort studies take place within a well-defined cohort, and often some cheaply measured covariates are available for all individuals in the cohort while expensive covariate measurements are only available for the cases and controls/subcohort. Chapters 20 and 21 discuss methods that use all the available information for the full cohort; multiple imputation is considered in Chapter 20 while maximum likelihood estimation is discussed in Chapter 21. Part IV concludes with a chapter on the self-controlled case series method; a method that may be used to evaluate the association between an adverse event and a time-varying exposure.

Bibliography

Andersen, P. K. and Gill, R. D. (1982). Cox's regression model for counting processes: A large sample study. *Annals of Statistics*, **10**, 1100–1120.

Barlow, W. E. (1994). Robust variance estimation for the case-cohort design. *Biometrics*, **50**, 1064–1072.

Barlow, W. E., Ichikawa, L., Rosner, D., and Izumi, S. (1999). Analysis of case-cohort designs. *Journal of Clinical Epidemiology*, **52**, 1165–1172.

Borgan, Ø. and Olsen, E. F. (1999). The efficiency of simple and counter-matched nested case-control sampling. *Scandinavian Journal of Statistics*, **26**, 493–509.

Borgan, Ø., Goldstein, L., and Langholz, B. (1995). Methods for the analysis of sampled cohort data in the Cox proportional hazards model. *Annals of Statistics*, **23**, 1749–1778.

Borgan, Ø., Langholz, B., Samuelsen, S. O., Goldstein, L., and Pogoda, J. (2000). Exposure stratified case-cohort designs. *Lifetime Data Analysis*, **6**, 39–58.

Carpenter, J. R. and Kenward, M. G. (2013). *Multiple Imputation and its Application*. Wiley, Chichester.

Chen, K. (2001). Generalized case-cohort estimation. *Journal of the Royal Statistical Society: Series B (Statistical Methodology)*, **63**, 791–809.

Chen, K. and Lo, S.-H. (1999). Case-cohort and case-control analysis with Cox's model. *Biometrika*, **86**, 755–764.

Goldstein, L. and Langholz, B. (1992). Asymptotic theory for nested case-control sampling in the Cox regression model. *Annals of Statistics*, **20**, 1903–1928.

Horvitz, D. G. and Thompson, D. J. (1952). A generalization of sampling without replacement from a finite universe. *Journal of the American Statistical Association*, **47**, 663–685.

Kalbfleisch, J. D. and Lawless, J. F. (1988). Likelihood analysis of multi-state models for disease incidence and mortality. *Statistics in Medicine*, **7**, 149–160.

Kalbfleisch, J. D. and Prentice, R. L. (2002). *The Statistical Analysis of Failure Time Data*. Wiley, Hoboken, New Jersey, 2nd edition.

Kupper, L. L., McMichael, A. J., and Spirtas, R. (1975). A hybrid epidemiologic study design useful in estimating relative risk. *Journal of the American Statistical Association*, **70**, 524–528.

Langholz, B. and Borgan, Ø. (1995). Counter-matching: A stratified nested case-control sampling method. *Biometrika*, **82**, 69–79.

Langholz, B. and Jiao, J. (2007). Computational methods for case-cohort studies. *Biometrics*, **51**, 3737–3748.

Langholz, B. and Thomas, D. C. (1991). Efficiency of cohort sampling designs: Some surprising results. *Biometrics*, **47**, 1563–1571.

Lin, D. Y. and Ying, Z. (1993). Cox regression with incomplete covariate measurements. *Journal of the American Statistical Association*, **88**, 1341–1349.

Lin, D. Y. and Ying, Z. (1994). Semiparametric analysis of the additive risk model. *Biometrika*, **81**, 61–71.

Miettinen, O. (1982). Design options in epidemiologic research: An update. *Scandinavian Journal of Work, Environment & Health*, **8** (supplement 1), 7–14.

Prentice, R. L. (1986). A case-cohort design for epidemiologic cohort studies and disease prevention trials. *Biometrika*, **73**, 1–11.

Rubin, D. B. (1987). *Multiple Imputation for Nonresponse in Surveys*. Wiley, New York.

Rundle, A. G., Vineis, P., and Ahsan, H. (2005). Design options for molecular epidemiology research within cohort studies. *Cancer Epidemiology, Biomarkers & Prevention*, **14**, 1899–1907.

Saarela, O., Kulathinal, S., Arjas, E., and Läärä, E. (2008). Nested case-control data utilized for multiple outcomes: A likelihood approach and alternatives. *Statistics in Medicine*, **27**, 5991–6008.

Samuelsen, S. O. (1989). *Two incompleted data problems in life-history analysis: Double censoring and the case-cohort design*. Ph.D. thesis, University of Oslo.

Samuelsen, S. O. (1997). A pseudolikelihood approach to analysis of nested case-control studies. *Biometrika*, **84**, 379–394.

Samuelsen, S. O., Ånestad, H., and Skrondal, A. (2007). Stratified case-cohort analysis of general cohort sampling designs. *Scandinavian Journal of Statistics*, **34**, 103–119.

Scheike, T. H. and Juul, A. (2004). Maximum likelihood estimation for Cox's regression model under nested case-control sampling. *Biostatistics*, **5**, 193–206.

Scheike, T. H. and Martinussen, T. (2004). Maximum likelihood estimation for Cox's regression model under case-cohort sampling. *Scandinavian Journal of Statistics*, **31**, 283–293.

Self, S. G. and Prentice, R. L. (1988). Asymptotic distribution theory and efficiency results for case-cohort studies. *Annals of Statistics*, **16**, 64–81.

Therneau, T. M. and Li, H. (1999). Computing the Cox model for case-cohort designs. *Lifetime Data Analysis*, **5**, 99–112.

Thomas, D. C. (1977). Addendum to: "Methods of cohort analysis: Appraisal by application to asbestos mining," by F. D. K. Liddell, J. C. McDonald and D. C. Thomas. *Journal of the Royal Statistical Society: Series A (General)*, **140**, 469–491.

Zeng, D. and Lin, D. Y. (2014). Efficient estimation of semiparametric transformation models for two-phase cohort studies. *Journal of the American Statistical Association*, **109**, 371–383.

Zeng, D., Lin, D. Y., Avery, C. L., North, K. E., and Bray, M. S. (2006). Efficient semiparametric estimation of haplotype-disease associations in case-cohort and nested case-control studies. *Biostatistics*, **7**, 486–502.

17

Survival Analysis of Case-Control Data: A Sample Survey Approach

Norman E. Breslow and Jie Kate Hu

University of Washington

17.1   Introduction

Large cohort (follow-up) studies, including those of patients in randomized clinical trials, provide the most definitive evidence of the effect of treatments on clinical outcomes and of exposure to risk factors on disease outcomes. The Atherosclerosis Risk in Communities (ARIC) study, for example, ascertained nearly 16,000 subjects to investigate the impact of environmental and genetic risk factors on cardiovascular disease (Williams, 1989). The Women's Health Initiative (WHI) randomized over 26,000 women to hormone therapy or placebo in clinical trials for women with and without an intact uterus (Anderson *et al.*, 2003). In view of logistic and financial constraints associated with measurement of biomarkers on tens of thousands of subjects, both ARIC and WHI selected random samples, termed a cohort random sample and a subcohort, respectively, for whom routine bioassays of selected biomarkers were performed. Sampling was stratified on demographic factors in order to achieve desired minority representation. In a series of substudies, biomarkers were assayed using stored serum samples for additional subjects who developed one of several disease outcomes of interest. Data from the cohort sample and from disease cases outside the sample were combined using specialized techniques based on the Cox model to estimate disease risks (Prentice, 1986). However, this approach ignored large quantities of information on baseline factors available for main cohort members who were not also a disease case or in the cohort sample.

This chapter presents a general sample survey approach to survival analysis of case-control data. By considering properties of the sampling design separately from those of the assumed model, it accommodates a variety of parametric and semiparametric models, in particular the Cox (1972) proportional and Lin-Ying (1994) additive hazards models. Stratification of the case-control sample may be based on any information available for the entire cohort, with the goal to select the most informative subjects. For example, stratification on a correlate of exposure can increase the variation of the true exposure in the sample and thus enhance the precision of the corresponding regression coefficient (Borgan *et al.*, 2000). Sampling of cases as well as controls is permitted, which is important when studying more common disease outcomes or when damaged serum samples or failed bioassays result in missing biomarker data for both cases and controls. Recovery of information lost by ignoring baseline covariates for nonsampled subjects is facilitated.

In the next section we present a data set on radiation and breast cancer that will be used to illustrate the methodology in this and the following four chapters. We then, in Section 17.3, explain how the case-control data may be viewed as a two-phase sample, where the cohort data correspond to the Phase I sample and the case-control data to the Phase II sample. Section 17.4 summarizes statistical methods to estimate relative (log hazard ratio) and absolute (cumulative hazard) risks when fitting the Cox model to full cohort data and to two-phase samples, and in Section 17.5 these methods are illustrated for the data on radiation and breast cancer. In Section 17.6, we review how estimation is performed in the Lin-Ying additive hazards model, and Section 17.7 gives estimates for the radiation and breast cancer data. A few concluding comments are given in Section 17.8.

17.2   Example: Radiation and breast cancer

Women treated for tuberculosis between 1930 and 1956 at one of two Massachusetts sanatoria were followed for the occurrence of breast cancer (BC) through 1980 (Hrubec *et al.*, 1989). A version of the data from this study, originally distributed with the Epicure computer program (Preston *et al.*, 1993), is used for illustration throughout this and the following four chapters. A majority of the 1,720 women in the cohort received radiation exposure to the breast from multiple fluoroscopies used for diagnostic X-ray in conjunction with lung collapse therapy for their tuberculosis; those not examined by fluoroscopy were considered unexposed. Cumulative doses of radiation to the breast (Gy) were estimated from the number of fluoroscopies, a reconstruction of exposure conditions, absorbed dose calculations and other available data.

For this cohort, radiation doses have been estimated for all 1,720 women. But the workload of exposure data collection would have been reduced if the investigators had used a cohort sampling design. Therefore, to illustrate the methods of this chapter, two random samples were drawn to simulate case-control studies in which the actual dose (the "expensive" covariate) was measured only for the breast cancer cases and a sample of controls. The fact that dose actually was known for the entire cohort allowed results obtained from the case-control analyses to be compared, for illustrative purposes, with results of fitting the same models to the entire cohort.

Note that we have referred to the two simulated studies as "case-control" studies rather than as "case-cohort" studies. From the viewpoint of survey sampling we regard the two designs as equivalent, and both terms are used in the sequel. The cases in a case-cohort study consist of all cases ascertained by the time of data analysis, whether or not they happened to have been sampled for the cohort random sample (subcohort). The controls consist of all noncases sampled for the subcohort. Since the subcohort was randomly sampled (possibly with stratification) from the main cohort, the controls consist of a random sample of noncases in the main cohort. All cases are sampled. The main difference between the two designs is that, in some applications involving a partially missing time-dependent covariate, the value of this covariate may be known only at the time of occurrence of cases that occur outside the subcohort, which would rule out the sample survey approach we describe. Other methods of analysis that include such cases only in the "risk set" corresponding to the time of its occurrence are required; see Prentice (1986), Borgan *et al.* (2000), and Chapter 16.

17.2.1   Description of the study cohort

Table 17.1 shows the frequency distributions of the 75 cases and 1,645 controls according to three major risk factors. One is interested in studying the effect of radiation on breast cancer risk, and whether women first irradiated early in life had higher rates of BC, at the same dose level and attained age, compared with those irradiated later.

Participants were followed from the date of discharge following their first hospitalization for tuberculosis, which was usually shortly after the onset of treatment, until the earliest of death, BC diagnosis or study closure. These events were recorded as of the ages at which they occurred. From the viewpoint of survival analysis, therefore, age at BC was left truncated at entry to the cohort and right censored at exit. Age was the fundamental time variable in the models; hence baseline hazards correspond to baseline age-specific rates.

A simple random sample (subcohort) of 150 of the 1,720 women, including by chance 7 of the 75 BC cases, was first drawn to simulate the standard case-cohort design. In an attempt to increase design efficiency for estimation of the effects of age at first treatment,

TABLE 17.1
Risk factors in the breast cancer study.

	Cases (BC)	Controls	Totals
Totals	75	1645	1720
Attained age (years)			
0-39	10	244	254
40-59	51	435	486
60-93	14	966	980
Radiation dose (Gy)			
0	21	677	698
< 2	46	858	904
≥ 2	8	110	118
Age at first treatment (years)			
0-19	33	621	654
20-29	28	609	637
30+	14	415	429

a second stratified random subcohort was drawn of 50 women from each of the three categories of age at first treatment shown in Table 17.1. Since, again by chance, 6 of the 75 BC cases were included in the stratified sample, the simple and stratified studies differed only slightly in terms of total sample size: 218 and 219, respectively. Radiation doses were considered unknown for subjects who were neither cases nor in the respective sample. Comparisons of the results obtained using the full cohort data with those for the two case-cohort samples, simple and stratified, are presented in Sections 17.5 and 17.7 for the proportional and additive hazards models. We consider first, however, how these data are best viewed from a sample survey perspective and outline the methods of analysis used to make the comparisons.

17.3 Two-phase sampling

Two-phase (or double) sampling was originally proposed for estimation of the finite population total of some target variable that is difficult to measure. A Phase I sample is first drawn from the finite population. Readily available information on some correlate of the target variable is ascertained for all Phase I subjects and used to stratify the sampling of a Phase II subsample. Multiplying together the Phase I and Phase II sampling probabilities for each Phase II subject, the population total is estimated by inverse probability weighting of the Phase II observations (Lumley, 2012, §8.1).

17.3.1 The case-control study as a two-phase design

The case-control study is profitably viewed as a two-phase design. Here the population is a probability model (superpopulation) and the goal is estimation of model parameters. The Phase I sample (cohort) is regarded as a series of independent and identically distributed (i.i.d) observations drawn from the model. If these were completely observed, inference would proceed simply by fitting the model to the cohort data following the usual paradigm

TABLE 17.2
Two-phase stratified sampling.

	Stratum				
	1	2	$\cdots$	J	Total
Phase I (cohort)	N_1	N_2	$\cdots$	N_J	N
Phase II (subsample)	n_1	n_2	$\cdots$	n_J	n
Sampling fractions	$\frac{n_1}{N_1}$	$\frac{n_2}{N_2}$	$\cdots$	$\frac{n_J}{N_J}$	$\frac{n}{N}$

of model based inference. However, a portion of the observations, e.g., the biomarkers, is in general only available for subjects in a Phase II subsample.

Let $\mathbf{Z}$ denote a generic observation from the probability model. For survival analyses with left truncation or a series of intermittent observation periods, $\mathbf{Z} = (Y, T, \Delta, \mathbf{X})$, where $Y = Y(t)$ is the "at risk" indicator of whether or not the subject is under observation at t, Δ is a censoring indicator for the survival time T and $\mathbf{X}$ is a vector of covariates, of which only a portion $\widetilde{\mathbf{X}}$ is fully observed at Phase I. When time is simply time on study, $Y(t) = \mathbf{1}(T \geq t)$.

The parameter is $(\boldsymbol{\beta}, \Lambda_0)$ where $\boldsymbol{\beta}$ are regression coefficients, interpretable as log hazard ratios, excess hazards or otherwise depending on the survival model, and Λ_0 is the baseline cumulative hazard function. We denote by $\mathbf{V} = (Y, T, \Delta, \widetilde{\mathbf{X}}, \mathbf{W}) \in \mathcal{V}$ the variables that are fully observable for the entire cohort, including possibly a vector $\mathbf{W}$ of auxiliary variables, i.e., variables that are not wanted in the model but may be useful for stratification of the Phase II subsample or otherwise to improve efficiency. Let $\mathcal{V} = \mathcal{V}_1 \cup \cdots \cup \mathcal{V}_J$ denote a partition of the range of the fully observed variables into J strata. For each of N Phase I subjects, define $R_i = 1/0$, $i = 1, \ldots, N$ to be the indicator of whether or not the ith subject is selected for the Phase II subsample. There are two possibilities for how the Phase II sampling may be performed.

17.3.2 Finite population stratified sampling (FPSS)

If the $\mathbf{V}$'s were available simultaneously for everyone in the cohort, we could count the numbers N_j in each of the J strata and use simple random sampling without replacement to sample n_j of them for Phase II (Table 17.2). Since the sampling indicators satisfy $\sum_{i=1}^{N} R_i \mathbf{1}(\mathbf{V}_i \in \mathcal{V}_j) = n_j \leq N_j$, where the n_j are fixed, they are dependent random variables, although exchangeable within strata and independent from stratum to stratum. The dependence complicates the asymptotic theory, for which reason most researchers prefer to develop the theory to preserve the i.i.d. structure of the data.

17.3.3 Bernoulli sampling

Alternatively, suppose the $\mathbf{V}_i$ became available sequentially and that a sampling indicator was drawn independently for each one according to $P(R_i = 1) = \pi_0(\mathbf{V}_i)$. Here $\pi_0(\mathbf{v})$ is a known function that is bounded away from zero; for stratified sampling, $\pi_0(\mathbf{v}) = p_j$ for $\mathbf{v} \in \mathcal{V}_j$ for p_j known *a priori*. In this case the Phase II sample sizes are random variables and n_j/N_j would converge in probability to p_j as $N \to \infty$. In Section 17.4.3 we explain how apparent differences between the two sampling schemes can be resolved by calibration of the sampling weights to the stratum totals N_j.

17.3.4   Example: Radiation and breast cancer

The two-phase design corresponding to the standard case-cohort study had just two strata, one comprising the cases sampled at 100% ($n_1 = N_1 = 75$) and the second the controls with $n_2 = 143, N_2 = 1645$. The four strata for the stratified study were the cases ($n_1 = N_1 = 75$) and the three control samples stratified by age at first treatment with, respectively, $n_2 = 44, N_2 = 621$, $n_3 = 50, N_3 = 609$ and $n_4 = 50, N_4 = 415$. Compare Tables 17.1 and 17.2.

17.4   Estimation of parameters in the Cox model

This section summarizes statistical methods that have been developed to estimate both relative (log hazard ratio) and absolute (cumulative hazard) risks when fitting the Cox model to full cohort data and to two-phase samples. The theoretical basis for the methodology relies heavily on empirical processes and semiparametric inference, for which a detailed discussion is beyond the scope of this handbook (van der Vaart and Wellner, 1996; van der Vaart, 1998). Hence some readers may find it advisable to proceed directly to the next section, on applications of the methods to the radiation and breast cancer study, referring back to the formulas presented in this section as needed to understand how the various estimates, standard errors and related quantities shown there were actually calculated from the data.

Under the Cox model, the cumulative hazard at t for the ith subject with covariates $\mathbf{X}_i$ is $\Lambda_i(t; \boldsymbol{\beta}, \Lambda_0) = e^{\mathbf{X}_i^{\mathrm{T}}\boldsymbol{\beta}}\Lambda_0(t)$, where the $\boldsymbol{\beta}$ are log hazard ratios corresponding to unit changes in the covariates and Λ_0 is the baseline cumulative hazard. This is assumed to be continuously differentiable on a finite time interval $[0, \tau]$ such that $P(Y(\tau) = 1) > 0$. Were the covariates fully observable for all Phase I subjects, $\boldsymbol{\beta}$ would be estimated by solving the partial likelihood score equations $\widetilde{\mathbf{U}}(\widetilde{\boldsymbol{\beta}}_N) = \sum_{i=1}^{N} \widetilde{\mathbf{U}}(\mathbf{Z}_i; \widetilde{\boldsymbol{\beta}}_N) = 0$ for $\widetilde{\boldsymbol{\beta}}_N$ (Cox, 1972), where

$$\widetilde{\mathbf{U}}(\mathbf{Z}; \boldsymbol{\beta}) = \Delta \left[\mathbf{X} - \widetilde{\mathbf{m}}(T; \boldsymbol{\beta}) \right], \tag{17.1}$$

and

$$\widetilde{\mathbf{m}}(t; \boldsymbol{\beta}) = \frac{\sum_{i=1}^{N} \mathbf{X}_i e^{\mathbf{X}_i^{\mathrm{T}}\boldsymbol{\beta}} Y_i(t)}{\sum_{i=1}^{N} e^{\mathbf{X}_i^{\mathrm{T}}\boldsymbol{\beta}} Y_i(t)} \tag{17.2}$$

denotes the weighted mean of the covariates of subjects "at risk" at t, weighting each by its hazard ratio. Asymptotic properties of estimators like $\widetilde{\boldsymbol{\beta}}_N$ are usually derived from asymptotic expansions for its normalized difference from the true value of the parameter, here $\sqrt{N}(\widetilde{\boldsymbol{\beta}}_N - \boldsymbol{\beta})$.

17.4.1   Expansion via the efficient influence function

Denote by $\mathbb{N}_i(t) = \mathbf{1}(T_i \le t, \Delta_i = 1)$ the standard counting process, by

$$\widetilde{\Lambda}_N(t; \boldsymbol{\beta}) = \sum_{i=1}^{N} \frac{\Delta_i \mathbf{1}(T_i \le t)}{\sum_{j=1}^{N} e^{\mathbf{X}_j^{\mathrm{T}}\boldsymbol{\beta}} Y_j(T_i)}$$

the Breslow estimate of $\Lambda_0(t; \boldsymbol{\beta})$, by

$$\widetilde{\mathbf{U}}^*(\mathbf{Z}; \boldsymbol{\beta}) = \int_0^{\tau} \left[\mathbf{X} - \widetilde{\mathbf{m}}(t; \boldsymbol{\beta}) \right] Y(t) \left(d\mathbb{N}(t) - e^{\mathbf{X}^{\mathrm{T}}\boldsymbol{\beta}} d\Lambda_0(t; \boldsymbol{\beta}) \right), \tag{17.3}$$

the semiparametric efficient score that corrects for estimation of Λ_0, and by

$$\tilde{\mathbf{I}}(\boldsymbol{\beta}) = -\frac{\partial \mathrm{E}\left[\tilde{\mathbf{U}}^*(\mathbf{Z};\tilde{\boldsymbol{\beta}})\right]}{\partial \tilde{\boldsymbol{\beta}}^{\mathrm{T}}}\Bigg|_{\tilde{\boldsymbol{\beta}}=\boldsymbol{\beta}} \tag{17.4}$$

$$= \int_0^\tau \left[\frac{\mathrm{E}\mathbf{X}^{\otimes 2}e^{\mathbf{X}^{\mathrm{T}}\boldsymbol{\beta}}Y(t)}{\mathrm{E}e^{\mathbf{X}^{\mathrm{T}}\boldsymbol{\beta}}Y(t)} - \left(\frac{\mathrm{E}\mathbf{X}e^{\mathbf{X}^{\mathrm{T}}\boldsymbol{\beta}}Y(t)}{\mathrm{E}e^{\mathbf{X}^{\mathrm{T}}\boldsymbol{\beta}}Y(t)}\right)^{\otimes 2}\right] \mathrm{E}e^{\mathbf{X}^{\mathrm{T}}\boldsymbol{\beta}}Y(t)\,d\Lambda_0(t;\boldsymbol{\beta}),$$

the efficient information. Then

$$\sqrt{N}\left(\tilde{\boldsymbol{\beta}}_N - \boldsymbol{\beta}\right) = \frac{1}{\sqrt{N}}\sum_{i=1}^N \tilde{\ell}(\mathbf{Z}_i;\boldsymbol{\beta}) + o_p(1) \tag{17.5}$$

with $\tilde{\ell}(\mathbf{Z}_i;\boldsymbol{\beta}) = \tilde{\mathbf{I}}^{-1}(\boldsymbol{\beta})\tilde{\mathbf{U}}^*(\mathbf{Z}_i;\boldsymbol{\beta})$ denoting the contribution to the efficient influence function for the ith subject (Cox, 1972; van der Vaart, 1998, §25.12.1).

17.4.2 Inverse probability weighted estimate

The survey estimator $\widehat{\boldsymbol{\beta}}_N$ (Binder, 1992; Lin, 2000) solves an inverse probability weighted (IPW) version of the Phase II score equations (17.1) and (17.2), namely

$$\widehat{\mathbf{U}}(\widehat{\boldsymbol{\beta}}_N) = \sum_{i=1}^N \frac{R_i}{\pi_i}\int_0^\tau \left[\mathbf{X}_i - \widehat{\mathbf{m}}(t;\widehat{\boldsymbol{\beta}}_N)\right]Y_i(t)d\mathbb{N}_i(t) = 0,$$

with

$$\widehat{\mathbf{m}}(t,\boldsymbol{\beta}) = \frac{\sum_{i=1}^N \frac{R_i}{\pi_i}\mathbf{X}_i e^{\mathbf{X}_i^{\mathrm{T}}\boldsymbol{\beta}}Y_i(t)}{\sum_{i=1}^N \frac{R_i}{\pi_i}e^{\mathbf{X}_i^{\mathrm{T}}\boldsymbol{\beta}}Y_i(t)}.$$

Here the π_i are the sampling probabilities used to select the Phase II sample ($R_i = 1$) based on the variables $\mathbf{V}_i$ known at Phase I. An asymptotic expansion for $\widehat{\boldsymbol{\beta}}_N$ that follows from the work of Lin (2000) and others is

$$\sqrt{N}\left(\widehat{\boldsymbol{\beta}}_N - \boldsymbol{\beta}\right) = \sqrt{N}\left(\tilde{\boldsymbol{\beta}}_N - \boldsymbol{\beta}\right) + \sqrt{N}\left(\widehat{\boldsymbol{\beta}}_N - \tilde{\boldsymbol{\beta}}_N\right)$$

$$= \frac{1}{\sqrt{N}}\sum_{i=1}^N \left[\frac{R_i}{\pi_i}\tilde{\ell}(\mathbf{Z}_i;\boldsymbol{\beta})\right] + o_p(1) \tag{17.6}$$

$$= \frac{1}{\sqrt{N}}\sum_{i=1}^N \left[\tilde{\ell}(\mathbf{Z}_i;\boldsymbol{\beta}) + \left(\frac{R_i - \pi_i}{\pi_i}\right)\tilde{\ell}(\mathbf{Z}_i;\boldsymbol{\beta})\right] + o_p(1).$$

These equations lead to several important insights:

1. The normalized difference between the IPW (Phase II) estimator and the true value equals the normalized difference between the (unobservable) Phase I estimator $\tilde{\boldsymbol{\beta}}_N$ and the true value plus the normalized difference between the Phase I and Phase II estimators. The first term in the expansion shown on the bottom line of (17.6) is the term corresponding to the Phase I estimator (17.5).

2. Since $\mathrm{E}\left(R_i|\mathbf{Z}_i\right) = \pi_i$, the two components of this expansion are uncorrelated, hence asymptotically independent. Thus

$$\text{Total Variance} = \text{Phase I Variance} + \text{Phase II Variance}.$$

3. The Phase I variance Var $\widetilde{\ell}(\mathbf{Z}; \boldsymbol{\beta})$, due to i.i.d. sampling from the superpopulation, is not affected by the choice of Phase II design. The Phase II variance, which represents the loss of information from not having complete data at Phase I, is affected, e.g., by stratification. It is the normalized error arising from IPW estimation of an unknown finite population total, namely, the total of the influence function contributions $\widetilde{\ell}(\mathbf{Z}_i; \boldsymbol{\beta})$ for all Phase I subjects. It is best viewed as *design based*, with the randomness stemming exclusively from the sampling indicators R_i, with the Phase I observations $\mathbf{Z}_i$ being regarded as fixed.

For finite population stratified sampling (FPSS) of the Phase II sample from the cohort (Table 17.2), $\pi_i = n_j/N_j$ if the ith subject is in stratum j, i.e., if $\mathbf{V}_i \in \mathcal{V}_j$. Given the Phase I data

$$\text{Phase II Variance} = \sum_{j=1}^{J} \frac{N_j}{N} \frac{N_j - n_j}{n_j} \widehat{\text{Var}}_j \left[\widetilde{\ell}(\mathbf{Z}; \boldsymbol{\beta}) \right], \tag{17.7}$$

where $\widehat{\text{Var}}_j$ denotes the finite population variance of the influence function contributions $\widetilde{\ell}(\mathbf{Z}_i; \boldsymbol{\beta})$ observed for stratum j in the Phase II sample. Strata sampled at 100% ($n_j = N_j$) do not contribute to the Phase II variance. See Chen and Lo (1999) for the simple case-cohort design ($J = 1$), Borgan *et al.* (2000) for the stratified case-cohort design and Breslow and Wellner (2007) for the general two-phase stratified design. The generality of the latter is important since it covers situations where the cases may also be selected by stratified sampling with sampling fractions less than 100%.

17.4.3   Calibration of the sampling weights

Survey samplers (Deville and Särndal, 1992) improve estimates of finite population totals by calibrating the design weights to known population totals of auxiliary variables that are highly correlated with the variable whose total is to be estimated. This technique may also improve the efficiency of IPW estimators. Suppose $\mathbf{C} = \mathbf{C}(\mathbf{V}) = (C_1(\mathbf{V}), \ldots, C_K(\mathbf{V}))^{\mathrm{T}}$, where the calibration variables $C_k(\mathbf{V})$ are known for the entire Phase I sample and $\mathrm{E}(\mathbf{CC}^{\mathrm{T}})$ is nonsingular. We consider calibration for Bernoulli sampling (Section 17.3.3). This implies the Phase II sample is an i.i.d. random sample from the superpopulation based on known selection probabilities $\pi_0(\mathbf{V}_i)$. The calibrated weights w_i are chosen to be as close as possible to the design weights $d_i = 1/\pi_0(\mathbf{V}_i)$ in terms of a distance measure G and also to satisfy the calibration equations $\sum_{i=1}^{N} C_k(\mathbf{V}_i) = \sum_{i=1}^{N} R_i w_i C_k(\mathbf{V}_i)$ whereby the IPW estimator exactly estimates the Phase I totals for $k = 1, \ldots, K$. The standard constrained optimization procedure involves calculation of a K-vector $\widehat{\boldsymbol{\lambda}}_N$ of Lagrange multipliers for the calibration equations. Choosing the Poisson deviance $G(w, d) = w\log(w) - w + d$ as the distance measure leads to a procedure known as "raking" that guarantees nonnegative weights: $w_i = \exp\left[-\widehat{\boldsymbol{\lambda}}_N^{\mathrm{T}} \mathbf{C}(\mathbf{V}_i)\right] \Big/ \pi_0(\mathbf{V}_i)$ (Lumley, 2012, §7.4).

Calibration generally results in a reduction in the limiting Phase II variance that may or may not be realized in finite samples. With $\widehat{\boldsymbol{\beta}}_N(\widehat{\boldsymbol{\lambda}}_N)$ denoting the estimator with calibrated weights, the asymptotic variance of $\sqrt{N} \left(\widehat{\boldsymbol{\beta}}_N(\widehat{\boldsymbol{\lambda}}_N) - \boldsymbol{\beta} \right)$ equals

$$\text{Var}\left[\widetilde{\ell}(\mathbf{Z}; \boldsymbol{\beta}) \right] + \mathrm{E}\left\{ \left(\frac{1 - \pi_0(\mathbf{V})}{\pi_0(\mathbf{V})} \right) \left[\widetilde{\ell}(\mathbf{Z}; \boldsymbol{\beta}) - \Pi_{\mathbf{C}} \widetilde{\ell}(\mathbf{Z}; \boldsymbol{\beta}) \right]^{\otimes 2} \right\} \tag{17.8}$$

where $\Pi_{\mathbf{C}} \widetilde{\ell} = \mathrm{E}(\widetilde{\ell}\mathbf{C}^{\mathrm{T}})(\mathbf{ECC}^{\mathrm{T}})^{-1}\mathbf{C}$ denotes population least squares projection of the influence function on $(C_1, \ldots, C_K)$ (Breslow *et al.*, 2009a). Since we are effectively attempting to estimate the unknown Phase I totals of this influence function, a good choice for the calibration variables would be $\mathbf{C} = \mathrm{E}(\widetilde{\ell}|\mathbf{V})$. This yields the optimal member of the class of augmented inverse probability weighted (AIPW) estimators of Robins *et al.* (1994); see Lumley *et al.* (2011). One method of approximating this optimal $\mathbf{C}$ is considered in the example in the next section.

It is instructive to consider calibration to the Phase I stratum totals by selecting $C_j(\mathbf{V}) = \mathbf{1}[\mathbf{V} \in \mathcal{V}_j]$ for $j = 1, \ldots, J$. The calibrated weights are inverses of the actual sampling fractions n_j/N_j, the design weights inverses of the *a priori* p_j. Since the projection onto $(C_1, \ldots, C_J)$ yields stratum specific means, the limiting Phase II variance of the calibrated estimator, i.e., the second term in (17.8), equals

$$\sum_{j=1}^{J} P(\mathcal{V}_j) \frac{1 - p_j}{p_j} \mathrm{Var}_j \left[\widetilde{\ell}(\mathbf{Z}; \boldsymbol{\beta}) \right] \tag{17.9}$$

where Var_j denotes the variance based on the restriction of the probability distribution of $\mathbf{Z}$ to the jth stratum. Without calibration the terms $\mathrm{Var}_j[\widetilde{\ell}(\mathbf{Z}; \boldsymbol{\beta})]$ are replaced by $\mathrm{E}_j \left[\widetilde{\ell}(\mathbf{Z}; \boldsymbol{\beta})^{\otimes 2} \right]$ where E_j denotes the corresponding expectation. Hence the gain from calibration would be greatest if the influence function contributions varied strongly by strata. Note that (17.9) is the limit of (17.7). Hence calibration allows one to reconcile the apparent differences between the FPSS and Bernoulli sampling schemes. After fitting the model assuming Bernoulli sampling with *a priori* weights, one could calibrate to the stratum frequencies to obtain correct standard errors under the more realistic FPSS sampling scheme.

In actual practice, as illustrated in the next section, one would start with design weights for FPSS and calibrate using variables $\mathbf{C}(\mathbf{V})$ thought to be highly correlated with $\widetilde{\ell}(\mathbf{Z}; \boldsymbol{\beta})$ to increase the precision of the standard survey estimator described in Section 17.4.2. Consideration of the related Bernoulli sampling scheme and (17.8) serves primarily to understand why $\mathbf{C}(\mathbf{V}) = \mathrm{E}(\widetilde{\ell}|\mathbf{V})$ might be a good choice. See, however, Saegusa and Wellner (2013).

17.4.4 Estimation of the cumulative hazard

The survey estimator of the baseline cumulative hazard function is the IPW version of the Breslow estimator

$$\widehat{\Lambda}_N(t; \boldsymbol{\beta}) = \sum_{i=1}^{N} \frac{\frac{R_i}{\pi_0(\mathbf{V}_i)} \Delta_i \mathbf{1}(T_i \leq t)}{\sum_{j=1}^{N} \frac{R_j}{\pi_0(\mathbf{V}_j)} e^{\mathbf{X}_j^{\mathrm{T}} \boldsymbol{\beta}} Y_j(T_i)}, \tag{17.10}$$

which depends on the log hazard ratios $\boldsymbol{\beta}$ (Lin, 2000; Breslow *et al.*, 2015). This is combined with $\widehat{\boldsymbol{\beta}}_N$ to estimate the cumulative hazard over the interval between times t_0 and t_1 for a subject with covariates $\mathbf{x}_0$, assuming the subject is "at risk" for the entire interval. The estimate is

$$e^{\mathbf{x}_0^{\mathrm{T}} \widehat{\boldsymbol{\beta}}_N} \left(\widehat{\Lambda}_N(t_1; \widehat{\boldsymbol{\beta}}_N) - \widehat{\Lambda}_N(t_0; \widehat{\boldsymbol{\beta}}_N) \right). \tag{17.11}$$

Therneau and Grambsch (2000, §10.2) discussed how the cumulative hazard may be interpreted as an estimate of "expected" survival over the interval.

17.4.5 Model misspecification

Most of the results stated in this section remain valid even if the Cox model does not strictly hold. As usual under general misspecification, the parameters $(\boldsymbol{\beta}, \Lambda_0)$ being estimated are those for the Cox model that is closest, in the sense of Kullback-Leibler distance, to the probability distribution generating the data. The only change is that the limiting Phase I variance, i.e., the asymptotic variance of $\sqrt{N}(\widehat{\boldsymbol{\beta}}_N - \boldsymbol{\beta})$, rather than being the inverse of the efficient information (17.4), is instead the "robust sandwich" version $\widetilde{\mathbf{I}}^{-1}\mathrm{E}\left[\widetilde{\mathbf{U}}^*\left(\widetilde{\mathbf{U}}^*\right)^{\mathrm{T}}\right]\widetilde{\mathbf{I}}^{-1}$, where $\widetilde{\mathbf{U}}^*$ denotes the efficient score (17.3) for a generic subject. Expressions derived under the model for the asymptotic expansion of the IPW Breslow estimator (17.10), which allow calculation of its asymptotic variance, continue to hold off the model (Breslow *et al.*, 2015, §6.1).

17.4.6   Time-dependent covariates

The expressions shown in this section for scores, efficient scores, efficient information, etc., are easily extended to accommodate time-dependent covariates, replacing $\mathbf{X}$ by $\mathbf{X}(t)$ or $\mathbf{X}(T)$ as the case may be. Interpretation of the results of analyses of such time-dependent data, however, is another matter. It is relatively straightforward when the covariates are "external" in the sense of Kalbfleisch and Prentice (2002, §6.3); results may be highly subject to misinterpretation otherwise.

In practice, time-dependent covariates are most easily handled by splitting the follow-up record for each subject at the times at which the covariate values change and using the "counting process" form of the Cox model (Therneau and Grambsch, 2000, §§3.7, 5.6). Contributions to the scores and information from each of the split records for a given subject are aggregated into a single contribution per subject before being inserted into the expressions shown here.

17.5   Cox model analysis of radiation and breast cancer

Here we apply the methods outlined in the last section to the analysis of the data on radiation and cancer described in Section 17.2. The data and computer code needed to perform these analyses are available from the handbook website. The code is written for the freely available statistical programming language R. It includes an updated version of the `cch` command found in the R `survival` package. This suffices for estimation of hazard ratios using data from simple and stratified case-cohort studies, where cases are sampled at 100%. For estimation of cumulative hazards we used commands from Lumley's (2012) `survey` package, which applies more generally to two-phase study designs where not all cases need be sampled.

17.5.1   Preliminary graphical analyses

To provide some insight into the basic structure of the data, we first estimated in Figure 17.1, panels A-C, cumulative hazards from the full cohort data using the `survfit` command in the `survival` package. Risk categories for radiation dose and age at first treatment correspond to those in Table 17.1. The estimates in panel C, with time-on-study rather than age as the basic time variable, were also estimated in panel D from the simple case-cohort data using the `svykm` command in the `survey` package. The two show good agreement. As of this writing, `svykm` was not implemented for "counting process" survival data as needed to handle the left truncation of age at entry into the cohort (panels A-B). In principle, however, these cumulative hazards are also estimable from two-phase study data.

The cumulative hazards in panel A were plotted on the log scale. If the hazards for the three dose groups were exactly proportional, one would therefore expect to see a constant vertical distance between the three curves. While the middle curve for the 0-2 Gy group did

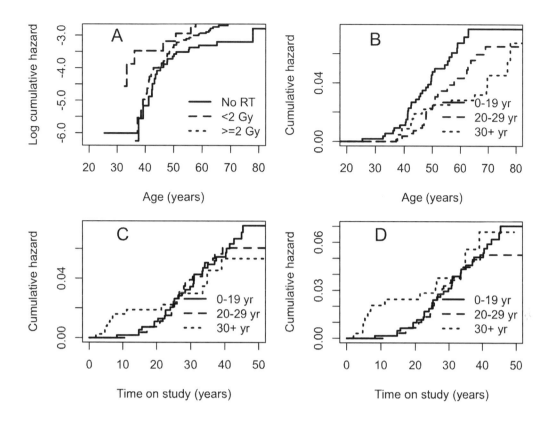

FIGURE 17.1
Cumulative hazards by radiation dose and age at first treatment. See text for interpretation of each panel.

not fall precisely between the other two, overall the assumption of proportionality seems reasonable. This is not so clear for age at first treatment (panel B), where the plot of the cumulative hazard itself offered a slightly different perspective. While the curves for the first two age at treatment categories (0-19 and 20-29 years) appeared proportional, that for the last category (30+ years) was not proportional to either of the others. This was due to a handful of BC cases that occurred within 20 years among women who started tuberculosis treatments after 30 years of age. For women irradiated earlier in life, time since first radiation largely determined the evolution of BC risk during the next decade or two. For women irradiated later, however, additional age-dependent risk factors may have started to exert their influence. Radiation treatment may have accelerated the appearance of cancers that would have occurred later anyway. This idea is reinforced by the plots in panel C, where the cumulative hazards according to time since start of radiation overlapped for those who were treated early, but started to rise sooner for those first treated at a later age. These remarks are of course highly speculative, given the relatively few BC events observed, especially for women first treated after 30 years of age. With a larger sample, it is possible that the three curves would overlap when plotted against time on study.

In spite of the questionable proportionality for age at first treatment, the analyses that

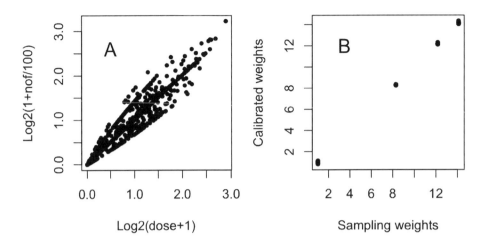

FIGURE 17.2
Results of calibration: A. Calibration variable by dose variable. B. Calibrated weights by
sampling weights.

follow assume that the proportional hazards model holds for underlying *continuous* versions
of these two risk factors.

17.5.2 Model for radiation and breast cancer

In view of radiobiological evidence of low dose linearity of radiation effects, radiation
epidemiologists often choose the excess relative risk version of the proportional haz-
ards model, where $\mathrm{RR}(\mathbf{X}; \boldsymbol{\beta}) = 1 + \mathbf{X}^{\mathrm{T}}\boldsymbol{\beta}$, rather than the standard exponential term
$\mathrm{RR}(\mathbf{X}; \boldsymbol{\beta}) = \exp(\mathbf{X}^{\mathrm{T}}\boldsymbol{\beta})$, multiplies the baseline cumulative hazard. Due to limitations in
software available for two-phase studies, however, and to be able to illustrate the stan-
dard Cox model, we instead followed Borgan and Samuelsen (2013) and used a log transform of radiation dose with the standard model. The covariates were $\mathbf{x} = (x_1, x_2)$ with
$x_1 = \log_2(\mathrm{dose} + 1)$ and $x_2 = \mathrm{ageRx}/10$, where ageRx denotes age at first treatment. This
implies the age-specific BC risk was multiplied by a *power* of (dose+1). Division by 10
ensured that the regression coefficient for ageRx represented the change in log hazard associated with a decade long rather than yearly change. It also had the effect of equalizing
the magnitudes of the regression coefficients for the two covariates. The model fitted to the
data for the cumulative hazard of a subject with $t =$ attained age and covariates $\mathbf{x}$ was thus

$$\Lambda(t, \mathbf{x}; \boldsymbol{\beta}, \Lambda_0) = \exp(x_1\beta_1 + x_2\beta_2)\Lambda_0(t), \qquad (17.12)$$

with $\Lambda_0(t)$ the baseline ($\mathbf{x} = 0$) cumulative hazard at age t. We fit model (17.12) to three
different data sets as described in Section 17.2.1: the entire set of cohort data, the simple case-cohort sample and the stratified (on ageRx) case-cohort sample. The case-cohort
analyses, however, failed to take advantage of all the information available for subjects in
the main cohort. Hence we considered the total number of fluoroscopies (nof) per subject,
which was used to reconstruct the radiation dose, to be an auxiliary variable known for all
Phase I subjects that served as a surrogate for dose. There was a very high correlation of
0.98 between log transforms of the two measurements (Figure 17.2, panel A) and the availability of such a strong surrogate exposure would be rare in actual practice. Nonetheless, its

use here illustrated the principle that efficiency gains are possible by using a good surrogate exposure to calibrate the weights.

17.5.3   Calibration and post-stratification

As described in Section 17.4.3, the idea behind the calibration method we employed was to modify the IPW design weights so that the Phase I totals of the calibration variable(s) $\mathbf{C} = \mathbf{C}(\mathbf{V})$ were exactly estimated by the IPW estimator, keeping the two sets of weights as close together as possible according to the Poisson deviance distance measure. The "insights" developed in Section 17.4.3 suggested that the optimal calibration variable was the conditional expectation of the influence function given all the main cohort variables $\mathbf{V}$. Since this was unknown, we needed to approximate it. Given the availability of a strong surrogate, one way to do this was simply to fit model (17.12) to the Phase I data, substituting $x_1 = \log_2(1 + \text{nof}/100)$ for $x_1 = \log_2(\text{dose} + 1)$. Estimates of the influence function contributions are extracted with the `dfbeta` option for the `residual` function applied to the model fit resulting from the call to `coxph` in the `survival` package. There are two components of the vector of influence function contributions, one for each covariate, and these are used as the calibration variables. Calibration resulted in only minor changes to the weights (Figure 17.2, panel B), but substantial gains in efficiency (see Section 17.5.4).

Gains from calibration depend heavily on the correlations between the calibration variables and those included in the model. They will be nil for biomarkers like genotype, known only at Phase II, that are not at all related to the Phase I variables. When the model contains adjustment variables, such as baseline risk factors known for all, calibration to the 'dfbetas' for these variables can increase substantially the precision of their regression coefficients. It may also have a modest effect on the precision of estimation of interaction effects between exposures known only at Phase II and adjustment variables known for everyone at Phase I.

If a strong exposure surrogate is not available, one may first fit an imputation model using IPW to the Phase II data (Kulich and Lin, 2004). Regression coefficients from the imputation model are then used to predict exposures for Phase I subjects who lack them, i.e., for those not included in the Phase II sample. The exposures for all Phase I subjects, whether observed or imputed, are next used together with the adjustment variables to fit a calibration model from which the 'dfbetas' are extracted. Finally, the 'dfbetas' are used as the calibration variables to adjust the design weights in an IPW analysis of the two-phase data. In other circumstances, it may be more efficacious simply to try to bring additional Phase I information to bear on the analysis by calibrating to variables, such as frequencies in a cross-classification, that summarize the marginal association between auxiliary Phase I variables and outcomes. See Breslow *et al.* (2009a,b, 2013) for examples of each of these approaches.

Post-stratification is an alternative to calibration for bringing into the analysis additional Phase I information. Rather than restricting the partition of the Phase I sample to the strata actually used for sampling, a finer partition based on additional (necessarily discrete) Phase I variables is used for the analysis. For example, the partition we chose based on categories of age at first treatment, which was used to stratify the sample, could have been based instead on the cross-classification of age at first treatment by number of fluoroscopies, e.g., in the three categories (i) none, (ii) 1-149, and (iii) 150+ considered by Borgan and Samuelsen (2013). For a nonstratified Phase II design, post-stratification to a set of stratum frequencies is equivalent to calibration using those same frequencies and avoids having to solve the calibration equations, an advantage since the need for specialized software may be avoided.

TABLE 17.3

Comparison of results for four designs. Robust standard errors.
(See text for explanations of column names.)

Model term	Coef.	SE1	SE2	SE	Z	p
A. Entire cohort						
$\log_2(\text{dose} + 1)$	0.469	0.153	NA	0.153	3.057	0.0022
ageRx/10	-0.242	0.144	NA	0.144	-1.677	0.0936
B. Simple case-cohort sample						
$\log_2(\text{dose} + 1)$	0.519	0.146	0.142	0.204	2.541	0.0111
ageRx/10	-0.111	0.159	0.106	0.191	-0.579	0.5629
C. Stratified case-cohort sample						
$\log_2(\text{dose}+1)$	0.559	0.185	0.162	0.246	2.273	0.0230
ageRx/10	-0.244	0.143	0.069	0.159	-1.537	0.1244
D. Stratified case-cohort sample with calibrated weights						
$\log_2(\text{dose}+1)$	0.440	0.182	0.0311	0.184	2.387	0.0170
ageRx/10	-0.250	0.140	0.0082	0.140	-1.781	0.0749

17.5.4 Results of the analyses: Regression coefficients

Regression coefficients and standard errors estimated by each model fit are shown in Table 17.3. Here Z denotes the equivalent normal deviate used by the Wald test, on which p is based. The column labeled SE1 contains the robust estimate of the Phase I standard error, that due to sampling of the cohort data from the superpopulation, as described above in Sections 17.4.2 and 17.4.5. Entries in column SE2 are the estimated Phase II standard errors, found by taking the square root in equation (17.7), and those in column SE the total standard errors. Note that $\text{SE1}^2 + \text{SE2}^2 = \text{SE}^2$.

Results for the entire cohort (Table 17.3, Part A) were obtained using `survfit` in the `survival` package, something made possible because radiation dose was in fact known for all Phase I subjects. They suggest that the age-specific risk of BC increased by a factor of $\exp(0.469) = 1.60$ with each doubling of (dose+1), whereas the risk decreased by a factor of $\exp(-0.242) = 0.79$ with each ten year increase in age at first treatment. The latter result, however, was subject to substantial sampling error. Considerably greater uncertainty, even in the coefficient for dose, was apparent when fitting the model to the simple case-cohort sample using the `LinYing` option with the `cch` function (Table 17.3, Part B). The uncertainty in the coefficient for dose due to sampling from the cohort (SE2 = 0.142) was nearly as large as that due to sampling the cohort from the population (SE1 = 0.146). Even for age at first treatment the two standard errors were of comparable magnitude. A substantial reduction in the Phase II standard error for ageRx was achieved by using the `II.Borgan` option for `cch` with data from the stratified case-cohort design (Table 17.3, Part C). The main difference between the two designs was that the relatively small number of controls (29) in the highest ageRx category (30+ years) that resulted from simple random sampling was increased to 50 by stratification on ageRx, with concomitant reductions in controls for the first two categories. Only 14 BC cases were observed for ageRx of 30 years or more. The additional controls in this category increased the information regarding risk at high ageRx and this lowered the standard error of the regression coefficient.

The most dramatic changes in Phase II standard errors followed calibration of the stratified sampling weights (see Section 17.5.3) using the estimated influence function contributions, which had components both for the surrogate dose measurement $\log_2(1 + \text{nof}/100)$ and for ageRx (Table 17.3, Part D). Phase II contributions to the total SE were negligible

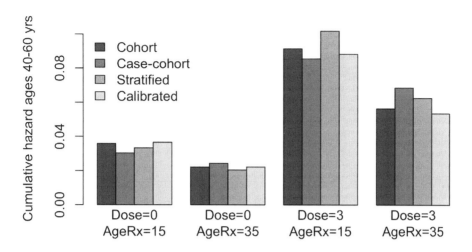

FIGURE 17.3
Expected numbers of breast cancers (cumulative hazards) between 40 and 60 years of age depending on covariate values.

in comparison to those for Phase I and results obtained from the calibrated design closely paralleled those obtained using the entire cohort.

One surprising feature of Table 17.3 was the variability in SE1 for $\log_2(\text{dose}+1)$ depending on the method of analysis, with values ranging from 0.146 to 0.185. All were estimating the same Phase I standard error. Since robust standard errors are notoriously variable, we reanalyzed the data using the options for model based standard errors and found SE1 for $\log_2(\text{dose}+1)$ of, respectively, 0.161, 0.157 and 0.178 for the models fitted to the entire cohort, to the simple case-cohort sample and to the stratified case-cohort sample. (The `survey` package provides only robust standard errors.) While the model based SE1 were indeed closer together, the high value of 0.178 for the stratified case-cohort sample is a reminder of the variability to be expected with relatively small Phase II samples.

17.5.5 Results of the analyses: Expected breast cancer risk

Figure 17.3 shows the expected numbers of BC between 40 and 60 years of age estimated for four configurations of covariate values. Two subjects received no radiation and two a dose of 3 Gy $[\log_2(\text{dose}+1) = 2]$ while at each radiation dose one started tuberculosis treatments (ageRx) at 15 years of age and one at age 35. The expected numbers were estimated from Equation (17.11) with $(t_0, t_1) = (40, 60)$ and $\mathbf{x}_0$, respectively, $(0, 1.5)$, $(0, 3.5)$, $(2, 1.5)$ and $(2, 3.5)$. The calculations were implemented using the `predict` command with type option `expected`, which is available in both the `survival` (for the full cohort analysis) and `survey` (for the case-cohort analyses) packages. Hence they represent cumulative hazards for these four covariate configurations, assuming that the women were at risk for the entire interval between 40 and 60 years of age. The four designs, designated Cohort, Case-cohort, Stratified and Calibrated, correspond to those described in detail in Section 17.5.4. The corresponding regression coefficients and standard errors are as shown in Table 17.3, Parts A-D.

Using data from the full cohort, the expected number of BC cases between ages 40 and 60 for a woman who started treatment for tuberculosis at age 15 but received no radiation was 3.6%. This declined to 2.2% for a nonirradiated woman who started tuberculosis treatment at age 35. The estimated risks were considerably higher (9.1% and 5.6%, respectively) at a radiation dose of 3 Gy. Taking the full cohort estimates as the "gold standard," overall those for the case-cohort analyses were as anticipated: worst for the simple case-cohort design, better for the stratified case-cohort design and best for the stratified design with calibration of the weights (Figure 17.3). In fact, the estimated risks using calibration were quite close to those estimated from the full cohort data, at 3.7%, 2.2%, 8.8% and 5.4% for the four covariate configurations.

17.6   The additive hazards model

In the two preceding sections, we have considered estimation in the Cox model for both cohort and case-control data and illustrated the methods for the data on radiation and breast cancer. We will now present similar results for the Lin-Ying additive hazards (AH) model (Lin and Ying, 1994). In this section we describe in general terms how we estimate the parameters of the AH model from cohort and case-control data, and in Section 17.7 we illustrate the use of these estimators for the data on radiation and breast cancer. As the results of this section rely heavily on empirical processes and semiparametric inference (van der Vaart and Wellner, 1996; van der Vaart, 1998), some readers may find it advisable to proceed directly to Section 17.7 on applications of the methods to the radiation and breast cancer study, referring back to the formulas presented in this section as needed to understand how the various estimates, standard errors and related quantities shown there were actually calculated from the data.

The AH model specifies the hazard function of a censored failure time T as a sum of a baseline hazard function $\lambda(\cdot)$, defined on a finite time interval $[0, \tau]$, and a regression function of $\mathbf{X}$:

$$\lambda(t|\mathbf{X}) = \lambda(t) + \mathbf{X}^T \boldsymbol{\theta}. \tag{17.13}$$

Unlike the Cox model, which gives approximate estimates of relative risk, the AH model provides the approximate estimates of excess risk. It offers a different perspective on the association between covariates and an outcome. In the context of public health, the AH model tells how much the absolute risk could be reduced if a risk factor were removed from the population. This interpretation could be useful for public health planning and prevention.

17.6.1   Estimation of parameters

As described in Section 17.3.1, we may view a case-control study as a two-phase design. The Phase I sample (cohort) is regarded as a series of independent and identically distributed (i.i.d) observations drawn from the probability model (cf. Section 17.3.1), and the Phase II sample is obtained by finite population stratified sampling (FPSS) or Bernoulli sampling from the cohort. In order to use the AH model in practice, our estimation methods need to cover a sequence of problems. These include estimating the regression parameter $\boldsymbol{\theta}$, the cumulative baseline hazard $\Lambda(\cdot) = \int_0^\cdot \lambda(t)dt$, as well as the individual cumulative hazards from both cohort and case-control data.

To estimate $\boldsymbol{\theta}$ and $\Lambda(\cdot)$ for cohort data, we consider an estimating equation of i.i.d.

functions:

$$\sum_{i=1}^{N} \psi_{\boldsymbol{\theta},\Lambda,h}(\mathbf{Z}_i) = 0, \quad h \in \mathcal{H}, \tag{17.14}$$

where $\mathbf{Z}_i = (Y_i, T_i, \Delta_i, \mathbf{X}_i)$ as in Section 17.3.1, $h = (h_1, h_2)$ and $\psi_{\boldsymbol{\theta},\Lambda,h} = \psi_{1,\boldsymbol{\theta},\Lambda,h_1} + \psi_{2,\boldsymbol{\theta},\Lambda,h_2}$ with

$$\psi_{1,\boldsymbol{\theta},\Lambda,h_1}(\mathbf{Z}) = h_1^T \int_0^{\tau} \mathbf{X}\{d\mathbb{N}(t) - Y(t)d\Lambda(t) - Y(t)\mathbf{X}^T\boldsymbol{\theta}dt\},$$

$$\psi_{2,\boldsymbol{\theta},\Lambda,h_2}(\mathbf{Z}) = \int_0^{\tau} \{h_2(t)d\mathbb{N}(t) - h_2(t)Y(t)d\Lambda(t) - h_2(t)Y(t)\mathbf{X}^T\boldsymbol{\theta}dt\}.$$

Following the notations introduced in Section 17.3.1, $\mathbf{X}$ is a vector of covariates, $\mathbb{N}(t)$ the standard counting process and $Y(t)$ the at-risk process. h and $\mathcal{H}$ are introduced for technical reasons. We can ignore the detail and the meaning of them in the discussion of the main ideas here, but note that for this estimation problem, we choose $h = (h_1, h_2)$, where h_1 is a vector of the same dimension as $\mathbf{X}$ (and $\boldsymbol{\theta}$) and h_2 is a function of t. Further, $\psi_{\boldsymbol{\theta},\Lambda,h}$ is motivated from the likelihood equation for the AH model but not exactly the same (see Chapter 3.6 in Hu (2014)). By carefully choosing h and solving equations (17.14) one obtains the cohort estimators $\tilde{\boldsymbol{\theta}}$ and $\tilde{\Lambda}(\cdot)$.

Depending on whether Phase II subsamples are obtained by FPSS or Bernoulli sampling, the estimating procedures for two-phase sampling estimators would be different. FPSS introduces dependency to Phase II subsamples. We only discuss estimation with Bernoulli sampling here, because according to Section 17.4.3, the calibration technique could reconcile the apparent differences between FPSS and Bernoulli sampling. We will leave the development of two-phase FPSS estimators to the discussion of calibrated two-phase sampling estimators instead.

To estimate $\boldsymbol{\theta}$ and $\Lambda(\cdot)$ with two-phase Bernoulli sampling, we consider a weighted estimating equation of i.i.d. functions:

$$\sum_{i=1}^{N} \frac{R_i}{\pi_0(\mathbf{V}_i)} \psi_{\boldsymbol{\theta},\Lambda,h}(\mathbf{Z}_i) = 0, \tag{17.15}$$

where $\mathbf{V}_i$ is a vector of the variables that are fully available for each individual in the cohort, and $R_i = 1/0$ is the Phase II membership indicator that follows a Bernoulli distribution with the selection probability $\pi_0(\mathbf{V}_i) = P(R_i = 1|\mathbf{V}_i)$. With the same choice of h as for the cohort estimators, solving equations (17.15) yields the two-phase Bernoulli estimators

$$\hat{\boldsymbol{\theta}} = \left(\sum_{i=1}^{N} \frac{R_i}{\pi_0(\mathbf{V}_i)} \int_0^{\tau} \left\{\mathbf{X}_i - \frac{\sum_{i=1}^{N} \frac{R_i}{\pi_0(\mathbf{V}_i)}\mathbf{X}_i Y_i(t)}{\sum_{i=1}^{N} \frac{R_i}{\pi_0(\mathbf{V}_i)}Y_i(t)}\right\}^{\otimes 2} Y_i(t)dt\right)^{-1}$$

$$\times \sum_{i=1}^{N} \frac{R_i}{\pi_0(\mathbf{V}_i)} \int_0^{\tau} \left\{\mathbf{X}_i - \frac{\sum_{i=1}^{N} \frac{R_i}{\pi_0(\mathbf{V}_i)}\mathbf{X}_i Y_i(t)}{\sum_{i=1}^{N} \frac{R_i}{\pi_0(\mathbf{V}_i)}Y_i(t)}\right\} d\mathbb{N}_i(t),$$

$$\hat{\Lambda}(s) = \int_0^s \frac{\sum_{i=1}^{N} \frac{R_i}{\pi_0(\mathbf{V}_i)}[Y_i(t)d\mathbb{N}_i(t)]}{\sum_{i=1}^{N} \frac{R_i}{\pi_0(\mathbf{V}_i)}Y_i(t)} - \int_0^s \frac{\sum_{i=1}^{N} \frac{R_i}{\pi_0(\mathbf{V}_i)}[\mathbf{X}_i^T Y_i(t)]}{\sum_{i=1}^{N} \frac{R_i}{\pi_0(\mathbf{V}_i)}Y_i(t)}\hat{\boldsymbol{\theta}}dt,$$

where $s \in [0, \tau]$. The cohort estimators $\tilde{\boldsymbol{\theta}}$ and $\tilde{\Lambda}(s)$ take the same form as $\hat{\boldsymbol{\theta}}$ and $\hat{\Lambda}(s)$ except that $R_i/\pi_0(\mathbf{V}_i)$ is replaced by 1.

In Section 17.4.3, we introduced calibration as a technique to further improve two-phase Bernoulli sampling estimators by incorporating auxiliary information embedded in Phase I that has not been fully exploited. Here we use the same technique to improve estimators $\hat{\boldsymbol{\theta}}$ and $\hat{\Lambda}(s)$, and call these improved estimators [denoted $\hat{\boldsymbol{\theta}}^*$ and $\hat{\Lambda}^*(s)$] calibrated two-phase sampling estimators. It turns out that by following the procedure explained in Section 17.4.3, mainly the standard constrained optimization technique, the calibrated two-phase sampling estimators also take the form of $\hat{\boldsymbol{\theta}}$ and $\hat{\Lambda}(s)$ except $\frac{R_i}{\pi_0(\mathbf{V}_i)}$ is replaced by $\frac{R_i}{\pi_0(\mathbf{V}_i)} \exp(-\hat{\boldsymbol{\lambda}}_N^T \tilde{\mathbf{V}}_i)$. Here $\tilde{\mathbf{V}}_i$ is a function of $\mathbf{V}_i$, in other words some summary or part of the information available in Phase I. Further, $\hat{\boldsymbol{\lambda}}_N$ are the calculated Lagrange multipliers for the additional calibration equations from the added constraints we enforced while performing weight calibration.

17.6.2 Asymptotic properties of the estimators

The asymptotic studies of these estimators are conducted using the Z-estimation system (Hu, 2014, Chapter 2). Z-estimation refers to methods for Z-estimators, the solutions to zero-valued estimating equations (van der Vaart and Wellner, 1996), previously called M-estimation. Our cohort estimators, two-phase sampling estimators, and calibrated two-phase sampling estimators, which were introduced in the previous section, are all Z-estimators. Therefore, we can consider using Z-estimation for the asymptotic studies of these estimators. In addition, their corresponding estimating equations are all about the same function $\psi_{\boldsymbol{\theta},\Lambda,h}$ and in the same form of the summation of i.i.d. functions of $\psi_{\boldsymbol{\theta},\Lambda,h}$. The i.i.d. functions for these estimators are different but are closely related to each other through $\psi_{\boldsymbol{\theta},\Lambda,h}$. This systematic structure makes it possible to employ the Z-estimation system. We follow the procedures and theorems in the Z-estimation system to derive the asymptotic properties of all the estimators. This system is built upon the Z-estimation theorem of van der Vaart (1998), an extension of Huber's (1967) Z-estimation theorem and draws upon techniques from the modern empirical process theory (van der Vaart and Wellner, 1996).

In the end we are able to show that the joint distribution of the estimators of $\boldsymbol{\theta}$ and $\Lambda(\cdot)$ are Gaussian no matter if the estimators are obtained from cohort data or two-phase sampling with or without calibration. The asymptotic variance formulas are as follows:

$$\text{Var}_A \left\{ \dot{\Psi}_0 \sqrt{N} \left(\begin{array}{c} \tilde{\boldsymbol{\theta}} - \boldsymbol{\theta}_0 \\ \tilde{\Lambda} - \Lambda_0 \end{array} \right) h \right\} = \text{E}\psi_{\boldsymbol{\theta}_0,\Lambda_0,h}^2, \quad h \in \mathcal{H}, \qquad (17.16)$$

$$\text{Var}_A \left\{ \dot{\Psi}_0 \sqrt{N} \left(\begin{array}{c} \hat{\boldsymbol{\theta}} - \boldsymbol{\theta}_0 \\ \hat{\Lambda} - \Lambda_0 \end{array} \right) h \right\} = \text{E}\psi_{\boldsymbol{\theta}_0,\Lambda_0,h}^2 + \text{E}\left[\frac{1-\pi_0(\mathbf{V})}{\pi_0(\mathbf{V})} \psi_{\boldsymbol{\theta}_0,\Lambda_0,h}^2 \right], \quad h \in \mathcal{H}, \quad (17.17)$$

and

$$\text{Var}_A \left\{ \dot{\Psi}_0 \sqrt{N} \left(\begin{array}{c} \hat{\boldsymbol{\theta}}^* - \boldsymbol{\theta}_0 \\ \hat{\Lambda}^* - \Lambda_0 \end{array} \right) h \right\} \qquad (17.18)$$

$$= \text{E}\psi_{\boldsymbol{\theta}_0,\Lambda_0,h}^2 + \text{E}\left[\frac{1-\pi_0(\mathbf{V})}{\pi_0(\mathbf{V})} \left\{ \psi_{\boldsymbol{\theta}_0,\Lambda_0,h} - \Pi(\psi_{\boldsymbol{\theta}_0,\Lambda_0,h}|\tilde{\mathbf{V}}) \right\}^2 \right], \quad h \in \mathcal{H},$$

where $(\boldsymbol{\theta}_0, \Lambda_0)$ are the true values of the parameters we are estimating, $\dot{\Psi}_0$ is the Fréchet derivative of $\text{E}\psi_{\boldsymbol{\theta},\Lambda,h}$ at $(\boldsymbol{\theta}_0, \Lambda_0)$ and $\Pi(\cdot|\tilde{\mathbf{V}})$ is population least squares projection on the space spanned by the calibration variables $\tilde{\mathbf{V}}$: $\Pi(\cdot|\tilde{\mathbf{V}}) = \text{E}\{\cdot\tilde{\mathbf{V}}^T\}(\text{E}\tilde{\mathbf{V}}\tilde{\mathbf{V}}^T)^{-1}\tilde{\mathbf{V}}$.

The estimates for the regression parameters and the individual cumulative hazard then can be developed based on the joint distributions. The model-based variances and robust variances under model misspecification can be developed immediately depending on whether the expectation $E(\cdot)$ is taken under the model assumption or not.

Notice that the findings from the above results are consistent with the insights gained from the methods development for the Cox model in Section 17.4.2. Namely, 1) total variance of a two-phase sampling estimator is the sum of the Phase I variance you would observe if $\mathbf{X}$ were observable for every Phase I subject and the Phase II variance; 2) The Phase I variance is not affected by the choice of Phase II design; 3) The variance of our calibrated two-phase sampling Z-estimators is generally reduced by a factor that is the least squares projection of the influence function for the parameters on $\tilde{\mathbf{V}}$.

17.6.3   Finite population stratified sampling estimators

Now we come back to the discussion of FPSS estimators. In Section 17.4.3 it was explained how calibration is able to reconcile the differences between FPSS and Bernoulli sampling schemes. This connection suggests an approach of using calibration to obtain correct standard errors under the FPSS scheme without invoking any new estimation methods. The approach is that we calibrate the design weights calculated from Bernoulli sampling to the strata frequencies by using stratum membership as our calibration variables. The resulting two-phase calibrated estimators are the desired FPSS estimators. We implement this procedure in the R package `addhazard`. Users can directly request FPSS or Bernoulli sampling estimators from this R Package.

17.7   Additive hazards model analysis for radiation and breast cancer

In Section 17.2 we introduced a cohort on radiation and breast cancer (BC) and two two-phase sampling data sets that were simulated from the cohort data, mimicking the case-cohort and stratified case-cohort studies. In Section 17.5, we fit the Cox model to these three data sets. In this section, we instead apply the methods outlined in Section 17.6 and use the Lin-Ying additive hazards (AH) model (Lin and Ying, 1994) to reanalyze these data sets. When analyzing the stratified case-cohort data, we use both standard and calibrated weights. The calibrated weights may further improve the precision in estimation by incorporating additional cohort information. All the analyses are performed with the freely available R package `addhazard` (Hu *et al.*, 2015), and the code is available from the handbook website. Phase II subsamples are treated as obtained by FPSS throughout the analyses. Our choice of the AH model is introduced in Section 17.7.1. Results on the estimates for covariate coefficients and the expected BC risk are provided in Sections 17.7.3 and 17.7.4.

17.7.1   The additive hazards model for radiation and breast cancer

In our AH model, the cumulative hazard for BC of a woman with covariates $\mathbf{x}$ and $t =$ attained age is modeled as

$$\Lambda(t, \mathbf{x}; \beta, \Lambda_0) = \Lambda_0(t) + (x_1\beta_1 + x_2\beta_2)t, \tag{17.19}$$

where $\mathbf{x} = (x_1, x_2)$ with $x_1 =$ dose and $x_2 =$ ageRx/10. Compared to the Cox model we assumed in Section 17.5, dose x_1 was modeled directly without a log transformation, due

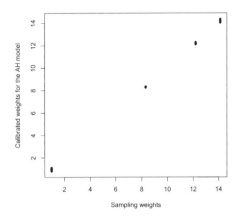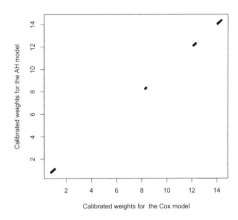

FIGURE 17.4
Results of weight calibration for the AH model. Left panel: Calibrated weights by sampling weights. Right panel: Calibrated weights for the AH model by calibrated weights for the Cox model.

to the radiobiological evidence that dose-response effect is usually linear at low radiation levels.

17.7.2 Calibration

Section 17.4.3 and formula (17.18) suggested the optimal calibration variables to adjust design weights are the conditional expectation of the influence function, $\dot{\Psi}_0^{-1}\psi_{\boldsymbol{\theta},\Lambda,h}(\mathbf{z})$, on all the Phase I information. Because only a subset of the Phase I members have dose measurements in the stratified case-cohort sample data, the dose variable x_1 in $\mathbf{z}$ is partially missing in Phase I. Thus, we approximated the optimal calibration variables by substituting $x_1' =$ total number of fluoroscopies/100, which was available for all the cohort members, for $x_1 =$ dose. We first fit an AH model to the Phase I data using x_1' and $x_2 =$ ageRx/10 as covariates. We obtained the (integrated) martingale residuals for the two covariates, which could be extracted from the model fit by the `addhazard` package. These residuals are highly correlated with $\psi_{\boldsymbol{\theta},\Lambda,h}$ and thus would effectively reduce the second term in the asymptotic variance formula (17.18) for the calibrated two-phase sampling estimators. Therefore, we chose these martingale residuals as our calibration variables. Note the correlation coefficient between x_1 and x_1' was as high as 0.966. It is rare to find such a surrogate in real applications but nevertheless our results will show the precision gain for estimates by finding a strong surrogate.

From the left-hand panel of Figure 17.4 we observe that the calibrated weights are similar to the original design weights. The right-hand panel of the figure shows that the calibrated weights based on the AH model are almost the same as the ones calculated based on the Cox model in Section 17.5.3. In the result section, we will see how much estimation precision can be improved by this slight change of design weights in the estimating procedure.

17.7.3 Results of the analyses: Regression coefficients

Table 17.4 shows the estimates of covariate coefficients and their model-based standard errors from four different study designs. Analyzing the entire cohort (Table 17.4 A) using the AH model shows that the age-specific risk of BC increases by 0.478×10^{-3} per person-year for 1 Gy increase in radiation dose, and if young women could receive radiation 10 years later in their treatment for tuberculosis, their age-specific risk of BC would decrease by 0.363×10^{-3} per person-year. The stratified case-cohort study gives very similar results when we calibrated weights using additional cohort information. Note that the conclusions drawn from fitting the AH model can be generally interpreted as an inference on the absolute risk change of a population attributable to a risk factor, for example, the approximate change of BC risk by reducing radiation dose. It is convenient for public health policy makers to use these statistical results to make a population-wise statement about a risk factor. Thus, this model may assist them make intervention decisions about a risk factor among a population.

TABLE 17.4

Comparison of results for four designs using additive hazards models. Model-based standard errors.(See Section 17.5.4 for the explanations of column names.)

Model term	Coef. $(\times 10^{-3})$	SE1 $(\times 10^{-3})$	SE2 $(\times 10^{-3})$	SE $(\times 10^{-3})$	Z	p
A. Entire Cohort						
dose	0.478	0.210	NA	0.210	2.272	0.0231
ageRx/10	-0.363	0.200	NA	0.200	-1.811	0.0701
B. Simple case-cohort sample, FPSS						
dose	0.477	0.190	0.209	0.282	1.690	0.0911
ageRx/10	-0.180	0.219	0.145	0.263	-0.685	0.4935
C. Stratified case-cohort sample, FPSS						
dose	0.716	0.286	0.246	0.377	1.900	0.0574
ageRx/10	-0.343	0.193	0.091	0.213	-1.609	0.1075
D. Stratified case-cohort sample with calibrated weights, FPSS						
dose	0.517	0.262	0.132	0.294	1.759	0.0787
ageRx/10	-0.365	0.192	0.036	0.195	-1.871	0.0613

We then look at the standard errors, and first examine the standard errors of the regression coefficients in Table 17.4 B and C. We find that SE for ageRx/10 becomes smaller in the stratified case-cohort study than in the case-cohort study, 0.213×10^{-3} compared to 0.263×10^{-3}, even though the absolute value of the ageRx/10 coefficient estimate is higher in the stratified the case-cohort study, -0.343×10^{-3} compared to -0.180×10^{-3}. As a result, the p-value is reduced from 0.4935 to 0.1075. This improvement in precision may be due to the more balanced amount of information among different categories of ageRx when we switched from selecting our subcohort by random sampling to by stratified sampling based on ageRx. The Phase II subsamples changed from 91, 84, and 43 for low, middle, and high ageRx categories to 77, 78, and 64, respectively, after the switch. We do not see this much precision improvement attributable to the stratified case-cohort design for the dose effect. This is probably because the stratification variable ageRx has a low correlation with dose. The correlation coefficient is only -0.0872 (based on the full cohort data). The precision of our estimation about dose effect is unlikely to be improved by using irrelevant information.

Next we compare the standard errors of regression coefficients in Table 17.4 D to C. Here SE1 and SE2 denote the estimated Phase I and Phase II standard errors. After calibrating

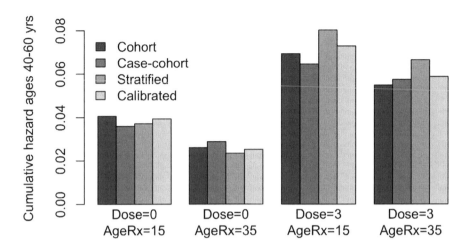

FIGURE 17.5
Cumulative hazards of breast cancer between age 40 and 60 predicted based on the AH model.

design weights, SE2 is reduced from 0.246×10^{-3} to 0.132×10^{-3} for the dose effect estimate and from 0.091×10^{-3} to 0.036×10^{-3} for ageRx/10. The p-value for ageRx/10 is further reduced from 0.1075 to 0.0613, while p-value for dose does not decrease because its coefficient estimate concurrently decreases.

By analyzing estimation results for dose and ageRx from different study designs, we learn that a thoughtful use of stratification and calibration can greatly improve estimation precision. Comparing the stratified case-cohort to the full cohort study design, although we miss 87.3% $[100 \cdot (1720 - 219)/1720]$ of dose measurements by design in the stratified case-cohort study, the precision of the dose effect estimation was not reduced this much (SE $= 0.294 \times 10^{-3}$ in Table 17.4 D versus SE $= 0.210 \times 10^{-3}$ in Table 17.4 A). Our result is consistent with the corresponding Cox model results (SE $= 0.184$ in Table 17.3 D for dose to SE $= 0.153$ in Table 17.3 A). When both the stratification variables and the calibration variables are highly correlated with the covariate we aim to make inference on, ageRx/10 in this case, the gain of precision can be substantial. These two methods together make the estimation of age at first treatment's effect from a subsample of only 219 subjects almost as precise as the entire cohort of 1,720 subjects (SE $= 0.195 \times 10^{-3}$ in Table 17.4 D versus SE $= 0.200 \times 10^{-3}$ in Table 17.4 A). A similar result was shown in the Cox model analysis (SE $= 0.140$ in Table 17.3 D compared to SE $= 0.144$ in Table 17.3 A).

17.7.4 Results of the analyses: Expected breast cancer risk

Based on the fitted AH model, we predicted the expected BC risk under the same four configurations of covariate values as Section 17.5.5. Figure 17.5 shows the predicted BC risk for four women between 40 to 60 years of age. Among them, two subjects received no radiation and two a dose of 3 Gy radiation. For each scenario, one started tuberculosis treatment at age 15 and one at age 35. The analysis was performed by using the `predict` command within the R package `addhazard`. Figure 17.5 follows the same pattern revealed in Figure 17.3 where the prediction was based on the Cox model. A woman who received a radiation dose of 3 Gy and started treatment at age 15 had the highest risk (cumulative hazard). As age at first treatment increased to 35, the BC risk of a woman declined. The same effect of ageRx is also observed in women without radiation. The full cohort analysis shows that by switching from a radiation dose of 3 Gy to no radiation, the risks were greatly reduced from 6.9% to 4.1% for women with ageRx at 15 and from 5.5% to 2.6% for women with ageRx at 35.

Suppose results from the full cohort analysis were treated as the "gold standard." We observe the predicted values from the three two-phase design analyses are all similar to the gold standard. Among them, the stratified samples with calibrated weights have the best predicted values. In the order of the plots in Figure 17.5, these values are 3.9%, 2.5%, 7.3% and 5.9% while the estimated risks from the full cohort are 4.1%, 2.6%, 6.9% and 5.5%, correspondingly. In addition, these four estimated risks from the full cohort based on the AH model are very close to the risks predicted based on the Cox models reported in Section 17.5.5.

17.8   Concluding remarks

In this chapter we presented a survey sampling approach to analyzing survival data from case-control studies and introduced several recently developed analyzing tools motivated by this approach. In this perspective, cohort data is regarded as a Phase I sample drawn from a superpopulation; case-control data is considered as a Phase II subsample. Some expensive exposures, e.g., biomarkers, in general are only available for the Phase II subsample. This perspective facilitates separation of the development of methods for sampling designs from the models for the cohort data. As a result, general estimation methods for handling different design properties could accommodate various survival models and vice versa.

We introduced several methods on sampling design. First, we showed that calibration techniques from survey sampling can be used to incorporate a large amount of auxiliary information, which is often ignored, into estimation procedures and enhance precision in estimation. Second, we demonstrated that calibration techniques can be used to resolve differences between FFPS and Bernoulli sampling. As a result, estimation methods that are developed for Bernoulli sampling can be adapted to FPSS, a more realistic sampling scheme, without invoking new methods. Third, by stratification on a surrogate of the expensive variable at Phase I, more informative Phase II subjects can be selected, and in consequence precision in regression coefficients estimates will be improved without increasing Phase II sample sizes.

In the discussion of survival models we introduced estimation methods for the Cox model and the Lin-Ying additive hazards (AH) models. The two estimation methods are slightly different, the former starting from the partial score function for regression coefficients and the latter from a set of estimating equations for both regression coefficients and the baseline cumulative hazard. Nevertheless, both methods rely on semiparametric inference and the modern empirical processes theory. These theoretical tools make the estimating procedures general enough to handle case-control studies with and without calibration.

All the methods in this chapter were implemented in freely available R softwares. To illustrate their applications, we performed survival analysis on three data sets on radiation and breast cancer. We fitted the Cox and the AH models to cohort, case-cohort and stratified case-cohort data for regression coefficient estimation and risk prediction. We demonstrated calibration techniques and estimation under FPSS. All the R codes are available on the handbook website. With these new tools, survival analysis for case-control studies has become more transparent and convenient. Researchers are encouraged to apply them to survival outcome data with case-control designs for risk factors studies and risk prediction.

Bibliography

Anderson, G. L., Manson, J., Wallace, R., Lund, B., Hall, D., Davis, S., Shumaker, S., Wang, C.-Y., Stein, E., and Prentice, R. L. (2003). Implementation of the Women's Health Initiative study design. *Annals of Epidemiology*, **13**, S5–S17.

Binder, D. A. (1992). Fitting Cox's proportional hazards model from survey data. *Biometrika*, **79**, 139–147.

Borgan, Ø. and Samuelsen, S. O. (2013). Nested case-control and case-cohort studies. In J. P. Klein, H. C. van Houwelingen, J. G. Ibrahim, and T. H. Scheike, editors, *Handbook of Survival Analysis*, pages 343–367. Chapman and Hall/CRC, Boca Raton, FL.

Borgan, Ø., Langholz, B., Samuelsen, S. O., Goldstein, L., and Pogoda, J. (2000). Exposure stratified case-cohort designs. *Lifetime Data Analysis*, **6**, 39–58.

Breslow, N. E. and Wellner, J. A. (2007). Weighted likelihood for semiparametric models and two-phase stratified samples, with application to Cox regression. *Scandinavian Journal of Statistics*, **34**, 86–102. Correction **35**, 186–192.

Breslow, N. E., Lumley, T., Ballantyne, C. M., Chambless, L. E., and Kulich, M. (2009a). Improved Horvitz-Thompson estimation of model parameters from two-phase stratified samples: Applications in epidemiology. *Statistics in Biosciences*, **1**, 32–49.

Breslow, N. E., Lumley, T., Ballantyne, C. M., Chambless, L. E., and Kulich, M. (2009b). Using the whole cohort in the analysis of case-cohort data. *American Journal of Epidemiology*, **169**, 1398–1405.

Breslow, N. E., Amorim, G., Pettinger, M. B., and Rossouw, J. (2013). Using the whole cohort in the analysis of case-control data. Application to the Women's Health Initiative. *Statistics in Biosciences*, **5**, 232–249.

Breslow, N. E., Hu, J., and Wellner, J. A. (2015). Z-estimation and stratified samples. Application to survival models. *Lifetime Data Analysis*, **21**, 493–516.

Chen, K. N. and Lo, S. H. (1999). Case-cohort and case-control analysis with Cox's model. *Biometrika*, **86**, 755–764.

Cox, D. R. (1972). Regression models and life-tables (with discussion). *Journal of the Royal Statistical Society (Series B)*, **34**, 187–220.

Deville, J. C. and Särndal, C. E. (1992). Calibration estimators in survey sampling. *Journal of the American Statistical Association*, **87**, 376–382.

Hrubec, Z., Boice, J. D., Monson, R. R., and Rosenstein, M. (1989). Breast-cancer after multiple chest fluoroscopies - 2nd follow-up of Massachusetts women with tuberculosis. *Cancer Research*, **49**, 229–234.

Hu, J. (2014). *A Z-estimation System for Two-phase Sampling with Applications to Additive Hazards Models and Epidemiologic Studies*. Ph.D. thesis, University of Washington.

Hu, J. K., Breslow, N. E., and Chan, G. (2015). *addhazard: Fit Additive Hazards Models for Survival Analysis*. R package version 1.0.0.

Huber, P. J. (1967). The behavior of maximum likelihood estimates under nonstandard conditions. In *Proceedings of the Fifth Berkeley Symposium on Mathematical Statistics and Probability, Volume 1: Statistics*, Fifth Berkeley Symposium on Mathematical Statistics and Probability, pages 221–233. University of California Press.

Kalbfleisch, J. D. and Prentice, R. L. (2002). *The Statistical Analysis of Failure Time Data*. Wiley, Hoboken, NJ, 2nd edition.

Kulich, M. and Lin, D. Y. (2004). Improving the efficiency of relative-risk estimation in case-cohort studies. *Journal of the American Statistical Association*, **99**, 832–844.

Lin, D. Y. (2000). On fitting Cox's proportional hazards model to survey data. *Biometrika*, **87**, 37–47.

Lin, D. Y. and Ying, Z. (1994). Semiparametric analysis of the additive risk model. *Biometrika*, **81**, 61–71.

Lumley, T. (2012). *Complex Surveys: A Guide to Analysis Using R*. Wiley, Hoboken, NJ.

Lumley, T., Shaw, P. A., and Dai, J. Y. (2011). Connections between survey calibration estimators and semiparametric models for incomplete data. *International Statistical Review*, **79**, 200–220.

Prentice, R. L. (1986). A case-cohort design for epidemiologic cohort studies and disease prevention trials. *Biometrika*, **73**, 1–11.

Preston, D. L., Lubin, J. H., Pierce, D. A., and McConney, M. D. (1993). *Epicure Users Guide*. Hirosoft International Corporation, Seattle, WA.

Robins, J. M., Rotnitzky, A., and Zhao, L. P. (1994). Estimation of regression-coefficients when some regressors are not always observed. *Journal of the American Statistical Association*, **89**, 846–866.

Saegusa, T. and Wellner, J. A. (2013). Weighted likelihood estimation under two-phase sampling. *Annals of Statistics*, **41**, 269–295.

Therneau, T. M. and Grambsch, P. M. (2000). *Modeling Survival Data: Extending the Cox Model*. Springer, New York.

van der Vaart, A. W. (1998). *Asymptotic Statistics*. Cambridge University Press, Cambridge, UK.

van der Vaart, A. W. and Wellner, J. A. (1996). *Weak Convergence and Empirical Processes with Applications in Statistics*. Springer, New York.

Williams, O. D. (1989). The Atherosclerosis Risk in Communities (ARIC) study - design and objectives. *American Journal of Epidemiology*, **129**, 687–702.

18

Nested Case-Control Studies: A Counting Process Approach

Ørnulf Borgan

University of Oslo

18.1   Introduction

For cohort data, estimation in Cox's regression model is based on a partial likelihood, which at each observed death or disease occurrence (generically denoted "failure") compares the covariate values of the failing individual to those of all individuals at risk at that time. Therefore, standard use of Cox regression requires collection of covariate information on all individuals in a cohort even when only a small fraction of them actually fails. This may be very expensive, or even logistically impossible, for large cohorts. Cohort sampling techniques, where covariate information is collected for all individuals who fail ("cases"), but only for a sample of the individuals who do not fail ("controls"), then offer useful alternatives that may drastically reduce the resources that need to be allocated to a study. Further, as most of the statistical information is contained in the cases, such studies may still

329

be sufficient to give reliable answers to the questions of interest. There are two important classes of cohort sampling designs: nested case-control sampling and case-cohort sampling. An overview of the two types of sampling designs is given in Chapter 16, and in Chapter 17 a detailed study of case-cohort sampling is provided. In this chapter we focus on nested case-control sampling.

For cohort data, it is well known that counting processes are useful for studying Cox regression and other methods for failure time data (e.g. Andersen *et al.*, 1993; Aalen *et al.*, 2008). But counting processes also provide a useful framework for nested case-control sampling (Borgan *et al.*, 1995). The counting process formulation of nested case-control studies allows for quite general sampling designs for the controls, including the classical case with simple random sampling of the controls (Thomas, 1977) and counter-matched control sampling (Langholz and Borgan, 1995). Moreover, the approach is key to deriving a number of statistical methods for Cox's regression model with nested case-control data, including partial likelihood inference, estimation of cumulative hazards and methods for model checking. The aim of the chapter is to give an overview of these results.

The chapter is organized as follows. In Section 18.2 we give a brief summary of Cox's regression model for cohort data, and describe how cohort data may be given a counting process formulation. We also review how the regression coefficients in Cox's model are estimated by a partial likelihood, and we mention estimation of the baseline cumulative hazard and model checking using martingale residuals. The purpose of Section 18.2 is to provide a background for the following sections, where similar methods are given for nested case-control data. Sections 18.3 and 18.4 present a general framework for control sampling in nested case-control studies and describe how nested case-control data may be given a counting process formulation. A partial likelihood for nested case-control data is derived in Section 18.5, and estimation of cumulative hazards is discussed in Section 18.6. In Section 18.7 we show how one may define martingale residuals for nested case-control data and discuss how cumulative sums of martingale residuals may be used for model checking. In nested case-control studies, it is quite common that the controls are matched to the cases on a number of variables. In Section 18.8 we discuss how the methods of the previous sections should be modified in the presence of such additional matching. Some concluding comments are given in the final Section 18.9.

Throughout the chapter we will without further references use standard results for counting processes, intensity processes and martingales (e.g. Andersen *et al.*, 1993; Aalen *et al.*, 2008). The data on radiation and breast cancer introduced in Section 17.2 of Chapter 17 will be used for illustration.

18.2   Cox regression for cohort data

In this section we describe how Cox's regression model may be formulated by means of counting processes, and we indicate how counting process theory (with corresponding intensity processes and martingales) is useful for deriving statistical methods and studying their properties. The aim of the section is to provide a background for the following sections on nested case-control data, where similar counting process arguments will be used.

We have a cohort of N independent individuals, and we want to study the risk of death of a particular cause or the occurrence of a specific disease. The term "failure" is used as a generic term for death or the occurrence of a disease. We let $\lambda_i(t)$ be the hazard rate (or failure rate) for the ith individual with vector of (possibly) time-dependent covariates $\mathbf{x}_i(t) = (x_{i1}(t), \ldots, x_{ip}(t))^{\mathrm{T}}$. The time variable t may be age, time since the onset of a disease, or some other time scale relevant to the problem at hand. Throughout we assume that $t \in [0, \tau]$ for a given terminal study time τ. We also assume that the time-dependent covariates (if any) are external (or exogeneous); cf. Kalbfleisch and Prentice (2002, section 6.3). Thus we do not allow for internal (or endogenous) time-dependent covariates like biomarkers measured for the individuals during follow-up.

We assume that the covariates of individual i are related to its hazard rate by Cox's regression model:

$$\lambda_i(t) = \lambda(t \mid \mathbf{x}_i) = \exp\{\boldsymbol{\beta}^\mathrm{T} \mathbf{x}_i(t)\} \lambda_0(t). \tag{18.1}$$

Here $\boldsymbol{\beta}$ is a vector of regression coefficients describing the effects of the covariates, while the baseline hazard rate $\lambda_0(t)$ corresponds to the hazard rate of an individual with all covariates equal to zero. We make no assumptions on the form of the baseline hazard rate, so model (18.1) is semi-parametric.

The individuals in the cohort may be followed over different periods of time, from an entry time to an exit time corresponding to failure or censoring. We denote by $t_1 < t_2 < \cdots$ the times when failures are observed and, assuming no tied failure times, we let i_j denote the individual who fails at t_j.

18.2.1 Counting processes, intensity processes and martingales

We may represent the observations for the individuals in the cohort by counting processes $\mathbb{N}_i(t)$ and at-risk processes $Y_i(t)$; $i = 1, \ldots, N$. Here $Y_i(t) = 1$ if individual i is under observation (i.e., at risk) just before time t, otherwise $Y_i(t) = 0$, and the process

$$\mathbb{N}_i(t) = \sum_{j \geq 1} I\{t_j \leq t; \, i_j = i\} \tag{18.2}$$

counts the number of failures for individual i in $[0, t]$. In this chapter we consider survival data, where a failure can happen at most once for each individual. Hence $\mathbb{N}_i(t) = 1$ if individual i has been observed to fail by time t; otherwise $\mathbb{N}_i(t) = 0$.

We also introduce the "cohort history" $\mathcal{H}_{t-}$, which contains the information that is available to the researcher in a cohort study on events, censorings, late entries and covariates up to, but not including, time t. We may define an *intensity process* $\widetilde{\lambda}_i(t)$ of the counting process $\mathbb{N}_i(t)$ relative to the cohort history $\mathcal{H}_{t-}$. Informally, this is given by

$$\widetilde{\lambda}_i(t)dt = P(d\mathbb{N}_i(t) = 1 \mid \mathcal{H}_{t-}),$$

where $d\mathbb{N}_i(t)$ is the number of jumps of the counting process in $[t, t + dt)$. Thus $d\mathbb{N}_i(t) = 1$ if a failure is observed for individual i in $[t, t + dt)$, and $d\mathbb{N}_i(t) = 0$ otherwise. Since $d\mathbb{N}_i(t)$ is a binary variable, we may alternatively write $\widetilde{\lambda}_i(t)dt = E(d\mathbb{N}_i(t) \mid \mathcal{H}_{t-})$. If we introduce the process

$$\mathbb{M}_i(t) = \mathbb{N}_i(t) - \int_0^t \widetilde{\lambda}_i(u)du, \tag{18.3}$$

we then have

$$E(d\mathbb{M}_i(t) \mid \mathcal{H}_{t-}) = E(d\mathbb{N}_i(t) \mid \mathcal{H}_{t-}) - \widetilde{\lambda}_i(t)dt = 0,$$

which shows heuristically that $\mathbb{M}_i(t)$ is a *martingale*.

We will assume throughout that late entries and censorings are independent in the sense that the additional knowledge of which individuals have entered the study or have been censored before time t does not carry information on the risks of failure at t; cf. Kalbfleisch and Prentice (2002, Sections 1.3 and 6.2). Then the intensity process takes the form

$$\widetilde{\lambda}_i(t) = Y_i(t)\lambda_i(t) = Y_i(t)\exp\{\boldsymbol{\beta}^\mathrm{T}\mathbf{x}_i(t)\}\lambda_0(t), \tag{18.4}$$

i.e., it equals the hazard rate (18.1) if individual i is at risk, and it is zero otherwise.

18.2.2   Cox's partial likelihood

The semi-parametric nature of Cox's model (18.1) makes it impossible to use ordinary likelihood methods to estimate the regression coefficients $\boldsymbol{\beta}$. Instead one has to resort to a partial likelihood. We will outline how this can be derived, essentially following Cox's original argument (Cox, 1975). To this end we introduce the aggregated counting process $\mathbb{N}_{\boldsymbol{\cdot}}(t) = \sum_{\ell=1}^{N} \mathbb{N}_\ell(t)$, registering failures among all individuals in the cohort, and note that the aggregated counting process has intensity process

$$\widetilde{\lambda}_{\boldsymbol{\cdot}}(t) = \sum_{\ell=1}^{N} \widetilde{\lambda}_\ell(t) = \sum_{\ell=1}^{N} Y_\ell(t) \exp\{\boldsymbol{\beta}^{\mathrm{T}} \mathbf{x}_\ell(t)\} \lambda_0(t). \tag{18.5}$$

The intensity process of $\mathbb{N}_i(t)$ may now be factorized as $\widetilde{\lambda}_i(t) = \widetilde{\lambda}_{\boldsymbol{\cdot}}(t)\, \pi(i|t)$, where

$$\pi(i|t) = \frac{\widetilde{\lambda}_i(t)}{\widetilde{\lambda}_{\boldsymbol{\cdot}}(t)} = \frac{Y_i(t) \exp\{\boldsymbol{\beta}^{\mathrm{T}} \mathbf{x}_i(t)\}}{\sum_{\ell=1}^{N} Y_\ell(t) \exp\{\boldsymbol{\beta}^{\mathrm{T}} \mathbf{x}_\ell(t)\}} \tag{18.6}$$

is the conditional probability of observing a failure for individual i at time t, given the cohort history $\mathcal{H}_{t-}$ and given that a failure is observed at that time (for any individual).

The partial likelihood for $\boldsymbol{\beta}$ is obtained by multiplying together the conditional probabilities (18.6) over all failure times t_j with corresponding failing individuals i_j. So the partial likelihood becomes

$$L_{\mathrm{full}}(\boldsymbol{\beta}) = \prod_{t_j} \pi(i_j|t_j) = \prod_{t_j} \frac{Y_{i_j}(t_j) \exp\{\boldsymbol{\beta}^{\mathrm{T}} \mathbf{x}_{i_j}(t_j)\}}{\sum_{\ell=1}^{N} Y_\ell(t_j) \exp\{\boldsymbol{\beta}^{\mathrm{T}} \mathbf{x}_\ell(t_j)\}}.$$

If we introduce the notation $\mathcal{R}_j = \{\ell \,|\, Y_\ell(t_j) = 1\}$ for the risk set at t_j, the partial likelihood may be written in the more familiar form

$$L_{\mathrm{full}}(\boldsymbol{\beta}) = \prod_{t_j} \frac{\exp\{\boldsymbol{\beta}^{\mathrm{T}} \mathbf{x}_{i_j}(t_j)\}}{\sum_{\ell \in \mathcal{R}_j} \exp\{\boldsymbol{\beta}^{\mathrm{T}} \mathbf{x}_\ell(t_j)\}}. \tag{18.7}$$

The maximum partial likelihood estimator $\widehat{\boldsymbol{\beta}}$ is the value of $\boldsymbol{\beta}$ that maximizes (18.7). Using results for counting processes, intensity processes and martingales, Andersen and Gill (1982) showed that $\widehat{\boldsymbol{\beta}}$ enjoys similar large sample properties as ordinary maximum likelihood estimators; see also Andersen *et al.* (1993, section VII.2.2) and Aalen *et al.* (2008, section 4.1.5). In particular, in large samples, $\widehat{\boldsymbol{\beta}}$ is approximately multivariate normally distributed around the true value of $\boldsymbol{\beta}$ with a covariance matrix that may be estimated by the inverse information matrix.

In Section 18.5 we will use similar arguments as those above to derive a partial likelihood for nested case-control data.

18.2.3   The Breslow estimator and martingale residuals

We then consider the cumulative baseline hazard $\Lambda_0(t) = \int_0^t \lambda_0(u)du$. This may be estimated by the Breslow estimator

$$\widehat{\Lambda}_{0,\mathrm{full}}(t) = \sum_{t_j \le t} \frac{1}{\sum_{\ell \in \mathcal{R}_j} \exp\{\widehat{\boldsymbol{\beta}}^{\mathrm{T}} \mathbf{x}_\ell(t_j)\}}. \tag{18.8}$$

Andersen and Gill (1982) used results on counting processes, intensity processes and martingales to study the statistical properties of the Breslow estimator; see also Andersen *et al.*

(1993, section VII.2.2) and Aalen *et al.* (2008, section 4.1.6). From the Breslow estimator one may obtain estimates of the cumulative hazard corresponding to given values of the covariates. We return to this in connection with nested case-control data in Section 18.6.

The Breslow estimator also plays a role in the derivation of martingale residuals for Cox's regression model. By (18.3) and (18.4) we have that the processes

$$\mathbb{M}_i(t) = \mathbb{N}_i(t) - \int_0^t Y_i(u) \exp\{\boldsymbol{\beta}^{\mathrm{T}} \mathbf{x}_i(u)\} \lambda_0(u) du, \tag{18.9}$$

$i = 1, \ldots, N$, are martingales. If we in (18.9) replace $\boldsymbol{\beta}$ by $\widehat{\boldsymbol{\beta}}$ and $\lambda_0(u) du$ by $d\widehat{\Lambda}_{0,\text{full}}(u)$, we obtain the martingale residual processes

$$\begin{aligned}
\widehat{\mathbb{M}}_i(t) &= \mathbb{N}_i(t) - \int_0^t Y_i(u) \exp\{\widehat{\boldsymbol{\beta}}^{\mathrm{T}} \mathbf{x}_i(u)\} d\widehat{\Lambda}_{0,\text{full}}(u) \\
&= \mathbb{N}_i(t) - \sum_{t_j \leq t} \frac{Y_i(t_j) \exp\{\widehat{\boldsymbol{\beta}}^{\mathrm{T}} \mathbf{x}_i(t_j)\}}{\sum_{\ell \in \mathcal{R}_j} \exp\{\widehat{\boldsymbol{\beta}}^{\mathrm{T}} \mathbf{x}_\ell(t_j)\}}.
\end{aligned}$$

If we evaluate the martingale residual processes at $t = \tau$, where τ is the upper time limit for the study, we arrive at the *martingale residuals* $\widehat{\mathbb{M}}_i = \widehat{\mathbb{M}}_i(\tau)$ first considered by Barlow and Prentice (1988). Plots of the martingale residuals are useful for checking the assumptions of Cox regression; see, e.g., Therneau and Grambsch (2000, section 5.7). Not all the methods for cohort data based on martingale residuals may be extended to nested case-control data. So for the purpose of this chapter, we will focus on the methods of Lin *et al.* (1993) based on cumulative sums of martingale residuals; cf. Section 18.7.

18.3   A general framework for nested-case control sampling

By using a counting process formulation, we may derive results for nested case-control data that are similar to the ones for the full cohort. Before we show how this may be done, we will in this section present a general framework for the sampling of controls in a nested case-control study and give three examples of specific sampling schemes for the controls.

For a nested case-control study, one selects, whenever a failure occurs, a small number of controls among those at risk. The set consisting of these controls together with the individual who fails (i.e., the case) is called a *sampled risk set*. Covariate information is collected for the individuals in the sampled risk sets but is not needed for the other individuals in the cohort.

Figure 18.1 illustrates the basic features of a nested case-control study for a hypothetical cohort of seven individuals when one control is selected per case. Note that the selection of controls is done independently at the different failure times. Thus subjects may serve as controls for multiple cases, and a case may serve as control for other cases that failed when the case was at risk. For example, the case at time t_4 in the figure had been selected as control at the earlier time t_1.

The sampling of controls may be performed in different ways. In Chapter 16 we discussed the classical nested case-control design, where the controls are selected by simple random sampling, and the counter-matched nested case-control design. In this chapter we will describe a general framework for the selection of controls that contains the classical and counter-matched nested case-control designs as special cases; cf. Sections 18.3.1 and 18.3.2.

We will describe in probabilistic terms how the sampling of controls is performed. To

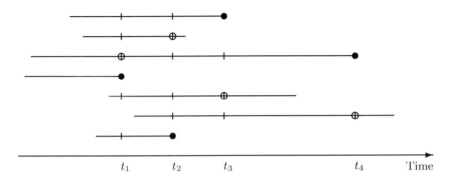

FIGURE 18.1

Illustration of nested case-control sampling, with one control per case, from a hypothetical cohort of seven individuals. Each individual is represented by a line starting at an entry time and ending at an exit time corresponding failure or censoring. Failure times are indicated by dots (•), potential controls are indicated by bars (|), and the sampled controls are indicated by circles (∘).

this end we need to introduce the "cohort and sampling history" $\mathcal{F}_{t-}$, which contains information about the cohort (described by the "cohort history" $\mathcal{H}_{t-}$), as well as on the sampling of controls, up to, but not including, time t. Based on the parts of this history that are available to the researcher, one decides a sampling plan for the controls.

Such a sampling plan may be specified as follows. Let $\mathcal{P}$ be the collection of all subsets of $\{1, 2, \ldots, N\}$. Then, given $\mathcal{F}_{t-}$, if individual i fails at time t, one selects the set $\mathbf{r} \in \mathcal{P}$ as the sampled risk set with (known) probability $\pi(\mathbf{r} \,|\, t, i)$. We assume that $\pi(\mathbf{r} \,|\, t, i) = 0$ if $i \notin \mathbf{r}$, so that only subsets containing i may be selected. For notational simplicity we let $\pi(\mathbf{r} \,|\, t, i) = 0$ if $Y_i(t) = 0$, and note that

$$\sum_{\mathbf{r} \in \mathcal{P}} \pi(\mathbf{r} \,|\, t, i) = Y_i(t)$$

since $\pi(\mathbf{r} \,|\, t, i)$ is a probability distribution if $Y_i(t) = 1$, and 0 otherwise.

It will be useful to have a factorization of the sampling probabilities $\pi(\mathbf{r} \,|\, t, i)$. To this end we write $n(t) = \sum_{i=1}^{N} Y_i(t)$ for the number of individuals at risk just before time t and introduce

$$\pi(\mathbf{r} \,|\, t) = \frac{\sum_{\ell=1}^{N} \pi(\mathbf{r} \,|\, t, \ell)}{\sum_{\ell=1}^{N} Y_\ell(t)} = n(t)^{-1} \sum_{\ell=1}^{N} \pi(\mathbf{r} \,|\, t, \ell). \tag{18.10}$$

That is, $\pi(\mathbf{r} \,|\, t)$ is the average of $\pi(\mathbf{r} \,|\, t, \ell)$ over all ℓ. Note that

$$\sum_{\mathbf{r} \in \mathcal{P}} \pi(\mathbf{r} \,|\, t) = n(t)^{-1} \sum_{\ell=1}^{N} \sum_{\mathbf{r} \in \mathcal{P}} \pi(\mathbf{r} \,|\, t, \ell) = n(t)^{-1} \sum_{\ell=1}^{N} Y_\ell(t) = 1. \tag{18.11}$$

Thus $\pi(\mathbf{r} \,|\, t)$ is a probability distribution over sets $\mathbf{r} \in \mathcal{P}$. We then introduce the weights

$$w_i(t, \mathbf{r}) = \frac{\pi(\mathbf{r} \,|\, t, i)}{\pi(\mathbf{r} \,|\, t)} \tag{18.12}$$

and get the factorization

$$\pi(\mathbf{r} \,|\, t, i) = w_i(t, \mathbf{r}) \, \pi(\mathbf{r} \,|\, t). \tag{18.13}$$

Note that the framework allows the sampling probabilities to depend in an arbitrary way on events in the past, that is, on events that are contained in $\mathcal{F}_{t-}$. The sampling probabilities may, however, not depend on events in the future. For example, one may not exclude as a potential control for a current case an individual that subsequently fails. A basic assumption throughout is that not only the truncation and censoring, but also the sampling of controls, are independent in the sense that the additional knowledge of which individuals have entered the study, have been censored, or have been selected as controls before time t do not carry information on the risks of failures at t.

18.3.1 Simple random sampling of controls

The most common nested case-control design is *simple random sampling*, the classical nested case-control design of Thomas (1977). For this design, if individual i fails at time t, one selects m controls by simple random sampling from the $n(t) - 1$ potential controls in the risk set $\mathcal{R}(t) = \{\ell \,|\, Y_\ell(t) = 1\}$. In probabilistic terms the design is given by

$$\pi(\mathbf{r} \,|\, t, i) = \binom{n(t) - 1}{m}^{-1} I\left\{ i \in \mathbf{r}, \, |\mathbf{r}| = m + 1, \, \mathbf{r} \subset \mathcal{R}(t) \right\}.$$

Here $|\mathbf{r}|$ is the number of elements in the set $\mathbf{r}$. The factorization (18.13) applies with

$$\pi(\mathbf{r} \,|\, t) = \binom{n(t)}{m + 1}^{-1} I\left\{ |\mathbf{r}| = m + 1, \, \mathbf{r} \subset \mathcal{R}(t) \right\}$$

and

$$w_i(t, \mathbf{r}) = \frac{n(t)}{m + 1} I\left\{ i \in \mathbf{r}, \, |\mathbf{r}| = m + 1, \, \mathbf{r} \subset \mathcal{R}(t) \right\}. \tag{18.14}$$

Thus for simple random sampling, the weights (18.14) are the same for all $i \in \mathbf{r}$.

18.3.2 Counter-matching

To select a simple random sample, the only piece of information needed from $\mathcal{F}_{t-}$ is the at-risk status of the individuals. Often, however, some additional information is available for all cohort members; for example, a surrogate measure of the exposure of main interest may be available for everyone. Langholz and Borgan (1995) have developed a stratified nested case-control design, which makes it possible to incorporate such information into the sampling process in order to obtain a more informative sample of controls.

For this design, which is called *counter-matching*, one applies the additional piece of information from $\mathcal{F}_{t-}$ to classify each individual at risk into one of, say, S, strata. We denote by $\mathcal{R}_s(t)$ the subset of the risk set $\mathcal{R}(t)$ that belongs to stratum s, and let $n_s(t) = |\mathcal{R}_s(t)|$ be the number at risk in this stratum just before time t. If individual i fails at t, we want to sample our controls such that the sampled risk set contains a prespecified number m_s of individuals from each stratum s; $s = 1, \ldots, S$. This is achieved as follows. Assume that the case i belongs to stratum $s(i)$. Then for $s \neq s(i)$ one samples randomly without replacement m_s controls from $\mathcal{R}_s(t)$. From the case's stratum $s(i)$ only $m_{s(i)} - 1$ controls are sampled. The case is, however, included in the sampled risk set so this contains a total of m_s from each stratum. Even though it is not made explicit in the notation, we note that the classification into strata may be time-dependent. A crucial assumption, however, is that the information on which the stratification is based has to be known before time t.

In probabilistic terms, counter-matched sampling may be described as follows. For any set $\mathbf{r} \in \mathcal{P}$ that contains i, is a subset of $\mathcal{R}(t)$, and satisfies $|\mathbf{r} \cap \mathcal{R}_s(t)| = m_s$ for $s = 1, \ldots, S$, we have

$$\pi(\mathbf{r} \,|\, t, i) = \left\{ \binom{n_{s(i)}(t) - 1}{m_{s(i)} - 1} \prod_{s \neq s(i)} \binom{n_s(t)}{m_s} \right\}^{-1}.$$

Here the factorization (18.13) applies, with

$$\pi(\mathbf{r} \,|\, t) = \left\{ \prod_{s=1}^{S} \binom{n_s(t)}{m_s} \right\}^{-1}$$

and

$$w_i(t, \mathbf{r}) = \frac{n_{s(i)}(t)}{m_{s(i)}}. \tag{18.15}$$

Note that for counter-matched sampling, the weights (18.15) are inversely proportional to the proportion of an individual's stratum that is in the sampled risk set.

18.3.3 Quota sampling and other sampling schemes

Suppose that we are interested in the effect of a binary exposure variable that is unknown for the individuals in the cohort, but is recorded for the cases and their controls. Then sampled risk sets where the case and its controls are concordant, i.e., all exposed or all unexposed, will contribute no information on the effect of the exposure. If a surrogate for the exposure is available for everyone, one may use counter-matching to reduce the probability of obtaining concordant sampled risk sets. Another option is to use quota sampling. One then selects new controls until there is at least one control that has a different value of the exposure variable than the case. More generally, with categorical exposure variables, one could continue sampling controls until specified quotas of controls attain the different values of the exposure variable.

For quota sampling, expressions for $\pi(\mathbf{r} \,|\, t, i)$, $\pi(\mathbf{r} \,|\, t)$ and $w_i(t, \mathbf{r})$ have been derived by Borgan *et al.* (1995, example 4). Other examples of nested case-control samplings schemes are discussed by Borgan *et al.* (1995), Langholz and Goldstein (1996), and Langholz (2007).

18.4 Counting process formulation of nested case-control data

It turns out to be convenient to use counting processes to describe data from a nested case-control study. As described in Section 18.2, we denote by $t_1 < t_2 < \cdots$ the times when failures are observed, and assuming that there are no tied failures, we let i_j be the individual who fails at t_j. Further, we denote by $\widetilde{\mathcal{R}}_j$ the sampled risk set at time t_j. This consists of the case i_j and its sampled controls.

For $\mathbf{r} \in \mathcal{P}$ and $i \in \mathbf{r}$ we now introduce the process

$$\mathbb{N}_{i,\mathbf{r}}(t) = \sum_{j \geq 1} I\{t_j \leq t, \, i_j = i, \, \widetilde{\mathcal{R}}_j = \mathbf{r}\} \tag{18.16}$$

that counts failures for individual i in $[0, t]$ with associated sampled risk set $\mathbf{r}$. Note that we may aggregate the processes $\mathbb{N}_{i,\mathbf{r}}(t)$ over sets $\mathbf{r} \in \mathcal{P}$ to recover the counting process

$$\mathbb{N}_i(t) = \sum_{\mathbf{r} \in \mathcal{P}} \mathbb{N}_{i,\mathbf{r}}(t) = \sum_{j \geq 1} I\{t_j \leq t,\, i_j = i\}; \qquad (18.17)$$

cf. (18.2). In a similar manner, for a set $\mathbf{r} \in \mathcal{P}$, we may aggregate over individuals $\ell \in \mathbf{r}$ to obtain the process

$$\mathbb{N}_{\mathbf{r}}(t) = \sum_{\ell \in \mathbf{r}} \mathbb{N}_{\ell,\mathbf{r}}(t) = \sum_{j \geq 1} I\{t_j \leq t,\, \widetilde{\mathcal{R}}_j = \mathbf{r}\} \qquad (18.18)$$

counting the number of times in $[0, t]$ that the sampled risk set equals the set $\mathbf{r}$.

The assumption that not only truncation and censoring, but also the sampling of controls, are independent ensures that the intensity process of the counting process $\mathbb{N}_i(t)$ is given by (18.4), not only with respect to the "cohort history" $\mathcal{H}_{t-}$, but also with respect to the "cohort and sampling history" $\mathcal{F}_{t-}$. From this, (18.4), and (18.13) it follows that the intensity process $\widetilde{\lambda}_{i,\mathbf{r}}(t)$ of the counting process (18.16) takes the form

$$\widetilde{\lambda}_{i,\mathbf{r}}(t) = \widetilde{\lambda}_i(t)\,\pi(\mathbf{r}\,|\,t, i) = Y_i(t)\,\exp\{\boldsymbol{\beta}^{\mathrm{T}}\mathbf{x}_i(t)\}w_i(t, \mathbf{r})\,\pi(\mathbf{r}\,|\,t)\,\lambda_0(t), \qquad (18.19)$$

while

$$\widetilde{\lambda}_{\mathbf{r}}(t) = \sum_{\ell \in \mathbf{r}} \widetilde{\lambda}_{\ell,\mathbf{r}}(t) = \sum_{\ell \in \mathbf{r}} Y_\ell(t)\,\exp\{\boldsymbol{\beta}^{\mathrm{T}}\mathbf{x}_\ell(t)\}w_\ell(t, \mathbf{r})\,\pi(\mathbf{r}\,|\,t)\,\lambda_0(t) \qquad (18.20)$$

is the intensity process of the counting process $\mathbb{N}_{\mathbf{r}}(t)$.

18.5   Partial likelihood for nested case-control data

Estimation of $\boldsymbol{\beta}$ for nested case-control data may be based on a partial likelihood that is derived in a similar manner as for the full cohort (cf. Section 18.2.2). We note that the intensity process (18.19) may be factorized as

$$\widetilde{\lambda}_{i,\mathbf{r}}(t) = \widetilde{\lambda}_{\mathbf{r}}(t)\,\pi(i\,|\,t, \mathbf{r}),$$

where

$$\pi(i\,|\,t, \mathbf{r}) = \frac{\widetilde{\lambda}_{i,\mathbf{r}}(t)}{\widetilde{\lambda}_{\mathbf{r}}(t)} = \frac{Y_i(t)\,\exp\{\boldsymbol{\beta}^{\mathrm{T}}\mathbf{x}_i(t)\}\,w_i(t, \mathbf{r})}{\sum_{\ell \in \mathbf{r}} Y_\ell(t)\,\exp\{\boldsymbol{\beta}^{\mathrm{T}}\mathbf{x}_\ell(t)\}\,w_\ell(t, \mathbf{r})} \qquad (18.21)$$

is the conditional probability that individual i fails at time t, given the past $\mathcal{F}_{t-}$ and given that a failure is observed for an individual in the set $\mathbf{r}$ at that time.

The partial likelihood for $\boldsymbol{\beta}$ is obtained by multiplying together the conditional probabilities (18.21) over all observed failure times t_j, cases i_j, and sampled risk sets $\widetilde{\mathcal{R}}_j$. Thus the partial likelihood for nested case-control data becomes

$$L_{\mathrm{ncc}}(\boldsymbol{\beta}) = \prod_{t_j} \pi(i_j\,|\,t_j, \widetilde{\mathcal{R}}_j) = \prod_{t_j} \frac{\exp\{\boldsymbol{\beta}^{\mathrm{T}}\mathbf{x}_{i_j}(t)\}w_{i_j}(t_j)}{\sum_{\ell \in \widetilde{\mathcal{R}}_j} \exp\{\boldsymbol{\beta}^{\mathrm{T}}\mathbf{x}_\ell(t)\}w_\ell(t_j)}, \qquad (18.22)$$

where we for short write $w_\ell(t_j)$ for $w_\ell(t_j, \widetilde{\mathcal{R}}_j)$. We note that (18.22) is similar to the full cohort partial likelihood (18.7). But in (18.22) we only sum over the sampled risks sets, and weights are included to reflect the properties of the control sampling design.

For simple random sampling of the controls, the weights (18.14) are the same for all individuals in a sampled risk set, and hence they cancel from (18.22). We are then left with the partial likelihood given by formula (16.3) in Chapter 16. For counter-matched sampling, the weights (18.15) are inversely proportional to the proportion of an individual's stratum that is in the sampled risk set, and the partial likelihood is given by formula (16.4) in Chapter 16. For all sampling designs, one may use standard software for Cox regression, formally treating the label of the sampled risk sets as a stratification variable in the model and using the logarithms of the weights "offsets." Alternatively, one may use ordinary Cox regression (i.e., without stratification) and pretend that the individuals in a sampled risk set enter the study just before the case's failure time, and that the controls are censored at the failure time.

The maximum partial likelihood estimator $\widehat{\boldsymbol{\beta}}$ is the value of $\boldsymbol{\beta}$ that maximizes (18.22). Using results for counting processes, intensity processes, and martingales, one may use arguments paralleling the ones for the full cohort (Andersen and Gill, 1982) to show that $\widehat{\boldsymbol{\beta}}$ enjoys similar large sample properties as ordinary maximum likelihood estimators; details are given by Borgan *et al.* (1995). In particular, in large samples, $\widehat{\boldsymbol{\beta}}$ is approximately multivariate normally distributed around the true value of $\boldsymbol{\beta}$ with a covariance matrix that may be estimated by $\mathbf{I}_{\mathrm{ncc}}(\widehat{\boldsymbol{\beta}})^{-1}$, where

$$\mathbf{I}_{\mathrm{ncc}}(\boldsymbol{\beta}) = -\frac{\partial^2}{\partial\boldsymbol{\beta}\partial\boldsymbol{\beta}^{\mathrm{T}}} \log L_{\mathrm{ncc}}(\boldsymbol{\beta})$$

is the observed information matrix.

The efficiency of the maximum partial likelihood estimator for nested case-control data with simple random sampling of the controls has been studied by a number of authors. In particular, Goldstein and Langholz (1992) showed that, when $\boldsymbol{\beta} = \mathbf{0}$, the asymptotic covariance matrix of the nested case-control estimator equals $(m+1)/m$ times the asymptotic covariance matrix of the full cohort estimator, independent of censoring and covariate distributions. Thus the efficiency of the simple nested case-control design relative to the full cohort is $m/(m+1)$ for testing associations between single exposures and disease. When $\boldsymbol{\beta}$ departs from zero, and when more than one regression coefficient has to be estimated, the efficiency of the nested case-control design may be quite a bit lower than given by the "$m/(m+1)$ efficiency rule" (e.g., Goldstein and Langholz, 1992; Borgan and Olsen, 1999).

Counter-matching may give an appreciable improvement in statistical efficiency for estimation of a regression coefficient of particular importance compared to simple nested case-control sampling. Intuitively, this is achieved by increasing the variation in the covariate of interest within each sampled risk set. The efficiency gain has been documented by asymptotic relative efficiency calculations (e.g., Langholz and Borgan, 1995; Borgan and Olsen, 1999) and empirical studies. For example, in a study of a cohort of gold miners, Steenland and Deddens (1997) found that a counter-matched design (with stratification based on duration of exposure) with three controls per case had the same statistical efficiency for estimating the effect of exposure to crystalline silica as a simple nested case-control study using ten controls.

18.5.1   Radiation and breast cancer

For illustration we will use the data on radiation and breast cancer introduced in Section 17.2 of Chapter 17. The data consist of a cohort of 1,720 female patients who were discharged from two tuberculosis sanatoria in Massachusetts between 1930 and 1956. Radiation doses have been assessed for the 1,022 women who received radiation exposure to the chest from X-ray fluoroscopy lung examinations. The remaining 698 women in the cohort received treatments that did not require fluoroscopic monitoring and were radiation unexposed. The

TABLE 18.1

Comparison of estimates for the radiation and breast cancer data.

Model term	Parameter estimate	Standard error	Wald test statistic	P-value
A. Full cohort				
$\log_2(\text{dose} + 1)$	0.469	0.161	2.91	0.004
ageRx/10	-0.242	0.149	-1.62	0.105
B. Simple nested case-control				
$\log_2(\text{dose} + 1)$	0.549	0.232	2.37	0.018
ageRx/10	-0.179	0.207	-0.86	0.388
C. Counter-matched nested case-control				
$\log_2(\text{dose} + 1)$	0.501	0.180	2.78	0.006
ageRx/10	-0.173	0.210	-0.83	0.408

patients have been followed up until the end of 1980, by which time 75 breast cancer cases were observed (Hrubec *et al.*, 1989).

For this cohort, radiation data have been collected for all 1,720 women. But the workload of exposure data collection would have been reduced if the investigators had used a cohort sampling design. In Chapter 17 the data were used to illustrated case-cohort sampling. In this chapter we will use the data to illustrate nested case-control studies. To this end we selected two nested case-control data sets with two controls per case. For the first data set, the two controls were selected by simple random sampling. For the second data set, the controls were selected by counter-matched sampling. Information on the number of fluoroscopic examinations is available for each woman in the cohort and may be used as a surrogate for radiation exposure. For the counter-matched sampling we stratify the cohort into three strata: (i) the 698 women with no fluoroscopic examinations, (ii) the 765 women with 1-149 examinations, and (iii) the 257 women with 150 examinations or more. We then select the controls such that the sampled risk sets contain one woman from each of the three strata, e.g., if the case is from stratum (ii), we select at random one control from each of stratum (i) and stratum (iii).

As in Section 17.5.2 of Chapter 17 we fit a Cox regression model of the form

$$\lambda(t \mid x_1, x_2) = \exp\{\beta_1 x_1 + \beta_2 x_2\}\lambda_0(t). \tag{18.23}$$

Here t is attained age, and the covariates are $x_1 = \log_2(\text{dose} + 1)$ and $x_2 = \text{ageRx}/10$, where "dose" is radiation dose (Gy) and "ageRx" denotes age at first treatment. Table 18.1 gives the estimated regression coefficients with corresponding standard errors, Wald test statistics, and P-values for the full cohort and the two nested case-control data sets. The estimates for the effect of dose are somewhat higher for the two nested case-control studies than for the full cohort, while the opposite is the case for the estimates of the effect of age at first treatment. But the differences between the estimates are small compared with their standard errors. The empirical efficiency of the estimates for the simple nested case control design relative to the full cohort is about 50%, which is lower than than the 67% given by the "$m/(m+1)$ efficiency rule." The efficiency gain obtained by counter-matching on a surrogate for an exposure depends on the correlation between the surrogate and the exposure. For the radiation data the number of fluoroscopic examinations is highly correlated with dose, and the relative efficiency of the estimate for dose is increased to 80%. One should be aware that it is not common to have available such a strong surrogate for an exposure.

18.6   Estimation of cumulative hazards

For nested case-control data we may estimate the cumulative baseline hazard $\Lambda_0(t) = \int_0^t \lambda_0(u)du$ in a similar way as for the full cohort; cf. Section 18.2.3. Specifically, the estimator is given by

$$\widehat{\Lambda}_{0,\mathrm{ncc}}(t) = \sum_{t_j \leq t} \frac{1}{\sum_{\ell \in \widetilde{\mathcal{R}}_j} \exp\{\widehat{\boldsymbol{\beta}}^{\mathrm{T}}\mathbf{x}_\ell(t_j)\}w_\ell(t_j)}. \tag{18.24}$$

This has the same form as the Breslow estimator (18.8) for the full cohort, except that we only sum over individuals in the sampled risk sets, and we have to weight their relative risks according to the sampling design for the controls.

We will indicate how one may use counting process theory to study the statistical properties of the Breslow type estimator (18.24). To this end we note that the estimator may be given as $\widehat{\Lambda}_{0,\mathrm{ncc}}(t) = \widehat{\Lambda}_{0,\mathrm{ncc}}(t; \widehat{\boldsymbol{\beta}})$, where

$$\begin{aligned}
\widehat{\Lambda}_{0,\mathrm{ncc}}(t; \boldsymbol{\beta}) &= \sum_{t_j \leq t} \frac{1}{\sum_{\ell \in \widetilde{\mathcal{R}}_j} \exp\{\boldsymbol{\beta}^{\mathrm{T}}\mathbf{x}_\ell(t_j)\}w_\ell(t_j)} \\
&= \sum_{\mathbf{r} \in \mathcal{P}} \int_0^t \frac{d\mathbb{N}_{\mathbf{r}}(u)}{\sum_{\ell \in \mathbf{r}} Y_\ell(u) \exp\{\boldsymbol{\beta}^{\mathrm{T}}\mathbf{x}_\ell(u)\}w_\ell(u, \mathbf{r})}.
\end{aligned} \tag{18.25}$$

Now we have the decomposition

$$d\mathbb{N}_{\mathbf{r}}(u) = \widetilde{\lambda}_{\mathbf{r}}(t)dt + d\mathbb{M}_{\mathbf{r}}(u),$$

where $d\mathbb{M}_{\mathbf{r}}(u)$ is a martingale increment; cf. (18.3). Using this result and (18.20), we may write

$$\begin{aligned}
\widehat{\Lambda}_{0,\mathrm{ncc}}(t; \boldsymbol{\beta}) &= \int_0^t \sum_{\mathbf{r} \in \mathcal{P}} \pi(\mathbf{r} \mid u)\lambda_0(u)du + \sum_{\mathbf{r} \in \mathcal{P}} \int_0^t \frac{d\mathbb{M}_{\mathbf{r}}(u)}{\sum_{\ell \in \mathbf{r}} Y_\ell(u) \exp\{\boldsymbol{\beta}^{\mathrm{T}}\mathbf{x}_\ell(u)\}w_\ell(u, \mathbf{r})} \\
&= \int_0^t \lambda_0(u)du + \sum_{\mathbf{r} \in \mathcal{P}} \int_0^t \frac{d\mathbb{M}_{\mathbf{r}}(u)}{\sum_{\ell \in \mathbf{r}} Y_\ell(u) \exp\{\boldsymbol{\beta}^{\mathrm{T}}\mathbf{x}_\ell(u)\}w_\ell(u, \mathbf{r})},
\end{aligned} \tag{18.26}$$

where the last equality follows by (18.11). The second term on the right-hand side of (18.26) is a sum of stochastic integrals, and hence it has mean zero. It follows that $\widehat{\Lambda}_{0,\mathrm{ncc}}(t; \boldsymbol{\beta})$ has mean $\Lambda_0(t) = \int_0^t \lambda_0(u)du$, so the estimator (18.24) is approximately unbiased.

If all the covariates are fixed, the cumulative hazard for an individual with a given covariate vector $\mathbf{x}_0$ is given by

$$\Lambda(t|\mathbf{x}_0) = \int_0^t \lambda(u|\mathbf{x}_0)du = \exp\{\boldsymbol{\beta}^{\mathrm{T}}\mathbf{x}_0\}\Lambda_0(u), \tag{18.27}$$

and this may be estimated by

$$\widehat{\Lambda}_{\mathrm{ncc}}(t|\mathbf{x}_0) = \exp\{\widehat{\boldsymbol{\beta}}^{\mathrm{T}}\mathbf{x}_0\}\widehat{\Lambda}_{0,\mathrm{ncc}}(t). \tag{18.28}$$

For models with external time-dependent covariates, it is usually not meaningful to estimate the cumulative hazard corresponding to a fixed value of the vector of covariates. What can be meaningfully estimated in such situations is the cumulative hazard over an interval

$[0, t]$ corresponding to a given covariate path $\mathbf{x}_0(s)$; $0 < s \leq t$. The cumulative hazard corresponding to such a path is

$$\Lambda(t|\mathbf{x}_0) = \int_0^t \exp\{\boldsymbol{\beta}^{\mathrm{T}}\mathbf{x}_0(u)\} \lambda_0(u)du, \tag{18.29}$$

which is estimated by

$$\widehat{\Lambda}_{\mathrm{ncc}}(t|\mathbf{x}_0) = \int_0^t \exp\{\widehat{\boldsymbol{\beta}}^{\mathrm{T}}\mathbf{x}_0(u)\} \, d\widehat{\Lambda}_{0,\mathrm{ncc}}(t) = \sum_{t_j \leq t} \frac{\exp\{\widehat{\boldsymbol{\beta}}^{\mathrm{T}}\mathbf{x}_0(t_j)\}}{\sum_{\ell \in \widetilde{\mathcal{R}}_j} \exp\{\widehat{\boldsymbol{\beta}}^{\mathrm{T}}\mathbf{x}_\ell(t_j)\}w_\ell(t_j)}. \tag{18.30}$$

In order to estimate the variance of (18.30), we introduce

$$\widehat{\omega}^2(t \,|\, \mathbf{x}_0) = \sum_{t_j \leq t} \left(\frac{\exp\{\widehat{\boldsymbol{\beta}}^{\mathrm{T}}\mathbf{x}_0(t_j)\}}{\sum_{\ell \in \widetilde{\mathcal{R}}_j} \exp\{\widehat{\boldsymbol{\beta}}^{\mathrm{T}}\mathbf{x}_\ell(t_j)\}w_\ell(t_j)} \right)^2,$$

and

$$\widehat{\mathbf{G}}(t \,|\, \mathbf{x}_0) = \sum_{t_j \leq t} \left\{ \frac{\mathbf{x}_0(t_j)\exp\{\widehat{\boldsymbol{\beta}}^{\mathrm{T}}\mathbf{x}_0(t_j)\}}{\sum_{\ell \in \widetilde{\mathcal{R}}_j} \exp\{\widehat{\boldsymbol{\beta}}^{\mathrm{T}}\mathbf{x}_\ell(t_j)\}w_\ell(t_j)} \right.$$
$$\left. - \frac{\exp\{\widehat{\boldsymbol{\beta}}^{\mathrm{T}}\mathbf{x}_0(t_j)\} \sum_{\ell \in \widetilde{\mathcal{R}}_j} \mathbf{x}_0(t_j)\exp\{\widehat{\boldsymbol{\beta}}^{\mathrm{T}}\mathbf{x}_\ell(t_j)\}w_\ell(t_j)}{\left(\sum_{\ell \in \widetilde{\mathcal{R}}_j} \exp\{\widehat{\boldsymbol{\beta}}^{\mathrm{T}}\mathbf{x}_\ell(t_j)\}w_\ell(t_j) \right)^2} \right\}.$$

Expanding (18.30) around the true value of $\boldsymbol{\beta}$ in a first order Taylor's series and applying standard counting process arguments [see Andersen *et al.* (1993, theorem VII.2.3 and corollaries VII.2.4-6) and Borgan *et al.* (1995, section 4 and theorem 3)] one may show that $\widehat{\Lambda}_{\mathrm{ncc}}(t|\mathbf{x}_0)$ is asymptotically normally distributed around its true value $\Lambda(t|\mathbf{x}_0)$, with a variance that may be estimated by

$$\widehat{\sigma}^2(t|\mathbf{x}_0) = \widehat{\omega}^2(t|\mathbf{x}_0) + \widehat{\mathbf{G}}(t|\mathbf{x}_0)^{\mathrm{T}}\mathbf{I}_{\mathrm{ncc}}(\widehat{\boldsymbol{\beta}})^{-1}\widehat{\mathbf{G}}(t|\mathbf{x}_0). \tag{18.31}$$

In (18.31) the first term on the right-hand side is due to the variability in estimating the hazard while the second term accounts for the variability due to estimation of $\boldsymbol{\beta}$.

18.6.1 Radiation and breast cancer

We now continue the analysis of the data on radiation and breast cancer. As described in Section 18.5.1, we for illustration consider data for the full cohort and two nested case-control data sets: one with simple random sampling of the controls and one with counter-matched control sampling. Figure 18.2 shows the estimated cumulative baseline hazard of the Cox regression model (18.23) for the three data sets. For the full cohort the Breslow estimate (18.8) is given, and for the two nested case-control data sets the estimates are obtained by (18.24). In the latter formula the weights are $w_\ell(t_j) = n(t_j)/3$ for the classical nested case-control data with simple random sampling of the controls, while for counter-matched sampling they are $w_\ell(t_j) = n_{s(\ell)}(t_j)$, where $s(\ell)$ is the stratum of individual ℓ. The three estimates of the cumulative baseline hazard are quite similar, but the two nested case-control estimates are a bit lower than the estimate for the full cohort.

Figure 18.3 shows the expected number of breast cancer cases between 40 and 60 years of age for the four configurations of covariate values considered in Section 17.5.5

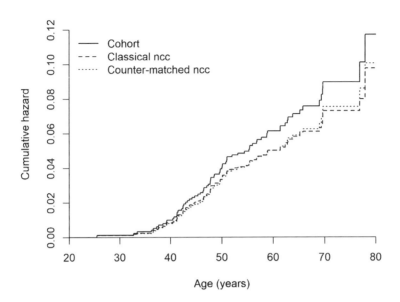

FIGURE 18.2
Estimated cumulative baseline hazards for the Cox regression model (18.23) based on cohort data and two nested case-control data sets. For the classical nested case-control data
("Classical ncc") the two controls are obtained by simple random sampling, and for the
counter-matched nested case-control data ("Counter-matched ncc") they are obtained by
stratified sampling as described in Section 18.5.1.

of Chapter 17. For a covariate configuration $\mathbf{x}_0 = (x_1, x_2)$, the estimates are given as
$\widehat{\Lambda}_{\mathrm{ncc}}(60|\mathbf{x}_0) - \widehat{\Lambda}_{\mathrm{ncc}}(40|\mathbf{x}_0)$ for the two nested case-control data sets [cf. (18.28)], and a similar formula applies for cohort data. The considered configurations of the covariates are no
radiation and 3 Gy, corresponding to $x_1 = \log_2(\mathrm{dose} + 1)$ equal to 0 and 2, and age at start
of treatment (ageRx) 15 years and 35 years, corresponding to $x_2 = \mathrm{ageRx}/10$ equal to 1.5
and 3.5. The estimates for the two nested case-control data sets are close to the estimates
for the full cohort, and they are comparable with the estimates obtained for case-cohort
data in Section 17.5.5 of Chapter 17.

18.7   Model checking

We now restrict attention to the situation where there are no time-dependent covariates.
So if $\mathbf{x}_i = (x_{i1}, \ldots, x_{ip})^{\mathrm{T}}$ is the vector of covariates for individual i, Cox's regression model
takes the form

$$\lambda_i(t) = \lambda(t \,|\, \mathbf{x}_i) = \exp\{\boldsymbol{\beta}^{\mathrm{T}} \mathbf{x}_i\} \lambda_0(t). \tag{18.32}$$

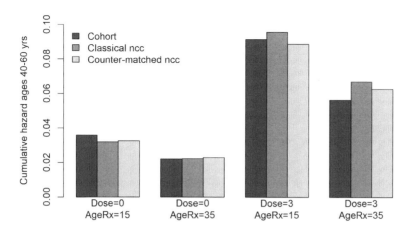

FIGURE 18.3
Expected number of breast cancers (cumulative hazards) between 40 and 60 years of age depending on covariate values.

Two crucial assumptions of model (18.32) are:

(i) Covariates have a *log-linear* effect, i.e., $\log\lambda(t\,|\,\mathbf{x}_i) = \boldsymbol{\beta}^{\mathrm{T}}\mathbf{x}_i + \log\lambda_0(t)$ is a linear function of the covariates $\mathbf{x}_i$.

(ii) Hazard rates are *proportional*, i.e., for individuals i and ℓ the hazard ratio $\lambda(t\,|\,\mathbf{x}_i)/\lambda(t\,|\,\mathbf{x}_\ell) = \exp\{\boldsymbol{\beta}^{\mathrm{T}}(\mathbf{x}_i - \mathbf{x}_\ell)\}$ does not depend on time t.

In this section we will outline how one may use cumulative sums of martingale residuals to check the two assumptions. The section is based on the work by Borgan and Zhang (2015) who extended the cohort methods of Lin *et al.* (1993) to nested case-control data.

18.7.1 Cumulative sums of martingale residuals

Our starting point is the counting processes (18.16) and the corresponding martingales

$$\mathbb{M}_{i,\mathbf{r}}(t) = \mathbb{N}_{i,\mathbf{r}}(t) - \widetilde{\Lambda}_{i,\mathbf{r}}(t); \quad \mathbf{r} \in \mathcal{P}, \, i \in \mathbf{r}, \tag{18.33}$$

where $\widetilde{\Lambda}_{i,\mathbf{r}}(t) = \int_0^t \widetilde{\lambda}_{i,\mathbf{r}}(u)du$; cf. (18.19). Borgan and Zhang (2015, appendix A and supplementary material) give an estimator of $\widetilde{\Lambda}_{i,\mathbf{r}}(t)$. If we denote this estimator by $\widehat{\Lambda}_{i,\mathbf{r}}(t)$, we obtain the *martingale residual processes*

$$\widehat{\mathbb{M}}_{i,\mathbf{r}}(t) = \mathbb{N}_{i,\mathbf{r}}(t) - \widehat{\Lambda}_{i,\mathbf{r}}(t); \quad \mathbf{r} \in \mathcal{P}, \, i \in \mathbf{r}. \tag{18.34}$$

The martingale residual processes (18.34) are of little use in their own right; in fact most of them will be zero. But they provide the building blocks for stochastic processes that are useful for checking the assumptions of Cox's model. To this end, we consider the multiparameter stochastic process

$$\mathbf{W}(t, \mathbf{x}) = \sum_{\mathbf{r}\in\mathcal{P}} \sum_{i\in\mathbf{r}} f(\mathbf{x}_i) I(\mathbf{x}_i \leq \mathbf{x})\widehat{\mathbb{M}}_{i,\mathbf{r}}(t). \tag{18.35}$$

Here f is a smooth and bounded p-variate function and the event $\{\mathbf{x}_i \leq \mathbf{x}\}$ means that all p components of $\mathbf{x}_i = (x_{i1}, \ldots, x_{ip})^{\mathrm{T}}$ are no larger than the corresponding components of $\mathbf{x} = (x_1, \ldots, x_p)^{\mathrm{T}}$. The process (18.35) is of similar form as the cumulative sum of martingale residuals for cohort data introduced by Lin *et al.* (1993, formula (2.1)). Borgan and Zhang (2015, appendix A and supplementary material) show that (18.35) may be written as

$$\mathbf{W}(t, \mathbf{x}) = \sum_{i=1}^N f(\mathbf{x}_i) I(\mathbf{x}_i \leq \mathbf{x}) \mathbb{N}_i(t) - \sum_{t_j \leq t} \frac{\sum_{i \in \tilde{\mathcal{R}}_j} f(\mathbf{x}_i) I(\mathbf{x}_i \leq \mathbf{x}) \exp\{\widehat{\boldsymbol{\beta}}^{\mathrm{T}} \mathbf{x}_i\} w_i(t_j)}{\sum_{\ell \in \tilde{\mathcal{R}}_j} \exp\{\widehat{\boldsymbol{\beta}}^{\mathrm{T}} \mathbf{x}_\ell\} w_\ell(t_j)}, \quad (18.36)$$

and that the process (18.36), standardized by $N^{-1/2}$, is asymptotically distributed as a Gaussian process under model (18.32).

The limiting Gaussian distribution has a complicated form. But it is shown by Borgan and Zhang (2015, appendix B and supplementary material) that we may approximate the distribution of $\mathbf{W}(t, \mathbf{x})$ by simulating a process $\mathbf{W}^*(t, \mathbf{x})$ that has the same limiting distribution as (18.36) when the Cox model is correctly specified. The simulation is performed by considering the process

$$\mathbf{W}^*(t, \mathbf{x}) = \sum_{t_j \leq t} \left\{ f(\mathbf{x}_{i_j}) I(\mathbf{x}_{i_j} \leq \mathbf{x}) - g(\widehat{\boldsymbol{\beta}}, t_j, \mathbf{x}) \right\} G_j \quad (18.37)$$

$$- \sum_{t_j \leq t} \frac{\sum_{i \in \tilde{\mathcal{R}}_j} f(\mathbf{x}_i) I(\mathbf{x}_i \leq \mathbf{x}) \left\{ \mathbf{x}_i - \widehat{\mathbf{E}}_j \right\}^{\mathrm{T}} \exp\{\widehat{\boldsymbol{\beta}}^{\mathrm{T}} \mathbf{x}_i\} w_i(t_j)}{\sum_{\ell \in \tilde{\mathcal{R}}_j} \exp\{\widehat{\boldsymbol{\beta}}^{\mathrm{T}} \mathbf{x}_\ell\} w_\ell(t_j)} \mathbf{I}_{\mathrm{ncc}}(\widehat{\boldsymbol{\beta}})^{-1} \sum_{t_j} \left\{ \mathbf{x}_{i_j} - \widehat{\mathbf{E}}_j \right\} G_j,$$

where we keep the observations fixed and only sample the G_j's from the standard normal distribution. Here

$$g(\widehat{\boldsymbol{\beta}}, t_j, \mathbf{x}) = \frac{\sum_{i \in \tilde{\mathcal{R}}_j} f(\mathbf{x}_i) I(\mathbf{x}_i \leq \mathbf{x}) \exp\{\widehat{\boldsymbol{\beta}}^{\mathrm{T}} \mathbf{x}_i\} w_i(t_j)}{\sum_{\ell \in \tilde{\mathcal{R}}_j} \exp\{\widehat{\boldsymbol{\beta}}^{\mathrm{T}} \mathbf{x}_\ell\} w_\ell(t_j)}, \quad (18.38)$$

and

$$\widehat{\mathbf{E}}_j = \frac{\sum_{i \in \tilde{\mathcal{R}}_j} \mathbf{x}_i \exp(\widehat{\boldsymbol{\beta}}^{\mathrm{T}} \mathbf{x}_i) w_i(t_j)}{\sum_{\ell \in \tilde{\mathcal{R}}_j} \exp(\widehat{\boldsymbol{\beta}}^{\mathrm{T}} \mathbf{x}_\ell) w_\ell(t_j)}. \quad (18.39)$$

This simulation technique is similar to the one given by Lin *et al.* (1993) for model checking for cohort data.

18.7.2   Check of log-linearity

Two special cases of (18.36) are of particular interest. If we let $f(\cdot) \equiv 1$, $t = \tau$ (the upper time limit of the study), $x_k = x$, and $x_\ell = \infty$ for $\ell \neq k$, we for each k obtain the process

$$W_k(x) = \sum_{i=1}^N I(x_{ik} \leq x) \mathbb{N}_i(\tau) - \sum_{t_j} \frac{\sum_{i \in \tilde{\mathcal{R}}_j} I(x_{ik} \leq x) \exp\{\widehat{\boldsymbol{\beta}}^{\mathrm{T}} \mathbf{x}_i\} w_i(t_j)}{\sum_{\ell \in \tilde{\mathcal{R}}_j} \exp\{\widehat{\boldsymbol{\beta}}^{\mathrm{T}} \mathbf{x}_\ell) w_\ell(t_j)}. \quad (18.40)$$

Note that $W_k(x)$ is the difference between the observed number of failures for individuals with a value of the kth covariate not larger than x and the corresponding expected number of failures when the model is correctly specified. Plots of (18.40) versus x may be used to check if log-linearity is satisfied for the kth covariate (assumed numeric). If the covariate is coded correctly, $W_k(x)$ will fluctuate around zero, while large deviations from zero indicate that one has assumed an incorrect functional form for the covariate. To assesses how large fluctuations one may expect by chance under a correctly specified model, one may use the simulation technique described in Section 18.7.1 and compare the process (18.40) obtained from the actual data with simulated realizations assuming a correctly specified model. To obtain a formal test, we may use $\sup_x |W_k(x)|$ as a measure of deviation from zero and obtain the P-value as the proportion of simulated processes that have a larger value of the supremum than the observed one.

18.7.3 Check of proportional hazards

If we in (18.36) let $f(\mathbf{x}_i) = \mathbf{x}_i$ and $x_\ell = \infty$ for all ℓ, we obtain

$$\mathbf{U}(\widehat{\boldsymbol{\beta}}, t) = \sum_{i=1}^{N} \mathbf{x}_i \mathbb{N}_i(t) - \sum_{t_j \leq t} \frac{\sum_{i \in \widetilde{\mathcal{R}}_j} \mathbf{x}_i \exp\{\widehat{\boldsymbol{\beta}}^{\mathrm{T}} \mathbf{x}_i\} w_i(t_j)}{\sum_{\ell \in \widetilde{\mathcal{R}}_j} \exp\{\widehat{\boldsymbol{\beta}}^{\mathrm{T}} \mathbf{x}_\ell\} w_\ell(t_j)}. \tag{18.41}$$

The process (18.41) is denoted a score process, since $\mathbf{U}(\widehat{\boldsymbol{\beta}}, \tau)$ is the vector of score functions obtained from the partial likelihood (18.22). Plots of the components $U_j(\widehat{\boldsymbol{\beta}}, t)$ of the score process versus t may be used to check the assumption of proportional hazards, and formal tests may be based on the supremum statistic $\sup_t |U_j(\widehat{\boldsymbol{\beta}}, t)|$.

18.7.4 Radiation and breast cancer

In Sections 18.5.1 and 18.6.1 we give results on estimation of regression coefficients and cumulative hazards for the radiation and breast cancer data. We will now show how one may use (18.40) to check log-linearity for the Cox model (18.23) and (18.41) to check proportional hazards. We only present results for the classical nested case-control data with two randomly selected controls per case. For these data the weights $w(t_j)$ are the same for all individuals in a sampled risk set [cf. (18.14)], and hence cancel in (18.40) and (18.41).

The plots in the upper panel of Figure 18.4 provide check of log-linearity of the covariates $x_1 = \log_2(\text{dose} + 1)$ (left) and $x_2 = \text{ageRx}/10$ (right). For both covariates, the observed process (18.40) fluctuates around zero, and neither the plots nor the formal tests (based on 1000 simulated processes) indicate deviation from log-linearity. The lower panel of Figure 18.4 gives plots of the score process (18.41) for the two covariates. In the left-hand plot the observed score process fluctuates around zero and indicates no deviation from proportional hazards for the covariate $x_1 = \log_2(\text{dose} + 1)$. For the covariate $x_2 = \text{ageRx}/10$, the observed score process deviates more from zero, so the proportional hazards assumption may be more questionable for this covariate (which is in agreement with the results of Section 17.5.1 in Chapter 17). However, the deviation from proportionality is not significant (P-value 8%).

The plots and P-values of Figure 18.4 have been obtained using the commands `cox.aalen` and `cum.residuals` in the `timereg` library in R; see the handbook website for a detailed description.

18.8 Additional matching

In order to keep the presentation as simple as possible, we have so far considered the proportional hazards model (18.1) where the baseline hazard rate is assumed to be the same for all individuals in the cohort. Sometimes this may not be reasonable, e.g., to control for

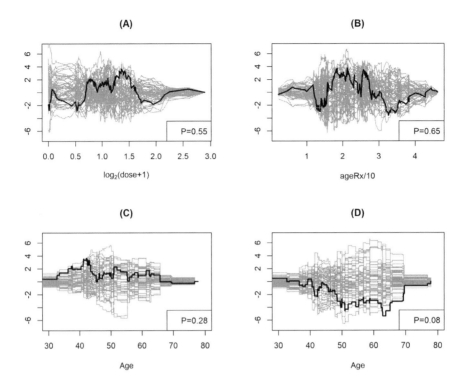

FIGURE 18.4
Cumulative martingale residual plots for the radiation and breast cancer data. In all plots the black line is for the actual data and the grey lines are 50 simulated processes assuming that the model is correctly specified. The two plots in the upper panel are for checking log-linearity of the covariates: (A) log-linearity of $\log_2(\text{dose} + 1)$, (B) log-linearity of ageRx/10. The two plots in the lower panel are for checking proportional hazards: (C) proportional hazards for $\log_2(\text{dose}+1)$, (D) proportional hazards for ageRx/10. The numbers in the lower right-hand corners of the plots are P-values of the supremum tests based on 1000 simulated processes.

the effect of one or more confounding factors, one may want to adopt a stratified version of (18.1) where the baseline hazard differs between population strata generated by the confounders. The regression coefficients are, however, assumed to be the same across these strata. Thus the hazard rate of an individual i from population stratum c is assumed to take the form

$$\lambda_i(t) = \lambda_{0c}(t) \exp\{\boldsymbol{\beta}^{\mathrm{T}} \mathbf{x}_i(t)\}. \tag{18.42}$$

When the stratified proportional hazards model (18.42) applies, the sampling of controls should be restricted to the individuals at risk who belong to the same population stratum as the case. We say that the controls are matched by the stratification variable(s).

More specifically, if individual i belongs to population stratum c, the sampling probabilities $\pi(\mathbf{r} \,|\, t, i)$ of Section 18.3 should be zero for all sets $\mathbf{r}$ that are not a subset of this population stratum. Further, in formula (18.10) the sums should be restricted to those individuals ℓ who belong to population stratum c and $n(t)$ should be replaced by $n_c(t)$, the number at risk in population stratum c just before time t. With these modifications, the weights are still given by (18.12) and the factorization (18.13) applies.

In particular for simple random sampling, if an individual in population stratum c fails at time t, one selects at random m controls from the $n_c(t) - 1$ nonfailing individuals at risk in this population stratum. The weights are then given by an expression similar to (18.14), but with $n(t)$ replaced by $n_c(t)$ and with the additional restriction that the set $\mathbf{r}$ should be a subset of population stratum c.

One may also combine matching and counter-matching by selecting the controls among those in the sampling strata used for counter-matching who belong to the population stratum of the case. [Here it is important to distinguish between the population strata that forms the basis for the stratified Cox model (18.42) and the sampling strata that are used for counter-matched sampling of the controls.] Then the weights (18.15) apply for subsets $\mathbf{r}$ of population stratum c if we replace $n_{s(i)}(t)$ by $n_{s(i),c}(t)$, where $n_{s,c}(t)$ is the number of individuals at risk in sampling stratum s who also belong to population stratum c.

Now the partial likelihood (18.22) applies for nested case-control data with additional matching provided one uses the weights $w_\ell(t_j)$ that are appropriate for the sampling design. The same hold for the methods for model checking discussed in Section 18.7. Further, when there is only a small number of strata, the stratum specific cumulative baseline hazard rates $\Lambda_{0c}(t) = \int_0^t \lambda_{0c}(u)du$ may be estimated using these weights by a slight modification of (18.24). All that is required is that the sum is restricted to those failure times t_j when a failure in the actual population stratum occurs. When there are many population strata, however, there may be too little information in each stratum to make estimation of the stratum specific cumulative baseline hazard rates meaningful.

18.9   Concluding remarks

In this chapter we have shown how a counting process formulation makes it possible to derive methods for nested case-control data that are similar to the ones for the full cohort. In the chapter we have focused on some important methods for Cox's regression model for failure time data: partial likelihood inference, estimation of cumulative hazards and model checking. But the counting process approach may also be used for other models and methods, and here we mention some of these.

The class of relative risk regression models is an extension of Cox's model, and it is given by

$$\lambda(t \mid \mathbf{x}_i) = r(\boldsymbol{\beta}, \mathbf{x}_i(t))\lambda_0(t), \qquad (18.43)$$

where $r(\boldsymbol{\beta}, \mathbf{x}_i(t))$ is a relative risk function. We assume that $r(\boldsymbol{\beta}, \mathbf{0}) = 1$, so the baseline hazard $\lambda_0(t)$ corresponds to the hazard of an individual with all covariates equal to zero. For Cox's regression model (18.1) we have the exponential relative risk function $r(\boldsymbol{\beta}, \mathbf{x}_i(t)) = \exp\{\boldsymbol{\beta}^{\mathrm{T}}\mathbf{x}_i(t)\}$. Other relative risk functions include the linear relative risk function $r(\boldsymbol{\beta}, \mathbf{x}_i(t)) = 1 + \boldsymbol{\beta}^{\mathrm{T}}\mathbf{x}_i(t)$ and the excess relative risk model $r(\boldsymbol{\beta}, \mathbf{x}_i(t)) = \prod_{j=1}^{p}\{1 + \beta_j x_{ij}(t)\}$.

The results on partial likelihood estimation (Section 18.5) continue to hold with only minor modifications for the general relative risk regression models (18.43); see Aalen *et al.* (2008, section 4.3.4) for a summary and Borgan and Langholz (2007, sections 3.3 and 5.1) for a detailed account. But note that one now ought to use the inverse of the *expected* information matrix for estimation of the covariance matrix of the maximum partial likelihood estimator. (For Cox's model the observed and expected information matrices coincide.) Also the results on estimation of cumulative hazards (Section 18.6) continue to hold with only minor modifications for general relative risk regression models (e.g. Langholz and Borgan, 1997). But the methods for model checking (Section 18.7) are specific for Cox's regression model, and may not immediately be generalized to general relative risk functions. However, model checking for general relative risk models may be performed by means of grouped martingale residual processes (Borgan and Langholz, 2007).

In this chapter we have considered failure time data, where the focus is on a single event of interest (disease occurrence or death). But nested case-control methods may also be used for relative and absolute risk estimation for competing risks (Langholz and Borgan, 1997) and more general multi-state models (Borgan, 2002).

Bibliography

Aalen, O. O., Borgan, Ø., and Gjessing, H. K. (2008). *Survival and Event History Analysis: A Process Point of View*. Springer, New York.

Andersen, P. K. and Gill, R. D. (1982). Cox's regression model for counting processes: A large sample study. *The Annals of Statistics*, **10**, 1100–1120.

Andersen, P. K., Borgan, Ø., Gill, R. D., and Keiding, N. (1993). *Statistical Models Based on Counting Processes*. Springer, New York.

Barlow, W. E. and Prentice, R. L. (1988). Residuals for relative risk regression. *Biometrika*, **75**, 65–74.

Borgan, Ø. (2002). Estimation of covariate-dependent Markov transition probabilities from nested case-control data. *Statistical Methods in Medical Research*, **11**, 183–202.

Borgan, Ø. and Langholz, B. (2007). Using martingale residuals to assess goodness-of-fit for sampled risk set data. In V. Nair, editor, *Advances in Statistical Modeling and Inference. Essays in Honor of Kjell A Doksum*, pages 65–90. Word Scientific Publishing, Singapore.

Borgan, Ø. and Olsen, E. F. (1999). The efficiency of simple and counter-matched nested case-control sampling. *Scandinavian Journal of Statistics*, **26**, 493–509.

Borgan, Ø. and Zhang, Y. (2015). Using cumulative sums of martingale residuals for model checking in nested case-control studies. *Biometrics*, **71**, 696–703.

Borgan, Ø., Goldstein, L., and Langholz, B. (1995). Methods for the analysis of sampled cohort data in the Cox proportional hazards model. *The Annals of Statistics*, **23**, 1749–1778.

Cox, D. R. (1975). Partial likelihood. *Biometrika*, **62**, 269–276.

Goldstein, L. and Langholz, B. (1992). Asymptotic theory for nested case-control sampling in the Cox regression model. *The Annals of Statistics*, **20**, 1903–1928.

Hrubec, Z., Boice, Jr., J. D., Monson, R. R., and Rosenstein, M. (1989). Breast cancer after multiple chest fluoroscopies: Second follow-up of Massachusetts women with tuberculosis. *Cancer Research*, **49**, 229–234.

Kalbfleisch, J. D. and Prentice, R. L. (2002). *The Statistical Analysis of Failure Time Data*. Wiley, Hoboken, New Jersey, 2nd edition.

Langholz, B. (2007). Use of cohort information in the design and analysis of case-control studies. *Scandinavian Journal of Statistics*, **34**, 120–136.

Langholz, B. and Borgan, Ø. (1995). Counter-matching: A stratified nested case-control sampling method. *Biometrika*, **82**, 69–79.

Langholz, B. and Borgan, Ø. (1997). Estimation of absolute risk from nested case-control data. *Biometrics*, **53**, 767–774. Correction **59**, 451.

Langholz, B. and Goldstein, L. (1996). Risk set sampling in epidemiologic cohort studies. *Statistical Science*, **11**, 35–53.

Lin, D. Y., Wei, L. J., and Ying, Z. (1993). Checking the Cox model with cumulative sums of martingale-based residualss. *Biometrika*, **80**, 557–572.

Steenland, K. and Deddens, J. A. (1997). Increased precision using countermatching in nested case-control studies. *Epidemiology*, **8**, 238–242.

Therneau, T. M. and Grambsch, P. M. (2000). *Modeling Survival Data: Extending the Cox Model*. Springer-Verlag, New York.

Thomas, D. C. (1977). Addendum to: "Methods of cohort analysis: Appraisal by application to asbestos mining" By Liddell, F. D. K., McDonald, J. C., and Thomas, D. C. *Journal of the Royal Statistical Society: Series A (General)*, **140**, 469–491.

19

Inverse Probability Weighting in Nested Case-Control Studies

Sven Ove Samuelsen

University of Oslo

Nathalie Støer

Oslo University Hospital

19.1 Introduction

The nested case-control (NCC) study, originally suggested by Thomas (1977) and described in detail in Chapters 16 and 18, is a cost-effective and efficient design. The basic feature of the design is that at each event time, t_i, we sample m_i controls from those still at risk at that time. We say that the m_i controls are matched to the case at t_i. In addition, the controls may be matched on potential confounders. Usually equal number of controls, $m_i = m$, are sampled for each case and the number is typically small, i.e., less than 10, and often $m = 1$ or 2. The sampled data is then traditionally analyzed with Cox regression using a partial likelihood approach which in practical terms can be described as Cox regression stratified on case-control sets or alternatively as conditional logistic regression.

The other major case-control design with time to event data is the case-cohort design

(CCH) suggested by Prentice (1986) and discussed in Chapters 16 and 17. Here, a subcohort is sampled from the full cohort and exposure variables are obtained both for the cases and for the individuals in the subcohort. The CCH design is similar to NCC in terms of cost-effectiveness and efficiency (Langholz and Thomas, 1991; Kim, 2015), but a partial likelihood method for analyzing the data has not been developed. Instead the data are usually analyzed by maximizing an inverse inclusion probability weighted (IPW) likelihood. This, in fact, has the great advantage that the same subcohort can be used as controls for cases of different types. If one were to investigate a new type of case, the economical savings can then be huge as only covariate information from the new cases is required. An additional advantage of the IPW approach is that it can readily be adapted to many kinds of analysis methods in addition to proportional hazards regression.

In Chapter 17, Breslow and Hu discuss the case-cohort design in terms of a two-phase case-control study. It is also possible to view nested case-control studies as two-phase studies only with a somewhat more complex sampling strategy for the controls. As discussed below, it is frequently also possible to calculate inclusion probabilities with NCC data and then analyze the data using the IPW approach. This is sometimes referred to as breaking the matching or, more positively phrased, as reusing the controls. One consequence is that controls sampled for a particular type of case can be used as controls for other types of cases in the same way as in a case-cohort study (Saarela *et al.*, 2008; Salim *et al.*, 2009). Another advantage is that the modelling flexibility of case-cohort studies is transferred to NCC studies.

One approach for calculating inclusion probabilities with NCC data is based on explicit consideration of the sampling design. This was first suggested by one of us (Samuelsen, 1997), but the same approach was soon after presented by Suissa *et al.* (1998) in order to calculate standardized mortality ratios. We will in the following refer to these probabilities as design based, but also, due to the formula for the inclusion probability, as the Kaplan-Meier (KM) method.

Another possibility, inspired by methods for analyzing missing data, is to propose a working model for the indicator variables of being sampled and regress them on observed variables such as length of follow-up. This suggestion has been discussed in a number of publications (Pugh *et al.*, 1993; Robins *et al.*, 1994; Chen, 2001; Mark and Katki, 2006; Samuelsen *et al.*, 2007; Saarela *et al.*, 2008) and we will refer to this type of weights as working model weights.

In this chapter we will present the weight estimators in Section 19.2 and the weighted Cox regression in Section 19.3. Section 19.4 concerns the multiple endpoints situation, where the IPW estimators have been shown to improve efficiency. When the matching of NCC data is broken, other models than the Cox model, and other time scales than the original can be accommodated and this is discussed in Section 19.5. Calibration of weights, which is an idea from the survey sampling literature (cf. Chapters 13 and 17), with the potential of increasing the efficiency of the IPW estimators, is presented in Section 19.6. In Section 19.7 we discuss complications that may arise (with regards to modelling and weight estimation) when controls are matched on possible confounders in addition to at-risk status. Finally, in Section 19.8 miscellaneous issues are briefly mentioned.

19.2   Inverse probability weights

The background for inverse probability weighting of (nested) case-control data is that the cases and controls form a biased sample from the cohort. By weighting the included individuals with the inverse of their probability of being sampled, they can be considered to represent a number of nonsampled subjects in the cohort equal to the weights. This idea traces back to the survey sampling literature and is referred to as the Horvitz-Thompson estimator (Horvitz and Thompson, 1952).

Central to survey sampling is the concept of two-phase studies and the nested case-control study can be considered in a two-phase sampling framework. The first phase consists of sampling the cohort data from a super-population, and the second phase consists of selecting the nested case-control sample from the cohort. To perform the nested case-control sampling we need to know which individuals became cases and which individuals were available as controls at the event times of the cases. We will only consider right censored and possibly left truncated data where individual i has an entry time v_i and a right censoring or event time t_i. Knowledge of the $(v_i, t_i]$ and event indicators δ_i amounts to knowledge of the indicator functions $Y_i(t)$ of being under observation and the counting process $\mathbb{N}_i(t)$ of events for each individual i in the cohort, $i = 1, \ldots, N$. In Samuelsen (1997) this Phase I information was referred to as the skeleton of the cohort. In addition, the Phase I data could consist of some covariates as well as some auxiliary variables known for all individuals, but for the following exposition we assume that the Phase I data is summarized by $\{(Y_i(t), \mathbb{N}_i(t)); i = 1, \ldots, N\}$. We will in later sections consider modifications involving more complex Phase I data. The Phase II data is then composed of the Phase I data along with covariate data for all cases and their matched controls. As mentioned above, the sampling weights can be estimated, given the Phase I data, using one of two approaches: design based weights and working model weights. The design based weights directly build on the survey sampling framework and we describe them first.

19.2.1 Design based weights

As described in the introduction, the NCC study consists of sampling a specified number of controls m_i at each event time t_i without replacement from the risk set $\mathcal{R}(t_i)$ excluding the case at that time. Let $n(t_i)$ be the number at risk at t_i and let i be the label of the subject who fails at time t_i. Then the conditional probability that individual $j \neq i$ is sampled as a control at t_i, given the Phase I data, becomes $\pi_{j0}(t_i) = m_i/[n(t_i) - 1]$ if individual j is at risk at t_i and zero otherwise. An individual can be sampled as a control at several event times and previous inclusions as a control will not change the probability of being sampled at t_i.

Thus with $\mathcal{D}$ denoting the set of all cases and $\mathcal{P}_i = \mathcal{R}(t_i) \setminus \{i\}$ the set of all eligible controls for the case at time t_i, we have that the probability of ever sampling subject j as a control, conditional on the Phase I information, is given by

$$\pi_{j0} = 1 - \prod_{i \in \mathcal{D}, j \in \mathcal{P}_i} \left(1 - \frac{m_i}{n(t_i) - 1}\right), \tag{19.1}$$

as suggested in Samuelsen (1997). It was then proposed to weight data according to $w_j = 1/\pi_j$, where $\pi_j = \pi_{j0}(1 - \delta_j) + \delta_j$ and δ_j is a binary indicator that individual j is (ever) a case. The rationale for this being that we assume that all cases are sampled. Since the formula for π_{j0} resembles the Kaplan-Meier estimator, we sometimes refer to the weights as KM-weights.

19.2.2 Working model weights

With case-control data, and more generally data that are missing by design, the mechanism for observing individuals will be known, as discussed above for the NCC data. For missing data in general such a mechanism can usually not be specified and what is often done is to postulate some working model for the probability of observing complete information for an individual, and for convenience a logistic regression is often applied (Tsiatis, 2006). This approach may also be used for case-control data.

To formalize, we introduce sampling indicators R_j, which equal 1 if subject j is included in the NCC study. We have assumed that covariates are obtained for all cases and so, conditional on the Phase I data, $\mathrm{P}(R_j = 1 \,|\, \Delta_j = 1) = 1$ where random variables Δ_j indicate events. The probability of sampling a noncase subject j will depend on the at-risk function $Y_j(t)$ which we have assumed equals one in the interval $(v_j, t_j]$. The working model can then be stated as

$$\pi_j = \mathrm{P}(R_j = 1 \,|\, t_j, v_j, \Delta_j = 0) = \frac{\exp(\xi_0 + f(t_j, v_j))}{1 + \exp(\xi_0 + f(t_j, v_j))} \tag{19.2}$$

for some function $f(t_j, v_j)$ and an intercept ξ_0. The simplest model possible is the logistic regression with no interactions in which

$$f(t_j, v_j) = f_1(t_j) + f_2(v_j) = \xi_1 t_j + \xi_2 v_j. \tag{19.3}$$

A more flexible version is the generalized additive model (GAM) (Hastie and Tibshirani, 1990, Chap. 9) with logit-link, in which f_1 and f_2 are smooth functions.

A seemingly different approach is local averaging (Chen, 2001), lightly modified to allow for left truncation in Støer and Samuelsen (2012). The method consists of partitioning the intervals where left-truncation times and censoring times occur into subintervals, and calculating the proportion of controls sampled among all noncases in each combination of left-truncation and censoring subintervals. This proportion is then used as the inclusion probability. It should be noted that Chen (2001) allowed for sampling of cases as well as other sampling strategies than NCC.

The local averaging approach can be put on the form (19.2) with the function $f(t_j, v_j)$ as a two-dimensional step function constant at combinations of left truncation and censoring intervals, or in other terms, as a logistic regression with factor variable that indicates combinations of the intervals. We note that there may be practical issues regarding the choice of intervals. Furthermore, as pointed out in Samuelsen *et al.* (2007), local averaging corresponds to post-stratification on the truncation and censoring intervals.

19.2.3   Comparison

The estimators described in Sections 19.2.1 and 19.2.2 generally give fairly similar results, both with regards to the weights themselves, and the estimated regression coefficients from the weighted Cox regression, described in Section 19.3. An example of estimated sampling probabilities is given in Figure 19.1 which displays the estimated probabilities in a synthetic NCC study from a data set on radiation and breast cancer described in Chapter 17 and Section 19.3.1 of this chapter. This NCC study was sampled with $m = 2$ controls per case and time since inclusion in the study as underlying time variable. Note that our results presented in the next subsections use another NCC data set sampled from the same cohort, namely the same as used in Chapter 18 with attained age as the time variable (and thus left truncated at age at inclusion). The reason for using time since inclusion in Figure 19.1 is that comparison between different types of inclusion probabilities becomes simpler when they only depend on one variable.

Since the number of times an individual can be sampled increases with follow-up time, so will generally the sampling probabilities. The design based inclusion probabilities are always nondecreasing. Flexible working model probabilities may, however, have local maxima and

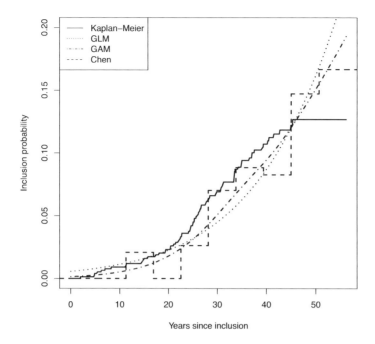

FIGURE 19.1
Estimated sampling probabilities as a function time since inclusion. Controls were sampled from risk sets based on time since inclusion and $m = 2$ controls were obtained from these risk sets with simple random sampling at each event time.

minima, as is seen for local averaging probabilities in Figure 19.1. A difference between the approaches is that the working model probabilities estimate the actual sampling of controls, whereas the design based probabilities reflect the sampling that on average will occur if the control sampling is repeated.

19.3 Weighted Cox regression

Under the proportional hazards model the hazard of individual i is given as

$$\lambda_i(t) = \lambda_0(t) \exp(\boldsymbol{\beta}^\mathsf{T} \mathbf{x}_i),$$

where $\lambda_0(t)$ is a baseline hazard and $\boldsymbol{\beta}$ regression parameters. Using the inclusion probabilities π_i and weights $w_i = 1/\pi_i$ described in either Section 19.2.1 or Section 19.2.2 we may then estimate $\boldsymbol{\beta}$ by maximizing a weighted likelihood, i.e., a weighted version of the Cox partial likelihood (Samuelsen, 1997; Chen, 2001; Saarela *et al.*, 2008)

$$L_w(\boldsymbol{\beta}) = \prod_{i \in \mathcal{D}} \frac{\exp(\boldsymbol{\beta}^\mathsf{T} \mathbf{x}_i)}{\sum_{j \in \mathcal{S}_i} \exp(\boldsymbol{\beta}^\mathsf{T} \mathbf{x}_j) w_j}, \tag{19.4}$$

where $\mathcal{S}_i$ is the set of all sampled subjects, both controls and cases, at risk at time t_i. Alternatively $L_w(\boldsymbol{\beta})$ is sometimes referred to as a pseudo-likelihood.

The weighted likelihood can be maximized with software that allows for weights in the Cox regression. The likelihood contributions in $L_w(\boldsymbol{\beta})$ will be dependent, thus the inverse of the information matrix cannot be used to estimate the standard errors. Such naive standard errors correspond to standard errors for cohort data and are therefore smaller than valid standard errors for the sampled data. For KM- and Chen-weights there exist variance estimators (Samuelsen, 1997; Chen, 2001; Samuelsen *et al.*, 2007); see also the next section. Another option usable for all weight estimators is robust variances (Lin and Wei, 1989; Barlow, 1994), although these are theoretically conservative (Samuelsen *et al.*, 2007; Cai and Zheng, 2012).

The weighted likelihood (19.4) can be maximized with $w_i = 1/\pi_i$ for the estimated inclusion probabilities π_i described in Sections 19.2.1 and 19.2.2 using the function wpl in the R package multipleNCC (see Støer and Samuelsen, 2016). This function also allows for reporting estimated standard errors for design based weights and Chen-weights, discussed in Section 19.3.2, and robust standard errors otherwise. The package also includes functions for calculating the different inclusion probabilities.

19.3.1   Data example: Radiation and breast cancer

As an illustration we will consider the radiation and breast cancer cohort used in Chapters 17 and 18. The cohort consists of 1,720 women followed from discharge from hospital after a tuberculosis diagnosis, with many patients treated by radiation, until diagnosis of breast cancer, death or end of study. The cases are 75 women who were diagnosed with breast cancer during the study period. We consider the same NCC data as in Chapter 18, with two controls per case, to allow for direct comparison. The time variable is age, left-truncated at time of inclusion in the study, with follow-up until first occurrence of cancer or censoring. These data were analyzed under a proportional hazards model with covariates measured radiation dose transformed by $x_1 = \log_2(\text{dose} + 1)$ and age at first treatment divided by 10, $x_2 = \text{ageRx}/10$.

A control in a NCC study can be matched to several cases and eventually also become a case. In the analysis file for a partial likelihood such individuals will be represented equally many times as they are sampled. In contrast, for the weighted analysis each subject will appear only once in the data set. For this particular (synthetic) NCC study 5 controls later became cases and 9 subjects were sampled as controls twice. For those controls who later became a case, the "case-entry" is kept in the analysis file while the "control-entry" is removed. For the controls sampled multiple times, only one of the entries is kept while the others are removed, resulting in 211 unique study subjects of whom 136 are controls.

Table 19.1 displays the results from the full cohort analysis and the nested case-control analyses. The estimates are fairly similar across estimation methods. The standard errors of the weighted estimators are somewhat smaller than the standard error of the traditional estimator, but this may simply be a reflection of slightly smaller estimates of regression parameters. The estimates are also close to those of Breslow and Hu in Chapter 17 for case-cohort data with simple random sampling of the subcohort.

For the variable $\log_2(\text{dose}+1)$ the robust standard errors shown in the table are in close agreement with the standard errors estimated as described in Section 19.3.2. These were 0.208 for design based weights and 0.206 for Chen-weights. For the variable ageRx/10 the estimated standard error for design based weights is also close to the robust standard error with a value of 0.184, but for Chen-weights we obtain the smaller value 0.164. We note that ageRx is strongly correlated (0.96) with the left truncation time and comment on the

TABLE 19.1

Comparison of results of cohort and NCC analyses for breast cancer data. Robust standard errors except for the traditional NCC estimate.

Model term	Coef.	SE	Z	p
	Entire cohort			
$\log_2(\text{dose}+1)$	0.469	0.153	3.06	0.002
ageRx/10	-0.242	0.144	-1.68	0.094
	Traditional NCC			
$\log_2(\text{dose}+1)$	0.549	0.232	2.37	0.018
ageRx/10	-0.179	0.207	-0.86	0.388
	KM-weights			
$\log_2(\text{dose}+1)$	0.482	0.204	2.37	0.018
ageRx/10	-0.152	0.187	-0.81	0.416
	GLM-weights			
$\log_2(\text{dose}+1)$	0.507	0.205	2.47	0.014
ageRx/10	-0.328	0.196	-1.68	0.094
	GAM-weights			
$\log_2(\text{dose}+1)$	0.505	0.203	2.48	0.013
ageRx/10	-0.278	0.181	-1.54	0.124
	Chen-weights			
$\log_2(\text{dose}+1)$	0.491	0.204	2.41	0.016
ageRx/10	-0.152	0.184	-0.83	0.408

finding at the end of Section 19.3.2. Note also that robust standard errors are reported for the cohort to be in agreement with Breslow and Hu in Chapter 17.

19.3.2 Outline of large sample properties

Maximization of $L_w(\boldsymbol{\beta})$ in (19.4) is equivalent to solving weighted score equations

$$\mathbf{U}_w(\boldsymbol{\beta}) = \sum_{i \in \mathcal{D}} [\mathbf{x}_i - \widetilde{\mathbf{m}}(\boldsymbol{\beta}; t_i)] = \mathbf{0} \tag{19.5}$$

where

$$\widetilde{\mathbf{m}}(\boldsymbol{\beta}; t_i) = \frac{\sum_{j \in \mathcal{S}_i} \mathbf{x}_j \exp(\boldsymbol{\beta}^\mathsf{T} \mathbf{x}_j) w_j}{\sum_{j \in \mathcal{S}_i} \exp(\boldsymbol{\beta}^\mathsf{T} \mathbf{x}_j) w_j}.$$

In this section we will outline the development of the large sample properties of the maximizer $\hat{\boldsymbol{\beta}}_w$ of (19.4) with the design based weights (19.1) from Section 19.2.1. Largely the derivation follows Samuelsen (1997) who conjectured the results, but we will fill in details from Lu and Liu (2012) who completed the proofs in the more general setting of linear transformation models. For asymptotics see also the supplement of Cai and Zheng (2012) who are addressing general estimating equations. The presentation is also parallel to the outline of large sample results for case-cohort studies discussed in Chapter 17. In particular we may, with $\mathbf{U}_C(\boldsymbol{\beta})$ denoting the score function for the full cohort data, expand the weighted score function as

$$\mathbf{U}_w(\boldsymbol{\beta}) = \mathbf{U}_C(\boldsymbol{\beta}) + \mathbf{U}_w(\boldsymbol{\beta}) - \mathbf{U}_C(\boldsymbol{\beta}) = \mathbf{U}_C(\boldsymbol{\beta}) + \sum_{i=1}^{N} \left[\frac{R_i}{\pi_i} - 1 \right] \mathbf{W}_i + o_p(n^{\frac{1}{2}}), \qquad (19.6)$$

where

$$\mathbf{W}_i = \int [\mathbf{x}_i - \mathbf{m}(\boldsymbol{\beta}, t)] Y_i(t) \exp(\boldsymbol{\beta}^{\mathsf{T}} \mathbf{x}_i) \lambda_0(t) dt$$

and

$$\mathbf{m}(\boldsymbol{\beta}; t) = \frac{\sum_{j \in \mathcal{R}(t)} \mathbf{x}_j \exp(\boldsymbol{\beta}^{\mathsf{T}} \mathbf{x}_j)}{\sum_{j \in \mathcal{R}(t)} \exp(\boldsymbol{\beta}^{\mathsf{T}} \mathbf{x}_j)}.$$

The expected value of the sampling indicator R_i will, conditional on the Phase I information, equal π_i. Furthermore as the sampling only depends on the Phase I information and not the additional full cohort data, the conditional expectation of R_i given the full cohort also equals π_i. It follows that both essential terms on the right-hand side of (19.6) have expectation zero and are uncorrelated.

It is standard theory for the Cox estimator that $N^{-\frac{1}{2}} \mathbf{U}_C(\boldsymbol{\beta})$ converges in distribution to a normal distribution with mean zero and a covariance matrix $\boldsymbol{\Sigma}_1$ which can be estimated from the information matrix of $\mathbf{U}_C(\boldsymbol{\beta})$ in the standard fashion. Furthermore, as conjectured in Samuelsen (1997) and proved in Lu and Liu (2012),

$$N^{-\frac{1}{2}} \sum_{i=1}^{N} [R_i/\pi_i - 1] \mathbf{W}_i$$

will converge to a normal distribution with mean zero and a covariance matrix $\boldsymbol{\Sigma}_2$. Here Lu and Liu (2012) relied on a weak convergence result for dependent variables $[R_i/\pi_i - 1] \mathbf{W}_i$. Consequently $N^{-\frac{1}{2}} \mathbf{U}_w(\boldsymbol{\beta})$ converges to a normal distribution with mean zero and covariance matrix $\boldsymbol{\Sigma}_1 + \boldsymbol{\Sigma}_2$ and $\sqrt{N}(\hat{\boldsymbol{\beta}}_w - \boldsymbol{\beta})$ converges to a normal distribution with mean zero and covariance matrix $\boldsymbol{\Sigma}_1^{-1} + \boldsymbol{\Sigma}_1^{-1} \boldsymbol{\Sigma}_2 \boldsymbol{\Sigma}_1^{-1}$.

The matrix $\boldsymbol{\Sigma}_2$ can be split into two parts, $\boldsymbol{\Sigma}_{2a}$ and $\boldsymbol{\Sigma}_{2b}$, where the first term is the limit of

$$\frac{1}{N} \sum_{i=1}^{N} \frac{1 - \pi_i}{\pi_i} \mathbf{W}_i \mathbf{W}_i^{\mathsf{T}}.$$

Here $(1 - \pi_i)/\pi_i$ is the variance of $R_i/\pi_i - 1$ conditional on the Phase I information. The second term relates to the covariance terms between R_i and R_j and is obtained as the limit of

$$\frac{2}{N} \sum_{i<j} \frac{\mathrm{Cov}_{ij}}{\pi_i \pi_j} \mathbf{W}_i \mathbf{W}_j^{\mathsf{T}},$$

where Cov_{ij} is the covariance between R_i and R_j conditional on the Phase I information. This covariance is nonpositive since sampling individual i at a particular time reduces the chance of sampling individual j. An expression for the covariance is developed in Samuelsen (1997), and in particular it was shown that the covariance is of order $O_p(N^{-1})$. Thus, the second term $\boldsymbol{\Sigma}_{2b}$ can in general not be ignored. However, as argued by Cai and Zheng (2012), it will always be conservative to omit this term.

A variance estimator for $\hat{\boldsymbol{\beta}}_w$ is obtained using the information matrix from $L_w(\boldsymbol{\beta})$ in place of $\boldsymbol{\Sigma}_1$. Next for the terms corresponding to $\boldsymbol{\Sigma}_2 = \boldsymbol{\Sigma}_{2a} + \boldsymbol{\Sigma}_{2b}$ one replaces the $\mathbf{W}_i$ by the individual score contributions routinely calculated by software for Cox regression. The second term involves a sum over indices i and j and is sometimes considered numerically hard, but with the matrix representation in Støer and Samuelsen (2016) the computation time can be reduced.

Alternatively, a theoretically conservative variance estimator is obtained by ignoring the second term. This approach will be asymptotically equivalent to using a robust variance estimator. Several simulation studies indicate that for practical use the robust variance is adequate (Samuelsen *et al.*, 2007; Saarela *et al.*, 2008; Støer and Samuelsen, 2012, 2013; Kim and Kaplan, 2013). The published examples (Samuelsen, 1997; Chen, 2001; Samuelsen *et al.*, 2007), where the robust variance is seriously conservative, all involve covariates that are strongly correlated to the censoring time. A third option for obtaining variance estimators is the resampling technique developed by Cai and Zheng (2013).

For the local averaging weights with right censored data (and possibly sampling of cases) the inclusion probabilities are estimated as the proportion of sampled individuals among those with censoring times (or events times) in each subinterval. Chen (2001) obtained large sample results for such estimators under the assumption that the number of subintervals increases to infinity at a rate so that the number of sampled individuals with follow-up times in all subintervals also goes to infinity at a rate $o_p(N^{\frac{1}{2}})$. This implies that the inclusion probabilities can be estimated consistently.

With a specified number of subintervals for censoring and truncation times the post-stratification argument of Samuelsen *et al.* (2007) gives a simple method for estimating variances using results from stratified case-cohort design as discussed in Chapters 16 and 17. Samuelsen *et al.* (2007) furthermore found that the variance of coefficient estimates for covariates strongly correlated to the right censoring time were smaller than robust variances and estimated without visible bias. It was interesting to observe that when we applied this variance estimator to the breast cancer data in Section 19.3.1 we found that these were smaller than the robust variances for the variable ageRx, corresponding to the strong correlation between this covariate and the left truncation time.

19.4 Multiple endpoints

Collecting exposure information, for instance biomarkers or genetic information, is often very expensive and using such information in the most efficient way possible should be a priority. In this respect there is a drawback with traditional analysis of nested case-control data due to the matching of controls to cases. For instance in a competing risk setting where the same exposures are of interest for two (or more) types of cases (e.g., different cancers) one will have to sample new controls for each type of case, and due to the matching it is not possible to reuse controls sampled for one type when analyzing the association with another type of case. Since the inverse probability weighted approach of analysing nested case-control data allows for breaking the matching between cases and controls, the above mentioned issues are no longer a problem as all sampled controls can be utilized for any type of case.

Some publications have investigated this benefit of the weighted estimator. One of these is Saarela *et al.* (2008) that considers using controls selected for one type of case as controls for cases of another type, either instead of or in addition to controls specifically sampled for the other type. Mathematically it will be acceptable not to collect new controls for the other type of case, but in particular with biomarker data there may be practical problems with such an approach. We give some comments in the Miscellaneous issues section (Section 19.8). Another point discussed by Salim *et al.* (2012) is that reusing a number of controls sampled for another type of case could be less informative than sampling the corresponding number of controls for the new type of case. They found this aspect more pronounced in the presence of additional matching.

In a somewhat different example Salim *et al.* (2009) considered a situation where two nested case-control studies have been sampled from overlapping cohorts. They proposed a method for calculating combined inclusion probabilities depending on separate inclusion probabilities in each study. This allowed for a pooled analysis of the nested case-control studies leading to more efficient results than those in the separate NCCs.

Furthermore Støer and Samuelsen (2013) considered sub-endpoints and a secondary endpoint. The situation was a nested case-control study with controls sampled for incident prostate cancer cases. This endpoint was later divided into local cancer, advanced cancer and unknown cancer status and three separate analyses were carried out using all sampled controls in all three analyses. This corresponds to a competing risk situation and is frequently of interest. For instance, Støer and Samuelsen (2016) list several papers where such sub-analyses were performed without taking advantage of the possiblity of reusing controls.

In addition, Støer and Samuelsen (2013) consider a secondary analysis where cases are the individuals who were observed to die of the prostate cancer, again using all sampled controls. If this analysis were to be carried out using the traditional estimator, only the controls for cases in question could have been included and the efficiency would have been much lower. This example shows that the reuse technique can be of interest in more situations than competing risk.

It should be noted that the efficiency of NCC studies compared to cohort studies increases when the number of controls is increased. Often $m/(m+1)$ is a good approximation to the efficiency. Thus if the number of controls m for each case is large, the gain in breaking the matching will be moderate. However, with $m = 1$ or 2 it can be substantial. Furthermore, some types of cases are often more frequent than others. With the same m for all types of cases, higher efficiency gains will be observed for the less frequent types since they are provided with a large number of controls from the other more frequent types.

19.4.1   Data example: Causes of death

To illustrate the use of the weighted Cox regression with multiple endpoints we will use a data set from Aalen *et al.* (2008) which is included in the R package `multipleNCC` (`data(CVD_Accidents)`). The data is a cohort of 3,933 men and women above the age of 40 who participated in cardiovascular health screenings in 1974-1978 in three counties in Norway. The cause of death is recorded and grouped into four broad categories: (i) cancer, (ii) cardiovascular disease (CVD), (iii) alcohol abuse, liver disease, accidents and violence (ALAV) and (iv) other causes. Information on several covariates, including systolic blood pressure (SBP), is recorded. We will use death from CVD and ALAV as our endpoints and sample one control for each CVD and ALAV case. Death from CVD is relatively common with 236 cases while death from ALAV is less common, 60 cases. We will consider SBP categorized as hypertension, i.e., above 140 mm Hg, compared to normal SBP below 140 mm Hg as the exposure variable (and ignore the other covariates for our illustrative purposes). The estimates and their standard errors can be found in Table 19.2. We only show the results with the design based weights as the other weighting methods gave almost identical estimates and standard errors. We note that there is a large efficiency gain from weighting for the rare outcome ALAV making these close to efficient compared to the cohort. For the more frequent outcome CVD, however, the improvement is marginal.

TABLE 19.2
Comparison of estimators using Causes of Death
data. Estimates are effect of high systolic blood
pressure ($\geq$140) on death from CVD and ALAV.
Estimated standard error for weighted analyses.

	CVD		ALAV	
Method	Coef.	SE	Coef.	SE
Cohort	0.927	0.130	0.783	0.259
Traditional NCC	0.770	0.182	0.647	0.372
Weighted KM	0.883	0.178	0.711	0.286

19.5 Other models and estimators than proportional hazards

The idea behind inverse probability weighting is that every sampled individual i represents $w_i = 1/\pi_i$ subjects in the cohort. Thus with the weighting, we obtain a data set that corresponds to aggregated population data. It will then be possible to modify virtually any method developed for cohort data so that it can be used on sampled weighted data. This, for instance, enables estimation of absolute risk, of fitting models outside the proportional hazards model and of using alternative time scales. We discuss such possibilities in the following subsections.

19.5.1 Weighted estimating equations

In order to fit general parametric survival models for case-cohort and related data, Kalbfleisch and Lawless (1988) presented weighted maximum likelihood estimators. Specifically if $l_i(\boldsymbol{\theta})$ are log-likelihood contributions of independent individuals in the cohort and $w_i = 1/\pi_i$ inverse probability weights, one may estimate $\boldsymbol{\theta}$ on the case-control data by maximizing $\tilde{l}(\boldsymbol{\theta}) = \sum_{i \in \mathcal{S}} w_i l_i(\boldsymbol{\theta})$ where $\mathcal{S}$ is the set of all sampled individuals. This idea was further discussed by Samuelsen (1997) using a weighted likelihood with design based weights for NCC data. Similarly Cai and Zheng (2012) discuss weighted versions $\sum_{i \in \mathcal{S}} w_i \mathbf{u}_i(\boldsymbol{\theta}) = \mathbf{0}$ of unbiased estimating equations $\sum_{i=1}^{N} \mathbf{u}_i(\boldsymbol{\theta}) = \mathbf{0}$ also in the context of NCC data. Other examples include those of Lu and Liu (2012) and Chen *et al.* (2012) on linear transformation models.

A careful examination may be needed in each specific case, but the derivations of Cai and Zheng (2012) show that under regularity assumptions one may develop large sample results along similar lines as those outlined in Section 19.3.2. For example Zheng *et al.* (2012) investigated a multiplicative-additive model with hazards, given covariates $\mathbf{z}$ and $\mathbf{x}$, $\lambda(t|\mathbf{x}, \mathbf{z}) = \lambda_0(t)h(\boldsymbol{\gamma}^\mathsf{T}\mathbf{z}) + \boldsymbol{\beta}^\mathsf{T}\mathbf{x}$ for NCC data with design based weights and presented the large sample distribution of the weighted estimator $\hat{\boldsymbol{\theta}}$ for $\boldsymbol{\theta} = (\boldsymbol{\gamma}^\mathsf{T}, \boldsymbol{\beta}^\mathsf{T})^\mathsf{T}$. If there is no component $\mathbf{z}$ this model reduces to a Ling-Ying additive model $\lambda(t|\mathbf{x}) = \lambda_0(t) + \boldsymbol{\beta}^\mathsf{T}\mathbf{x}$ (Lin and Ying, 1994).

The Lin-Ying additive model can be fitted using the R-library `timereg` which allows for weights and robust variance estimation. In Table 19.3 we present results from fitting Lin-Ying additive models to both the complete cohort and the sampled NCC data used in Section 19.3.1 with covariates $\log_2(\text{dose}+1)$ and ageRx/10. For the NCC data we use design based weights calculated in `multipleNCC` with the function `KMprob`. Although no

TABLE 19.3
Results from Lin-Ying additive model using breast cancer data.
Robust standard errors for weighted analysis.

Model term	Coef.	Naive SE	Robust SE	Z	p
		Entire cohort			
$\log_2(\text{dose}+1)$	0.000700	0.000263	0.000264	2.65	0.008
ageRx/10	-0.000366	0.000199	0.000199	-1.84	0.066
		KM-weights			
$\log_2(\text{dose}+1)$	0.000590	0.000219	0.000284	2.08	0.037
ageRx/10	-0.000191	0.000190	0.000228	-0.84	0.401

examination of the validity of using robust standard errors in this particular case has been done, we present these as well as the naive standard errors for both data sets.

The NCC estimates are slightly closer to zero compared to the cohort estimates. However, when calculating the ratio of the robust standard errors for the cohort and the NCC estimates we find that these are strikingly similar to the ratios for the proportional hazards model in Table 19.1.

19.5.2 Estimation of absolute risks

After the regression parameters in a proportional hazard model have been estimated, it will often be of importance to consider absolute risks quantities of different kinds. In particular one may want to estimate a cumulative baseline hazard $\Lambda_0(t) = \int_0^t \lambda_0(s)ds$ or the probability of event before time t with a specified covariate value $\mathbf{x}$ which is expressed as

$$F_{\mathbf{x}}(t) = 1 - \exp(-\exp(\boldsymbol{\beta}^{\mathsf{T}}\mathbf{x})\Lambda_0(t)).$$

A modification of the Breslow estimator for the cumulative baseline hazard using an IPW approach is given by

$$\widehat{\Lambda}_0(t) = \int_0^t \frac{d\mathbb{N}_\cdot(s)}{\widehat{S}_0(\widehat{\boldsymbol{\beta}}_w, s)},$$

where $\mathbb{N}_\cdot(s) = \sum_{i=1}^N \mathbb{N}_i(s)$ and

$$\widehat{S}^{(0)}(\widehat{\boldsymbol{\beta}}_w, s) = \sum_{i \in \mathcal{D}} w_i Y_i(s) \exp(\widehat{\boldsymbol{\beta}}_w^{\mathsf{T}} \mathbf{x}_i).$$

This suggests

$$\hat{F}_{\mathbf{x}}(t) = 1 - \exp(-\exp(\widehat{\boldsymbol{\beta}}_w^{\mathsf{T}} \mathbf{x})\widehat{\Lambda}_0(t))$$

as an estimator for $F_{\mathbf{x}}(t)$. Theory for $\widehat{\Lambda}_0(t)$ and $\hat{F}_{\mathbf{x}}(t)$ builds on results from Lin (2000) and has been presented in for instance Cai and Zheng (2012) and Lu and Liu (2012). Under regularity assumptions these give that the estimators are consistent and with weak convergence of $\sqrt{N}(\widehat{\Lambda}_0(t) - \Lambda_0(t))$ to a Gaussian process with mean zero and covariance function

$$\phi(t,s) = \int_0^{\min(t,s)} \frac{\lambda_0(r)dr}{s^{(0)}(\boldsymbol{\beta}, r)} + \mathbf{r}(s, \boldsymbol{\beta})^{\mathsf{T}} \mathbf{D}^{-1} \mathbf{r}(t, \boldsymbol{\beta}),$$

where $\mathbf{D} = \boldsymbol{\Sigma}_1^{-1} + \boldsymbol{\Sigma}_1^{-1}\boldsymbol{\Sigma}_2\boldsymbol{\Sigma}_1^{-1}$ is the limiting covariance matrix of $\sqrt{N}(\hat{\boldsymbol{\beta}}_w - \boldsymbol{\beta})$, and $s^{(0)}(\boldsymbol{\beta}, s)$ and $\mathbf{r}(s, \boldsymbol{\beta})$ are the limits in probability of $S^{(0)}(\boldsymbol{\beta}, s) = (1/N)\sum_{i=1}^N Y_i(s)\exp(\boldsymbol{\beta}^{\mathsf{T}}\mathbf{x}_i)$ and $(1/N)\int_0^s \tilde{\mathbf{m}}(\boldsymbol{\beta}; r)d\mathbb{N}_\cdot(r)$, where $\tilde{\mathbf{m}}(\boldsymbol{\beta}; r)$ is defined right below formula (19.5).

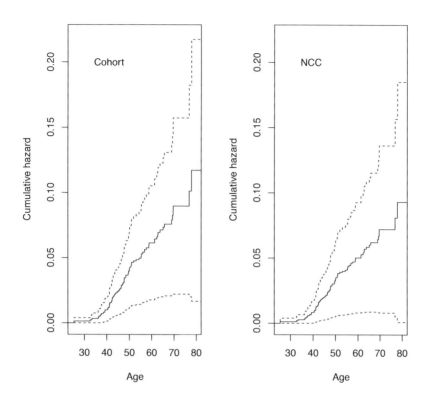

FIGURE 19.2
Estimated cumulative baseline from proportional hazards model for cohort and nested case-control data using breast cancer data with 95% pointwise confidence limits.

Such results can be used as intermediate steps, for instance when developing predictive measures and ROC-curves; see, for instance, Cai and Zheng (2011, 2012) and Ganna *et al.* (2012). Another application is the goodness-of-fit tests for the proportional hazards assumption suggested for cohort data using martingale residuals by Lin *et al.* (1993) and modified to weighted NCC by Lu *et al.* (2014). Furthermore, in a competing risk setting Rebora *et al.* (2016) develop estimators from case-cohort and weighted NCC data of cumulative incidence based on a Fine-Gray approach (Fine and Gray, 1999).

The cumulative baseline in the breast cancer data estimated using the full cohort and the NCC-sample is plotted in Figure 19.2 and they follow each other quite closely.

One could also attempt estimation of the cumulative intercept or baseline function $\Lambda_0(t) = \int_0^t \lambda_0(s)ds$ for the Lin-Ying additive model discussed in Section 19.5.1. Both the cohort and the weighted NCC estimates with 95% confidence intervals using robust variances can be obtained using the R-library `timereg`. We plot these two functions in Figure 19.3. The cumulative intercept function for the NCC data is somewhat smaller than that of the cohort. However, the confidence interval is considerably wider for the NCC estimate.

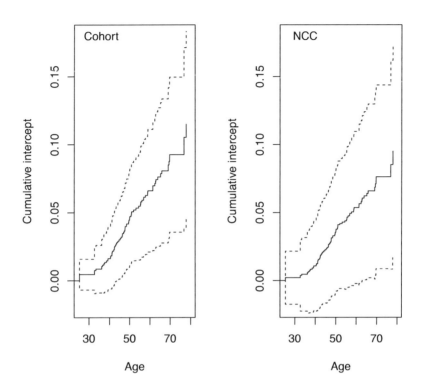

FIGURE 19.3
Estimated intercept function from Lin-Ying additive model using breast cancer data with
95% pointwise confidence limits.

19.5.3   Alternative time scales

It is not always obvious which time scale should be used for analysis. In this and previous
chapters when analysing the breast cancer data from Section 19.3.1 we used attained age
left-truncated at age at inclusion in the study. An alternative could be time since inclusion.
Also calendar time might be the most relevant time scale in some applications.

When discussing properties of inclusion probabilities in Section 19.2.3, we selected a
nested case-control sample where risk sets were determined using time from inclusion. Then
one can estimate hazard ratios relating to a proportional hazards model on this time scale
using the partial likelihood method for NCC. However, since controls are matched to cases
one can not switch between time scales with this traditional method. With the IPW approach on the other hand we are free to choose any time scale in the same way as with
cohort data.

In Table 19.4 we present results from fitting a proportional hazards model on time since
inclusion and covariates (as before) $\log_2(\text{dose}+1)$ and ageRx/10 both on the full cohort
data and on the NCC data with controls sampled using attained age as time scale and with
inclusion probabilities calculated according to this time scale. For $\log_2(\text{dose}+1)$ the results
are close to those using attained age (Table 19.1), but the coefficients for ageRx/10, which
is strongly correlated to age at entry to the study, change sign.

TABLE 19.4
Comparison of estimators under proportional hazards model
using breast cancer data and time since inclusion as time
variable.

Model term	Coef.	Naive SE	Robust SE	Z	p
		Entire cohort			
$\log_2(\text{dose}+1)$	0.470	0.161	0.154	3.06	0.002
ageRx/10	0.035	0.139	0.140	0.25	0.803
		KM-weights			
$\log_2(\text{dose}+1)$	0.481	0.160	0.201	2.39	0.017
ageRx/10	0.102	0.147	0.187	0.54	0.586

19.6 Calibration

Frequently the Phase I information consists of information additional to the at-risk function $Y_i(t)$ and the event counting process $N_i(t)$. This information could be some covariates $\tilde{\mathbf{x}}_{i0}$ and auxiliary information $\mathbf{Z}_i$. It could possibly be used for improving precision of estimators, compared to only using weights based on initial inclusion probabilities. For case-cohort data Breslow and Hu in Chapter 17 discuss this potential by applying calibration techniques (Särndal *et al.*, 1992). With this technique one modifies the initial weights such that weighted estimates of population totals equal the known population totals, but at the same time keeping the modified weights close to the original.

In the previous sections we have presented results from weighted analyses with initial weights from NCC data. Inspired by results of Breslow *et al.* (2009a,b) and Lumley (2010), we (Støer and Samuelsen, 2012) attempted calibration of these NCC weights. Recently, Rivera and Lumley (2016a,b) refined this technique both for standard NCC data and for counter-matched studies. For counter-matched data in general, see Langholz and Borgan (1995) and Chapters 16 and 18. Some more comments on IPW for this design are given in Section 19.7.1.

The approach in Støer and Samuelsen (2012) to obtain standard errors relied on the local averaging weights of Chen (2001) using their interpretation from Samuelsen *et al.* (2007) as post-stratification on truncation and censoring subintervals. Then we followed the recipe in Lumley (2010) and Breslow *et al.* (2009b) for stratified case-cohort studies. We have here applied the same approach to calibration of the breast cancer data analyzed in Section 19.3.1 and in previous chapters.

Our data is the NCC sample used in Section 19.3.1 and in Chapter 18, and we have assumed that the covariate age of first radiation (ageRx) is known in the full cohort. In addition, the auxiliary variable total number of fluoroscopies `nof` is also assumed known in the cohort, and the correlation between the variable $\log_2(1+\text{dose})$ and $\log_2(1+\text{nof}/100)$ is as noted in Chapter 17 as high as 0.98. We caution the reader that such a high correlation between a surrogate and the true exposure will be rare in practice.

Table 19.5 displays the results from the nested case-control analyses using calibration under the same model as used for Table 19.1. The estimates are fairly similar across estimation methods. The standard errors of both calibration estimators are considerably smaller than the corresponding standard errors of the weighted estimator using initial weights for the variable ageRx. However, the standard error of $\log_2(1+\text{dose})$ is only reduced when calibrating on both nof and ageRx, but then the reduction is substantial.

TABLE 19.5
Nested case-control analyses of breast cancer
data using calibration.

Model term	Coef.	SE	Z	p
Calibrated on nof and ageRx				
$\log_2(\text{dose}+1)$	0.442	0.167	2.65	0.008
ageRx/10	-0.272	0.162	-1.68	0.094
Calibrated on ageRx only				
$\log_2(\text{dose}+1)$	0.496	0.210	2.36	0.019
ageRx/10	-0.334	0.170	-1.97	0.049

19.7   Additional matching

A common way of handling confounders is to adjust for them in the regression model. Another approach sometimes possible is to require that the controls have the same or similar confounder values as the case. This is known as matching, or in the context of NCC data, where there is always matching on at-risk status, as *additional matching*. Matching will balance the data with respect to these confounders and can have the advantage of more efficient estimation.

Matching can be carried out in different ways, but in this chapter we will consider the two main methods: category and caliper matching (Cochran and Rubin, 1973) relating, respectively, to categorical and continuous matching variables. With category matching the cases and controls are required to match exactly on the given variable. Examples of this can be sex or county of residence. With caliper matching, the matching variable of a potential control must lie within a specified interval around the matching variable of the case. Examples of such matching can be date of birth $\pm$ 12 months or BMI ± 2 kg/m^2.

With the traditional estimator for NCC data, the sum in the denominator of the partial likelihood is over the sampled risk set. Thus the subjects in each risk set will have equal, or similar, values of the matching variables. With category matching, the matching variables will cancel out of the partial likelihood and is therefore not included in the regression model. The matching variables are perhaps also sometimes ignored with caliper matching, but then omission can lead to biased estimation.

Using the weighted approach with additionally matched controls requires two adaptations compared to controls only matched on time. The most important modification is that the matching variables should always be adjusted for in the regression model since their contributions do not cancel out even with exact matching. Secondly, matching will affect the sampling probabilities and it would be prudent to also account for the matching criteria when estimating weights.

For the design based weights, we may use the same formula as equation (19.1), but with the modification that all eligible controls for case i, $\mathcal{P}_i$, will now be those at risk at t_i with matching variables sufficiently close to the matching variables of the case (Salim *et al.*, 2009; Cai and Zheng, 2012; Støer and Samuelsen, 2013). The working model weights given in (19.2) can be modified by including the matching variables in the regression model for the inclusion probabilities (Støer and Samuelsen, 2013).

The effect of additional matching has been explored in Støer and Samuelsen (2013) and they show through simulations that adjusting the weights for the matching variables need not be essential, while adjusting for the matching variables in the regression model is mandatory.

We have here assumed that it is possible to quantify the matching variable. There may be situations where this is difficult, for instance when matching on neighbourhoods. Similar problems occur when the matched controls are relatives of the case, i.e., family studies, but such studies should perhaps not be considered as nested case-control studies.

19.7.1 Counter-matching

Counter-matching was described in Chapter 16 and 18. It can be considered as stratified sampling for nested case-control studies. Specifically, suppose there is an auxiliary categorical variable Z known for every individual in the Phase I study. If case i with event time at t_i has the value $Z_i = z$, one will sample $m_z - 1$ controls from those at risk with $Z_j = z$ and $m_{z'}$ controls from those at risk with other values $Z_j = z'$. Here the values of the m_z are fixed. For such data Langholz and Borgan (1995) developed a partial likelihood and showed that when Z is predictive of an exposure, this design can give more efficient estimates compared to a standard NCC for the exposure variable. This gain may, however, be at the cost of reduced precision for other covariates.

Samuelsen *et al.* (2007) suggested both design based and working model weights for counter-matched studies, but in their examples they found that the weighted Cox regression was not as efficient as the partial likelihood approach. Recently Rivera and Lumley (2016a,b) investigated (design based) weighting for counter-matched studies both without and with calibration on the auxiliary Z. Indeed, as Z is supposed to be predictive of the exposure and must be known in the Phase I study, counter-matching is an ideal situation for calibration of weights. Rivera and Lumley (2016b) also show examples where crude weighting does not improve on the partial likelihood estimator, but in virtually all their examples the calibrated estimator gives more precise estimates than the partial likelihood estimator.

19.7.2 Quota-matching

With a binary exposure variable one will obtain several concordant case-control sets, that is, where both the case and the controls are all exposed or nonexposed. Such case-control sets will with the traditional analysis contribute no information on the association between the exposure and the outcome. As a remedy one could sample new controls until there is at least one control with a different value of the exposure variable than the case. More generally, with categorical exposure variables, one could continue sampling controls until specified quotas of control attain the different values of the exposure variable. This sampling strategy is referred to as quota sampling and is described, for instance, in Keogh and Cox (2014). Borgan *et al.* (1995) developed a partial likelihood method for analyzing this variant of a nested case-control design. Zheng *et al.* (2013) point out that it is possible to calculate probabilities of ever being sampled as a control also under this design. This then allows for fitting weighted likelihoods (19.4) as well as reusing the controls for other outcomes or analyzing models outside the realm of proportional hazards.

19.8 Miscellaneous issues

Inverse probability weighting for nested case-control studies should now be considered an established method for analyzing the data and, at least essentially, large sample properties have been developed. The main advantage of the method is that it is a numerically simple method allowing for reusing controls towards other endpoints and for analyzing other survival models than the proportional hazards model.

We have emphasized the application of inclusion probabilities directly with a Horvitz-Thompson approach. But there are also methods available that allow for using background information available at the Phase I of the study such as calibration. Perhaps these are in particular useful when the main focus in a study is such a Phase I variable, but where it is realized that it is essential to adjust for data obtained in the second phase. Then calibration should give essential improvements over the more crude IPW method. An alternative to calibration for improving precision is augmented inverse probability weighting; see, e.g., Tsiatis (2006) and Mark and Katki (2006), which could work well also for NCCs. However, we are not aware of any studies that have yet investigated this possibility carefully.

The focus of comparison in this chapter has been the traditional partial likelihood estimator for NCC. Other alternatives to this method are treated in Chapter 20 on multiple imputation and in Chapter 21 on maximum likelihood methods. A main advantage of IPW to these approaches is that it is numerically quite simple and requires relatively few assumptions about Phase II data. For instance, regarding multiple imputation, which is the most easily implemented alternative, there is a need to develop a sensible imputation model. Furthermore we note that since complete cohort data are imputed the analysis file can be quite large compared to IPW which only require a file containing the cases and sampled controls. Also the computational time may be considerably longer when multiple imputation is used for large cohorts.

In all our examples we have considered survival outcomes with the same follow-up scheme as the original study. We have some reservations against using these weights for other applications, say estimating population means of exposures. This is due to the fact that individuals with short follow-up will have small inclusion probabilities leading to large weights and this could give unstable estimates. As an example consider a biomarker like Vitamin D obtained from blood samples. With the interest of estimating the population mean of this biomarker using weights as described in this chapter one might encounter the unfortunate situation that an individual with an extreme biomarker measurement has been followed for a very short period and thus have a very large weight which will have a large effect on the estimate. For survival situations, however, we consider this problem to be modest, since individuals with short follow-up also are at risk at few event times and hence have a small influence to score contributions and estimates.

Some practical issues involved in using weighting techniques for NCC data have not been discussed thoroughly. When considering reuse of controls for other endpoints in Section 19.4 we noted that there may be practical problems in only obtaining biomarker data for new cases and only relying on measurements for previously measured controls. As discussed by Rundle *et al.* (2005) the new and old measurements may be systematically different, for instance, due to different lengths of storage of biological specimens and differences relating to laboratory handling. Langseth *et al.* (2010) give the advice that some new controls should always be included. Another issue is that the biomarkers are often analyzed in batches and there may be systematical differences between batches. If these batch effects are additive, meaning that the whole batch is shifted from the true value with the same amount, they will effectively be taken care of with the traditional analysis if the cases and its matched controls are placed on the same batch. With the weighting technique, however, Støer and Samuelsen (2013) and Borgan and Keogh (2015) showed that bias can occur. There is therefore a need to develop and investigate methods for handling the batch effects.

Bibliography

Aalen, O. O., Borgan, Ø., and Gjessing, H. K. (2008). *Survival and Event History Analysis: A Process Point of View*. Springer-Verlag, New York.

Barlow, W. E. (1994). Robust variance estimation for the case-cohort design. *Biometrics*, **50**, 1064–1072.

Borgan, Ø. and Keogh, R. (2015). Nested case-control studies: Should one break the matching? *Lifetime Data Analysis*, **21**, 517–541.

Borgan, Ø., Goldstein, L., and Langholz, B. (1995). Methods for the analysis of sampled cohort data in the Cox proportional hazards model. *Annals of Statistics*, **23**, 1749–1778.

Breslow, N. E., Lumley, T., Ballantyne, C. M., Chambless, L. E., and Kulich, M. (2009a). Improved Horvitz-Thompson estimation of model parameters for two-phase stratified samples: Applications in epidemiology. *Statistics in Bioscience*, **1**, 32–49.

Breslow, N. E., Lumley, T., Ballantyne, C. M., Chambless, L. E., and Kulich, M. (2009b). Using the whole cohort in the analysis of case-cohort data. *American Journal of Epidemiology*, **169**, 1398–1405.

Cai, T. and Zheng, Y. (2011). Nonparametric evaluation of biomarker accuracy under nested case-control studies. *Journal of the American Statistical Association*, **106**, 569–580.

Cai, T. and Zheng, Y. (2012). Evaluating prognostic accuray of biomarkers in nested case-control studies. *Biostatistics*, **13**, 89–100.

Cai, T. and Zheng, Y. (2013). Resampling procedures for making inference under nested case-control studies. *Journal of the American Statistical Association*, **108**, 1532–1544.

Chen, K., Sun, L., and Tong, X. (2012). Analysis of cohort survival data with transformation model. *Statistica Sinica*, **22**, 489–508.

Chen, K. N. (2001). Generalized case-cohort sampling. *Journal of the Royal Statistical Society: Series B (Methodological)*, **63**, 791–809.

Cochran, W. G. and Rubin, D. B. (1973). Controlling bias in observational studies: A review. *Sankhyā: The Indian Journal of Statistics, Series A*, **35**, 417–446.

Fine, J. P. and Gray, R. J. (1999). A proportional hazards model for the subdistribution of a competing risk. *Journal of the American Statistical Association*, **94**, 496–509.

Ganna, A., Reilly, M., Faire, U., Pedersen, N., Magnussson, P., and Ingelsson, E. (2012). Risk prediction measures for case-cohort and nested case-control designs: An application to cardiovascular diseases. *American Journal of Epidemiology*, **175**, 715–724.

Hastie, T. J. and Tibshirani, R. J. (1990). *Generalized Additive Models*. Chapman & Hall, London.

Horvitz, D. G. and Thompson, D. J. (1952). A generalization of sampling without replacement from a finite universe. *Journal of the American Statistical Association*, **47**, 663–685.

Kalbfleisch, J. D. and Lawless, J. F. (1988). Likelihood analysis of multi-state models for disease incidence and mortality. *Statistics in Medicine*, **7**, 149–160.

Keogh, R. H. and Cox, D. R. (2014). *Case-Control Studies*. Cambridge University Press, Cambridge.

Kim, R. S. (2015). A new comparison of nested case-control and case-cohort designs and methods. *European Journal of Epidemiology*, **30**, 197–207.

Kim, R. S. and Kaplan, R. C. (2013). Analysis of secondary outcomes in nested case-control study designs. *Statistics in Medicine*, **33**, 4215–4226.

Langholz, B. and Borgan, Ø. (1995). Counter-matching: A stratified nested case-control sampling method. *Biometrika*, **82**, 69–79.

Langholz, B. and Thomas, D. C. (1991). Efficiency of cohort sampling designs: Some surprising results. *Biometrics*, **47**, 1563–1571.

Langseth, H., Luostarinen, T., Bray, F., and Dillner, J. (2010). Ensuring quality in studies linking cancer registries and biobanks. *Acta Oncologica*, **49**, 368–377.

Lin, D. Y. (2000). On fitting Cox's proportional hazards model to survey data. *Biometrika*, **87**, 37–47.

Lin, D. Y. and Wei, L. J. (1989). The robust inference for the Cox proportional hazards model. *Journal of the American Statistical Association*, **84**, 1074–1078.

Lin, D. Y. and Ying, Z. (1994). Semiparametric analysis of the additive risk model. *Biometrika*, **81**, 61–71.

Lin, D. Y., Wei, L. J., and Ying, Z. (1993). Checking the Cox model with cumulative sums of martingale based residuals. *Biometrika*, **80**, 557–572.

Lu, W. and Liu, M. (2012). On estimation of linear transformation models with nested case-control sampling. *Lifetime Data Analysis*, **18**, 80–93.

Lu, W., Liu, M., and Chen, Y. H. (2014). Testing goodness-of-fit for the proportional hazards model based on nested case-control data. *Biometrics*, **70**, 845–851.

Lumley, T. (2010). *Complex Surveys: A Guide to Analysis Using R*. Wiley, New York.

Mark, S. D. and Katki, H. A. (2006). Specifying and implementing nonparametric and semiparametric survival estimators in two-stage (nested) cohort studies with missing case data. *Journal of the American Statistical Association*, **101**, 460–471.

Prentice, R. L. (1986). A case-cohort design for epidemiologic cohort studies and disease prevention trials. *Biometrika*, **73**, 1–11.

Pugh, M., Robins, J., Lipsitz, S., and Harrington, D. (1993). Inference in the Cox proportional hazards model with missing covariate data. http://www.biostat.harvard.edu/robins/pugh-robins.pdf.

Rebora, P., Antolini, L., Glidden, D. V., and Valsecchi, G. (2016). Crude incidence in two-phase designs in the presence of competing risks. *BMC Medical Research Methodology*, **16:5**.

Rivera, C. and Lumley, T. (2016a). Using the entire history in the analysis of nested case cohort samples. *Statistics in Medicine*, **35**, 3213–3228.

Rivera, C. and Lumley, T. (2016b). Using the whole cohort in the analysis of countermatched samples. *Biometrics*, **72**, 382–391.

Robins, J. M., Rotnitzky, A., and Zhao, L. P. (1994). Estimation of regression coefficients when some regressors are not always observed. *Journal of the American Statistical Association*, **89**, 846–866.

Rundle, A. G., Vineis, P., and Ashan, H. (2005). Design options in molecular epidemiology research within cohort studies. *Cancer Epidemiology, Biomarkers and Prevention*, **14**, 1899–1907.

Saarela, O., Kulathinal, S., Arjas, E., and Läärä., E. (2008). Nested case-control data utilized for multiple outcomes: A likelihood approach and alternatives. *Statistics in Medicine*, **27**, 5991–6008.

Salim, A., Hultman, C., Sparén, P., and Reilly, M. (2009). Combining data from 2 nested case-control studies of overlapping cohorts to improve efficiency. *Biostatistics*, **10**, 70–79.

Salim, A., Yang, Q., and Reilly, M. (2012). The value of reusing prior nested case-control data in new studies with different outcome. *Statistics in Medicine*, **31**, 1291–1302.

Samuelsen, S. O. (1997). A pseudolikelihood approach to analysis of nested case-control studies. *Biometrika*, **84**, 379–394.

Samuelsen, S. O., Ånestad, H., and Skrondal, A. (2007). Stratified case-cohort analysis of general cohort sampling designs. *Scandinavian Journal of Statistics*, **34**, 103–119.

Särndal, C. E., Swensson, B., and Wretman, J. (1992). *Model Assisted Survey Sampling*. Springer-Verlag, New York.

Støer, N. C. and Samuelsen, S. O. (2012). Comparison of estimators in nested case-control studies with multiple outcomes. *Lifetime Data Analysis*, **18**, 261–283.

Støer, N. C. and Samuelsen, S. O. (2013). Inverse probability weighting in nested case-control studies with additional matching - a simulation study. *Statistics in Medicine*, **32**, 5328–5339.

Støer, N. C. and Samuelsen, S. O. (2016). multipleNCC: Inverse probability weighting of nested case-control data. *The R Journal*, **8/2**.

Suissa, S., Edwardes, M. D. D., and Boivin, J. F. (1998). External comparisons from nested case-control designs. *Epidemiology*, **9**, 72–78.

Thomas, D. C. (1977). Addendum to: "Methods of cohort analysis: Appraisal by application to asbestos mining" by F. D. K. Liddell, J. C. McDonald and D. C. Thomas. *Journal of the Royal Statistical Society: Series A (General)*, **140**, 469–491.

Tsiatis, A. A. (2006). *Semiparametric Theory and Missing Data*. Springer-Verlag, New York.

Zheng, M., Lin, R., Sun, Y., and Yu, W. (2012). Nested case-control analysis with general additive-multiplicative hazard models. *Applied Mathematics - A Journal of Chinese Universities: Series B*, **27**, 159–168.

Zheng, Y., Cai, T., and Pepe, M. (2013). Adopting nested case-control quota sampling designs for the evaluation of risk markers. *Lifetime Data Analysis*, **19**, 568–588.

Multiple Imputation for Sampled Cohort Data

Ruth H. Keogh

London School of Hygiene and Tropical Medicine

20.1   Introduction

Large prospective cohorts are widely used in epidemiology and other areas of research to investigate associations between putative risk factors and time-to-event outcomes, for example, disease diagnosis or death. To avoid the collection of expensive explanatory variables, such as biological measurements, on the full cohort a substudy can be sampled, within which all variables of interest for a particular investigation are then obtained. There are two main study designs which are used to obtain a sample within a full cohort; the nested case-control design and the case-cohort design. There is a large literature on the design and analysis of these studies; for overviews see Chapters 16–18 and Keogh and Cox (2014, Chapters 7 and

8). In both types of study, measures of explanatory variables of interest are obtained for all cases (individuals who have the event) and a subset of the noncases in the full cohort.

In a nested case-control study each case is matched to a small number of noncases sampled randomly from the risk set at the case's event time. In a case-cohort study a random sample of individuals from the underlying cohort is selected at the start of follow-up; this is referred to as the subcohort. The case-cohort sample is comprised of the subcohort plus all individuals in the rest of the cohort who become cases during follow-up. Both nested case-control and case-cohort studies are increasingly used. Sharp *et al.* (2014) give an overview of applications of case-cohort studies.

The traditional analyses of nested case-control and case-cohort studies use only data on sampled individuals. However, while expensive variable measurements are available only for sampled individuals, there may be other cheaply measured variables which are available for all individuals in the full cohort. In fact this is a very common situation, since many cheaply measured variables are routinely collected on the full cohort. The traditional analyses ignore any data on individuals in the full cohort not sampled for the substudy. However, the substudy plus the additional data available on the remainder of the full-cohort may be viewed as a full cohort study with a large missing data problem, in which the expensive measurements are only available in the substudy. The missing data occurs by design and is determined by the sampling scheme.

In regression analyses, missing data in explanatory variables can result in loss of efficiency and, depending on the mechanism by which the missingness arose, biased estimates of regression coefficients, if individuals with missing data are omitted from the analysis. Over recent years multiple imputation (MI) has become an increasingly popular approach to handling missing data. In this chapter we describe how MI can be used to make use of data available on the full cohort in the analysis of nested case-control and case-cohort studies, as an alternative to the traditional analyses. In the general presentation we focus on the situation of right-censored survival data. Extensions to incorporate left-truncation and stratified Cox regression are considered in Sections 20.7.3 and 20.7.4.

20.2   Example: Fibre intake and colorectal cancer

Here we introduce a motivating example, to which the methods are applied in Section 20.8. EPIC-Norfolk is a cohort of 25,639 individuals recruited during 1993-1997 from the population of individuals aged 45-75 years in Norfolk, UK (Day *et al.*, 1999). The cohort has been followed up for a range of disease outcomes. Participants provided information about their dietary intake in two main ways: using a food frequency questionnaire (FFQ) and using a 7-day diet diary. Diet diaries are often considered to give superior measurements of dietary intake compared with FFQs, but are more expensive to process. For this reason, some diet-disease associations have been studied using nested case-control samples within EPIC-Norfolk (and other UK cohorts) with diet diary measurements being obtained in the substudy (Dahm *et al.*, 2010).

The association between fibre intake and colorectal cancer was studied using a nested case-control sample within EPIC-Norfolk (Dahm *et al.*, 2010). The nested case-control sample comprised 318 cases of colorectal cancer and four controls per case. Controls were matched to cases on sex and age at recruitment to the cohort within 3 years. Diet diary measurements of average daily food and nutrient intakes were obtained for individuals in the nested case-control sample. Dahm *et al.* (2010) used a traditional analysis to investigate the association between average daily fibre intake and colorectal cancer risk, adjusting for exact age, weight, height, smoking status, social class, level of education, average daily alcohol intake (obtained from the FFQ) and three other dietary exposures obtained from the 7-day diet diary (average daily intakes of folate, energy from fat sources, and energy from nonfat sources). The main exposure and the last three adjustment variables were measured only in the nested case-control sample, while the remaining adjustment variables were available for the full cohort.

20.3   Traditional analysis of sampled cohort data

In this section we outline the traditional analyses of nested case-control and case-cohort studies. We let $\mathbf{X}$ denote a vector of variables which are expensive to measure and $\mathbf{Z}$ denote a vector of cheaply measured variables. Events are assumed to occur according to the Cox proportional hazards model (Cox, 1972) conditional on $\mathbf{X} = \mathbf{x}$ and $\mathbf{Z} = \mathbf{z}$

$$\lambda(t) = \lambda_0(t)e^{\mathbf{x}^{\mathrm{T}}\boldsymbol{\beta}+\mathbf{z}^{\mathrm{T}}\boldsymbol{\gamma}}, \tag{20.1}$$

where $\lambda_0(t)$ is the baseline hazard at time t and $\boldsymbol{\beta}$ and $\boldsymbol{\gamma}$ are vectors of log hazard ratios.

We consider a cohort $\mathcal{C} = \{1, \ldots, N\}$ of N independent individuals and suppose for a moment that both $\mathbf{X}$ and $\mathbf{Z}$ can be measured on the full cohort. The measures of $(\mathbf{X}, \mathbf{Z})$ for individual i are denoted $(\mathbf{x}_i, \mathbf{z}_i)$. Due to censoring, we do not observe the event times for all individuals. For each individual $i \in \mathcal{C}$ we observe (t_i, δ_i), where t_i is the minimum of the event time and a censoring time, and $\delta_i = 1$ if t_i equals the event time and $\delta_i = 0$ otherwise. We assume that censoring is independent (Kalbfleisch and Prentice, 2002, Sections 1.3 and 6.2), which implies that censoring may depend on $\mathbf{X}$ and $\mathbf{Z}$.

The risk set $\mathcal{R}(t) = \{i \mid t_i \geq t\}$ is the collection of all individuals who are under observation just before time t. We let $\mathcal{E} = \{i \mid \delta_i = 1\}$ denote the set of all cases. In an analysis of the full cohort the vectors of regression coefficients $\boldsymbol{\beta}$ and $\boldsymbol{\gamma}$ in (20.1) are estimated by the values that maximize Cox's partial likelihood (Cox, 1972)

$$L_{\mathrm{full}}(\boldsymbol{\beta}, \boldsymbol{\gamma}) = \prod_{i \in \mathcal{E}} \frac{e^{\mathbf{x}_i^{\mathrm{T}}\boldsymbol{\beta}+\mathbf{z}_i^{\mathrm{T}}\boldsymbol{\gamma}}}{\sum_{j \in \mathcal{R}(t_i)} e^{\mathbf{x}_j^{\mathrm{T}}\boldsymbol{\beta}+\mathbf{z}_j^{\mathrm{T}}\boldsymbol{\gamma}}}. \tag{20.2}$$

Nested case-control and case-cohort studies are traditionally analysed using modified versions of the partial likelihood in (20.2). In the traditional analysis of a nested case-control study each case is compared at its event time with m controls sampled at random from the risk set at that time. We let $\widetilde{\mathcal{R}}(t_i)$ denote the sampled risk set at time t_i which comprises the case at t_i and the m sampled controls. The modified partial likelihood used to analyse nested case-control data is

$$L_{\mathrm{ncc}}(\boldsymbol{\beta}, \boldsymbol{\gamma}) = \prod_{i \in \mathcal{E}} \frac{e^{\mathbf{x}_i^{\mathrm{T}}\boldsymbol{\beta}+\mathbf{z}_i^{\mathrm{T}}\boldsymbol{\gamma}}}{\sum_{j \in \widetilde{\mathcal{R}}(t_i)} e^{\mathbf{x}_j^{\mathrm{T}}\boldsymbol{\beta}+\mathbf{z}_j^{\mathrm{T}}\boldsymbol{\gamma}}}. \tag{20.3}$$

In the traditional analysis of a case-cohort study, each case is compared at its event time with individuals at risk in the subcohort at that time. We let $\mathcal{S}(t_i)$ denote the set of individuals in the subcohort who are at risk at time t_i, and let $\widetilde{\mathcal{S}}(t_i) = \mathcal{S}(t_i)$ if the case at time t_i is in the subcohort and $\widetilde{\mathcal{S}}(t_i) = \mathcal{S}(t_i) \bigcup \{i\}$ if the case at time t_i is not in the subcohort. The traditional analysis of the case-cohort data is using the pseudo-partial likelihood

$$L_{\text{ca-co}}(\boldsymbol{\beta}, \boldsymbol{\gamma}) = \prod_{i \in \mathcal{E}} \frac{e^{\mathbf{x}_i^{\mathrm{T}}\boldsymbol{\beta} + \mathbf{z}_i^{\mathrm{T}}\boldsymbol{\gamma}}}{\sum_{j \in \widetilde{\mathcal{S}}(t_i)} e^{\mathbf{x}_j^{\mathrm{T}}\boldsymbol{\beta} + \mathbf{z}_j^{\mathrm{T}}\boldsymbol{\gamma}}}. \tag{20.4}$$

Because (20.4) is a pseudo-likelihood the usual formulae for standard errors do not apply for making correct inferences about $\boldsymbol{\beta}$ and $\boldsymbol{\gamma}$. Correct inferences can be made by using robust standard errors, though other possibilities have been described (Therneau and Li, 1999). The form for the analysis of the case-cohort data in (20.4) is that which was suggested by Prentice (1986). Several variants have been proposed, which are summarized, for example, by Onland-Moret *et al.* (2007); see also Chapter 16

20.4   Multiple imputation (MI): an overview

The aim of this section is to give an outline summary of MI as a general approach to handling missing data in regression analyses. The original justification for MI was given by Rubin (1987). For an up-to-date account of the theory and application of MI see Carpenter and Kenward (2013).

In this section we use generic notation and in the next section this is set into the context of time-to-event data. We let $\mathbf{Y}$ denote a matrix representing the data, including both explanatory variables and outcome variables. $\mathbf{Y}$ is partitioned into $\mathbf{Y}_M$, the missing data, and $\mathbf{Y}_O$, the observed data. The 'substantive model' refers to the analysis model of interest, and we denote the parameters of the substantive model by $\boldsymbol{\beta}$. In our specific context the substantive model is the Cox regression model.

MI is usually carried out under the assumption that the data are missing at random (MAR), and we make this assumption here, which can be expressed as the assumption that $P(\mathbf{R}|\mathbf{y}_M, \mathbf{y}_O) = P(\mathbf{R}|\mathbf{y}_O)$, where $\mathbf{R}$ denotes a matrix of indicators of missingness associated with $\mathbf{Y}$, such that $R_{ij} = 1$ if the (i, j)th element of $\mathbf{Y}$ is observed and $R_{ij} = 0$ if it is missing. See Rubin (1987), Carpenter and Kenward (2013, Chapter 1) and Seaman *et al.* (2013) for detail on missingness mechanisms.

The procedure involves the following three steps (Carpenter and Kenward, 2013, p. 39):

1. The missing data are imputed from the distribution of the missing data given the observed data, $f(\mathbf{y}_M|\mathbf{y}_O)$. This is performed K times to obtain K 'complete' imputed data sets in which missing values in $\mathbf{Y}_M$ are filled in. The imputations should take into account all sources of uncertainty, including in the estimation of the parameters of $f(\mathbf{y}_M|\mathbf{y}_O)$ by obtaining draws of the parameters from their estimated posterior distribution and using these draws when obtaining imputed values of $\mathbf{Y}_M$.

2. The substantive model is fitted to each of the K imputed data sets to give K estimates of the parameters of the substantive model. We denote the estimates from the kth imputed data set $\hat{\boldsymbol{\beta}}_k$ $(k = 1, \ldots, K)$, with corresponding estimated variance-covariance matrix $\widehat{\mathrm{Var}}(\hat{\boldsymbol{\beta}}_k)$ $(k = 1, \ldots, K)$.

3. The estimates $\hat{\boldsymbol{\beta}}_k$ and their variance-covariance matrices $\widehat{\mathrm{Var}}(\hat{\boldsymbol{\beta}}_k)$ $(k = 1, \ldots, K)$ are combined using 'Rubin's rules' (see below) to give pooled estimates and a corresponding variance-covariance matrix.

The MI estimates of the substantive model parameters $\boldsymbol{\beta}$, which combine the estimates obtained across imputed data sets, are

$$\hat{\boldsymbol{\beta}}_{MI} = \frac{1}{K} \sum_{k=1}^{K} \hat{\boldsymbol{\beta}}_k \qquad (20.5)$$

and their variance-covariance matrix is estimated by

$$\widehat{\text{Var}}(\hat{\boldsymbol{\beta}}_{MI}) = \widehat{\mathbf{W}} + \left(1 + \frac{1}{K}\right) \widehat{\mathbf{B}} \qquad (20.6)$$

where

$$\widehat{\mathbf{W}} = \frac{1}{K} \sum_{k=1}^{K} \widehat{\text{Var}}(\hat{\boldsymbol{\beta}}_k), \quad \widehat{\mathbf{B}} = \frac{1}{K-1} \sum_{k=1}^{K} \left(\hat{\boldsymbol{\beta}}_k - \hat{\boldsymbol{\beta}}_{MI}\right) \left(\hat{\boldsymbol{\beta}}_k - \hat{\boldsymbol{\beta}}_{MI}\right)^{\text{T}} \qquad (20.7)$$

are, respectively, the average within-imputation variance-covariance matrix and the between imputation variance-covariance matrix. The formulae in (20.5) and (20.6) are referred to as Rubin's rules.

To obtain the imputations (step 1 above), we need to know (or be able to derive) the distribution of $\mathbf{Y}_M$ given $\mathbf{Y}_O$ and then be able to draw values from that distribution. The draws of $\mathbf{Y}_M$ should be proper 'Bayesian' draws (at least approximately) in the sense that they correctly represent the amount of information that is available from the observed data about the missing data. We do not go into the details of this aspect here, but below outline how it is achieved in our context.

20.5 MI in Cox regression

20.5.1 Introduction to MI in full-cohort studies

In this section we outline how MI can be applied in the context of analysing *full cohort* data using Cox regression. For simplicity and clarity we focus primarily on the situation of a single explanatory variable with missing data, denoted X. Let $\mathbf{Z}$ denote a vector of fully observed explanatory variables. Extensions to missing data in several variables are considered in Section 20.5.4. It is assumed that the data on event or censoring times are complete for all individuals.

In the notation of the preceding section, the missing values of X correspond to $\mathbf{Y}_M$, and $(\mathbf{Z}, T, \Delta)$ and the nonmissing values of X correspond to $\mathbf{Y}_O$, where T denotes the event or censoring time and Δ is the event indicator taking value 1 if T is the event time and 0 if T is the censoring time. We assume throughout that $(X_i, \mathbf{Z}_i, T_i, \Delta_i)$ $(i = 1, \dots, N)$ are independent and identically distributed. The aim is to impute missing values of X from the conditional distribution of X given $\mathbf{Z} = \mathbf{z}$, $T = t$ and $\Delta = \delta$, which can be written as

$$f(x|\mathbf{z}, t, \delta) = f(t, \delta|x, \mathbf{z}) f(x|\mathbf{z}) f(t, \delta|\mathbf{z})^{-1}. \qquad (20.8)$$

For what follows we make the assumptions of noninformative censoring and that the censoring time distribution is independent of X given $\mathbf{Z}$; the latter can be relaxed and is discussed in Section 20.7.1. Using these assumptions, under the Cox proportional hazards model in (20.1) the first factor on the right hand side of (20.8) takes the form

$$f(t, \delta|x, \mathbf{z}) \propto \left\{ \lambda_0(t) e^{x\beta + \mathbf{z}^{\text{T}} \gamma} \right\}^{\delta} \exp\left\{ -\Lambda_0(t) e^{x\beta + \mathbf{z}^{\text{T}} \gamma} \right\}, \qquad (20.9)$$

where $\Lambda_0(t)$ is the cumulative baseline hazard. The third factor of (20.8) does not depend on x and so we absorb this into a constant term $C(\mathbf{z}, t, \delta)$ in the following results. Using (20.8) and (20.9) it follows that

$$\log f(x|\mathbf{z}, t, \delta) = \log f(x|\mathbf{z}) + \delta\log\lambda_0(t) + \delta\left(x\beta + \mathbf{z}^{\mathrm{T}}\boldsymbol{\gamma}\right) - \Lambda_0(t)e^{x\beta + \mathbf{z}^{\mathrm{T}}\boldsymbol{\gamma}} + C(\mathbf{z}, t, \delta). \quad (20.10)$$

It is clear from this that in general the distribution $f(x|\mathbf{z}, t, \delta)$ is nonstandard. For example, it is not a normal distribution or some other common distribution from which we could easily draw in order to obtain imputed values.

Two approaches have been developed for imputation of missing data on explanatory variables in Cox regression which can be implemented in standard software. The first is that of White and Royston (2009) who derived an approximate imputation model. The second approach is that described by Bartlett *et al.* (2015), which uses rejection sampling to draw imputed values from $f(x|\mathbf{z}, t, \delta)$. For an overview see Carpenter and Kenward (2013, Chapter 8). Both methods assume that any censoring does not depend on X, though extensions to allow this are possible (see Section 20.7.1).

20.5.2   Using an approximate imputation model

White and Royston (2009) derived an approximate form for $f(x|\mathbf{z}, t, \delta)$ to give an imputation model for X which includes $\mathbf{z}$, δ and $\widehat{\Lambda}(t)$ as linear predictors, where $\widehat{\Lambda}(t)$ denotes the Nelson-Aalen estimate of the cumulative hazard at time t.

We give a sketch outline of the derivation for binary X. To specify a form for $f(x|\mathbf{z})$ we assume a logistic model for X given $\mathbf{z}$:

$$\mathrm{logit}\{P(X = 1|\mathbf{z})\} = \zeta_0 + \mathbf{z}^{\mathrm{T}}\boldsymbol{\zeta}_1.$$

Equation (20.10) then implies

$$\mathrm{logit}\{P(X = 1|\mathbf{z}, t, \delta)\} = \zeta_0 + \mathbf{z}^{\mathrm{T}}\boldsymbol{\zeta}_1 + \delta\beta + \Lambda_0(t)e^{\mathbf{z}^{\mathrm{T}}\boldsymbol{\gamma}} - \Lambda_0(t)e^{\beta + \mathbf{z}^{\mathrm{T}}\boldsymbol{\gamma}}. \quad (20.11)$$

The form of (20.11) implies that an appropriate imputation model for X is a logistic regression of X on $\mathbf{z}$, δ, $\Lambda_0(t)$ and $\mathbf{z} \times \Lambda_0(t)$. If $\mathbf{Z}$ includes numeric variables, this is an approximate result derived by approximating $e^{\mathbf{z}^{\mathrm{T}}\boldsymbol{\gamma}}$ by a linear expression in $\mathbf{z}$. White and Royston (2009) suggested using the Nelson-Aalen estimate of the cumulative hazard, $\widehat{\Lambda}(t)$, in place of $\Lambda_0(t)$ in the imputation model and this was found to work well in simulation studies. It has also been found that there is usually little to be gained from the inclusion of the interaction term $\mathbf{z} \times \widehat{\Lambda}(t)$ [see also Carpenter and Kenward (2013, Chapter 8, p. 174-176)]. To obtain imputed values we begin by fitting the imputation model for X in the subset of individuals with complete data,

$$\mathrm{logit}\{P(X_i = 1|\mathbf{z}_i, t_i, \delta_i)\} = \eta_0 + \boldsymbol{\eta}_1^{\mathrm{T}}\mathbf{z}_i + \eta_2\delta_i + \eta_3\widehat{\Lambda}(t_i), \quad (20.12)$$

to obtain estimates $\hat{\boldsymbol{\eta}} = (\hat{\eta}_0, \hat{\boldsymbol{\eta}}_1^{\mathrm{T}}, \hat{\eta}_2, \hat{\eta}_3)^{\mathrm{T}}$ and corresponding variance-covariance matrix $\mathbf{V} = \widehat{\mathrm{Var}}(\hat{\boldsymbol{\eta}})$. Next, K independent draws of the parameters, denoted $\boldsymbol{\eta}^{(k)} = (\eta_0^{(k)}, \boldsymbol{\eta}_1^{(k)\mathrm{T}}, \eta_2^{(k)}, \eta_3^{(k)})^{\mathrm{T}}$ $(k = 1, \ldots, K)$, are taken from a multivariate normal distribution with mean vector $\hat{\boldsymbol{\eta}}$ and variance-covariance matrix $\mathbf{V}$. The kth set of imputations of X is obtained by drawing from a Bernoulli distribution with probability

$$\mathrm{logit}\{P(X_i^{(k)} = 1|\mathbf{z}_i, t_i, \delta_i)\} = \eta_0^{(k)} + \boldsymbol{\eta}_1^{(k)\mathrm{T}}\mathbf{z}_i + \eta_2^{(k)}\delta_i + \eta_3^{(k)}\widehat{\Lambda}(t_i). \quad (20.13)$$

For continuous X, White and Royston (2009) assumed $X|\mathbf{z} \sim \mathrm{Normal}(\phi_0 + \boldsymbol{\phi}^{\mathrm{T}}\mathbf{z}, \sigma_{X|\mathbf{Z}}^2)$, giving the form for $f(x|\mathbf{z})$ to be used in (20.10). They showed that a suitable imputation model for X is (approximately) a linear regression of X on $\mathbf{z}$, δ, $\widehat{\Lambda}(t)$. We fit the imputation model in the subset of individuals with complete data,

$$X_i = \eta_0 + \boldsymbol{\eta}_1^{\mathrm{T}}\mathbf{z}_i + \eta_2\delta_i + \eta_3\widehat{\Lambda}(t_i) + \epsilon_i \tag{20.14}$$

where ϵ_i is a normally distributed residual term with mean 0 and variance σ_ϵ^2. After fitting the imputation model, random draws of the parameters are obtained from their estimated posterior distribution. As above, we let $\hat{\boldsymbol{\eta}} = (\hat{\eta}_0, \hat{\boldsymbol{\eta}}_1^{\mathrm{T}}, \hat{\eta}_2, \hat{\eta}_3)^{\mathrm{T}}$ denote the estimated regression coefficients from (20.14) with variance-covariance matrix $\mathbf{V}$, and let $\hat{\sigma}_\epsilon^2$ denote the estimated residual variance. Draws $\sigma_\epsilon^{(k)}$ are obtained using $\sigma_\epsilon^{(k)} = \hat{\sigma}_\epsilon\sqrt{(N_{\mathrm{obs}} - J)/g}$, where N_{obs} is the number of individuals with X observed, J is the length of the vector $\hat{\boldsymbol{\eta}}$ and g is a draw from a chi-squared distribution with $N_{\mathrm{obs}} - J$ degrees of freedom. Draws $\boldsymbol{\eta}^{(k)}$ are then obtained using $\boldsymbol{\eta}^{(k)} = \hat{\boldsymbol{\eta}} + \sigma_\epsilon^{(k)}\hat{\sigma}_\epsilon^{-1}\mathbf{u}^{\mathrm{T}}\mathbf{V}^{1/2}$, where $\mathbf{u}$ is a vector of random draws from a standard normal distribution and $\mathbf{V}^{1/2}$ denotes the Cholesky decomposition of $\mathbf{V}$ (White *et al.*, 2011). For the kth imputed data set, for a given individual with missing X an imputed value is obtained using

$$x_i^{(k)} = \eta_0^{(k)} + \boldsymbol{\eta}_1^{(k)\mathrm{T}}\mathbf{z}_i + \eta_2^{(k)}\delta_i + \eta_3^{(k)}\widehat{\Lambda}(t_i) + \epsilon_i^{(k)} \tag{20.15}$$

where $\epsilon_i^{(k)}$ is a random draw from a normal distribution with mean 0 and variance $\sigma_\epsilon^{2(k)}$.

20.5.3 Using rejection sampling

The second approach we outline was described by Bartlett *et al.* (2015). The distribution from which we wish to impute, $f(x|\mathbf{z}, t, \delta)$, is referred to as the 'target distribution'. As noted above, this distribution is in general nonstandard when the analysis model is a Cox regression. The basis of the rejection sampling approach is that we first draw a potential value for X from a so-called 'proposal distribution', and then use a 'rejection rule' to decide whether to accept the potential value as a draw from the target distribution. The proposal distribution is some standard distribution which is easy to draw values from. Bartlett *et al.* (2015) suggested using $f(x|\mathbf{z})$ as the proposal distribution, which might be assumed to be a Bernoulli (for binary X) or normal (for continuous X) distribution.

The steps used to obtain the kth imputed data set, after choosing starting values for the missing data, are as follows:

1. Fit the Cox proportional hazards model to the current 'complete' imputed data set (or, in the first instance, using the starting values) to obtain estimates $\hat{\beta}, \hat{\boldsymbol{\gamma}}$ and their estimated variance-covariance matrix $\widehat{\boldsymbol{\Sigma}}$. Draw values $\beta^{(k)}, \boldsymbol{\gamma}^{(k)}$ from a joint normal distribution with mean $\hat{\beta}, \hat{\boldsymbol{\gamma}}$ and variance-covariance matrix $\widehat{\boldsymbol{\Sigma}}$.

2. Obtain an estimate, denoted $\Lambda_0^{(k)}(t)$ (using Breslow's estimator (Breslow, 1972)), of the baseline cumulative hazard $\Lambda_0(t)$, evaluated using the drawn parameter values $\beta^{(k)}, \boldsymbol{\gamma}^{(k)}$.

3. Estimate the parameters of a model for the proposal distribution $f(x|\mathbf{z})$ and their variance-covariance matrix and draw parameter values from their estimated joint posterior distribution.

4. For each individual with X missing, draw a value x^* from the distribution $f(x|\mathbf{z})$, using the parameter values drawn at step 3.

5. Draw a value U from a uniform distribution on $[0, 1]$. Accept the value x^* if

$$\begin{cases} U \leq \exp\{-\Lambda_0^{(k)}(t)e^{\beta^{(k)}x^* + \mathbf{z}^{\mathrm{T}}\boldsymbol{\gamma}^{(k)}}\} & \text{if } \delta = 0 \\ U \leq \Lambda_0^{(k)}(t)\exp\{1 + \beta^{(k)}x^* + \boldsymbol{\gamma}^{(k)\mathrm{T}}\mathbf{z} - \Lambda_0^{(k)}(T)e^{\beta^{(k)}x^* + \mathbf{z}^{\mathrm{T}}\boldsymbol{\gamma}^{(k)}}\} & \text{if } \delta = 1. \end{cases}$$

$$(20.16)$$

6. Repeat steps 4 and 5 until a value x^* is accepted for each individual for whom it is missing.

7. Return to step 1 and iterate the whole procedure until the algorithm has converged to a stationary distribution and use these imputations for the kth imputed data set.

20.5.4 Missing data for several variables

Missingness in several variables $\mathbf{X} = (X_1, X_2, \ldots, X_p)$ may be nonmonotone or monotone, the latter meaning that if an individual has X_j missing then $X_{j+1}, \ldots, X_p$ are also missing. There are two approaches to imputing missing data in several variables: 'joint modelling' and 'full conditional specification' (FCS; also called 'multiple imputation by chained equations'). In the first, a joint model is specified for the set of variables with missing data conditional on the fully observed variables. In FCS a separate model is specified for each individual variable with missing data conditional on the fully observed variables *and* the other variables with missing data, and these models are fitted iteratively until convergence (see Van Buuren (2007) and White *et al.* (2011) for overviews). The two imputation methods described in the previous two sections have been extended to accommodate missingness in several variables using FCS (White and Royston, 2009; Bartlett *et al.*, 2015). This is simpler than joint modelling, especially when there are partially missing variables of different types (e.g., binary and numeric)

20.5.5 Software

Both imputation methods can be applied using packages available in standard software. The approximate MI approach can be implemented using the `mice` package in R (Van Buuren and Groothuis-Oudshoorn, 2011) or `mi impute` in Stata, and `PROC MI` in SAS. All this requires is pre-calculation of the estimated cumulative hazards, but this is straightforward. The rejection sampling approach has been implemented in R and Stata in packages called `smcfcs` ('Substantive model compatible - full conditional specification') (Bartlett and Morris, 2015).

20.6 Application of MI to sampled cohort data

20.6.1 Description of the methods

We return now to discuss the application of MI in the analysis of nested case-control and case-cohort studies. As before, X denotes an expensive variable which can only be measured in sampled individuals and $\mathbf{Z}$ denotes a vector of variables which are observed for all individuals in the full cohort. R denotes a sampling indicator and in this situation R is equivalent to the missing data indicator introduced in Section 20.4.

As outlined in Section 20.3, the traditional analyses of nested case-control and case-cohort studies are based only on sampled individuals ($R = 1$) and ignore data on ($\mathbf{Z}, T, \Delta$) which are available for nonsampled individuals in the full cohort ($R = 0$). The methods for MI in a full-cohort study outlined in the preceding section can be applied directly to impute missing values of X for individuals in the full cohort who were not sampled to the nested case-control or case-cohort study.

The use of MI in this setting for both nested case-control and case-cohort studies was described by Keogh and White (2013), who assessed the two imputation approaches using simulation studies. Use of MI in this way for case-cohort studies was previously considered by Marti and Chavance (2011), though they used an imputation model for X which included only $\mathbf{z}$ and δ, which is not recommended in general. Borgan and Keogh (2015) considered the approximate imputation approach (Section 20.5.2) for use in nested case-control studies as one way of enabling 'sharing' of controls across multiple cases.

There are two main ways in which the use of MI in this setting differs from its use in a more standard missing data setting. Firstly, in our situation the expensive variable is typically unmeasured for a very large proportion of the full cohort. This approach therefore involves imputing a large proportion of values for the expensive variable. One might expect that the consequences of misspecifying the imputation model could be severe in this situation. In Section 20.6.3 we summarize simulation study results which include assessments of the consequences of misspecifying the imputation model. Secondly, in our situation the data are missing by design. In the standard setting, the assumption that data are missing at random (MAR) is a crucial assumption that we cannot be certain is met. Here we do not have this concern and so in this sense the use of MI in this situation is 'safer' than in the standard setting.

The methods described extend to missingness in several variables $\mathbf{X}$. When data are missing only by design the missingness will be monotone. However, in many situations there will be additional missingness not by design. For example, although the variables $\mathbf{Z}$ are in principle measured in the full cohort, there may be missing data on $\mathbf{Z}$ for some individuals which is likely to result in nonmonotone missingness. The MI methods accommodate this using the FCS approach (Section 20.5.4), assuming MAR.

If all cases are used in the substudy then data will be missing only on noncases $\delta = 0$ and hence only one of the rejection rules in step 5 in Section 20.5.3 would be used. However, as an extension to the standard substudy designs a sample of cases may be used instead of the full set of cases, resulting in missing data in both cases and noncases in the full cohort.

20.6.2   Using auxiliary variables

So far we have assumed that there is no direct information about the expensive explanatory variable X for individuals in the full cohort but who are not in the nested case-control or case-cohort sample. However, in some studies there may be 'auxiliary' variables that are predictive of the expensive covariate but not used as predictors in the substantive model, here the Cox proportional hazards model. For example, when an expensive variable is a biological measurement obtained using a gold standard technique, cheaper but error-prone measurements may be available in the full cohort. In the example study of fibre intake and colorectal cancer (Section 20.2) the expensive variables were measures of dietary intake derived from 7-day diet diaries. However cheaper measures of dietary intake were available on the full cohort from food frequency questionnaires.

In the approximate imputation approach (Section 20.5.2) auxiliary variables can be included as additional variables in the imputation model. Auxiliary variables can also be incorporated in the rejection sampling approach (Section 20.5.3) (Bartlett *et al.*, 2015).

TABLE 20.1
Results from simulation studies. Analyses are based on nested case-control or case-cohort samples within a full cohort. Results are presented '*Est. (SD)*', where *Est.* and *SD* are the mean and standard deviation of the log hazard ratio estimates over 1000 simulations.

Nested case-control study	1 control per case		5 controls per case	
	β	γ	β	γ
Full-cohort analysis	0.693 (0.037)	0.692 (0.040)	0.693 (0.037)	0.692 (0.040)
Traditional analysis	0.698 (0.076)	0.696 (0.079)	0.694 (0.050)	0.693 (0.050)
MI without auxiliary variable				
Approximate	0.681 (0.065)	0.687 (0.046)	0.676 (0.045)	0.687 (0.042)
Rejection sampling	0.699 (0.070)	0.693 (0.047)	0.695 (0.047)	0.692 (0.041)
MI with auxiliary variable				
Approximate	0.685 (0.051)	0.690 (0.043)	0.683 (0.040)	0.691(0.040)
Rejection sampling	0.696 (0.054)	0.692 (0.043)	0.694 (0.041)	0.692 (0.040)
Case-cohort study	5% in subcohort		20% in subcohort	
	β	γ	β	γ
Full-cohort analysis	0.693 (0.037)	0.692 (0.040)	0.693 (0.037)	0.692 (0.040)
Traditional analysis	0.700 (0.077)	0.697 (0.082)	0.695 (0.049)	0.693 (0.050)
MI without auxiliary variable				
Approximate	0.683 (0.058)	0.685 (0.044)	0.677 (0.043)	0.687 (0.041)
Rejection sampling	0.692 (0.065)	0.693 (0.046)	0.691 (0.045)	0.693 (0.041)
MI with auxiliary variable				
Approximate	0.685 (0.049)	0.690 (0.042)	0.684 (0.039)	0.691 (0.041)
Rejection sampling	0.694 (0.053)	0.692 (0.043)	0.692 (0.042)	0.693 (0.040)

20.6.3   Assessment of the methods

The performance of MI analyses to make use of full-cohort data in nested case-control and case-cohort studies was assessed by Keogh and White (2013) using detailed simulation studies. Here we summarize a subset of their results to demonstrate the main points.

Data were simulated for a full cohort of 25,000 individuals. Two variables X and Z were generated from a bivariate normal distribution with correlation 0.5 and event times were generated using a hazard model of the form in (20.1) with constant baseline hazard and log hazard ratios $\beta = \gamma = \log 2$. Approximately 5% of individuals had the event before the end of follow-up, 10% were randomly censored, and the remainder were administratively censored at the end of follow-up. Nested case-control samples (with 1 or 5 controls per case) and case-cohort samples (with a random subcohort of 5% or 20% of the full cohort) were selected within the full cohort. X was assumed to be an expensive variable measured only in the substudy, while Z was measured in the full cohort. An auxiliary variable, assumed to be observed in the full cohort, was generated for X so that the correlation between X and the auxiliary variable was 0.8. 1000 simulated data sets were generated.

The following analyses were performed on each simulated data set: (i) a full-cohort analysis, assuming X and Z were observed for all individuals; (ii) a traditional nested case-control or case-cohort analysis; (iii) MI analyses performed with and without using the auxiliary variable and using both the approximate and rejection sampling approaches.

The results are shown in Table 20.1. As expected, the traditional analyses give larger standard errors relative to the full-cohort analysis. Both MI approaches give good gains in efficiency relative to the traditional analyses. The reduction in the standard deviation is greater for γ than for β because Z is observed in the full cohort. Using the auxiliary variable brings further substantial reductions in the standard deviations for β. MI using an approximate imputation model gives some very minor downward bias in the estimates of β, due to the approximation. The bias is much reduced for smaller effect sizes. Using MI with rejection sampling gives unbiased estimates. When the size of the substudy increases (5 controls per case or 20% in the subcohort), the gains from using MI are smaller, but still nonnegligible, especially for the parameter γ, and for β when a good auxiliary variable is available. Similar results were found by Borgan and Keogh (2015).

MI using the approximate imputation model requires an assumption about the distribution of X given $Z, \Delta, \widehat{\Lambda}(T)$ and the rejection sampling approach requires an assumption about the distribution of X given Z. Keogh and White (2013) investigated the potential impact of misspecification of the imputation models using a simulation in which X and Z were generated from a bivariate log normal distribution but the imputation methods were carried out assuming normal distributions for X given $Z, \Delta, \widehat{\Lambda}(T)$ in the approximate method and for X given Z in the rejection sampling method. This resulted in some bias in the estimates. For example, for parameter β the mean estimate (and standard deviation) across 1000 simulations was 0.697 (0.064) using the traditional nested case-control analysis, 0.623 (0.043) using the MI approximate approach, and 0.753 (0.053) using the MI rejection sampling approach. The biases are nonnegligible but not very severe even for this large effect size and quite extreme model misspecification. Borgan and Keogh (2015) investigated a similar form of misspecification and found similar results.

20.7 Some extensions

20.7.1 More than one endpoint

The MI methods can be extended to accommodate competing risks analysed using cause-specific hazards. Borgan and Keogh (2015) show that for a competing risks setting with two endpoints, in which both cause-specific hazard models may depend on X and $\mathbf{Z}$, a suitable approximate imputation model is (for continuous X, for example)

$$X_i = \eta_0 + \boldsymbol{\eta}_1^{\mathrm{T}} \mathbf{z}_i + \boldsymbol{\eta}_2^{\mathrm{T}} \boldsymbol{\delta}_i + \boldsymbol{\eta}_3^{\mathrm{T}} \widehat{\boldsymbol{\Lambda}}(t_i) + \epsilon_i \qquad (20.17)$$

where $\boldsymbol{\delta}_i = (\delta_{1i}, \delta_{2i})^{\mathrm{T}}$ is a vector of event type indicators and $\widehat{\boldsymbol{\Lambda}}(t_i) = (\widehat{\Lambda}_1(t_i), \widehat{\Lambda}_2(t_i))^{\mathrm{T}}$ is a vector of Nelson-Aalen estimates of the cumulative hazards for the two endpoints. The rejection sampling approach, including the software, has also been extended to competing risks (Bartlett and Taylor, 2016). These methods can also be used when the censoring depends on X given $\mathbf{Z}$, which both imputation methods as described earlier assume is not the case.

20.7.2 Imputing transformed variables

For a continuous variable X it is often of interest to include nonlinear terms in the hazard model, e.g., X^2, and interaction terms, e.g., $X \times Z$. To incorporate such terms in the imputation is not trivial, because an imputation model which is compatible with the Cox substantive model (referred to as congeniality (Meng, 1994)) may be difficult to derive and/or difficult to draw from. Carpenter and Kenward (2013, Chapters 6 and 7) give an overview of methods of imputation which have been considered for handling nonlinear and interaction terms. See also Seaman *et al.* (2012). The approximate MI method does not extend to allow nonlinear predictors or interactions in the substantive model (Keogh and White, 2013). However, the rejection sampling approach naturally accommodates nonlinear predictors and interactions because ensuring compatibility between the imputation model and the specified substantive model is an inherent part of the algorithm (Bartlett *et al.*, 2015). It has been verified that this approach performs well for interaction terms in our setting (Keogh and White, 2013).

20.7.3 Left-truncation

Event times are sometimes subject to left-truncation. In particular this occurs when the time scale for the analysis is age, but individuals were followed up from the age at which they joined the cohort rather than from birth. When there is left-truncation, the distribution from which we wish to draw imputed values is $f(x|\mathbf{z}, t, \delta, T \geq t_L)$, where t_L denotes the left-truncation time. In the approximate MI approach left-truncation can be accommodated by replacing $\widehat{\Lambda}(t)$ by $\widehat{\Lambda}(t) - \widehat{\Lambda}(t_L)$. The rejection sampling algorithm can also be extended similarly; currently this is accommodated in Stata but not R.

20.7.4 Stratified Cox regression

In stratified Cox regression there is a separate baseline hazard for each level of a categorical covariate, and this is used when the effects of the levels of the covariate do not meet the proportional hazards assumption. When the population is stratified in this way, in a nested case-control study the controls are selected from the same stratum as the case. In other words, controls are matched to cases on the stratifying variables. The traditional analysis of nested case-control studies is unaffected by the matching, and the traditional case-cohort analysis uses a stratified pseudo-partial likelihood. In the MI methods, the assumed population stratification should be accounted for in the imputation model. In the approximate MI approach the imputation model should include stratum-specific intercepts and stratum-specific estimated cumulative hazards $\hat{\Lambda}_s(t)$ (in place of $\hat{\Lambda}(t)$). The rejection sampling procedure can also be extended to accommodate a stratified Cox model by using $f(x|\mathbf{z}, s)$ as the proposal distribution, where s denotes the stratum, and replacing $\Lambda_0(t)$ by a stratum-specific version $\Lambda_{0s}(t)$. However, the software does not yet accommodate this.

A different issue is that of the use of stratified sampling in nested case-control and case-cohort studies, in which the sampling strata are typically based on a surrogate of an exposure of main interest, with the aim of obtaining a sample which is more informative for the main exposure. For nested case-control studies, stratified sampling is denoted 'counter-matching' (Langholz and Borgan, 1995) and is discussed in Chapters 16 and 18. For case-cohort studies, stratified sampling is discussed in Chapters 16 and 17; see also Borgan *et al.* (2000). Although the use of MI in studies which have used stratified sampling has not been considered in detail, the methods described in this chapter should extend to this setting because the missingness is by design.

20.8 Example: Fibre intake and colorectal cancer

The approximate MI approach described in Section 20.5.2 was applied to the example data from the EPIC-Norfolk cohort, introduced in Section 20.2. The nested case-control sampling used matching on age and sex and we obtained the Nelson-Aalen estimator separately in strata defined by sex and 5-year age groups for use in the imputation model. The analysis performed on each imputed full-cohort data set was a Cox proportional hazards model stratified by sex and age group and adjusted for the variables given in Section 20.2. The

TABLE 20.2

EPIC-Norfolk example. Results from a traditional analysis of the nested case-control study and MI analyses. Coef is the log hazard ratio for colorectal cancer for a 6 grams per day increase in fibre intake, adjusted for age, sex, weight, height, smoking status, education, social class, exercise level, alcohol intake, energy intake from fat and nonfat sources, folate intake.

Method	Coef.	SE	95% CI
Traditional analysis	-0.173	0.104	(-0.377,0.030)
MI analysis: without auxiliary variable	-0.162	0.097	(-0.353,0.029)
MI analysis: with auxiliary variable	-0.140	0.096	(-0.328,0.047)

rejection sampling approach was not used because the software does not currently accommodate stratified Cox models.

A small percentage of individuals in the full cohort had missing values for the variables that were in principle measured on the full cohort. This was handled using the FCS approach. The approximate imputation models included exact age and sex as predictors, in addition to the other adjustment variables included in the Cox regression model, the event indicator and the stratum-specific Nelson-Aalen estimates of the cumulative hazard. The main exposure and three of the dietary adjustment variables were measured only in the nested case-control sample since the measurements were obtained using 7-day diet diaries which are expensive to process. However, auxiliary variables are available from FFQ measures of intakes of these four variables. MI was performed with and without the auxiliary variables.

The results for the main exposure (fibre intake, in units of 6 grams per day) are shown in Table 20.2. The estimated coefficients from the traditional analysis and the MI analyses are similar, indicating an inverse association between fibre intake and colorectal cancer risk. The MI analysis gives a reduction in the standard error. Using the auxiliary variables was not helpful in this example, which is not unexpected since the correlation between the auxiliary variables and the main measures was not very high.

It should be noted that 7-day diet diary measurements have become available over time for a large proportion of individuals in the EPIC-Norfolk cohort, but for the purposes of this illustration, we assumed they were only available in the nested case-control sample.

20.9 Worked example: Radiation and breast cancer study

20.9.1 Description

We also illustrate the methods described in this chapter using data from a study of radiation and breast cancer (Hrubec *et al.*, 1989), which was considered earlier (Chapters 17 and 18). The full cohort contains 1,720 women, of whom 75 were diagnosed with breast cancer over the course of follow-up. For this illustration we will investigate the effect of radiation on breast cancer risk, and also if women first irradiated early in life had a higher risk of breast cancer.

As described in Chapters 17 and 18, two sub-studies were sampled within the full cohort: a nested case-control study with 2 controls per case and a case-cohort study with 150 individuals in the subcohort.

20.9.2 Analysis

The data and computer code needed to perform the analyses are available from the Handbook website. The code is written for the freely available statistical programming language R.

For the substudy analyses we pretend that the information on radiation dose is available only for individuals in the substudy. Information on age at commencement of treatment is assumed available in the full cohort. An additional variable recording the total number of fluoroscopies (nof), which was used to calculate the radiation dose, is treated as an auxiliary variable in the MI analyses and is assumed available in the full cohort.

The MI analyses are based on the approximate method because the R software for the rejection sampling approach does not yet accommodate left-truncation. We used the `mice` function (Van Buuren and Groothuis-Oudshoorn, 2011) in R and 100 imputed data sets were used. For discussions of the choice of number of imputations see White *et al.* (2011) and Carpenter and Kenward (2013, Chapter 2, p. 54-55). The imputation model for $\log_2(\text{dose} + 1)$ included as predictors ageRx/10, where ageRx is age at first TB treatment, the indicator of breast cancer status at the end of follow-up, and the difference between the cumulative hazard at the end of follow-up and the cumulative hazard at the start of follow-up $(\widehat{\Lambda}(t) - \widehat{\Lambda}(t_L))$. We additionally performed an analysis which included the auxiliary variable $\log_2(1 + \text{nof}/100)$ in the imputation model. This variable is very highly correlated with $\log_2(\text{dose} + 1)$ (correlation 0.98).

20.9.3 Results

The results from the full-cohort analysis (assuming all variables were observed in the full cohort), the traditional analyses and MI analyses are shown in Table 20.3.

The MI estimates are similar to those obtained under the full-cohort analysis, with the MI estimates tending to be a little further from zero. The MI analyses not using the auxiliary variable show a substantial reduction in the standard error for the estimated log hazard ratio for the variable ageRx/10, which is observed in the full cohort, compared to the traditional analyses. In fact, the standard errors for ageRx/10 from the MI analyses are close to the standard error obtained in the full-cohort analysis. For the variable which is assumed only observed in the substudy, $\log_2(\text{dose} + 1)$, the MI analysis using the case-cohort sample gives a slight gain in the standard error, while the standard error from the MI analysis using the nested case-control sample is a little reduced. However, including the auxiliary variable as a predictor in the imputation model for $\log_2(\text{dose} + 1)$ results in a large reduction in the standard error for the log hazard ratio parameter associated with $\log_2(\text{dose} + 1)$. The reduced standard error is similar to that obtained from the full-cohort analysis.

When imputing values of $\log_2(\text{dose}+1)$ we assumed a normal distribution for $\log_2(\text{dose} + 1)$ conditional on ageRx/10, the event indicator, and $\widehat{\Lambda}(T) - \widehat{\Lambda}(T_L)$ (and $\log_2(1 + \text{nof}/100)$ in the MI analysis using the auxiliary variable). Further investigations suggest that this assumption is not met. The variable $\log_2(\text{dose}+1)$ itself has a nonnormal distribution, with a peak at the point where dose $= 0$ (698/1720 individuals in the full cohort have a dose of 0). However, the fact that the MI analyses gave similar estimates to those found from the full-cohort analysis suggests that a violation of the assumption of normality has not had an important impact on the results.

As discussed in Section 20.7.2 the rejection sampling MI approach enables imputation of a variable on a transformed scale, followed by a transformation of the variable to the scale of interest for the substantive analysis. However, in this example it was difficult to find a suitable transformation for $\log_2(\text{dose} + 1)$.

TABLE 20.3

Results from the radiation and breast cancer study using different analyses.

Model term	Coef.	SE	Z	p
A. Full cohort				
$\log_2(\text{dose} + 1)$	0.469	0.161	2.914	0.0036
ageRx/10	-0.242	0.149	-1.622	0.1048
B. Case-cohort				
$\log_2(\text{dose} + 1)$	0.515	0.206	2.504	0.0123
ageRx/10	-0.112	0.191	-0.586	0.5580
C. Nested case-control				
$\log_2(\text{dose} + 1)$	0.549	0.232	2.365	0.018
ageRx/10	-0.179	0.207	-0.863	0.388
D. Case-cohort: MI without auxiliary variable				
$\log_2(\text{dose} + 1)$	0.574	0.221	2.601	0.0095
ageRx/10	-0.249	0.148	-1.684	0.0922
E. Nested case-control: MI without auxiliary variable				
$\log_2(\text{dose} + 1)$	0.484	0.203	2.377	0.0176
ageRx/10	-0.263	0.148	-1.773	0.0763
F. Case-cohort: MI with auxiliary variable				
$\log_2(\text{dose} + 1)$	0.470	0.162	2.910	0.0036
ageRx/10	-0.245	0.150	-1.636	0.1018
G. Nested case-control: MI with auxiliary variable				
$\log_2(\text{dose} + 1)$	0.427	0.161	2.662	0.0078
ageRx/10	-0.244	0.150	-1.632	0.1027

20.10   Concluding remarks

The nested case-control and case-cohort study designs enable time-to-event analyses to be performed when explanatory variables that are expensive to measure can only be obtained on a sample of the full cohort. The traditional analyses of these sub-studies ignore information on covariates measured for individuals in the full cohort who were not sampled for the substudy. It is very common for such full-cohort data to be available. When the number of controls per case is large in a nested case-control study, or when the subcohort used in a case-cohort study is large, the traditional analyses give very good efficiency relative to a full-cohort analysis. However, it has been thought that gains in efficiency could be made by making use of data available in the full cohort, which could be especially important when the proportion of individuals sampled to the substudy is small.

In this chapter we have described how MI can enable use of data available on the full cohort in the analysis of nested case-control and case-cohort studies. A number of authors have now investigated this, including Keogh and White (2013), Borgan and Keogh (2015), and Marti and Chavance (2011). Related work has been carried out by Noma and Tanaka (2012, 2017) in the context of two-stage case-control sampling and analyses based on logistic regression. Use of MI has been found via simulation studies, summarized in Section 20.6.3, to offer potentially important gains in efficiency relative to the traditional analyses. There are particular gains to be made when there is a small number of controls per case or the subcohort is small relative to the full cohort, and by making use of auxiliary variables measured in the full cohort.

The use of MI to make use of full-cohort data in this setting is attractive because it exploits a large body of work on the use of MI in a general missing data context and the availability of well-developed software. The MI approach not only handles missingness by design due to the nested case-control or case-cohort sampling; it also easily accommodates missingness not by design in several variables.

Other methods have been developed for enabling more efficient analyses of nested case-control and case-cohort data by making use of full-cohort data. Full likelihood analyses for nested case-control and case-cohort studies which make use of full-cohort data were described by Scheike and Juul (2004), Scheike and Martinussen (2004) and Saarela *et al.* (2008). Recent progress on maximum likelihood estimation for nested case-control and case-cohort data is summarized in Chapter 21. As described in Chapter 19, inverse probability weighting (IPW) has also been proposed as a way of enabling more efficient analysis of nested case-control studies (Samuelsen, 1997; Støer and Samuelsen, 2013). The weights are obtained using full-cohort data. Borgan and Keogh (2015) found that the MI approach tended to outperform IPW in terms of efficiency gains. Methods using IPW have also been devised for case-cohort studies, by Borgan *et al.* (2000), Breslow *et al.* (2009) and Kulich and Lin (2004) (see Chapters 16 and 17). Keogh and White (2013) performed some comparisons between the IPW method and the MI method for case-cohort studies, again finding MI to be more efficient. The IPW analyses for both nested case-control and case-cohort studies use data available on the full cohort only in the estimation of the weights, whereas the full-cohort information is used more explicitly in the MI approach.

The methods summarized in this chapter come from an area of research which is still relatively new. More research is merited to further investigate the performance of MI relative to alternative methods, notably use of IPW, in particular to compare the robustness of the two approaches to different forms of model misspecification. Gains in efficiency from using MI may come at the expense of additional costs in terms of model assumptions. Other areas for further work include extensions of the MI approach used in this setting to handle time-dependent variables and variables with time-varying effects.

Bibliography

Bartlett, J. W. and Morris, T. P. (2015). Multiple imputation of covariates by substantive-model compatible fully conditional specification. *The Stata Journal*, **15**, 437–456.

Bartlett, J. W. and Taylor, J. M. G. (2016). Missing covariates in competing risks analysis. *Biostatistics*, **17**, 751–763.

Bartlett, J. W., Seaman, S. R., White, I. R., and Carpenter, J. R. (2015). Multiple imputation of covariates by fully conditional specification: Accommodating the substantive model. *Statistical Methods in Medical Research*, **24**, 462–487.

Borgan, Ø. and Keogh, R. H. (2015). Nested case-control studies: Should one break the matching? *Lifetime Data Analysis*, **21**, 517–541.

Borgan, Ø., Langholz, B., Samuelsen, S. O., Goldstein, L., and Pogoda, J. (2000). Exposure stratified case-cohort designs. *Lifetime Data Analysis*, **6**, 39–58.

Breslow, N. E. (1972). Contribution to the discussion of the paper by D.R. Cox. *Journal of the Royal Statistical Society. Series B*, **34**, 216–217.

Breslow, N. E., Lumley, T., Ballantyne, C. M., Chambless, L. E., and Kulich, M. (2009). Using the whole cohort in the analysis of case-cohort data. *American Journal of Epidemiology*, **169**, 1398–1405.

Carpenter, J. R. and Kenward, M. G. (2013). *Multiple Imputation and its Application*. Wiley, Chichester.

Cox, D. R. (1972). Regression models and life tables (with discussion). *Journal of the Royal Statistical Society. Series B*, **34**, 187–202.

Dahm, C. C., Keogh, R. H., Spencer, E. A., Greenwood, D. C., Key, T. J., Fentiman, I. S., Shipley, M. J., Brunner, E. J., Cade, J. E., Burley, V. J., Mishra, G., Stephen, A. M., Kuh, D., White, I. R., Luben, R., Lentjes, M. A. H., Khaw, K. T., and Rodwell (Bingham), S. A. (2010). Dietary fiber and colorectal cancer risk: A nested case-control study using food diaries. *Journal of the National Cancer Institute*, **102**, 614–626.

Day, N. E., Oakes, S., Luben, R., Khaw, K.-T., Bingham, S., Welch, A., and Wareham, N. (1999). EPIC in Norfolk: Study design and characteristics of the cohort. *British Journal of Cancer*, **80** (Suppl. 1), 95–103.

Hrubec, Z., Boice, J. D., Monson, R. R., and Rosenstein, M. (1989). Breast cancer after multiple chest fluoroscopies: Second follow-up of Massachusetts women with tuberculosis. *Cancer Research*, **49**, 229–234.

Kalbfleisch, J. D. and Prentice, R. L. (2002). *The Statistical Analysis of Failure Time Data*. Wiley, Hoboken, 2nd edition.

Keogh, R. H. and Cox, D. R. (2014). *Case-Control Studies*. Cambridge University Press, Cambridge.

Keogh, R. H. and White, I. R. (2013). Using full-cohort data in nested case-control and case-cohort studies by multiple imputation. *Statistics in Medicine*, **32**, 4021–4043.

Kulich, M. and Lin, D. Y. (2004). Improving the efficiency of relative-risk estimation in case-cohort studies. *Journal of the American Statistical Association*, **99**, 832–844.

Langholz, B. and Borgan, Ø. (1995). Counter-matching: A stratified nested case-control sampling method. *Biometrika*, **82**, 69–79.

Marti, H. and Chavance, M. (2011). Multiple imputation analysis of case-cohort studies. *Statistics in Medicine*, **30**, 1595–1607.

Meng, X. (1994). Multiple-imputation inferences with uncongenial sources of input. *Statistical Science*, **9**, 538–558.

Noma, H. and Tanaka, S. (2012). Multiple imputation analysis of two-stage case control studies. *Japanese Journal of Applied Statistics*, **41**, 79–95.

Noma, H. and Tanaka, S. (2017). Analysis of case-cohort designs with binary outcomes: Improving efficiency using whole-cohort auxiliary information. *Statistical Methods in Medical Research*, **26**, 691–706.

Onland-Moret, N. C., van der A, D. L., van der Schouw, Y. T., Buschers, W., Elias, S. G., van Gils, C. H., Koerselman, J., Roest, M., Grobbee, D. E., and Peeters, P. H. M. (2007). Analysis of case-cohort data: A comparison of different methods. *Journal of Clinical Epidemiology*, **60**, 350–355.

Prentice, R. L. (1986). A case-cohort design for epidemiologic cohort studies and disease prevention trials. *Biometrika*, **73**, 1–11.

Rubin, D. B. (1987). *Multiple Imputation for Nonresponse in Surveys*. Wiley, New York.

Saarela, O., Kulathinal, S., Arjas, E., and Läärä, E. (2008). Nested case-control data utilized for multiple outcomes: A likelihood approach and alternatives. *Statistics in Medicine*, **27**, 5991–6008.

Samuelsen, S. O. (1997). A pseudolikelihood approach to analysis of nested case-control studies. *Biometrika*, **84**, 379–394.

Scheike, T. H. and Juul, A. (2004). Maximum likelihood estimation for Cox's regression model under nested case-control sampling. *Biostatistics*, **5**, 193–206.

Scheike, T. H. and Martinussen, T. (2004). Maximum likelihood estimation for Cox's regression model under case-cohort sampling. *Scandinavian Journal of Statistics*, **31**, 283–293.

Seaman, S., Bartlett, J., and White, I. (2012). Multiple imputation of missing covariates with non-linear effects and interactions: An evaluation of statistical methods. *BMC Medical Research Methodology*, **12**, 46.

Seaman, S., Galati, J., Jackson, D., and Carlin, J. (2013). What is meant by "missing at random"? *Statistical Science*, **28**, 257–268.

Sharp, S. J., Poulaliou, M., Thompson, S. J., White, I. R., and Wood, A. M. (2014). A review of published analyses of case-cohort studies and recommendations for future reporting. *PLoS ONE*, **9**, e101176.

Støer, N. C. and Samuelsen, S. O. (2013). Inverse probability weighting in nested case-control studies with additional matching – a simulation study. *Statistics in Medicine*, **32**, 5328–5339.

Therneau, T. M. and Li, H. (1999). Computing the Cox model for case cohort designs. *Lifetime Data Analysis*, **5**, 99–112.

Van Buuren, S. (2007). Multiple imputation of discrete and continuous data by fully conditional specification. *Statistical Methods in Medical Research*, **16**, 219–242.

Van Buuren, S. and Groothuis-Oudshoorn, K. (2011). mice: Multivariate imputation by chained equations in R. *Journal of Statistical Software*, **45**, Issue 3.

White, I. R. and Royston, P. (2009). Imputing missing covariate values for the Cox model. *Statistics in Medicine*, **28**, 1982–1998.

White, I. R., Royston, P., and Wood, A. (2011). Multiple imputation using chained equations: Issues and guidance for practice. *Statistics in Medicine*, **30**, 377–399.

21

Maximum Likelihood Estimation for Case-Cohort and Nested Case-Control Studies

Donglin Zeng and Dan-Yu Lin

University of North Carolina at Chapel Hill

21.1 Introduction

In epidemiological cohort studies, the occurrences of major clinical events, such as cancer, cardiovascular disease, and death, are typically infrequent, such that large cohorts are required to provide reliable information about the effects of exposures or other covariates on the event times or failure times. The covariates of interest often involve biomarker assay, genome sequencing, medical imaging, or extraction of detailed exposure histories and thus are prohibitively expensive to measure on all cohort members in a large study. A cost-effective solution to this problem is to measure the covariates on all cases, i.e., the subjects who have developed the event of interest during the follow-up, and a subset of controls, i.e., those who have not developed the event of interest by the end of the study. There are two commonly used sampling schemes for selecting controls: case-cohort sampling selects a random subcohort of the original cohort (Prentice, 1986); nested case-control sampling selects a small number of controls, usually between 1 and 5, for each observed failure time (Thomas, 1977). Such sampling schemes can drastically reduce the cost of conducting large epidemiological cohort studies while incurring little loss of statistical efficiency relative to full-cohort sampling.

In virtually all epidemiological cohort studies, there exist inexpensive covariates, such as demographic factors, environmental conditions, and basic clinical variables, that are readily measured on all cohort members. Such covariates can be used as stratification variables to improve the efficiency of the case-cohort or nested case-control design. Thus, case-cohort and nested case-control studies can be regarded as two-phase studies. In the first phase, the data on the duration of follow-up, case-control status, and inexpensive covariates are collected for all cohort members; in the second phase, the data collected in the first phase are used to determine which cohort members are selected for measurements of expensive covariates.

Inexpensive covariates may also be used in the analysis stage to adjust for confounding or to evaluate interactions between expensive and inexpensive covariates.

There is a large body of statistical literature on case-cohort studies. Much of the work is devoted to the original design of Prentice (1986), under which the subcohort is selected by simple random sampling and the data on the first-phase covariates for unselected subjects are disregarded in the analysis. For this design, Prentice (1986) and Self and Prentice (1988) derived pseudo-partial likelihood functions for the proportional hazards model (Cox, 1972) by replacing the risk sets of the whole cohort in the partial likelihood function (Cox, 1975) with their subcohort counterparts. Kalbfleisch and Lawless (1988) weighted individuals' contributions to the partial likelihood function by their inverse probabilities of selection. Barlow (1994), Chen and Lo (1999), Borgan *et al.* (2000) and Chen (2001) studied similar weighted estimators. Kong *et al.* (2004) and Lu and Tsiatis (2006) constructed weighted estimators for the class of linear transformation models, which includes the proportional hazards model as a special case. Similar estimators were developed by Kulich and Lin (2000), Nan *et al.* (2006) and Kong and Cai (2009) for the additive hazards and accelerated failure time models.

The aforementioned estimators are not asymptotically efficient. To improve efficiency, Kulich and Lin (2004), Qi *et al.* (2005), Breslow *et al.* (2009), and Luo *et al.* (2009) adjusted the sampling weights by using auxiliary variables along the lines of Robins *et al.* (1994). In addition, efficient estimation of the proportional hazards model was studied by Chen and Little (1999) and Martinussen (1999) under parametric covariate distributions, by Nan (2004) for discrete covariates, and by Scheike and Martinussen (2004) under the original case-cohort design.

There are quite a few statistical papers on nested case-control sampling. Specifically, Goldstein and Langholz (1992) established the asymptotic theory of the maximum partial likelihood estimator for the proportional hazards model. Langholz and Borgan (1995) proposed a stratified nested case-control sampling method via counter-matching to improve efficiency. Scheike and Juul (2004) studied nonparametric maximum likelihood estimation (NPMLE) for a proportional hazards model stratified by the first-phase covariates. Zeng *et al.* (2006) studied NPMLE for semiparametric transformation models (Zeng and Lin, 2007) under both nested case-control and case-cohort sampling by assuming the independence of inexpensive covariates with expensive covariates. Cai and Zheng (2011, 2012) constructed weighted estimators for nested case-control studies.

Recently, Zeng and Lin (2014) studied efficient estimation of semiparametric transformation models under general two-phase designs. They allowed inexpensive covariates to be continuous and correlated with expensive covariates and did not parameterize the distribution of covariates. It is challenging to deal with this general situation because the likelihood function involves the conditional density functions given continuous variables. To overcome this challenge, Zeng and Lin (2014) incorporated kernel functions for conditional density functions into the nonparametric likelihood function and developed a semiparametric EM algorithm to maximize the modified likelihood function. They established the consistency, asymptotic normality, and asymptotic efficiency of the resulting estimators. Much of the exposition in this chapter is based on the general framework of Zeng and Lin (2014), which covers prior NPMLE work as special cases.

21.2 Methods

21.2.1 Data, models and likelihood

Let T denote the failure time, i.e., time to the occurrence of the clinical event of interest. There are two types of covariates: inexpensive ones that are measured on all cohort members in the first-phase, and expensive ones that are measured on a subset of cohort members in the second phase. We distinguish inexpensive covariates that are correlated with expensive covariates from those that are independent of expensive covariates. Notationally, let $\mathbf{X}$ denote the set of expensive covariates, $\mathbf{Z}$ denote the set of inexpensive covariates that is potentially correlated with $\mathbf{X}$, and $\mathbf{W}$ denote the set of inexpensive covariates that is known to be independent of $\mathbf{X}$. We specify that the hazard function of T conditional on $\mathbf{X} = \mathbf{x}$, $\mathbf{Z} = \mathbf{z}$ and $\mathbf{W} = \mathbf{w}$ satisfies the proportional hazards model (Cox, 1972)

$$\lambda(t|\mathbf{x}, \mathbf{z}, \mathbf{w}) = \lambda_0(t)e^{\boldsymbol{\beta}^{\mathrm{T}}\mathbf{x}+\boldsymbol{\gamma}^{\mathrm{T}}\mathbf{z}+\boldsymbol{\eta}^{\mathrm{T}}\mathbf{w}}, \tag{21.1}$$

where $\lambda_0(\cdot)$ is an unspecified baseline hazard function, and $\boldsymbol{\beta}$, $\boldsymbol{\gamma}$ and $\boldsymbol{\eta}$ are unknown regression parameters. The linear predictor in (21.1) can be modified to include products between $\mathbf{x}$, $\mathbf{z}$ and $\mathbf{w}$.

To accommodate nonproportional hazards structures, we consider a class of semiparametric transformation models, under which the cumulative hazard function of T conditional on $\mathbf{X} = \mathbf{x}$, $\mathbf{Z} = \mathbf{z}$ and $\mathbf{W} = \mathbf{w}$ takes the form

$$\Lambda(t|\mathbf{x}, \mathbf{z}, \mathbf{w}) = G\left\{\Lambda(t)e^{\boldsymbol{\beta}^{\mathrm{T}}\mathbf{x}+\boldsymbol{\gamma}^{\mathrm{T}}\mathbf{z}+\boldsymbol{\eta}^{\mathrm{T}}\mathbf{w}}\right\}, \tag{21.2}$$

where G is a known increasing function, and $\Lambda(\cdot)$ is an unspecified positive increasing function (Zeng and Lin, 2007). It is useful to adopt the class of Box-Cox transformations $G(x) = \{(1+x)^\rho - 1\}/\rho$ ($\rho \geq 0$) and the class of logarithmic transformations $G(x) = \log(1+rx)/r$ ($r \geq 0$) (Chen *et al.*, 2002). The choices of $\rho = 1$ or $r = 0$ and $\rho = 0$ or $r = 1$ correspond to the proportional hazards and proportional odds models, respectively. If G is not the identity function, then the regression parameters in (21.2) have different meanings than those of (21.1) and the cumulative baseline hazard function is $G\{\Lambda(t)\}$ rather than $\Lambda(t)$.

Suppose that T is subject to right censoring by C, such that we observe Y and Δ instead of T, where $Y = \min(T, C)$, $\Delta = I(T \leq C)$, and $I(\cdot)$ is the indicator function. Let N denote the total number of subjects in the cohort, and let $\mathbf{O}$ denote the first-phase data $(Y_i, \Delta_i, \mathbf{Z}_i, \mathbf{W}_i)$ ($i = 1, \ldots, N$). In addition, let R_i indicate, by the values 1 versus 0, whether the ith subject is selected for the measurement of $\mathbf{X}$ in the second phase. Write $\mathcal{S} = \{i : R_i = 1\}$ and $\overline{\mathcal{S}} = \{i : R_i = 0\}$.

We make two assumptions:

(A.1) The censoring time C is independent of T conditional on $(\mathbf{X}, \mathbf{Z}, \mathbf{W})$ for $R = 1$ and independent of T and $\mathbf{X}$ conditional on $(\mathbf{Z}, \mathbf{W})$ for $R = 0$.

(A.2) The sampling vector $(R_1, \ldots, R_N)$ is independent of $(\mathbf{X}_1, \ldots, \mathbf{X}_N)$ conditional on $\mathbf{O}$.

Remark 1. Assumption (A.1) is the standard coarsening-at-random assumption. Under Assumption (A.2), the selection of a subject for the measurement of $\mathbf{X}$ may depend on any first-phase data. This assumption is clearly satisfied by the original case-cohort design, where R_i depends only on Δ_i, and by the original nested case-control design, where R_i depends on Δ_i and the risk sets.

Let $\boldsymbol{\theta} = (\boldsymbol{\beta}^{\mathrm{T}}, \boldsymbol{\gamma}^{\mathrm{T}}, \boldsymbol{\eta}^{\mathrm{T}})^{\mathrm{T}}$, and let $P(\cdot|\cdot)$ denote a conditional density function. Under

Assumption (A.2), the sampling probabilities can be omitted from the likelihood function in estimating $\boldsymbol{\theta}$ and Λ. For a subject in $\mathcal{S}$, the likelihood contribution is the density of $(Y, \Delta, \mathbf{X}, \mathbf{Z}, \mathbf{W})$; for a subject in $\overline{\mathcal{S}}$, the likelihood contribution is the density of $(Y, \Delta, \mathbf{Z}, \mathbf{W})$. Thus, the log-likelihood function concerning $\boldsymbol{\theta}$, Λ and $P(\mathbf{x}|\mathbf{z})$, conditional on $(\mathbf{Z}_i, \mathbf{W}_i), i = 1, \ldots, N$, takes the form

$$\sum_{i \in \mathcal{S}} \left\{ \log P(Y_i, \Delta_i | \mathbf{X}_i, \mathbf{Z}_i, \mathbf{W}_i) + \log P(\mathbf{X}_i | \mathbf{Z}_i) \right\} + \sum_{i \in \overline{\mathcal{S}}} \log \int P(Y_i, \Delta_i | \mathbf{x}, \mathbf{Z}_i, \mathbf{W}_i) P(\mathbf{x} | \mathbf{Z}_i) d\mathbf{x}.$$

(21.3)

Under Assumption (A.1), $P(Y_i, \Delta_i | \mathbf{X} = \mathbf{x}, \mathbf{Z}_i, \mathbf{W}_i)$ (for $i \in \overline{\mathcal{S}}$) is the product of

$$\left[\Lambda'(Y_i) e^{\boldsymbol{\beta}^{\mathrm{T}}\mathbf{x} + \boldsymbol{\gamma}^{\mathrm{T}}\mathbf{Z}_i + \boldsymbol{\eta}^{\mathrm{T}}\mathbf{W}_i} G' \left\{ \Lambda(Y_i) e^{\boldsymbol{\beta}^{\mathrm{T}}\mathbf{x} + \boldsymbol{\gamma}^{\mathrm{T}}\mathbf{Z}_i + \boldsymbol{\eta}^{\mathrm{T}}\mathbf{W}_i} \right\} \right]^{\Delta_i} \exp \left[-G \left\{ \Lambda(Y_i) e^{\boldsymbol{\beta}^{\mathrm{T}}\mathbf{x} + \boldsymbol{\gamma}^{\mathrm{T}}\mathbf{Z}_i + \boldsymbol{\eta}^{\mathrm{T}}\mathbf{W}_i} \right\} \right]$$

(21.4)

and a function that does not involve $\mathbf{x}$ or $(\boldsymbol{\theta}, \Lambda)$ and thus can be factored out of the integral in (21.3). Here and in the sequel, $f'(x) = df(x)/dx$ for any function f. In the special case of model (21.1), the likelihood function given in (21.4) simplifies to the familiar expression

$$\left[\lambda(Y_i) e^{\boldsymbol{\beta}^{\mathrm{T}}\mathbf{x} + \boldsymbol{\gamma}^{\mathrm{T}}\mathbf{Z}_i + \boldsymbol{\eta}^{\mathrm{T}}\mathbf{W}_i} \right]^{\Delta_i} \exp \left[-\int_0^{Y_i} e^{\boldsymbol{\beta}^{\mathrm{T}}\mathbf{x} + \boldsymbol{\gamma}^{\mathrm{T}}\mathbf{Z}_i + \boldsymbol{\eta}^{\mathrm{T}}\mathbf{W}_i} \lambda(t) dt \right]$$

(Kalbfleisch and Prentice, 2002, p. 54).

To maximize (21.3), we adopt the NPMLE approach (Johansen, 1983), under which both Λ and $P(\mathbf{x}|\mathbf{z})$ are nonparametric. Specifically, we let the estimator for Λ be a step function which jumps only at the observed Y_i with $\Delta_i = 1$ and replace (21.4) by

$$\left[\Lambda\{Y_i\} e^{\boldsymbol{\beta}^{\mathrm{T}}\mathbf{x} + \boldsymbol{\gamma}^{\mathrm{T}}\mathbf{Z}_i + \boldsymbol{\eta}^{\mathrm{T}}\mathbf{W}_i} G' \left\{ \Lambda(Y_i) e^{\boldsymbol{\beta}^{\mathrm{T}}\mathbf{x} + \boldsymbol{\gamma}^{\mathrm{T}}\mathbf{Z}_i + \boldsymbol{\eta}^{\mathrm{T}}\mathbf{W}_i} \right\} \right]^{\Delta_i} \exp \left[-G \left\{ \Lambda(Y_i) e^{\boldsymbol{\beta}^{\mathrm{T}}\mathbf{x} + \boldsymbol{\gamma}^{\mathrm{T}}\mathbf{Z}_i + \boldsymbol{\eta}^{\mathrm{T}}\mathbf{W}_i} \right\} \right],$$

where $\Lambda\{Y_i\}$ denotes the jump size of $\Lambda(\cdot)$ at Y_i. The estimator for $P(\mathbf{x}|\mathbf{z})$ depends on whether or not there are any continuous components in $\mathbf{Z}$. We consider those two cases separately.

21.2.2   Discrete inexpensive covariates

If $\mathbf{Z}$ is discrete, then $P(\mathbf{x}|\mathbf{z})$ can be estimated well. If there is no $\mathbf{Z}$, then $P(\mathbf{x}|\mathbf{z})$ is estimated simply by the empirical distribution function of $\mathbf{X}$. In those situations, maximization of (21.3) is relatively easy. Suppose that $\mathbf{Z}$ takes only a small number of discrete values, denoted by $\mathbf{z}_1, \ldots, \mathbf{z}_k$. For $l = 1, \ldots, k$, let the estimator for $P(\mathbf{x}|\mathbf{Z} = \mathbf{z}_l)$ be a discrete probability function on the distinct observed values of $\mathbf{X}$, denoted by $\mathbf{x}_1, \ldots, \mathbf{x}_{m_l}$, where m_l is the total number of distinct values of $\mathbf{X}$ among subjects with $\mathbf{Z} = \mathbf{z}_l$. Then the likelihood function (21.3) can be written as

$$\sum_{i \in \mathcal{S}} \left\{ \log P(Y_i, \Delta_i | \mathbf{X}_i, \mathbf{Z}_i, \mathbf{W}_i) + \sum_{l=1}^{k} \sum_{s=1}^{m_l} I(\mathbf{X}_i = \mathbf{x}_s, \mathbf{Z}_i = \mathbf{z}_l) \log p_{sl} \right\}$$

$$+ \sum_{i \in \overline{\mathcal{S}}} \sum_{l=1}^{k} I(\mathbf{Z}_i = \mathbf{z}_l) \log \left\{ \sum_{s=1}^{m_l} P(Y_i, \Delta_i | \mathbf{x}_s, \mathbf{Z}_i, \mathbf{W}_i) p_{sl} \right\},$$

where $p_{sl} = P(\mathbf{X} = \mathbf{x}_s | \mathbf{Z} = \mathbf{z}_l)$.

We maximize the above likelihood function through an EM algorithm, where we treat $\mathbf{X}_i$ for $i \in \overline{\mathcal{S}}$ as missing data. In the M-step, we maximize the following function

$$\sum_{i \in \mathcal{S}} \left\{ \log P(Y_i, \Delta_i | \mathbf{X}_i, \mathbf{Z}_i, \mathbf{W}_i) + \sum_{l=1}^{k} \sum_{s=1}^{m_l} I(\mathbf{X}_i = \mathbf{x}_s, \mathbf{Z}_i = \mathbf{z}_l) \log p_{sl} \right\}$$

$$+ \sum_{i \in \overline{\mathcal{S}}} \sum_{l=1}^{k} I(\mathbf{Z}_i = \mathbf{z}_l) \sum_{s=1}^{m_l} \{ w_{si} \log P(Y_i, \Delta_i | \mathbf{x}_s, \mathbf{Z}_i, \mathbf{W}_i) + \log p_{sl} \}$$

to update $\boldsymbol{\theta}$, Λ, and p_{sl}, where w_{si} is the conditional probability of $\mathbf{X}_i = \mathbf{x}_s$ given the observed data $(Y_i, \Delta_i, \mathbf{Z}_i)$ for $i \in \overline{\mathcal{S}}$. That is, we update $\boldsymbol{\theta}$ and the jump sizes of Λ by maximizing

$$\sum_{i \in \mathcal{S}} \log P(Y_i, \Delta_i | \mathbf{X}_i, \mathbf{Z}_i, \mathbf{W}_i) + \sum_{i \in \overline{\mathcal{S}}} \sum_{l=1}^{k} I(\mathbf{Z}_i = \mathbf{z}_l) \sum_{s=1}^{m_l} w_{si} \log P(Y_i, \Delta_i | \mathbf{x}_s, \mathbf{Z}_i, \mathbf{W}_i),$$

and we update p_{sl} $(s = 1, \ldots, m_l; l = 1, \ldots, k)$ by

$$p_{sl} = \frac{\sum_{i \in \mathcal{S}} I(\mathbf{X}_i = \mathbf{x}_s, \mathbf{Z}_i = \mathbf{z}_l) + \sum_{i \in \overline{\mathcal{S}}} w_{si} I(\mathbf{Z}_i = \mathbf{z}_l)}{\sum_{s=1}^{m_l} \left\{ \sum_{i \in \mathcal{S}} I(\mathbf{X}_i = \mathbf{x}_s, \mathbf{Z}_i = \mathbf{z}_l) + \sum_{i \in \overline{\mathcal{S}}} w_{si} I(\mathbf{Z}_i = \mathbf{z}_l) \right\}}.$$

In the E-step, we evaluate

$$w_{si} = \frac{\sum_{l=1}^{k} I(\mathbf{Z}_i = \mathbf{z}_l) p_{sl} P(Y_i, \Delta_i | \mathbf{x}_s, \mathbf{Z}_i, \mathbf{W}_i)}{\sum_{l=1}^{k} I(\mathbf{Z}_i = \mathbf{z}_l) \sum_{s=1}^{m_l} p_{sl} P(Y_i, \Delta_i | \mathbf{x}_s, \mathbf{Z}_i, \mathbf{W}_i)}.$$

We iterate between the E-step and M-step until convergence in the parameter estimates. Denote the resulting estimators for $\boldsymbol{\theta}$ and Λ as $\widehat{\boldsymbol{\theta}}$ and $\widehat{\Lambda}$, respectively. Also, denote the estimator for the distribution function of $\mathbf{X}$ given $\mathbf{Z} = \mathbf{z}_l$ as

$$\widehat{F}_l(\mathbf{x}) = \sum_{s=1}^{m_l} I(\mathbf{x}_s \le \mathbf{x}) \widehat{p}_{sl},$$

where $\widehat{p}_{sl}$ is the estimator for p_{sl} from the EM algorithm.

By the arguments of Zeng *et al.* (2006),

$$\sqrt{N}(\widehat{\boldsymbol{\theta}} - \boldsymbol{\theta}, \widehat{\Lambda} - \Lambda, \widehat{F}_1 - F_1, \ldots, \widehat{F}_k - F_k)$$

converges weakly to a zero-mean Gaussian process. In addition, the limiting covariance matrix of $\sqrt{N}(\widehat{\boldsymbol{\theta}} - \boldsymbol{\theta})$ attains the semiparametric efficiency bound.

We estimate the covariance matrix of $\widehat{\boldsymbol{\theta}}$ by inverting the observed-data information matrix, which is obtained via the Louis (1982) formula by treating $\boldsymbol{\theta}$, the jump sizes of Λ, and p_{sl} $(s = 1, \ldots, m_l; l = 1, \ldots, k)$ as parameters. The consistency of the covariance matrix estimator follows from the arguments of Zeng *et al.* (2006) and Zeng and Lin (2007).

21.2.3 Continuous inexpensive covariates

If some components of $\mathbf{Z}$ are continuous, then only a small number of observations on $\mathbf{X}$ are associated with each observed $\mathbf{Z}$, such that maximization of (21.3) becomes difficult. To address this challenge, we estimate the conditional distribution of $\mathbf{X}$ given $\mathbf{Z}$ by maximizing a kernel-smoothed local likelihood function. Specifically, we approximate $\log P(\mathbf{X}_i | \mathbf{Z}_i)$ and

$P(\mathbf{x}|\mathbf{Z}_i)$ in (21.3) by $\sum_{j=1}^{N} w_{ji}\log P(\mathbf{X}_i|\mathbf{Z} = \mathbf{Z}_j)$ and $\sum_{j=1}^{N} w_{ji}P(\mathbf{x}|\mathbf{Z} = \mathbf{Z}_j)$, respectively, where

$$w_{ji} = \frac{K\{(\mathbf{Z}_j - \mathbf{Z}_i)/a_N\}}{\sum_{j=1}^{N} K\{(\mathbf{Z}_j - \mathbf{Z}_i)/a_N\}},$$

$K(\cdot)$ is a symmetric kernel function, and a_N is a constant. Then expression (21.3) becomes

$$\sum_{i \in \mathcal{S}} \left\{ \log P(Y_i, \Delta_i|\mathbf{X}_i, \mathbf{Z}_i, \mathbf{W}_i) + \sum_{j=1}^{N} w_{ji}\log P(\mathbf{X}_i|\mathbf{Z}_j) \right\}$$

$$+ \sum_{i \in \overline{\mathcal{S}}} \log \left\{ \int P(Y_i, \Delta_i|\mathbf{x}, \mathbf{Z}_i, \mathbf{W}_i) \sum_{j=1}^{N} w_{ji}P(\mathbf{x}|\mathbf{Z}_j)d\mathbf{x} \right\}.$$

Denote the point mass of $P(\mathbf{X}|\mathbf{Z}_j)$ at $\mathbf{x}_s$ by p_{sj}. Our objective is to maximize the following function

$$l_N(\boldsymbol{\theta}, \Lambda, p_{sj}) = \sum_{i \in \mathcal{S}} \left\{ \log P(Y_i, \Delta_i|\mathbf{X}_i, \mathbf{Z}_i, \mathbf{W}_i) + \sum_{s=1}^{m} I(\mathbf{X}_i = \mathbf{x}_s) \sum_{j=1}^{N} w_{ji}\log p_{sj} \right\}$$

$$+ \sum_{i \in \overline{\mathcal{S}}} \log \left\{ \sum_{s=1}^{m} P(Y_i, \Delta_i|\mathbf{X} = \mathbf{x}_s, \mathbf{Z}_i, \mathbf{W}_i) \sum_{j=1}^{N} w_{ji}p_{sj} \right\} \tag{21.5}$$

under the constraints $\sum_{s=1}^{m} p_{sj} = 1$ and $p_{sj} \geq 0$ $(j = 1, \ldots, N)$. If $\mathbf{Z}$ is discrete, we can choose a_N sufficiently small such that $w_{ji} = I(j = i)$. Then (21.5) reduces to the original log-likelihood function with $P(\mathbf{X} = \mathbf{x}_s|\mathbf{Z} = \mathbf{Z}_l) = p_{sl}$, as given in Section 2.2.

As in the case of discrete $\mathbf{Z}$, it is natural to use an EM algorithm for maximizing the modified log-likelihood function given in (21.5). To make the second term in (21.5) more tractable, we artificially create a latent variable $\widetilde{\mathbf{Z}}$ that takes values on the observed $\mathbf{Z}_1, \ldots, \mathbf{Z}_N$ and satisfies the equations

$$P(\widetilde{\mathbf{Z}} = \mathbf{Z}_j|\mathbf{Z} = \mathbf{Z}_i, \mathbf{W}) = w_{ji},$$

$$P(\mathbf{X} = \mathbf{x}_s|\mathbf{Z} = \mathbf{Z}_i, \widetilde{\mathbf{Z}} = \mathbf{Z}_j, \mathbf{W}) = P(\mathbf{X} = \mathbf{x}_s|\widetilde{\mathbf{Z}} = \mathbf{Z}_j) = p_{sj},$$

and

$$P(Y, \Delta|\mathbf{X}, \mathbf{Z}, \mathbf{W}, \widetilde{\mathbf{Z}}) = P(Y, \Delta|\mathbf{X}, \mathbf{Z}, \mathbf{W}).$$

Then

$$P(\mathbf{X} = \mathbf{x}_s|\mathbf{Z} = \mathbf{Z}_i) = \sum_{j=1}^{N} w_{ji}p_{sj}$$

for subjects in $\overline{\mathcal{S}}$. It is easy to see that the second term in (21.5) is equivalent to the log-likelihood of $(Y_i, \Delta_i, \mathbf{Z}_i, \mathbf{W}_i)$ $(i \in \overline{\mathcal{S}})$ assuming that the complete data consist of $(Y_i, \Delta_i, \mathbf{X}_i, \mathbf{Z}_i, \mathbf{W}_i, \widetilde{\mathbf{Z}}_i)$ $(i \in \overline{\mathcal{S}})$ but both $\mathbf{X}_i$ and $\widetilde{\mathbf{Z}}_i$ are missing.

We now present an EM-type algorithm to maximize (21.5) by treating $(\mathbf{X}_i, \widetilde{\mathbf{Z}}_i)$ $(i \in \overline{\mathcal{S}})$ as missing data. The complete-data log-likelihood for subjects in $\overline{\mathcal{S}}$ can be written as

$$\sum_{i \in \overline{\mathcal{S}}} \left\{ \log P(Y_i, \Delta_i|\mathbf{X}_i, \mathbf{Z}_i, \mathbf{W}_i) + \log P(\mathbf{X}_i|\widetilde{\mathbf{Z}}_i) + \log P(\widetilde{\mathbf{Z}}_i|\mathbf{Z}_i) + \log P(\mathbf{Z}_i, \mathbf{W}_i) \right\}$$

$$= \sum_{i \in \overline{\mathcal{S}}} \left\{ \sum_{s=1}^{m} I(\mathbf{X}_i = \mathbf{x}_s)\log P(Y_i, \Delta_i|\mathbf{X} = \mathbf{x}_s, \mathbf{Z}_i, \mathbf{W}_i) + \sum_{j=1}^{N} \sum_{s=1}^{m} I(\mathbf{X}_i = \mathbf{x}_s, \widetilde{\mathbf{Z}}_i = \mathbf{Z}_j)\log p_{sj} \right\}$$

$$+ \sum_{j=1}^{N} I(\widetilde{\mathbf{Z}}_i = \mathbf{Z}_j) \mathrm{log} w_{ji} + \mathrm{log} P(\mathbf{Z}_i, \mathbf{W}_i) \bigg\}.$$

In the E-step, we calculate the conditional expectations of $I(\mathbf{X}_i = \mathbf{x}_s)$ and $I(\mathbf{X}_i = \mathbf{x}_s, \widetilde{\mathbf{Z}}_i = \mathbf{Z}_j)$ given the observed data for $i \in \overline{\mathcal{S}}$ and $j = 1, \ldots, N$ as

$$\widehat{q}_{is} = \frac{P(Y_i, \Delta_i | \mathbf{X} = \mathbf{x}_s, \mathbf{Z}_i, \mathbf{W}_i) \sum_{j=1}^{N} w_{ji} p_{sj}}{\sum_{s=1}^{m} P(Y_i, \Delta_i | \mathbf{X} = \mathbf{x}_s, \mathbf{Z}_i, \mathbf{W}_i) \sum_{j=1}^{N} w_{ji} p_{sj}},$$

and

$$\widehat{\psi}_{sji} = \frac{w_{ji} p_{sj}}{\sum_{j=1}^{N} w_{ji} p_{sj}} \widehat{q}_{is},$$

respectively. In the M-step, we update $\boldsymbol{\theta}$ and Λ by maximizing

$$\sum_{i \in \mathcal{S}} \mathrm{log} P(Y_i, \Delta_i | \mathbf{X}_i, \mathbf{Z}_i, \mathbf{W}_i) + \sum_{i \in \overline{\mathcal{S}}} \sum_{s=1}^{m} \widehat{q}_{is} \mathrm{log} P(Y_i, \Delta_i | \mathbf{X} = \mathbf{x}_s, \mathbf{Z}_i, \mathbf{W}_i). \qquad (21.6)$$

Because (21.6) is a weighted sum of the log-likelihood functions under the semiparametric transformation model, this optimization can be carried out by the algorithms of Zeng and Lin (2007). We update p_{sj} $(j = 1, \ldots, N; s = 1, \ldots, m)$ by maximizing

$$\sum_{i \in \mathcal{S}} \sum_{s=1}^{m} I(\mathbf{X}_i = \mathbf{x}_s) w_{ji} \mathrm{log} p_{sj} + \sum_{i \in \overline{\mathcal{S}}} \sum_{s=1}^{m} \widehat{\psi}_{sji} \mathrm{log} p_{sj},$$

such that

$$p_{sj} = \frac{\sum_{i \in \mathcal{S}} I(\mathbf{X}_i = \mathbf{x}_s) w_{ji} + \sum_{i \in \overline{\mathcal{S}}} \widehat{\psi}_{sji}}{\sum_{s=1}^{m} \left\{ \sum_{i \in \mathcal{S}} I(\mathbf{X}_i = \mathbf{x}_s) w_{ij} + \sum_{i \in \overline{\mathcal{S}}} \widehat{\psi}_{sji} \right\}}.$$

Setting the initial values of $\boldsymbol{\theta}$, $\Lambda\{\cdot\}$ and p_{sj} to $\mathbf{0}$, the inverse of the total number of cases, and m^{-1}, respectively, we iterate between the E-step and M-step until the differences of parameter estimates at two successive iterations are smaller than a certain threshold. Denote the resulting estimator of $\boldsymbol{\theta}$, Λ and p_{sj} by $\widehat{\boldsymbol{\theta}}$, $\widehat{\Lambda}$ and $\widehat{p}_{sj}$. Since the MLE for the distribution function of $\mathbf{Z}$ is the empirical distribution function based on $(\mathbf{Z}_1, \ldots, \mathbf{Z}_N)$, the joint distribution function of $(\mathbf{X}, \mathbf{Z})$, denoted by $F(\cdot, \cdot)$, can be estimated by the distribution function $\widehat{F}(\cdot, \cdot)$ with point mass $\widehat{p}_{sj}/N$ at $(\mathbf{x}_s, \mathbf{Z}_j)$ $(s = 1, \ldots, m; j = 1, \ldots, N)$.

Zeng and Lin (2014) established the asymptotic properties of $\widehat{\boldsymbol{\theta}}$ and $\widehat{\Lambda}$ under mild regularity conditions. Specifically, $\widehat{\boldsymbol{\theta}}$ and $\widehat{\Lambda}$ are strongly consistent in that

$$|\widehat{\boldsymbol{\theta}} - \boldsymbol{\theta}| + \sup_{[0,\tau]} |\widehat{\Lambda}(t) - \Lambda(t)| + \sup_{\mathbf{x}, \mathbf{z}} |\widehat{F}(\mathbf{x}, \mathbf{z}) - F(\mathbf{x}, \mathbf{z})| \to 0$$

almost surely. In addition, $\widehat{\boldsymbol{\theta}}$ is asymptotically normal and asymptotically efficient in that $N^{1/2}(\widehat{\boldsymbol{\theta}} - \boldsymbol{\theta})$ converges in distribution to a zero-mean normal random vector whose covariance matrix attains the semiparametric efficiency bound.

The limiting covariance matrix of $\widehat{\boldsymbol{\theta}}$ can be estimated by the negative inverse of the second-order difference of the profile likelihood function for $\boldsymbol{\theta}$ (Murphy and van der Vaart, 2000). Specifically, we hold $\boldsymbol{\theta}$ fixed in the EM algorithm and set the profile likelihood function $pf(\boldsymbol{\theta})$ to the value of $l_N(\boldsymbol{\theta}, \Lambda, p_{sj})$ at the convergence. Then we estimate the covariance matrix of $\widehat{\boldsymbol{\theta}}$ by the negative inverse of the matrix whose (k, l)th element is

$$h_N^{-2} \left\{ pf(\widehat{\boldsymbol{\theta}} + \mathbf{e}_k h_N + \mathbf{e}_l h_N) - pf(\widehat{\boldsymbol{\theta}} + \mathbf{e}_k h_N) - pf(\widehat{\boldsymbol{\theta}} + \mathbf{e}_l h_N) + pf(\widehat{\boldsymbol{\theta}}) \right\},$$

TABLE 21.1
Simulation results for simple case-cohort studies. EST denotes the mean of the parameter estimator; SE denotes the standard error of the parameter estimator; SEE denotes the mean of the standard error estimator; CP denotes the coverage probability of the 95% confidence interval.

N		NPMLE				Prentice	
		EST	SE	SEE	CP	EST	SE
1000	$\beta = -0.2$	-0.211	0.241	0.231	0.94	-0.213	0.261
	$\gamma = 0.5$	0.501	0.245	0.242	0.95	0.508	0.450
	$\eta = 0.8$	0.800	0.241	0.237	0.95	0.810	0.446
2000	$\beta = -0.2$	-0.206	0.165	0.163	0.95	-0.208	0.178
	$\gamma = 0.5$	0.497	0.171	0.170	0.95	0.495	0.311
	$\eta = 0.8$	0.807	0.167	0.167	0.95	0.810	0.308

where $\mathbf{e}_k$ is the kth canonical vector, and h_N is a perturbation constant that is typically set to a multiplier of $N^{-1/2}$.

Remark 2. In the kernel-smoothed local likelihood, the kernel function can be chosen to be Gaussian or Epanechnikov. We recommend to choose the bandwidth $a_N = N^{-1/(3+d_z)}$, where d_z is the dimension of $\mathbf{Z}$, such that the estimator for $P(\mathbf{x}|\mathbf{z})$ is under-smoothed. In evaluating the profile likelihood function for variance estimation, we recommend to use $h_N = N^{-1/2}$ or $5N^{-1/2}$ for the perturbation constant.

21.3   Simulation study

We conducted a simulation study to evaluate the performance of the NPMLE approach for two-phase studies. We generated the expensive covariate X from the Bernoulli distribution with success probability $0.2 + |Z - 0.5|$, where the inexpensive covariate Z is a discrete variable taking values 0, 0.1, 0.2, ..., 0.9 with equal probabilities. We also generated an inexpensive variable W from the standard uniform distribution. We then generated the failure time T from model (21.1) with $G(x) = x$, $\lambda_0(t) = 0.1t$, $\beta = -0.2, \gamma = 0.5$, and $\eta = 0.8$. In addition, we generated the censoring time C from the uniform $[0, 3]$ distribution, creating approximately 78% censored observations. Finally, we considered the cohort size of $N = 1,000$ or 2,000 and randomly selected 30% subjects as a subcohort under the case-cohort design, such that X is available for all cases and the subcohort.

For each simulated data set, we adopted the NPMLE approach for discrete Z to estimate all parameters. We applied the EM algorithm with initial values $\beta = \gamma = \eta = 0$ and the jump sizes of $\Lambda_0(\cdot)$ being $1/m$, where m is the total number of cases. To estimate the covariance matrix of the parameter estimators, we calculated the observed-data information matrix for all regression parameters, the jump sizes of $\Lambda_0(\cdot)$ and the conditional probabilities of X given each value of Z and then inverted this matrix.

Table 21.1 summarizes the results based on 10,000 replicates. The NPMLE approach performs well: the parameter estimator has little bias; the standard error estimator reflects very well the true variability; the confidence interval has correct coverage. We also evaluated the pseudo-partial likelihood approach of Prentice (1986). As shown in Table 21.1,

Example 399

TABLE 21.2

Risk factors in the radiation and breast cancer study.

Risk factor		Cases	Controls
Age at first treatment (years)	$0 - 19$	33	621
	$20 - 29$	28	609
	$30+$	14	415
Radiation dose (Gy)	0	21	677
	< 2	46	858
	≥ 2	8	110

the NPMLE tends to be more efficient than the pseudo-partial likelihood approach, with efficiency gain as much as 15% for estimating β and much higher for estimating γ and η.

21.4 Example

We consider a radiation and breast cancer study (Preston *et al.*, 1993). A total of 1,720 women were treated for tuberculosis between years 1930 and 1956 at one of two Massachusetts sanatoria and then followed for the occurrence of breast cancer through 1980. Most women had radiation exposure to the breast from multiple fluoroscopies used for diagnostic X-ray in conjunction with lung collapse therapy for their tuberculosis; those not examined by fluoroscopy were considered unexposed. Cumulative doses of radiation to the breast (Gy) were estimated from the number of fluoroscopies, a reconstruction of exposure conditions, absorbed dose calculations and other available data. It is of scientific interest to assess the association of breast cancer incidence with dose level of radiation exposure to the breast and age at first treatment. Table 21.2 displays the frequency distributions of the 75 cases and 1,645 controls according to these two risk factors.

Both radiation dose and age at first treatment were known for all women in the cohort. For illustrative purposes, we pretend that the radiation dose is an expensive covariate that was available through case-cohort or nested case-control sampling. The fact that dose actually was known for the entire cohort allows us to compare the results from the two-phase designs to the full-cohort results. In Chapter 17, Breslow and Hu created a simple case-cohort sample by drawing a random subcohort of 150 women and also a stratified case-cohort sample by drawing a random subcohort of 50 women for each of the three age groups at first treatment. In Chapter 18, Borgan created a nested case-control sample with two controls per case. We analyze those three data sets with the NPMLE approach and compare our results with what are reported in those two chapters.

Following the approach of Chapters 17 and 18, we fit the proportional hazards model with covariates $\log_2(\text{dose} + 1)$ and ageRx/10, where ageRx denotes age at first treatment. We also fit the proportional odds model. The results based on the full-cohort data are shown in the top block of Table 21.3. The risk of breast cancer increases with dose and decreases with age at first treatment, with p-values of 0.002 and 0.094, respectively, under the proportional hazards model.

We then analyze the case-cohort and nested case-control data, with $X = \log_2(\text{dose} + 1)$, $Z = \text{ageRx}/10$, and no W. We let X depend on age at first treatment rounded to the nearest integer (with a total of 59 unique values). Since the rounded age is discrete, the kernel function in the EM algorithm takes values of 1 and 0. We use the profile likelihood

TABLE 21.3

Results from the analysis of the radiation and breast cancer study.

Covariate	Proportional hazards model				Proportional odds model			
	Est	SE	Z-stat	*p*-value	Est	SE	Z-stat	*p*-value
Entire Cohort								
$\log_2(\text{dose} + 1)$	0.469	0.153	3.057	0.002	0.489	0.166	2.949	0.003
ageRx/10	-0.242	0.144	-1.677	0.094	-0.255	0.149	-1.719	0.086
Simple case-cohort								
$\log_2(\text{dose} + 1)$	0.594	0.202	2.942	0.003	0.623	0.214	2.911	0.002
ageRx/10	-0.237	0.146	-1.616	0.106	-0.251	0.150	-1.669	0.095
Stratified case-cohort								
$\log_2(\text{dose} + 1)$	0.688	0.227	3.027	0.003	0.714	0.237	3.009	0.003
ageRx/10	-0.231	0.147	-1.576	0.115	-0.47	0.151	-1.643	0.100
Nested case-control								
$\log_2(\text{dose} + 1)$	0.525	0.201	2.608	0.009	0.548	0.211	2.590	0.010
ageRx/10	-0.262	0.146	-1.799	0.072	-0.276	0.149	-1.847	0.065

function with the perturbation constant $h_N = 5/\sqrt{N}$ to estimate the covariance matrix. The results are shown in Table 21.3.

Compared to the full-cohort analysis, both the case-cohort analysis and nested case-control analysis yield slightly larger effect estimates and larger standard errors for dose, with comparable *p*-values. The standard errors for the age effect are almost identical between the full cohort analysis and the case-cohort or nested case-control analysis. The conventional method for analyzing the case-cohort data under the proportional hazards model, as reported in Chapter 17, yields a similar standard error for the dose effect but a very different standard error for the age effect. For the age effect, the conventional method provides an estimate of -0.111 with standard error 0.191. This result is considerably different from that of the full cohort analysis. For the stratified case-cohort data, the NPMLE for the dose effect is 0.688 with standard error 0.227. This result is much more significant than that of the conventional method (i.e., estimate 0.559 with standard error 0.246) and the method using calibrated weights (i.e., estimate 0.440 with standard error 0.184). For the nested case-control data, the partial likelihood approach (Chapter 18) yields the estimates 0.549 and -0.179 with standard errors 0.232 and 0.207 for the dose effect and age effect, respectively, both results being less significant than their NPMLE counterparts.

21.5 Remarks

We have described efficient maximum likelihood estimators for semiparametric transformation models under general two-phase designs, allowing the first-phase covariates to be continuous and correlated with expensive covariates. With continuous first-phase covariates, the likelihood function of interest is not tractable because it involves the conditional density function of expensive covariates given continuous first-phase covariates. We approximated the conditional density function by kernel smoothing; an alternative approach is B-splines.

In many two-phase studies, the sample sizes are very large and there are only a small number of distinct observed values for $\mathbf{Z}$. Then we can treat $\mathbf{Z}$ as discrete random variables and choose the bandwidth sufficiently small, such that the kernel estimation is essentially equivalent to the use of empirical probability functions, or, equivalently, we may use the method of Section 21.2.2. Then the computation is fast, and asymptotic approximations are accurate.

For continuous $\mathbf{Z}$, we estimate the covariance matrix of regression parameters through the profile likelihood. For discrete $\mathbf{Z}$, it is preferable to use the observed-data information matrix, which does not involve a perturbation constant. When there are a large number of distinct values, however, the information calculation may not be stable. In that case, we recommend to use the profile likelihood (even though $\mathbf{Z}$ is discrete), as we did in the real example.

The methods for both discrete $\mathbf{Z}$ and continuous $\mathbf{Z}$ are immune to the dimensionality of $\mathbf{X}$ because the estimator for $P(\mathbf{x}|\mathbf{z})$ takes probability masses at the distinct values of the observed $\mathbf{X}_i$. For the same reason, the method for discrete $\mathbf{Z}$ does not depend on the dimensionality of $\mathbf{Z}$ and the computational burden is only driven by the number of distinct values of $\mathbf{Z}$.

When $\mathbf{Z}$ has a continuous component, the NPMLE approach entails estimation of the conditional density of $P(\mathbf{x}|\mathbf{z})$ via kernel smoothing over $\mathbf{Z}$ and thus may suffer from the curse of dimensionality for $\mathbf{Z}$. Our numerical experience indicates that the estimation is numerically stable when the dimension of $\mathbf{Z}$ is no higher than three. When the dimension of $\mathbf{Z}$ is greater than three, we suggest to discretize $\mathbf{Z}$ and thus collapse the observed $\mathbf{Z}_i$ into a small number of categories and then apply the NPMLE method for discrete $\mathbf{Z}$. This data reduction leads to computationally efficient estimation and the resulting bias is ignorable if the number of collapsed categories is not too small.

We have focused on right-censored data. In some applications, subjects may be at risk over different time intervals due to, say, delayed entry. We can apply the NPMLE approach to this situation. The only change is to replace $\Lambda'(t)$ and $\Lambda(t)$ in the likelihood function (21.4) by $A(t)\Lambda'(t)$ and $\Lambda(t)$, respectively, where $A(t)$ indicates at-risk at time t.

We have assumed that the covariates are time-independent. The methods can be readily modified if there are external time-dependent covariates in $\mathbf{W}$. Generalization to the case of time-dependent $\mathbf{Z}$ is challenging due to the difficulties in estimating the conditional density of $\mathbf{X}$ given time-dependent covariates. One possible strategy is to jointly model the event time T and the latent trajectory of $\mathbf{Z}$ over time while allowing $\mathbf{X}$ to depend on the trajectory of $\mathbf{Z}$.

We have assumed that each study subject can experience only one event of interest. In many applications, each subject can potentially experience a given type of event repeatedly or multiple types of event, or the subjects are sampled in clusters (e.g., families, classrooms) such that the failure times within the same cluster are correlated. Weighted estimators for such multivariate failure time data under case-cohort designs have been proposed (Lu and Shih, 2006; Kang and Cai, 2009; Zhang *et al.*, 2011). The NPMLE methods presented in this chapter can be extended to the multivariate setting.

Bibliography

Barlow, W. E. (1994). Robust variance estimation for the case-cohort design. *Biometrics*, **50**, 1064–1072.

Borgan, Ø., Langholz, B., Samuelsen, S. O., Goldstein, L., and Pagoda, J. (2000). Exposure stratified case-cohort designs. *Lifetime Data Analysis*, **6**, 39–58.

Breslow, N. E., Lumbley, T., Ballantyne, C. M., Chambless, L. E., and Kulich, M. (2009).

Using the whole cohort in the analysis of case-cohort data. *American Journal of Epidemiology*, **169**, 1398–1405.

Cai, T. and Zheng, Y. (2011). Non-parametric evaluation of biomarker accuracy under nested case-control studies. *Journal of the American Statistical Association*, **106**, 569–580.

Cai, T. and Zheng, Y. (2012). Evaluating prognostic accuracy of biomarkers under nested case-control studies. *Biostatistics*, **13**, 89–100.

Chen, H. Y. and Little, R. J. A. (1999). Proportional hazards regression with missing covariates. *Journal of the American Statistical Association*, **94**, 896–908.

Chen, K. (2001). Generalized case-cohort sampling. *Journal of the Royal Statistical Society, Series B*, **63**, 791–809.

Chen, K. and Lo, S.-H. (1999). Case-cohort and case-control analysis with Cox's model. *Biometrika*, **86**, 755–764.

Chen, K., Jin, Z., and Ying, Z. (2002). Semiparametric analysis of transformation models with censored data. *Biometrika*, **89**, 659–668.

Cox, D. R. (1972). Regression models and life-tables (with discussion). *Journal of the Royal Statistical Society, Series B*, **34**, 187–220.

Cox, D. R. (1975). Partial likelihood. *Biometrika*, **62**, 269–276.

Goldstein, L. and Langholz, B. (1992). Asymptotic theory for nested case-control sampling in the Cox regression model. *The Annals of Statistics*, **20**, 69–79.

Johansen, S. (1983). An extension of Cox's regression model. *International Statistical Review*, **51**, 258–262.

Kalbfleisch, J. D. and Lawless, J. F. (1988). Likelihood analysis of multi-state models for disease incidence and mortality. *Statistics in Medicine*, **7**, 149–160.

Kalbfleisch, J. D. and Prentice, R. L. (2002). *The Statistical Analysis of Failure Time Data, 2nd edn.* Wiley, New York, NY.

Kang, S. and Cai, J. (2009). Marginal hazards model for case-cohort studies with multiple disease outcomes. *Biometrika*, **96**, 887–901.

Kong, L. and Cai, J. (2009). Case-cohort analysis with accelerated failure time model. *Biometrics*, **65**, 135–142.

Kong, L., Cai, J., and Sen, P. K. (2004). Weighted estimating equations for semiparametric transformation models with censored data from a case-cohort design. *Biometrika*, **91**, 305–319.

Kulich, M. and Lin, D. Y. (2000). Additive hazards regression for case-cohort studies. *Biometrika*, **87**, 73–87.

Kulich, M. and Lin, D. Y. (2004). Improving the efficiency of relative-risk estimation in case-cohort studies. *Journal of the American Statistical Association*, **99**, 832–844.

Langholz, B. and Borgan, Ø. (1995). Counter-matching: A stratified nested case-control sampling method. *Biometrika*, **82**, 69–79.

Louis, T. A. (1982). Finding the observed information matrix when using the EM algorithm. *Journal of the Royal Statistical Society, Series B*, **44**, 226–233.

Lu, S. E. and Shih, J. H. (2006). Case-cohort designs and analysis for clustered failure time data. *Biometrics*, **62**, 1138–1148.

Lu, W. and Tsiatis, A. A. (2006). Semiparametric transformation models for the case-cohort study. *Biometrika*, **93**, 207–214.

Luo, X., Tsai, W. Y., and Xu, Q. (2009). Pseudo-partial likelihood estimators for the Cox regression model with missing covariates. *Biometrika*, **96**, 617–633.

Martinussen, T. (1999). Cox regression with incomplete covariate measurements using the EM-algorithm. *Scandinavian Journal of Statistics*, **26**, 479–491.

Murphy, S. A. and van der Vaart, A. W. (2000). On the profile likelihood. *Journal of the American Statistical Association*, **95**, 449–465.

Nan, B. (2004). Efficient estimation for case-cohort studies. *Canadian Journal of Statistics*, **32**, 403–419.

Nan, B., Yu, M., and Kalbfleisch, J. D. (2006). Censored linear regression for case-cohort studies. *Biometrika*, **93**, 747–762.

Prentice, R. L. (1986). A case-cohort design for epidemiologic cohort studies and disease prevention trials. *Biometrika*, **73**, 1–11.

Preston, D. L., Lubin, J. H., Pierce, D. A., and McConney, M. D. (1993). *Epicure Users Guide*. Hirosoft International Corporation, Seattle, WA.

Qi, L., Wang, C. Y., and Prentice, R. L. (2005). Weighted estimators for proportional hazards regression with missing covariates. *Journal of the American Statistical Association*, **100**, 1250–1263.

Robins, J. M., Rotnitzky, A., and Zhao, L. P. (1994). Estimation of regression coefficients when some regressors are not always observed. *Journal of the American Statistical Association*, **89**, 846–866.

Scheike, T. H. and Juul, A. (2004). Maximum likelihood estimation for Cox's regression model under nested case-control sampling. *Biostatistics*, **5**, 193–206.

Scheike, T. H. and Martinussen, T. (2004). Maximum likelihood estimation for Cox's regression model under case-cohort sampling. *Scandinavian Journal of Statistics*, **31**, 283–293.

Self, S. G. and Prentice, R. L. (1988). Asymptotic distribution theory and efficiency results for case-cohort studies. *The Annals of Statistics*, **16**, 64–81.

Thomas, D. (1977). Addendum to "Methods of cohort analysis: Appraisal by application to asbestos mining" by F. D. K. Liddell, J. C. McDonald and D. C. Thomas. *Journal of the Royal Statistical Society, Series A*, **140**, 469–491.

Zeng, D. and Lin, D. Y. (2007). Maximum likelihood estimation in semiparametric regression models with censored data (with discussion). *Journal of the Royal Statistical Society, Series B*, **69**, 507–564.

Zeng, D. and Lin, D. Y. (2014). Efficient estimation of semiparametric transformation models for two-phase cohort studies. *Journal of the American Statistical Association*, **109**, 371–383.

Zeng, D., Lin, D. Y., Avery, C. L., North, K. E., and Bray, M. S. (2006). Efficient semiparametric estimation of haplotype-disease associations in case-cohort and nested case-control studies. *Biostatistics*, **7**, 486–502.

Zhang, H., Schaubel, D. E., and Kalbfleisch, J. D. (2011). Proportional hazards regression for the analysis of clustered survival data from case-cohort studies. *Biometrics*, **67**, 18–29.

22

The Self-Controlled Case Series Method

Paddy Farrington and Heather Whitaker

The Open University

22.1 Introduction

The self-controlled case series (SCCS) model uses only individuals with one or more events over the observation period. It may be derived from a Poisson cohort model by conditioning on the total number of events experienced by each individual. It automatically controls for all fixed confounders that act multiplicatively on the event intensity function (Farrington, 1995; Farrington and Whitaker, 2006).

The method was developed in the early 1990s to quantify the association between vaccination with certain types of measles, mumps and rubella (MMR) vaccines, and occurrences of aseptic meningitis in young children. Data on aseptic meningitis cases were obtained from hospital admission records, and linked to the children's vaccination histories, obtained from a different database. Evidence of a positive association between aseptic meningitis and MMR vaccines containing the Urabe mumps strain was sufficiently strong without a controlled epidemiological study to warrant the decision to replace these vaccines (Miller *et al.*, 2004). Nevertheless it was felt that a more formal quantification of the association was required. The nonrandom distribution of vaccinations in the population made it awkward to select suitable controls, and it was decided instead to seek a new method that exploited the information about the temporal association between exposures (MMR vaccination) and events (aseptic meningitis) within cases.

This led to the development of the SCCS method, which has since found many applications in the study of vaccine safety (Weldeselassie *et al.*, 2011) and in pharmacoepidemiology more widely. For a comprehensive account of the method see Farrington *et al.* (2018).

22.2   The self-controlled case series model

22.2.1   The SCCS likelihood

Suppose that an individual i is observed over the age period $(a_i, b_i]$, which may vary from individual to individual. Here 'age' refers to the natural timeline of analysis, which will often be age but may alternatively be calendar time, depending on circumstances. Suppose that, for individual i, events arise with intensity function $\lambda_i(t|v_i, \boldsymbol{x}_i)$ where t denotes age, v_i is the exposure history (for example, vaccination history) over the interval $(a_i, b_i]$ and $\boldsymbol{x}_i$ is a vector of time-invariant covariates.

Consider now just those n individuals within a cohort that experience one or more events within their observation period. Specifically, suppose that individual i, $i = 1, 2, \ldots, n$, observed over the observation period $(a_i, b_i]$, has r_i events in $(a_i, b_i]$, at ages $t_{i1}, t_{i2}, \ldots, t_{ir_i}$. The contribution to the SCCS likelihood for this individual is then

$$L_i = \frac{\prod_{j=1}^{r_i} \lambda_i(t_{ij}|v_i, \boldsymbol{x}_i)}{\left(\int_{a_i}^{b_i} \lambda_i(s|v_i, \boldsymbol{x}_i)ds \right)^{r_i}}.$$

The overall SCCS likelihood is the product of these n contributions:

$$L = \prod_{i=1}^{n} \frac{\prod_{j=1}^{r_i} \lambda_i(t_{ij}|v_i, \boldsymbol{x}_i)}{\left(\int_{a_i}^{b_i} \lambda_i(s|v_i, \boldsymbol{x}_i)ds \right)^{r_i}}.$$

The derivation of this likelihood, and the assumptions required in its derivation, will be considered in the next subsection. However, three key features emerge from this definition. First, only individuals having experienced one or more events within their observation period are required: in this sense, only cases are involved – no separate controls are needed. Second, as the likelihood is a ratio, any factors that act multiplicatively on the intensity function $\lambda_i(t|v_i, \boldsymbol{x}_i)$ cancel out. In particular, if

$$\lambda_i(t|v_i, \boldsymbol{x}_i) = h(\boldsymbol{x}_i)\lambda_{i0}(t|v_i)$$

for some function h, then the SCCS likelihood reduces to

$$L = \prod_{i=1}^{n} \frac{\prod_{j=1}^{r_i} \lambda_{i0}(t_{ij}|v_i)}{\left(\int_{a_i}^{b_i} \lambda_{i0}(s|v_i)ds \right)^{r_i}}.$$

In other words, time-invariant confounders acting multiplicatively on the intensity function are automatically adjusted for – and this, whether they are measured or not, and indeed whether or not they are known. Thus, while the SCCS method does not involve external controls, it does involve self-control, that is, by reference to nonevent ages within the observation periods.

These two features – only requiring cases, and self-control of multiplicative time-invariant confounders – are key properties of the SCCS method, which explain its name. These properties are shared with the case-crossover method (Chapter 7). The SCCS model differs from the case-crossover model in that the event (or event period) is random and the exposure history is regarded as fixed. In this sense, the SCCS design stems from cohort rather than case-control logic. The distinction between case-crossover and SCCS models is further explored in Vines and Farrington (2001) and Whitaker *et al.* (2007).

Note that the SCCS likelihood involves integrals

$$\int_{a_i}^{b_i} \lambda_i(s|v_i, \boldsymbol{x}_i)ds$$

which, unusually, involve ages s over the entire observation period $(a_i, b_i]$, including ages *after* the occurrence of any events. Furthermore, the method conditions on exposure histories over the entire observation period. This feature is the source of some constraints on the use of the method, to be clarified in the next section. When the event of interest affects subsequent exposures, it may be necessary to use a modification of the method. Such modifications are considered in Section 22.3.3.

22.2.2 Derivation of the SCCS model

In this subsection, the SCCS likelihood is derived from a cohort model. Suppose that events arise within a defined cohort of size N. For an individual i within this cohort, let $v_i(t)$ denote the time-varying exposure at age t, and $v_i^t = \{v_i(s) : s \leq t\}$ the exposure history to age t. Let $v_i = v_i^{b_i}$. Suppose that events for individual i arise in a counting process with intensity function $\lambda_i(t|v_i^t, \boldsymbol{x}_i)$, observed over an interval $(a_i, b_i]$. Our first assumption is that events arise in a nonhomogeneous Poisson process. The cohort likelihood that individual i experiences r_i events at ages $t_{i1}, t_{i2}, \ldots, t_{ir_i}$ in $(a_i, b_i]$, given the exposures, is then

$$L_{ci} = \prod_{j=1}^{r_i} \lambda_i(t_{ij}|v_i^{t_{ij}}, \boldsymbol{x}_i) \exp\left(-\int_{a_i}^{b_i} \lambda_i(s|v_i^s, \boldsymbol{x}_i)ds\right).$$

If individual i experiences $r_i = 0$ events in $(a_i, b_i]$, the product in this expression conventionally defaults to 1.

The SCCS likelihood is derived from this cohort likelihood contribution by conditioning on the observation period $(a_i, b_i]$, the exposure history $v_i = v_i^{b_i}$ up to the end of observation, and the total number of events r_i observed for individual i. What is not conditioned upon is the set of event ages $t_{i1}, t_{i2}, \ldots, t_{ir_i}$ when $r_i > 0$.

For inferences about the intensity functions $\lambda_i(t|v_i^t, \boldsymbol{x}_i)$ to be valid in the SCCS model, conditioning on the observation period $(a_i, b_i]$ and on the exposure history to b_i must not affect these intensities. Under these assumptions, we can write

$$\lambda_i(t|v_i^t, \boldsymbol{x}_i) = \lambda_i(t|v_i, \boldsymbol{x}_i),$$

where $v_i^t = \{v_i(s) : s \leq t\}$ is the exposure history up to t and $v_i = v_i^{b_i}$ is the exposure history up to the end of the observation period.

Then we have

$$L_{ci} = \prod_{j=1}^{r_i} \lambda_i(t_{ij}|v_i, \boldsymbol{x}_i) \exp\left(-\int_{a_i}^{b_i} \lambda_i(s|v_i, \boldsymbol{x}_i)ds\right)$$

and the probability that individual i experiences r_i events, given the exposure history and the observation period, is

$$\frac{1}{r_i!}\Big(\int_{a_i}^{b_i}\lambda_i(s|v_i,\boldsymbol{x}_i)ds\Big)^{r_i}\exp\Big(-\int_{a_i}^{b_i}\lambda_i(s|v_i,\boldsymbol{x}_i)ds\Big),$$

so the contribution to the conditional likelihood kernel is

$$L_i=\frac{\prod_{j=1}^{r_i}\lambda_i(t_{ij}|v_i,\boldsymbol{x}_i)}{\Big(\int_{a_i}^{b_i}\lambda_i(s|v_i,\boldsymbol{x}_i)ds\Big)^{r_i}}.$$

This is the SCCS likelihood contribution previously defined when $r_i > 0$; when $r_i = 0$ it reduces to 1: noncases need not be sampled.

22.3   Assumptions and modifications

In this section we revisit the assumptions of the SCCS model. We also briefly describe some modifications of the SCCS method to avoid some of these assumptions. To recapitulate, the three assumptions used in the derivation of Section 22.2.2 are:

1. Events arise in a nonhomogeneous Poisson process.

2. Exposures are not influenced by prior events.

3. The observation periods are not event-dependent.

As it turns out, all three assumptions may be weakened to some degree, or circumvented.

22.3.1   The Poisson assumption

The SCCS likelihood was derived under the assumption that events arise in a nonhomogeneous Poisson process. Under this assumption, events within individuals are potentially recurrent, and recurrence ages are independent within individuals. This assumption may fail in two ways: first, the event may not be recurrent, and second, if the event is recurrent, then recurrences within individuals may not be independent. For example, diagnosis of autism is not a recurrent event; and nonfatal myocardial infarctions (MI) may be potentially recurrent, but not independent within individuals: occurrence of a first MI increases the chance of a second.

The SCCS method may nevertheless be used without modification with nonrecurrent events, provided that these are rare. Suppose that the hazard for individual i is

$$\lambda_i(t|v_i,\boldsymbol{x}_i)=\phi\nu_i(t|v_i,\boldsymbol{x}_i).$$

The underlying cohort from which cases are sampled includes individuals i who have not experienced the event by age a_i, and are followed to age b_i. The cohort likelihood contribution of individual i is

$$L_{ci}=\{\phi\nu_i(t_i|v_i,\boldsymbol{x}_i)\}^{I_i}\exp\Big(-\phi\int_{a_i}^{c_i}\nu_i(s|v_i,\boldsymbol{x}_i)ds\Big),$$

where t_i is the age of event, I_i is an indicator equal to 1 if individual i has an event in $(a_i,b_i]$

and 0 otherwise, and $c_i = I_i t_i + (1 - I_i) b_i$. The probability that individual i experiences an event, given the exposure history and the observation period, is

$$\int_{a_i}^{b_i} \phi \nu_i(t|v_i, \boldsymbol{x}_i) \exp\left(-\phi \int_{a_i}^{t} \nu_i(s|v_i, \boldsymbol{x}_i) ds\right) dt$$

and so the conditional likelihood contribution for an individual with one event is

$$L_i = \frac{\nu_i(t_i|v_i, \boldsymbol{x}_i) \exp\left(-\phi \int_{a_i}^{t_i} \nu_i(s|v_i, \boldsymbol{x}_i) ds\right)}{\int_{a_i}^{b_i} \nu_i(t|v_i, \boldsymbol{x}_i) \exp\left(-\phi \int_{a_i}^{t} \nu_i(s|v_i, \boldsymbol{x}_i) ds\right) dt}.$$

When the event is rare, we approach the limit in which $\phi \to 0$, in which case the exponential terms in the above expression both tend to 1. Thus the likelihood contribution reduces to

$$L_i = \frac{\nu_i(t_i|v_i, \boldsymbol{x}_i)}{\int_{a_i}^{b_i} \nu_i(s|v_i, \boldsymbol{x}_i) ds} = \frac{\lambda_i(t_i|v_i, \boldsymbol{x}_i)}{\int_{a_i}^{b_i} \lambda_i(s|v_i, \boldsymbol{x}_i) ds},$$

which coincides with the SCCS likelihood contribution. Thus, the assumption that events are Poisson can be weakened to include rare unique events.

If events are recurrent but not independent within individuals, a simple analysis strategy is to repeat the analysis with just the first occurrence of the event in the observation period, provided that first occurrences are rare.

The analysis of recurrent, dependent events within an SCCS framework has been considered in Farrington and Hocine (2010). Simpson (2013) has developed a modified SCCS model to cater for situations in which each event increases the probability of occurrence of a subsequent event.

22.3.2 Event-dependent observation periods

It is a requirement of the SCCS method that events should not influence the observation period. This is violated if the event is death, or carries high event-associated mortality, and the observation period is curtailed at age of death. The assumption is required so that conditioning on the observation periods $(a_i, b_i]$ does not bias inferences about the association between exposures and events. If the event of interest is not associated with high mortality, observation periods may usually be assumed to be independent of the event.

In some circumstances, however, it is possible to redefine the observation periods so that they are necessarily independent of the event. In such circumstances, standard SCCS analyses may then be undertaken. Here are two examples where this has been done to handle deaths within the SCCS framework.

First, if the exposure is necessarily unique (as is the case, for example, with some childhood vaccinations, or if interest focuses on the initiation of a new therapy), the observation periods can be redefined as $(e_i, f_i]$ where e_i is the start of exposure and f_i is the age at which observation would have ceased had death not occurred. Note that then only exposed cases are included in the analysis, and their exposure history is known throughout the observation period. This approach has been used to investigate sudden deaths after the initiation of an anti-smoking therapy (Hubbard *et al.*, 2005).

Second, if exposures are not unique but occur with minimum known separations τ (as is the case with many multi-dose vaccinations), a standard SCCS analysis may be possible with observation period comprising the interval $(e_{k_i i}, e_{k_i i} + \tau]$ where $e_{k_i i}$ is the k_ith and final exposure start age for individual i; if the maximum number of exposures is known to be K, and $k_i = K$, we can use the observation period $(e_{K i}, f_i]$ where f_i is the age at which observation would have ceased had no event occurred. Again, the exposure history in this observation period is known, by definition. This approach was proposed to handle sudden infant deaths after hexavalent vaccines (Kuhnert et al., 2011).

When the event is not death but carries high mortality, a modified SCCS method may be used. This involves explicitly modelling the time from event until end of observation. The method is described in Farrington et al. (2011), with an application to stroke and antipsychotics. Finally, when the event is death, another modified SCCS method, described in Farrington et al. (2009), may sometimes be used.

22.3.3   Event-dependent exposures

A key assumption of the standard SCCS method is that events do not influence the probability of subsequent exposures. This is what makes it possible to condition on the exposure history in the observation periods $(a_i, b_i]$ without affecting inferences about the strength of association between the exposure and the event. The direction of the bias resulting from the failure of this assumption can be predicted. If occurrence of an event reduces the probability of subsequent exposure, then the relative risk for the association will be biased upwards, since fewer events then take place before exposure than would otherwise be the case. Similarly, if occurrence of an event increases the probability of subsequent exposure, the relative risk for the association will be biased downwards.

In certain situations, standard SCCS analyses can be undertaken that allow for event-dependent exposures. Here are two such situations; the first is similar to that described in Section 22.3.2. First, if the exposure is necessarily unique, the observation periods can be redefined as $(e_i, b_i]$ where e_i is the start of exposure. Since the exposure is unique, occurrence of an event in $(e_i, b_i]$ cannot influence subsequent exposures since no further exposures can occur.

Second, if the impact of the event on exposures is limited to a period of duration τ after the event, then this will be revealed by an atypical event frequency in the period $[-\tau, 0)$ before exposure. This can be investigated by redefining the exposure functions $v_i(t)$ to incorporate such a pre-exposure 'risk' period. This approach has been described in Farrington and Whitaker (2006); see also Sardiñas et al. (2001); Andrews (2002).

In other situations, notably when multiple exposures can occur for each individual with unspecified separations between them, and when the probability of exposure is modified permanently after the occurrence of an event, for example when the event itself is a contraindication to the exposure, a more complex modification of the SCCS method is required, described in Farrington et al. (2009). In this approach, the likelihood framework is replaced by a system of unbiased estimating equations.

22.3.4   Other requirements of the SCCS method

It is important to emphasize that the SCCS method should not generally be used with case series assembled because of a suspected association between exposure and event, as is common, for example, with voluntary adverse event reporting systems. The ascertainment of events and exposures should be independent. This requirement is not limited to SCCS studies: it is shared with all epidemiological designs. However, because the SCCS method is so easy to apply to any case series, it seems particularly important to emphasize this requirement in the present context. In some very specific circumstances, use of the SCCS method with nonindependently ascertained cases may be acceptable for investigating possible signals, but not for definitive confirmation of an association. These rather special circumstances are described in Escolano et al. (2013).

Finally, while the SCCS method controls for fixed confounders that act multiplicatively on the event intensity function, it does not control automatically for time-varying confounders. These need to be included explicitly in the model, like age. A common instance is when seasonal as well as age variation is important; see for example the application to oral polio vaccination in Cuba in Sardiñas *et al.* (2001).

22.4 Modelling with the SCCS method

In this section we present some SCCS models used in applications in epidemiology. In keeping with the terminology in this field, we shall use the term incidence to refer to the intensity function of the Poisson process of events (or the hazard function when events are nonrecurrent and rare). To keep matters simple, we assume that there is a single exposure which can take one of K levels, level 1 corresponding to no exposure. Thus, an individual i progresses through a sequence of control periods and periods at different levels of risk. The exposure is represented by a time-varying K-level factor denoted $\boldsymbol{v}_i(t)$.

We consider models of the proportional incidence form

$$\lambda_i(t|v_i, \boldsymbol{x}_i) = \phi_i \theta(t) \exp\{g_i(\boldsymbol{x}_i) + \boldsymbol{v}_i(t)^T \boldsymbol{\beta}\},$$

where ϕ_i is the incidence at some reference age, say $a = \min\{a_i, i = 1, \ldots, n\}$, $\theta(t)$ is the relative age-specific incidence, common to all individuals, with $\theta(a) = 1$, g_i is some unspecified function, and $\boldsymbol{\beta}$ is the vector of parameters of primary interest. The component β_k, for $k = 1, \ldots, K$, is the log relative incidence associated with exposure at level k, with $\beta_1 = 0$. Note that the terms ϕ_i and $\exp\{g_i(\boldsymbol{x}_i)\}$ act multiplicatively on the incidence, and so they are eliminated from the SCCS likelihood: they are not specified further.

Other models, in which exposure is represented by a spline function, are available (Ghebremichael-Weldeselassie *et al.*, 2016). More detailed modelling guides are available in Whitaker *et al.* (2006) and Farrington *et al.* (2018).

22.4.1 A simple model

In the simplest SCCS model, originally described in Farrington (1995), the age effect $\theta(t)$ is also represented by a step function on J intervals covering $(a, b]$ where $b = \max\{b_i\}$, parameterised as a factor with levels 1 to J and J parameters α_j, α_1 being set to 0. Combined with the partition in risk and control exposure periods, this results in a partition of $(a_i, b_i]$ into sets A_{ijk} including those ages t at which individual i is in age category j and exposure category k. Let e_{ijk} denote the time duration spent by individual i in A_{ijk}. The model may be written

$$\lambda_i(t|v_i, \boldsymbol{x}_i) = \phi_i \exp\{g_i(\boldsymbol{x}_i) + \alpha_j + \beta_k\} \qquad \text{for } t \in A_{ijk}.$$

Note that

$$\int_{a_i}^{b_i} \lambda_i(s|v_i, \boldsymbol{x}_i) ds = \phi_i \exp\{g_i(\boldsymbol{x}_i)\} \sum_{j=1}^{J} \sum_{k=1}^{K} \exp(\alpha_j + \beta_k) e_{ijk}.$$

Suppose that individual i has r_i events, r_{ijk} occurring in age group j and exposure group k. Suppose that the sth event falls within age group j_s and exposure group k_s. The SCCS likelihood contribution for individual i is

$$L_i = \frac{\prod_{s=1}^{r_i} \exp(\alpha_{j_s} + \beta_{k_s})}{\left(\sum_{j=1}^{J} \sum_{k=1}^{K} \exp(\alpha_j + \beta_k) e_{ijk}\right)^{r_i}}.$$

This is equivalent to a multinomial likelihood with index r_i, responses $\{r_{ijk}\}$ and probabilities

$$p_{iuv} = \frac{\exp(\alpha_u + \beta_v)e_{iuv}}{\sum_{j=1}^{J} \sum_{k=1}^{K} \exp(\alpha_j + \beta_k)e_{ijk}}.$$

Thus the full SCCS likelihood is equivalent to a product multinomial likelihood, and can therefore be maximised using standard software for loglinear Poisson models with offsets. The specification of the model is

$$r_{ijk} \sim \text{Poisson}(\nu_{ijk}e_{ijk}),$$
$$\log(\nu_{ijk}) = \alpha_j + \beta_k + \gamma_i,$$

where the γ_i represent a nuisance individual factor with levels $i = 1, 2, \ldots, n$, required to keep the marginal event totals equal to those observed. This individual factor must be included to guarantee the equivalence of the Poisson model to the intended multinomial likelihood, but is of no intrinsic interest. When n is large, model fitting strategies that circumvent the estimation of the γ_i (for example by absorption) are desirable.

The SCCS likelihood is also akin to the conditional logistic model for $1 : M$ matched case-control studies, see Breslow and Day (1980, Chapter 7). The likelihood contribution for an individual i may equivalently be written as

$$L_i \propto \prod_{s=1}^{r_i} L_{is},$$

with

$$L_{is} = \frac{\exp(\alpha_{j_s} + \beta_{k_s})e_{ij_sk_s}}{\sum_{j=1}^{J} \sum_{k=1}^{K} \exp(\alpha_j + \beta_k)e_{ijk}}.$$

Each term L_{is} has the form of an individual contribution of a $1 : M_i$ matched case-control set, in which the M_i 'controls' are the control periods for SCCS case i and the 'case' is the period in which the sth event (for the ith SCCS case) occurs. This connection means that software designed to fit conditional logistic regression models can also be coaxed into fitting SCCS models.

22.4.2   Semiparametric model

The SCCS model described in Section 22.4.1 requires the specification of age groups. Misspecification of these age groups may result in biased estimates of the exposure effects when exposures are age-related. In the semiparametric model, the age effect is unspecified and determined by the data, the exposure categories remaining under the control of the analyst. This semiparametric model is described further in Farrington and Whitaker (2006).

Let $\mathbb{E} = \{t_1, t_2, \ldots, t_E\}$ denote the set of E distinct event ages experienced by the n individuals. The nonparametric maximum likelihood estimator of the cumulative relative age function $\Theta(t) = \int_a^t \theta(s)ds$, $t \in (a, b]$, is selected within the family of nondecreasing step functions constant outside $\mathbb{E}$ and with jumps $\exp(\alpha_s)$ at t_s. Let α_{ij} be the value α_u corresponding to t_{ij} (so that $t_{ij} = t_u$), the jth event age of individual i, and let w_{iu} be the indicator function taking the value 1 if $t_u \in (a_i, b_i]$ and the value 0 otherwise. The semiparametric SCCS likelihood is then

$$L = \prod_{i=1}^{n} \prod_{j=1}^{r_i} \frac{\exp\{\alpha_{ij} + \boldsymbol{v}_i(t_{ij})^T \boldsymbol{\beta}\}}{\sum_{r=1}^{E} w_{ir} \exp\{\alpha_r + \boldsymbol{v}_i(t_r)^T \boldsymbol{\beta}\}}.$$

This is again of product multinomial form, and may be fitted via an associated Poisson model, as follows. Let r_{iu} denote the number of events experienced by individual i at age t_u. The associated model is then

$$
\begin{aligned}
r_{iu} &\sim \text{Poisson}(\nu_{iu}), \\
\text{weight}(r_{iu}) &= w_{iu}, \\
\log(\nu_{iu}) &= \alpha_{iu} + \boldsymbol{v}_i(t_u)^T \boldsymbol{\beta} + \gamma_i.
\end{aligned}
$$

The main difference with the model described in Section 22.4.1 is that the model includes no offset, but does include the weights w_{iu}. As before, estimation of the large-dimensional nuisance parameters γ_i can be avoided by absorption. However, the parameter $\{\alpha_{iu}\}$ is also high-dimensional, since typically $E = O(n)$. In consequence, fitting the semiparametric model can be computationally demanding for large data sets. The model may also be fitted using software for conditional logistic regression, as previously described. This can also be computationally demanding owing to the high-dimensional age parameter.

22.4.3 Other SCCS models

As noted in Section 22.4.2, the semiparametric model can be computationally demanding for large data sets. It can also result in some loss of efficiency, when the age effect in fact follows a simple functional form. Two alternative methods have been proposed in this setting.

In Lee and Carlin (2014) it is suggested that the piecewise-constant age effect of Section 22.4.1 be retained, but with a larger number of age categories than would normally be used with this method. However, instead of using a separate parameter for each age category, the levels for each category are linked with a suitably flexible but parsimoniously parameterised functional form, such as a fractional polynomial. Thus, the log relative age-specific incidences are of the form

$$
\alpha_j = f(j|\boldsymbol{\delta})
$$

with f a fractional polynomial with low-dimensional parameter $\boldsymbol{\delta}$. The model may still be fitted with an associated Poisson model as in Section 22.4.1, the linear predictor for the intensity for individual i in age group j and exposure category k now being of the form

$$
\log(\nu_{ijk}) = f(j|\boldsymbol{\delta}) + \beta_k + \gamma_i.
$$

An advantage of this approach is that it remains within the loglinear modelling framework. However, it still makes use of a piecewise-constant age effect. A contrasting approach is that of Ghebremichael-Weldeselassie *et al.* (2014), in which the piecewise-constant model is eschewed in favour of a spline function. Thus, the age-specific relative incidence function $\theta(t)$ is modelled as

$$
\theta(t) = \sum_{s=1}^{S} \eta_s^2 M_s(t),
$$

namely a nonnegative linear combination of S cubic splines $M_s(t)$. The $M_s(t)$ are M-splines, whose integrals are corresponding I-splines; these are chosen to facilitate the calculation of the SCCS likelihood, which involves integrations in its denominator. The approach closely follows that of Joly *et al.* (1998), and proceeds by maximising a penalised likelihood, the smoothing parameter being chosen using an approximation to the cross-validation score. An advantage of this approach is that it lends itself to further extension to model the relative incidence associated with exposures also by splines, thus resulting in a fully nonparametric spline-based SCCS model (Ghebremichael-Weldeselassie, 2014).

22.5   Designing an SCCS study

In Section 22.2.2, the SCCS likelihood was derived from a Poisson cohort model by conditioning on the numbers of events experienced by each individual in the cohort over the entire observation period. Inversely, the case data for an SCCS analysis may often be thought of as being derived from an underlying cohort study, in which only the cases – that is, the individuals with one or more events – have been retained. This perspective is fruitful when it comes to designing an SCCS study.

22.5.1   Relative efficiency and sample size

It is instructive to consider the asymptotic efficiency of an SCCS design, compared to that of the underlying cohort model, for estimating the log relative incidence associated with exposure. For simplicity, we assume that the exposure is binary so there is a single log relative incidence parameter β. The asymptotic limit considered here is that in which the cohort size N, and hence the number of cases n within it, grows large.

Let $\text{var}(\hat{\beta})$ denote the variance of the estimator of β from an SCCS design, and $\text{var}(\hat{\beta}_c)$ the variance of the estimator from the underlying cohort obtained from a Poisson cohort model. The asymptotic relative efficiency is then

$$\text{ARE} = \lim_{N \to \infty} \frac{\text{var}(\hat{\beta}_c)}{\text{var}(\hat{\beta})}.$$

Because the SCCS estimator is conditional, one can expect that $\text{ARE} \leq 1$. Key insights are apparent in the simple scenario in which each individual has the same observation period, there are no age effects, a proportion p of the cohort is exposed and the risk period is a fixed proportion s of the observation period (Farrington and Whitaker, 2006). In this scenario,

$$\text{ARE} = \frac{1 + ps \exp(\beta)/(1 - ps)}{1 + s \exp(\beta)/(1 - s)}.$$

The ARE is close to 1 when p is close to 1 and s is close to 0. Thus, the loss of efficiency is least for common exposures and short risk periods. These conditions are often met in the case of routine childhood vaccinations, for example. In some circumstances, notably when working with large electronic databases, relative efficiency may be less of an issue. In such circumstances, an SCCS analysis may be indicated even for uncommon exposures and long risk periods if, for example, there is concern about confounding bias. This may arise, for example, in the study of adverse reactions to pharmaceutical drugs potentially subject to indication bias.

In the simplified setting just described, an approximate sample size formula for an SCCS study is:

$$n_e = \frac{(z_{1-\alpha/2} + z_\gamma)^2}{4\{\arcsin(\sqrt{e^\beta s/(e^\beta s + 1 - s)}) - \arcsin(\sqrt{s})\}^2},$$

where n_e denotes the number of events required in individuals who have been exposed during their observation period, and z_p is the p-quantile of the standard normal distribution (Musonda *et al.*, 2006). This sample size formula is for a two-sided test of the null hypothesis $\beta = 0$ at significance level $100\alpha\%$ and power $100\gamma\%$. (Note that unexposed cases can also be included in an SCCS analysis, and contribute to the estimation of the age effects.)

Sample size formulas such as this are useful mainly for rough preliminary calculations.

Age effects can seriously affect the power. Though more general approximate sample size formulas are available that take age into account (Musonda *et al.*, 2006), it may be advisable to undertake realistic simulations to study the power in situations where the study size is likely to be limited.

22.5.2 Risk and observation periods

Two key decisions when undertaking an SCCS study are the choice of risk and observation periods. The choice of risk period is usually based on empirical evidence from other studies, on expert knowledge, or on a specific prior hypothesis. Several contiguous risk periods can be used, with different log relative incidence parameters if it is thought that the relative incidence varies with time since exposure, or if the precise duration of the risk period is uncertain. Multiple exposures for each individual can be accommodated. In this case the log relative incidence parameters can be identical at each exposure, or different if there is thought to be a dose effect, and the evidence in support of these choices can be assessed in log likelihood ratio tests. The choice of observation period will depend on the specificities of the application. Two factors to consider are the duration of the risk period, and the variability of age at exposure. If the risk periods of interest are long, it makes little sense to choose short observation periods. On the other hand, better identifiability of age and exposure effects is obtained if the observation period spans the ages at which exposures occur. In some circumstances it is not possible to reconcile these two requirements: in this case, the inclusion of cases that have had no exposure can help to separate the age and exposure effects (Musonda *et al.*, 2008). In an extreme, and in practice unlikely, scenario, if exposures were to occur in all individuals at exactly the same age, then age and exposure effects would be wholly confounded unless unexposed cases were included.

When working with electronic databases, a typical specification of the observation period is to include all ages between ages A and B and between calendar dates C and D. This results in individuals having observation periods of different durations. This poses no problem for the SCCS analysis. An individual's exposure history is needed for all ages within that individual's observation period. Thus, if an individual's observation period is $(a_i, b_i]$ and the risk period of interest is of duration d, then exposure information will be required in $(a_i - d, b_i]$ in order to determine the exposure status at all ages in $(a_i, b_i]$.

22.6 An example: MMR vaccine and blood disorders

We illustrate some of the methods described with a data set relating to measles, mumps and rubella (MMR) vaccine and idiopathic thrombocytopenic purpura (ITP), a bleeding disorder, in children. The study was reported in Miller *et al.* (2001), with a slightly different data set from that used here. The events are admissions to hospital for ITP.

The file `sccsexample.r`, available from the website associated with this book, contains R script including the data and analysis described here.

22.6.1 A baseline parametric SCCS model

The observation period included all days between 1st October 1991 and 30th September 1994, and between days 366 and 730 of age, inclusive. All events within two English health regions occurring within this period were identified and linked to vaccine histories. The data comprise 44 events in 35 children: five children were admitted twice and one child was

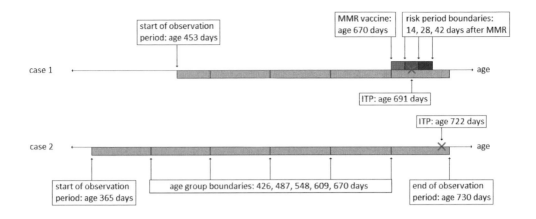

FIGURE 22.1
Schematic representation of the first two ITP cases.

admitted five times for ITP within the observation period. Time is measured in discrete days. To allow for variation in the incidence of ITP with age, the analysis uses six age groups: 366-426 days, 427-487 days, 488-548 days, 549-609 days, 610-670 days, and 671-730 days of age. In the primary analysis, three risk periods were used: 0-14 days, 15-28 days, and 29-42 days after MMR vaccination. Note that, in this analysis, the day of vaccination (day 0 after MMR) is included in the first risk period.

Figure 22.1 shows a diagrammatic representation of the first two cases. The first case is observed over the interval $(453, 730]$ days of age (and thus between days 454 and 730 inclusive), receives MMR vaccine at 670 days, and is admitted for ITP at 691 days. This being 21 days after MMR vaccination, the event occurs in the second risk period. The second case is observed over the interval $(365, 730]$ days of age, but only receives the MMR vaccine at 868 days of age. Thus no day of observation is included in a risk period. This case experiences the event at age 722 days.

The results for the baseline SCCS model described above are shown in Table 22.1. The relative incidence is greater than 1 in all three post-MMR risk periods, and is very significantly elevated in the 15-28 day risk period. However, the numbers of events in some of these risk periods is low. An analysis with all three risk periods combined into a single 0-42 day risk period gives a relative incidence of 3.23, 95% CI (1.53, 6.79). This suggests that there is a positive association between MMR vaccine and ITP.

22.6.2   Verifying the assumptions

We now investigate the robustness of the baseline model to the assumptions of the SCCS method. The method assumes that recurrences are independent within individuals. One way in which this may fail is if one event precipitates others; in an extreme form, events may be part of the same episode rather than genuinely distinct. One way to investigate this is to restrict the analysis to the 35 first events within the observation period; this is acceptable because ITP is a rare event. The results are in Table 22.2.

The point estimates are slightly higher than in the baseline analysis as all the recurrences

TABLE 22.1

Relative incidence (RI) and 95% confidence interval (CI) by risk period under the baseline model.

Risk period (days post-MMR)	Events	RI	95% CI
Unexposed	31	1.00	-
0 - 14	2	1.31	(0.30, 5.73)
15 - 28	8	5.95	(2.52, 14.1)
29 - 42	3	2.60	(0.75, 9.07)
0 - 42	13	3.23	(1.53, 6.79)

TABLE 22.2

Relative incidence (RI) and 95% confidence interval (CI) for first events only.

Risk period (days post-MMR)	Events	RI	95% CI
Unexposed	22	1.00	-
0 - 14	2	1.59	(0.36, 7.15)
15 - 28	8	7.19	(2.92, 17.7)
29 - 42	3	3.22	(0.89, 11.6)
0 - 42	13	3.94	(1.78, 8.72)

occurred in unexposed periods. However, the results convey essentially the same message as the baseline analysis. We conclude that the assumption of within-individual independence is not critical.

A second assumption is that events do not influence subsequent exposures. This may fail if, as is likely, occurrence of an ITP delays subsequent MMR vaccination. This may be examined by using a pre-MMR 'risk' period: if occurrence of ITP delays MMR vaccination, this will be reflected in a deficit of ITP admissions immediately prior to MMR vaccination. Table 22.3 presents the results of an analysis with a two-month pre-MMR 'risk' period, stretching from days 1 to 61 inclusive prior to receipt of the MMR vaccine.

The relative incidence for the 2-month period prior to MMR vaccination is indeed less than 1, though not significantly so. This provides weak support for the hypothesis that MMR vaccination is delayed after an ITP admission. As expected, the relative incidences for the three post-MMR risk periods, and for the combined risk period 0-42 days post MMR, are lower than those obtained for the baseline model, though not so substantially as

TABLE 22.3

Relative incidence (RI) and 95% confidence interval (CI) with a pre-MMR 'risk' period.

Risk period (days post-MMR)	Events	RI	95% CI
Unexposed	28	1.00	-
pre-MMR	3	0.49	(0.13, 1.85)
0 - 14	2	1.09	(0.24, 4.95)
15 - 28	8	5.02	(2.01, 12.5)
29 - 42	3	2.21	(0.61, 7.97)
0 - 42	13	2.72	(1.22, 6.09)

TABLE 22.4

Age effect for the baseline model: relative
incidence (RI) and 95% confidence interval.

Age group (days of age)	Events	RI	95% CI
366 - 426	16	1.00	-
427 - 487	11	0.66	(0.30, 1.46)
488 - 548	3	0.21	(0.06, 0.74)
549 - 609	4	0.29	(0.09, 0.90)
610 - 670	5	0.40	(0.14, 1.13)
671 - 730	5	0.40	(0.14, 1.15)

TABLE 22.5

Relative incidence (RI) and 95% confidence
interval (CI) by risk period under the
semiparametric model.

Risk period (days post-MMR)	Events	RI	95% CI
Unexposed	31	1.00	-
0 - 14	2	1.47	(0.32, 6.68)
15 - 28	8	5.52	(2.18, 13.9)
29 - 42	3	2.05	(0.56, 7.57)
0 - 42	13	3.03	(1.39, 6.63)

to alter the conclusions: the results are robust to short-term delay in vaccination following
an admission for ITP.

We now consider sensitivity to the choice of age groups. The baseline model used six
two-month age groups; the age effect in this model is shown in Table 22.4. This suggests
that the incidence of ITP (allowing for MMR vaccination) may vary with age. Fitting the
baseline model without any age effects produces a likelihood ratio test statistic of 10.28
on 5 degrees of freedom for the age effect: the corresponding p-value is 0.068. Thus, for
these data, the evidence for an age effect is weak. However, the estimated relative incidence
associated with MMR vaccination is moderately sensitive to age: if the age effect is omitted,
the relative incidence in the 0-42 day period increases from 3.23 to 4.53, 95% CI (2.27,
9.01). To investigate the robustness of the baseline model to the modelling of age, we fit
the semiparametric SCCS model. The results are shown in Table 22.5.

The results are only marginally different from those obtained using the baseline (parametric) model. We conclude that our conclusions are robust to our choice of age groups.
Note also that, with these data, use of the semiparametric model does not reduce markedly
the efficiency of the relative incidence estimates associated with MMR vaccination.

The final assumption of the SCCS model is that observation periods do not depend on
the event. In these data there is no censoring by death, or other occurrences that may be
associated with the event, and indeed all but six of the 35 cases have observation periods
spanning the maximum age duration, 366-730 days. Thus, this issue does not arise in the
present analysis.

22.6.3   Conclusions from the analysis

The overall conclusion from this analysis is that MMR vaccination in children aged one
year is associated with a three-fold increase in the risk of ITP admission in period 0-42

days following vaccination: the estimated relative incidence from the baseline parametric model is 3.23, 95% CI (1.53, 6.79). The relative risk appears to be highest in weeks 3 and 4 following MMR vaccination. There is some weak evidence that MMR vaccination is delayed after a hospital admission for ITP, but this does not substantially affect the conclusion.

22.7   Final remarks

The SCCS method works best for uncommon events that are not life changing. For such events, the assumptions of the SCCS model are often plausibly satisfied. For life-changing events, such as myocardial infarction and stroke, the SCCS method or its modifications may be useful when there is serious concern about potential confounding, notably confounding by indication. A good strategy is often to use and compare results from several methods of analysis, for example both a case-control analysis and an SCCS analysis based on the cases alone, as these methods rely on contrasting assumptions: for the case-control method, that all confounders have been included in the model; and for the SCCS method, that exposures are not event-related.

Bibliography

Andrews, N. J. (2002). Statistical assessment of the association between vaccination and rare adverse events post-licensure. *Vaccine*, **20**, S49–S53.

Breslow, N. E. and Day, N. E. (1980). *Statistical Methods in Cancer Research. Volume I: The Analysis of Case-Control Studies*. International Agency for Research on Cancer, Lyon.

Escolano, S., Hill, C., and Tubert-Bitter, P. (2013). A new self-controlled case series method for analyzing spontaneous reports of adverse events after vaccination. *American Journal of Epidemiology*, **20**, 1496–1504.

Farrington, C. P. (1995). Relative incidence estimation from case series for vaccine safety evaluation. *Biometrics*, **51**, 228–235.

Farrington, C. P. and Hocine, M. N. (2010). Within-individual dependence in self-controlled case series models for recurrent events. *Applied Statistics*, **59**, 457–475.

Farrington, C. P. and Whitaker, H. J. (2006). Semiparametric analysis of case series data (with discussion). *Journal of the Royal Statistical Society: Series C (Applied Statistics)*, **55**, 553–594.

Farrington, C. P., Whitaker, H. J., and Hocine, M. N. (2009). Case series analysis for censored, perturbed, or curtailed post-event exposures. *Biostatistics*, **10**, 3–16.

Farrington, C. P., Anaya-Izquierdo, K., Whitaker, H. J., Hocine, M. N., Douglas, I., and Smeeth, I. (2011). Self-controlled case series analysis with event-dependent observation periods. *Journal of the American Statistical Association*, **106**, 417–426.

Farrington, P., Whitaker, H., and Ghebremichael-Weldeselassie, Y. (2018). *Self-Controlled Case Series Studies: A modelling guide with R*. Chapman & Hall/CRC Press, Boca Raton.

Ghebremichael-Weldeselassie, Y. (2014). *Smooth Risk Functions for Self-Controlled Case Series Models*. PhD Thesis, The Open University, Milton Keynes.

Ghebremichael-Weldeselassie, Y., Whitaker, H. J., and Farrington, C. P. (2014). Self-controlled case series method with smooth age effect. *Statistics in Medicine*, **33**, 639–649.

Ghebremichael-Weldeselassie, Y., Whitaker, H. J., and Farrington, C. P. (2016). Flexible modelling of vaccine effect in self-controlled case series models. *Biometrical Journal*, **58**, 607–622.

Hubbard, R., Lewis, S., West, J., Smith, C., Godfrey, C., Smeeth, L., Farrington, P., and Britton, J. (2005). Bupropion and the risk of sudden death: A self-controlled case-series analysis using The Health Improvement Network. *Thorax*, **60**, 848–850.

Joly, P., Commenges, D., and Letenneur, L. (1998). Penalized likelihood approach for arbitrarily censored and truncated data: Application to age-specific incidence of dementia. *Biometrics*, **54**, 185–194.

Kuhnert, R., Hecker, H., Poethko-Muller, C., Schlaud, S., Vennemann, M., Whitaker, H. J., and Farrington, C. P. (2011). A modified self-controlled case series method to examine association between multidose vaccinations and death. *Statistics in Medicine*, **30**, 666–677.

Lee, K. J. and Carlin, J. B. (2014). Fractional polynomial adjustment for time-varying covariates in a self-controlled case series analysis. *Statistics in Medicine*, **33**, 105–116.

Miller, E., Waight, P., Farrington, P., Andrews, N., Stowe, J., and Taylor, B. (2001). Idiopathic thrombocytopenic purpura and MMR vaccine. *Archives of Disease in Childhood*, **84**, 227–229.

Miller, E., Goldacre, M., Pugh, S., Colville, A., Farrington, P., Flower, A., Nash, J., Macfarlane, L., and Tettmar, R. (2004). Risk of aseptic meningitis after measles, mumps and rubella vaccine in UK children. *Lancet*, **341**, 979–982.

Musonda, P., Farrington, C. P., and Whitaker, H. J. (2006). Sample sizes for self-controlled case series studies. *Statistics in Medicine*, **25**, 2618–2631. Erratum **27**, 4854–4856.

Musonda, P., Hocine, M. N., Whitaker, H. J., and Farrington, C. P. (2008). Self-controlled case series analyses: Small-sample performance. *Computational Statistics and Data Analysis*, **52**, 1942–1957.

Sardiñas, M. A. G., Cárdenas, A. Z., Coutin-Marie, G., Peña, M. S., Santiago, M. A., Sanchez, M. V., and Farrington, C. P. (2001). Lack of association between intussusception and oral polio vaccine in Cuban children. *Journal of the American Statistical Association*, **17**, 783–787.

Simpson, S. E. (2013). A positive dependence model for self-controlled case series with applications in postmarketing surveillance. *Biometrics*, **69**, 128–136.

Vines, S. K. and Farrington, C. P. (2001). Within-subject exposure dependency in case-crossover studies. *Statistics in Medicine*, **20**, 3039–3049.

Weldeselassie, Y. G., Whitaker, H. J., and Farrington, C. P. (2011). Use of the self-controlled case-series method in vaccine safety studies: Review and recommendations for best practice. *Epidemiology and Infection*, **139**, 1805–1817.

Whitaker, H., Hocine, M. N., and Farrington, C. P. (2007). On case-crossover methods for environmental time series data. *Environmetrics*, **18**, 157–171.

Whitaker, H. J., Farrington, C. P., Spiessens, B., and Musonda, P. (2006). Tutorial in biostatistics: The self-controlled case series method. *Statistics in Medicine*, **25**, 1768–1797.

Part V

Case-Control Studies in Genetic Epidemiology

23

Case-Control Designs for Modern Genome-Wide Association Studies: Basic Principles and Overview

Nilanjan Chatterjee

Johns Hopkins University

23.1   Background

Genetic linkage studies of highly affected families have long been used to identify genomic regions that harbor rare high penetrant mutations for various diseases and conditions (Botstein and Risch, 2003; Gusella *et al.*, 1983; Hall *et al.*, 1990; Kerem *et al.*, 1989; Nishisho *et al.*, 1991). The completion of the Human Genome Sequencing project (International Human Genome Sequencing Consortium *et al.*, 2001) in the beginning of this century and subsequent development of cost-effective large-scale genotyping and sequencing technologies ushered the era of genome-wide association studies (GWAS) in the last decade (Hirschhorn and Daly, 2005; McCarthy *et al.*, 2008; Wang *et al.*, 2005; Wellcome Trust Case Control Consortium *et al.*, 2007). These studies allowed studying association of a trait simultaneously with hundreds of thousands to millions of genetic markers across the genome by studying large number of individuals from the general population. Most GWAS to date have focused on common single nucleotide polymorphisms (SNPs), which are bi-allelic genetic markers that have minor allele frequency (MAF) 5% or higher in at least one major ethnic population. These studies have already led to the discovery of thousands of genetic susceptibility loci across a large variety of complex traits (MacArthur *et al.*, 2016; Visscher *et al.*, 2017). With the decreasing cost of sequencing technologies, GWAS are now beginning to shift its focus to low frequency ($0.5\% < \text{MAF} < 5\%$) and rare variants ($\text{MAF} < 0.5\%$) .

     The case-control study design has been widely popular for conducting GWAS for disease traits for multiple reasons. Unlike linkage studies, which focused on identification of high penetrant rare mutation, GWAS focus on discovery of more prevalent genetic variations that individually may have modest effects on the underlying diseases (Risch and Merikangas, 1996). In fact, recent analysis of genetic architecture shows that risks of complex diseases may be associated with thousands to tens of thousands of genetics markers, which, individually, may have very small effects, but in combination can explain substantial variation of disease-risk in the general population (Chatterjee *et al.*, 2016, 2013). Discovery of genetic loci that harbor disease predisposing variations with small effects requires comparing genetic profiles of large number of subjects with and without a disease, often in the order of tens of thousands. For relatively rare diseases, the case-control sampling design allows including a large number of diseased individuals in a study without incurring the cost associated with recruiting or/and genotyping/sequencing disproportionately large number of healthy individuals.

Case-control studies of genetic associations are also more immune to various types of biases that may otherwise arise for application of this design for investigation of epidemiologic risk factors (Clayton and McKeigue, 2001). First of all, inherited genetic variations, the main exposures of interest, are time invariant and thus can be ascertained in an objective fashion without concern about recall-bias and reverse causality that are typically faced in questionnaire administration or/and nongenetic biomarker evaluation in epidemiologic studies. Second, case-control studies can suffer from selection bias if cases and controls participate in a study in differential manner for reasons that are directly or indirectly related to the exposure of interest. As participants in epidemiologic studies are typically unaware of their genetic profiles, the concern of selection bias for studies of genetic association has been minimal to date. In the future, however, as genetic testing become more common, potential effect of selection bias may become a bigger concern (VanderWeele, 2010).

23.2   Study designs, quality control and bias corrections

GWAS require large scale ascertainment of genotypes across markers in the genome. For studies of common variants, GWAS have largely been carried out using various types of commercially available SNP-arrays which limits genotyping effort by taking advantage of the fact that physically proximal common SNPs are expected to show high-degree of linkage disequilibrium (Barrett and Cardon, 2006; Carlson *et al.*, 2004). In the early era, the arrays were designed to select a fixed number of SNP markers, typically in the range of 300K-1 million depending on ethnicity of the underlying population. These markers were selected in an agnostic but informative fashion so that a high proportion of all underlying ∼10 million common variants can be accurately "tagged," i.e., can be represented by surrogate markers in high correlation. Under such design, even if a true disease susceptibility marker is not genotyped, the underlying region could be identified through association testing using the tagging markers. More recent GWAS have used customized arrays that include promising SNPs identified from existing studies of groups of related traits, in addition to a backbone of tagging SNPs (Amos *et al.*, 2017; Cortes and Brown, 2011; Voight *et al.*, 2012).

As costs for sequencing technologies are decreasing rapidly, whole exome and whole genome sequencing technologies are now increasingly being used to conduct GWAS for rare variants (Cirulli and Goldstein, 2010; The UK10K Consortium *et al.*, 2015; Do *et al.*, 2012; Lee *et al.*, 2014; Zuk *et al.*, 2014). Unlike fixed-array genotyping, sequencing allows discovery of new rare variants in a population and simultaneous testing of their association with the underlying traits of interest. Population genetic theory predicts that there will be increasingly a large number of genetic variants with decreasing allele frequencies, and the number of rare genetic variants in a population, including those which may be unique to individuals, can be extremely large. While sequencing provides a more comprehensive catalog of genetic variations in the genome, there are number of challenges for using this technology for conducting GWAS. The noise associated with called genotypes in sequencing studies tend to be much higher than that is observed for genotype-based studies. Thus, chance for false positive findings due to differential errors between cases and controls is much higher. Further, power of these studies can be seriously limited due to multiplicity associated with testing large number of variants, sparsity of the individuals carrying rare variants and limited sample size for existing studies.

Case-control studies of genetic association can be affected by certain types of biases. Various types of uncertainty associated with variant calling can lead to differential misclassification between cases and controls (Clayton *et al.*, 2005). Differential error can arise due to different quality of biological samples, storage, processing, batching and calling algorithms. Imputation of untyped variants, a common practice for analysis of GWAS, can also cause differential error when genotyping platforms differ between cases and controls (Sinnott and Kraft, 2012). Differential misclassification, which can manifest to biased associations across large number of genetic markers, can cause serious problems in interpreting results from GWAS. The problem is best mitigated at the design stage so that the whole data generating process is as similar as possible between the selected cases and controls in the study. Further, after data generation is completed, strict quality control steps need to be followed to identify variants and individuals which may cause artifacts in the subsequent association analysis due to the poor quality of data.

Bias due to population stratification (PS), i.e., genetically heterogeneous substructures in the underlying population, could also be a major concern in case-control studies specially when cases and controls may not be selected from the same underlying study base (Cardon and Palmer, 2003; Pritchard and Donnelly, 2001; Thomas and Witte, 2002). While demographic information such as self-reported ethnicity and country of origin could be used as covariates to control for confounding bias in the usual manner, there remains concern for residual bias due to hidden substructure. Fortunately, as GWAS provide information on genetic markers across the whole genome, the high-dimensional genetic data itself can be used to detect and account for PS and some other types of systematic biases. The simplest of the methods is to adjust association test statistics across all the markers by a constant genomic-control (GC) factor λ_{GC}, which is defined as the median of the association statistics across SNPs divided by its theoretical value under the assumption of no associations (Devlin and Roeder, 1999). The advantage of GC method is that it can account for different types of structure in the data, including population structure due to recent genetic drift, family structure and cryptic relatedness, all of which is expected to lead to inflation in association statistics by a constant factor (Price *et al.*, 2010). The disadvantage is that the method can be overly conservative, especially in recent very large studies, where GC factors are expected to be large simply because of association signals associated with large number of polygenic effects.

Principal component analysis of genome-wide markers is also a popular method for adjustment of population-stratification and other types of structure that is expected to lead to long-distance linkage-disequilibrium or correlation across genetic markers (Price *et al.*, 2006). In this analysis, principal component analysis of the genetic markers is performed and a certain number of top eigenvectors are selected as covariates for subsequent association analysis. Intuitively, the top eigenvectors (EVs) are expected to capture directions across which large number of genetic markers will have significant co-variations in allele frequencies. As population stratification is expected to lead to large-scale variations in allele frequencies, adjustments of top EVs are expected to correct for hidden population structure. There are formal statistical tests available for selecting the eigenvectors based on statistical significance of the associated eigenvalues by evaluating against their expected null distribution under the assumption of no population structure (Johnstone, 2001).

Imputation has emerged as a powerful technique for increasing power for array-based genome-wide association studies (Howie *et al.*, 2012; Marchini and Howie, 2010). The technique allows inferring genotype status of markers that are not included in genotyping arrays by exploiting their linkage disequilibrium patterns with typed markers. Imputation algo-

TABLE 23.1
Example of genotype data represented as 2×3
contingency table.

	$G = AA(0)$	$G = Aa(1)$	$G = aa(2)$	Total
$D = 0$	r_0	r_1	r_2	r
$D = 1$	s_0	s_1	s_2	s
Total	n_0	n_1	n_2	n

rithms typically rely on a "reference sample" (The 1000 Genomes Project Consortium *et al.*, 2015; McCarthy *et al.*, 2016), which is assumed to have been sequenced for ascertainment of genotype profiles of participating individuals across all the underlying observable genetic variations. The reference sample is used as a training data set to build models for joint distribution of genotypes, taking into account population genetic theory of linkage disequilibrium patterns. These trained models are then used to make probabilistic prediction of genotype status of untyped markers based typed ones in GWAS. Imputation has been proven to be particularly powerful for testing association of low frequency and rare variants, which can be "tagged" or predicted accurately by combinations of, but not by individual, common variants included in the GWAS platforms. As the sample size for the reference data set increases, the algorithms become more precise for imputing increasingly rare variants.

23.3   Basic association analysis

Basic association analysis in case-control GWAS follows fairly standard techniques of hypothesis testing in the framework of contingency tables and logistic regression models. Genotype data for an individual bi-allelic SNP marker can be represented as a trinomial outcome corresponding to three possible combination of alleles an individual may carry in the pair of homologous chromosomes. Thus, for a given marker, if A and a denote the major, i.e., the more common form, and the minor allele, respectively, then the genotype (G) of an individual can take value AA, Aa or aa. Numerically, genotype data are often coded as 0, 1 or 2 corresponding to the number of a specific allele, say a, it contains. Thus, the available genotype data in a case-control study can be represented in 2×3 contingency tables of the form given in Table 23.1.

The null hypothesis of no association between case-control status D, taking value 1 for case and 0 for control, and genotype G can be tested based on standard two degrees-of-freedom chi-square test for independence for contingency tables (Agresti, 2013). A more powerful test, however, can be performed taking into account the natural ordering of the three genotype values using the Armitage-Cochran trend test statistics in the form (Armitage, 1955; Cochran, 1954)

$$Z^2 = \frac{\frac{r \times s}{n} \times \left[\sum_{k=0}^{2} x_k \times \left(\frac{r_k}{r} - \frac{s_k}{s} \right) \right]^2}{\left[\left(\sum_{k=0}^{2} x_k^2 \times \frac{n_k}{n} \right) - \sum_{k=0}^{2} x_k \times \frac{n_k}{n} \right]^2}, \tag{23.1}$$

where $(x_0, x_1, x_2) = (0, 0.5, 1)$ represent a dosage assigned to genotypes according to the model that assumes risk of the disease changes in a linear fashion per copy of an allele.

More generally, association testing with respect to individual markers in case-control studies is performed using a logistic regression model that includes SNP-genotype data as the main exposure of interest and additionally adjusts for covariates like principal components of population stratification. Typically, the model is specified as

$$\log\left(\frac{P(D=1)}{P(D=0)}\right) = \alpha + \beta G + \boldsymbol{\gamma}^T \boldsymbol{C}, \tag{23.2}$$

where G denotes the genotype data coded as 0, 1 or 2 and $\boldsymbol{C}$ is a vector of potential confounders. The null hypothesis of no association, which corresponds to $H_0 : \beta = 0$, can be tested using Wald, likelihood-ratio or score tests. In practice, the use of score tests is very popular as it requires fitting the null model, which is the same across all the markers, only once and thus avoids computational burdens associated with separate model fittings for hundreds of thousands to millions of genetic markers. Further, under score tests, markers with imputed genotypes can easily be handled by simply replacing genotype-dosage with its expected value calculated under assigned probabilities returned by the imputation algorithm. It is noteworthy that the Cochran-Armitage trend test described above can be derived also in the form of a score test under the logistic regression model when no additional covariates are involved.

Typically, the effect of case-control sampling can be ignored for standard single-variant association tests under the logistic regression model. When no assumptions are invoked regarding joint distribution of genotype (G) and covariates ($\boldsymbol{C}$), standard analysis based on the prospective likelihood is expected to be both valid and fully efficient because of the well-known equivalence of prospective and retrospective likelihood in this setting. More efficient analysis, however, is possible using a retrospective likelihood by invoking the Hardy-Weinberg equilibrium (HWE) model for genotype frequencies. In particular, it has been shown that testing for association under nonadditive models, such as those that could be obtained by dominant, recessive or saturated coding of the genotypes, can be improved substantially by incorporating the HWE assumption into the retrospective likelihood (Chen and Chatterjee, 2007; Luo *et al.*, 2009). The result is analogous to improvement in efficiency in analysis of gene-environment interactions based on the retrospective likelihood, a topic which has received detailed treatment in this book in Chapter 24.

23.4 Multi-marker association testing

Power for single-marker association tests may be low due to weak effects or/and low frequency of individual causal variants. To see this, we observe that the association test statistics for an individual variant (m) can be written in the form

$$Z_m^2 = \frac{T_m^2}{\text{Var}(T_m)}, \tag{23.3}$$

which follow one degree-of-freedom chi-square distribution with a noncentrality parameter in the form

$$nc_m = 2p_m(1-p_m)\beta_m^2 \times \frac{N_1 \times N_0}{N_1 + N_0}. \tag{23.4}$$

Above, the term $2p_m(1-p_m)$ corresponds to variance of genotype G_m under the assumption of Hardy-Weinberg equilibrium and allele frequency p_m, β_m denotes effect size, and $N_d, d = 0, 1$, denote the number of controls and cases, respectively.

A large number of methods have been proposed to improve power for detecting association for an underlying genomic region by aggregation of association signals across multiple markers (Derkach *et al.*, 2018; Lee *et al.*, 2012; Li and Leal, 2008; Lin and Tang, 2011; Madsen and Browning, 2009; Neale *et al.*, 2011; Wu *et al.*, 2011). Particularly popular are two classes of aggregated tests, sum-based tests and variance-component tests. Sum-based tests aggregate variant level association statistics by a linear combination in the forms $T_{ST} = \sum_{m=1}^{M} w_m T_m$ and variance component tests aggregate by quadratic combination in the form $T_{VC} = \sum_{m=1}^{M} w_m T_m^2$, where the w_ms are weights that take into account various extraneous information, including allele frequencies, on the marker, and the T_ms are the numerator of the association statistics, e.g., score statistics, as defined above, for the individual genetic markers ($m = 1, \ldots, M$). The sum-based test has standard distribution theory as it is defined by linear combinations of normal variates. The variance-component test follows a scaled mixture of chi-square distributions. For case-control studies, the underlying score statistics are typically derived from a logistic regression model and thus the effect of case-control sampling can be ignored given the known equivalence between prospective and retrospective likelihood under this model.

23.5   Fitting mixed models

Standard association analyses in GWAS to date have led to identification of dozens and sometimes hundreds of common susceptibility SNPs associated with individual diseases, such as breast cancer, heart disease and type-2 diabetes. It is yet possible that there are many SNPs, which may be associated with a given disease, but may not have reached stringent genome-wide significance level (typically $p = 0.5 \times 10^{-8}$) used for discovery, due to limited power of the current studies. Remarkably, fitting of mixed models in existing GWAS can allow one to estimate how much variation of the risk of a disease can potentially be explained by the whole GWAS-panel of SNPs, thus including effects of susceptibility SNPs yet to be discovered (Lee *et al.*, 2013; Yang *et al.*, 2010, 2011). Such quantification of "narrow sense" heritability, i.e., the degree of the variation of a trait that could be explained by the additive effects of a large panel of underlying variants, can be very useful for understanding the future potential of various types of GWAS, e.g., those based on common versus rare variants, to explain genetic basis of complex diseases (Gibson, 2012). Further, power for association testing for individual genetic markers can also be enhanced by fitting of mixed models that allows adjustment for effects of all underlying susceptibility markers simultaneously (Yang *et al.*, 2014; Zhou and Stephens, 2012).

Statistically speaking, inferring heritability requires fitting a joint model involving all SNPs in the GWAS through suitable regularization technique. A multi-SNP model for association, for example, can be defined based on the logistic regression model as

$$\log\left(\frac{P(D=1)}{P(D=0)}\right) = \alpha + \sum_{m=1}^{M} \beta_m G_m + \boldsymbol{\gamma}^T \boldsymbol{C}. \tag{23.5}$$

The most popular approach for regularization is to use an underlying random-effect model under the assumption that β_m's are independently and identically distributed as a normal random variable with mean 0 and variance σ^2. Under this model, if we assume genotypes are standardized so that $\mathrm{Var}(G_m) = 1$, then $\sigma^2 = E(\beta_m^2)$ can be interpreted as per SNP heritability (in the logit-scale) and $h^2 = M \times \sigma^2$ as the total heritability.

Fitting of mixed models to GWAS has been a major focus of research in the last decade. There are major computational bottlenecks in dealing with high dimensional genetic markers and large sample sizes simultaneously. As fitting of nonlinear mixed models is even more challenging, somewhat ad hoc methods have been proposed to fit linear mixed models for disease outcome data and then transforming parameters for obtaining estimate of heritability in a more interpretable scale. Moreover, for case-control studies, there are additional complexities in dealing with nonrandom sampling of subjects – the topic is addressed in detail in Chapter 27 of this book.

23.6   Conclusion

The case-control study design has been fundamental to success for recent GWAS in providing deep insight into the genetic basis of complex diseases. For studies of inherited genetic variations, the design is immune to certain types of biases, including those due to reverse causality and nondifferential selection, which usually are considered of major concern for conducting epidemiologic studies. Further, the large scale genetic data available in GWAS itself can be utilized to correct for other types of biases, such as those due to hidden population structure and batch effects. It can be anticipated the design will continue to play a critical role in the future as GWAS shifts focus from studies of common to low-frequency and rare variants.

This chapter provides a brief overview of basic design and analysis issues for case-control studies in genetic epidemiology. The remaining chapters in Part V of the handbook address various advanced topics for analysis. Chapters 24 and 25 address modern methods for analysis and exploration of gene-environment interactions under the case-control design. Chapter 26 addresses design and analysis issues for family-based case-control studies where cases and controls are sampled in a matched fashion from the same families. Chapter 27 addresses methods for fitting mixed models with high-dimensional genetic data under the case-control sampling scheme. Chapter 28 addresses methodological issues related to genetic association analysis of outcomes other than the primary disease endpoint under the case-control sampling scheme.

Bibliography

Agresti, A. (2013). *Categorical Data Analysis*. John Wiley & Sons, Hoboken, New Jersey.

Amos, C. I., Dennis, J., Wang, Z., Byun, J., Schumacher, F. R., Gayther, S. A., Casey, G., Hunter, D. J., Sellers, T. A., Gruber, S. B., *et al.* (2017). The OncoArray Consortium: A network for understanding the genetic architecture of common cancers. *Cancer Epidemiology and Prevention Biomarkers*, **26**, 126–135.

Armitage, P. (1955). Tests for linear trends in proportions and frequencies. *Biometrics*, **11**, 375–386.

Barrett, J. C. and Cardon, L. R. (2006). Evaluating coverage of genome-wide association studies. *Nature Genetics*, **38**, 659–662.

Botstein, D. and Risch, N. (2003). Discovering genotypes underlying human phenotypes: Past successes for Mendelian disease, future approaches for complex disease. *Nature Genetics*, **33**, 228–237.

Cardon, L. R. and Palmer, L. J. (2003). Population stratification and spurious allelic association. *The Lancet*, **361**, 598–604.

Carlson, C. S., Eberle, M. A., Rieder, M. J., Yi, Q., Kruglyak, L., and Nickerson, D. A. (2004). Selecting a maximally informative set of single-nucleotide polymorphisms for association analyses using linkage disequilibrium. *The American Journal of Human Genetics*, **74**, 106–120.

Chatterjee, N., Wheeler, B., Sampson, J., Hartge, P., Chanock, S. J., and Park, J.-H. (2013). Projecting the performance of risk prediction based on polygenic analyses of genome-wide association studies. *Nature Genetics*, **45**, 400–405.

Chatterjee, N., Shi, J., and García-Closas, M. (2016). Developing and evaluating polygenic risk prediction models for stratified disease prevention. *Nature Reviews Genetics*, **17**, 392–406.

Chen, J. and Chatterjee, N. (2007). Exploiting Hardy-Weinberg equilibrium for efficient screening of single SNP associations from case-control studies. *Human Heredity*, **63**, 196–204.

Cirulli, E. T. and Goldstein, D. B. (2010). Uncovering the roles of rare variants in common disease through whole-genome sequencing. *Nature Reviews Genetics*, **11**, 415–425.

Clayton, D. and McKeigue, P. M. (2001). Epidemiological methods for studying genes and environmental factors in complex diseases. *The Lancet*, **358**, 1356–1360.

Clayton, D. G., Walker, N. M., Smyth, D. J., Pask, R., Cooper, J. D., Maier, L. M., Smink, L. J., Lam, A. C., Ovington, N. R., Stevens, H. E., , Nutland, S., Howson, J. M. M., Faham, M., Moorhead, M., Jones, H. B., Falkowski, M., Hardenbol, P., Willis, T. D., and Todd, J. A. (2005). Population structure, differential bias and genomic control in a large-scale, case-control association study. *Nature Genetics*, **37**, 1243–1246.

Cochran, W. G. (1954). Some methods for strengthening the common chi-squared tests. *Biometrics*, **10**, 417–451.

Cortes, A. and Brown, M. A. (2011). Promise and pitfalls of the immunochip. *Arthritis Research and Therapy*, **13**, 101.

Derkach, A., Zhang, H., and Chatterjee, N. (2018). Power analysis for genetic association test (PAGEANT) provides insights to challenges for rare variant association studies. *Bioinformatics*, **34**, 1506–1513.

Devlin, B. and Roeder, K. (1999). Genomic control for association studies. *Biometrics*, **55**, 997–1004.

Do, R., Kathiresan, S., and Abecasis, G. R. (2012). Exome sequencing and complex disease: Practical aspects of rare variant association studies. *Human Molecular Genetics*, **21**, R1–R9.

Gibson, G. (2012). Rare and common variants: Twenty arguments. *Nature Reviews Genetics*, **13**, 135–145.

Gusella, J. F., Wexler, N. S., Conneally, P. M., Naylor, S. L., Anderson, M. A., Tanzi, R. E., Watkins, P. C., Ottina, K., Wallace, M. R., Sakaguchi, A. Y., Young, A. B., Shoulson, I., Bonilla, E., and Martin, J. B. (1983). A polymorphic DNA marker genetically linked to Huntington's disease. *Nature*, **306**, 234–238.

Hall, J. M., Lee, M. K., Newman, B., Morrow, J. E., Anderson, L. A., Huey, B., and King, M.-C. (1990). Linkage of early-onset familial breast cancer to chromosome 17q21. *Science*, **250**, 1684–1689.

Hirschhorn, J. N. and Daly, M. J. (2005). Genome-wide association studies for common diseases and complex traits. *Nature Reviews Genetics*, **6**, 95–108.

Howie, B., Fuchsberger, C., Stephens, M., Marchini, J., and Abecasis, G. R. (2012). Fast and accurate genotype imputation in genome-wide association studies through pre-phasing. *Nature Genetics*, **44**, 955–959.

International Human Genome Sequencing Consortium *et al.* (2001). Initial sequencing and analysis of the human genome. *Nature*, **409**, 860–921.

Johnstone, I. M. (2001). On the distribution of the largest eigenvalue in principal components analysis. *Annals of Statistics*, **29**, 295–327.

Kerem, B., Rommens, J. M., Buchanan, J. A., Markiewicz, D., Cox, T. K., Chakravarti, A., Buchwald, M., and Tsui, L.-C. (1989). Identification of the cystic fibrosis gene: Genetic analysis. *Science*, **245**, 1073–1080.

Lee, S., Wu, M. C., and Lin, X. (2012). Optimal tests for rare variant effects in sequencing association studies. *Biostatistics*, **13**, 762–775.

Lee, S., Abecasis, G. R., Boehnke, M., and Lin, X. (2014). Rare-variant association analysis: Study designs and statistical tests. *The American Journal of Human Genetics*, **95**, 5–23.

Lee, S. H., Yang, J., Chen, G.-B., Ripke, S., Stahl, E. A., Hultman, C. M., Sklar, P., Visscher, P. M., Sullivan, P. F., Goddard, M. E., and R., W. N. (2013). Estimation of SNP heritability from dense genotype data. *The American Journal of Human Genetics*, **93**, 1151–1155.

Li, B. and Leal, S. M. (2008). Methods for detecting associations with rare variants for common diseases: Application to analysis of sequence data. *The American Journal of Human Genetics*, **83**, 311–321.

Lin, D.-Y. and Tang, Z.-Z. (2011). A general framework for detecting disease associations with rare variants in sequencing studies. *The American Journal of Human Genetics*, **89**, 354–367.

Luo, S., Mukherjee, B., Chen, J., and Chatterjee, N. (2009). Shrinkage estimation for robust and efficient screening of single-SNP association from case-control genome-wide association studies. *Genetic Epidemiology*, **33**, 740–750.

MacArthur, J., Bowler, E., Cerezo, M., Gil, L., Hall, P., Hastings, E., Junkins, H., McMahon, A., Milano, A., Morales, J., Pendlington, Z. M., Welter, D., Burdett, T., Hindorff, L., Flicek, P., Cunningham, F., and Parkinson, H. (2016). The new NHGRI-EBI Catalog of published genome-wide association studies (GWAS catalog). *Nucleic Acids Research*, **45**, D896–D901.

Madsen, B. E. and Browning, S. R. (2009). A groupwise association test for rare mutations using a weighted sum statistic. *PLoS Genetics*, **5**, e1000384.

Marchini, J. and Howie, B. (2010). Genotype imputation for genome-wide association studies. *Nature Reviews Genetics*, **11**, 499–511.

McCarthy, M. I., Abecasis, G. R., Cardon, L. R., Goldstein, D. B., Little, J., Ioannidis, J. P., and Hirschhorn, J. N. (2008). Genome-wide association studies for complex traits: Consensus, uncertainty and challenges. *Nature Reviews Genetics*, **9**, 356–369.

McCarthy, S., Das, S., Kretzschmar, W., Delaneau, O., Wood, A. R., Teumer, A., Kang, H. M., Fuchsberger, C., Danecek, P., Sharp, K., *et al.* (2016). A reference panel of 64,976 haplotypes for genotype imputation. *Nature Genetics*, **48**, 1279–1283.

Neale, B. M., Rivas, M. A., Voight, B. F., Altshuler, D., Devlin, B., Orho-Melander, M., Kathiresan, S., Purcell, S. M., Roeder, K., and Daly, M. J. (2011). Testing for an unusual distribution of rare variants. *PLoS Genetics*, **7**, e1001322.

Nishisho, I., Nakamura, Y., Miyoshi, Y., Miki, Y., Ando, H., Horii, A., Koyama, K., Utsunomiya, J., Baba, S., and Hedge, P. (1991). Mutations of chromosome 5q21 genes in FAP and colorectal cancer patients. *Science*, **253**, 665–669.

Price, A. L., Patterson, N. J., Plenge, R. M., Weinblatt, M. E., Shadick, N. A., and Reich, D. (2006). Principal components analysis corrects for stratification in genome-wide association studies. *Nature Genetics*, **38**, 904–909.

Price, A. L., Zaitlen, N. A., Reich, D., and Patterson, N. (2010). New approaches to population stratification in genome-wide association studies. *Nature Reviews Genetics*, **11**, 459–463.

Pritchard, J. K. and Donnelly, P. (2001). Case–control studies of association in structured or admixed populations. *Theoretical Population Biology*, **60**, 227–237.

Risch, N. and Merikangas, K. (1996). The future of genetic studies of complex human diseases. *Science*, **273**, 1516–1517.

Sinnott, J. A. and Kraft, P. (2012). Artifact due to differential error when cases and controls are imputed from different platforms. *Human Genetics*, **131**, 111–119.

The 1000 Genomes Project Consortium *et al.* (2015). A global reference for human genetic variation. *Nature*, **526**, 68–74.

The UK10K Consortium *et al.* (2015). The UK10K project identifies rare variants in health and disease. *Nature*, **526**, 82–90.

Thomas, D. C. and Witte, J. S. (2002). Point: Population stratification: A problem for case-control studies of candidate-gene associations? *Cancer Epidemiology, Biomarkers and Prevention*, **11**, 505–512.

VanderWeele, T. (2010). Genetic self knowledge and the future of epidemiologic confounding. *The American Journal of Human Genetics*, **87**, 168–172.

Visscher, P. M., Wray, N. R., Zhang, Q., Sklar, P., McCarthy, M. I., Brown, M. A., and Yang, J. (2017). 10 years of GWAS discovery: Biology, function, and translation. *The American Journal of Human Genetics*, **101**, 5–22.

Voight, B. F., Kang, H. M., Ding, J., Palmer, C. D., Sidore, C., Chines, P. S., Burtt, N. P., Fuchsberger, C., Li, Y., Erdmann, J., *et al.* (2012). The Metabochip, a custom genotyping array for genetic studies of metabolic, cardiovascular, and anthropometric traits. *PLoS Genetics*, **8**, e1002793.

Wang, W. Y., Barratt, B. J., Clayton, D. G., and Todd, J. A. (2005). Genome-wide association studies: Theoretical and practical concerns. *Nature Reviews Genetics*, **6**, 109–118.

Wellcome Trust Case Control Consortium *et al.* (2007). Genome-wide association study of 14,000 cases of seven common diseases and 3,000 shared controls. *Nature*, **447**, 661–678.

Wu, M. C., Lee, S., Cai, T., Li, Y., Boehnke, M., and Lin, X. (2011). Rare-variant association testing for sequencing data with the sequence kernel association test. *The American Journal of Human Genetics*, **89**, 82–93.

Yang, J., Benyamin, B., McEvoy, B. P., Gordon, S., Henders, A. K., Nyholt, D. R., Madden, P. A., Heath, A. C., Martin, N. G., Montgomery, G. W., Goddard, M. E., and Visscher, P. M. (2010). Common SNPs explain a large proportion of the heritability for human height. *Nature Genetics*, **42**, 565–569.

Yang, J., Lee, S. H., Goddard, M. E., and Visscher, P. M. (2011). GCTA: A tool for genome-wide complex trait analysis. *The American Journal of Human Genetics*, **88**, 76–82.

Yang, J., Zaitlen, N. A., Goddard, M. E., Visscher, P. M., and Price, A. L. (2014). Advantages and pitfalls in the application of mixed-model association methods. *Nature Genetics*, **46**, 100–106.

Zhou, X. and Stephens, M. (2012). Genome-wide efficient mixed-model analysis for association studies. *Nature Genetics*, **44**, 821–824.

Zuk, O., Schaffner, S. F., Samocha, K., Do, R., Hechter, E., Kathiresan, S., Daly, M. J., Neale, B. M., Sunyaev, S. R., and Lander, E. S. (2014). Searching for missing heritability: Designing rare variant association studies. *Proceedings of the National Academy of Sciences*, **111**, E455–E464.

Analysis of Gene-Environment Interactions

Summer S. Han

Stanford University

Raymond J. Carroll

Texas A&M University & University of Technology Sydney

Nilanjan Chatterjee

Johns Hopkins University

24.1 Introduction

Understanding the interplay between genes (G) and environmental risk factors (E) is important to evaluate the etiology of complex disease; it is understood that genes do not operate in isolation but rather in complex networks and pathways influenced by environmental factors. In addition, the discovery of novel susceptibility loci for complex disease may be enhanced by identifying gene-environment interactions, where genetic effects are modified, and, sometimes, masked by the effects of environmental factors (Eichler *et al.*, 2010; Thompson, 1991; Ottman, 1996). Ignoring these interactions can lead to incorrect estimates of the proportions of a disease that are explained by the environment, genes, and their joint effect in epidemiological studies. Eventually, identifying gene-environment interaction may also help develop strategies for targeted intervention in public health and help implement personalized medicine; applying an intervention focusing on a subset of the population that is identified by gene-environment interactions can provide efficiency in disease prevention (Hutter *et al.*, 2013; Maas *et al.*, 2016; Wacholder *et al.*, 2002; Thomas, 2010; Clayton and McKeigue, 2001).

While a gene-environment interaction has various meanings in epidemiology, it can be generally defined as a joint effect of genetic and environmental risk factors that cannot be explained by their separate marginal effects (Thomas, 2010). A common statistical definition of interaction depends on the concept of a disease risk model that describes the relationship between a response disease outcome and genetic and environmental factors, which will be further described in Section 24.2. Statistically, an interaction can be measured as a departure from the underlying disease risk model, which can be tested by examining whether the cross product term based on genetic and environmental effects is zero or not.

There are several study designs for evaluating gene-environment interactions, including cohort studies, case-control study designs, and family-based studies. A prospective cohort study can be ideal for evaluating the interactions between genetic and environmental factors, which recruits healthy individuals and follows them over time to observe disease incidence (Chatterjee and Mukherjee, 2008). In particular, cohort studies allow objective pre-diagnostic measurement of environmental exposures, which, unlike genetic factors, can change over time and can be altered by the disease itself. However, cohort studies can be expensive for rare diseases because most of the subjects would remain disease-free during the study period, while collecting demographic and exposure information is needed for a very large number of participants for a long time. On the other hand, case-control studies can be more cost-effective by reducing the number of unaffected subjects included in the study (Chatterjee and Mukherjee, 2008). One disadvantage of case-control studies is that the estimate of environmental effect could be biased due to the presence of various types of differential recall in addition to selection and misclassification biases by case-control status and exposures of interest (Wacholder *et al.*, 1992a,b; Mandel *et al.*, 1992). As the inherited genetic susceptibility of individuals does not change over time and is unlikely to affect study participation, case-control studies have proven to be robust for studying genetic main effects through modern genome-wide association studies (GWAS). Moreover, it has been argued that case-control studies are expected to be robust for studying gene-environment interactions in the multiplicative scale even in the presence of various types of biases that may distort the main effect of environmental exposure (Wacholder *et al.*, 2002; Clayton and McKeigue, 2001).

In this chapter, we will focus on case-control design and review various methods of testing for gene-environment interactions. In Section 24.2, we will introduce several disease risk models for modeling the joint effects of genetic (G) and environmental (E) factors including multiplicative, additive, and liability threshold models. In Section 24.3, several methods for estimating interaction parameters (mainly using multiplicative and additive models) will be introduced, including the standard inference method using a prospective likelihood, case-only methods, log-linear models, and retrospective-likelihood methods, all of which incorporate an assumption of gene-environment independence, and an empirical Bayes-type method that can provide a bridge between alternative methods to balance a trade-off between bias and variance. The application of these methods will be illustrated with R code using an R package CGEN (https://bioconductor.org/packages/release/bioc/html/CGEN.html). In Section 24.4, we will describe various methods of testing for genetic associations in the presence of gene-environment interactions. The chapter concludes with an overall summary and a discussion about future challenges in Section 24.5.

Data description: NAT2 and smoking for bladder cancer

In order to illustrate various methods for detecting gene-environment interactions, we will use the National Cancer Institute (NCI) bladder cancer data for testing the interactions between a SNP genetic marker in the N-acetyltransferase 2 (NAT2) gene and smoking status (Rothman *et al.*, 2010). The interaction between smoking and NAT2 is one of the well-established gene-environment interactions, in which the NAT2 slow acetylation genotype has been shown to be associated with an elevated relative risk of bladder cancer in current/former smokers but not in never smokers (Garcia-Closas *et al.*, 2005). These data include 5,942 cases and 10,857 controls from five different studies conducted at NCI: the Prostate, Lung, Colorectal and Ovarian (PLCO) cancer screening trial, the Spanish Bladder Cancer Study (SPBC), the Alpha-Tocopherol, Beta-Carotene Cancer Prevention (ATBC) study, the New England Bladder Cancer Study, Maine and Vermont components (NEBCS-ME/VT), and the American Cancer Society Cancer Prevention Study II Nutrition Cohort (CPS-II). The details of the designs of these studies are already published (Rothman *et al.*, 2010; Figueroa *et al.*, 2014). We will investigate the interaction between the SNP rs1495741 in NAT2 and smoking status. All analyses will be adjusted for age, gender, and study site.

24.2 Models for gene-environment interaction

24.2.1 Multiplicative model and logistic regression to approximate multiplicative model

Interaction has diverse meanings in the epidemiologic literature (Cordell, 2002), and there has been a long-standing controversy concerning its definition and the selection of proper scales for measuring the presence of interactions (Rothman *et al.*, 1980; Walter and Holford, 1978). An interaction test based on the logistic model – which approximates the multiplicative risk for rare diseases – has been widely used for analyses of case-control studies of disease traits. A test for interaction under the logistic model corresponds to a test for interaction on the odds ratio scale.

24.2.1.1 Logistic regression for a multiplicative model under a rare disease assumption

Suppose that for subject i, G_i is a genotype of a single nucleotide polymorphism (SNP), E_i is an environmental risk factor, and D_i is the disease status. Additive effects of G_i and E_i on the logistic scale (or log odds ratio scale) are specified as:

$$\text{logit}\{P(D_i = 1|G_i, E_i)\} = \log\left(\frac{P(D_i = 1|G_i, E_i)}{1 - P(D_i = 1|G_i, E_i)}\right) = \beta_0 + \beta_G G_i + \beta_E E_i. \quad (24.1)$$

This is equivalent to multiplicative effects of G and E on the odds scale:

$$\frac{P(D_i = 1|G_i, E_i)}{1 - P(D_i = 1|G_i, E_i)} = \exp(\beta_0 + \beta_G G_i + \beta_E E_i) = \exp(\beta_0)\exp(\beta_G G_i)\exp(\beta_E E_i).$$

For rare diseases, $P(D_i = 1|G_i, E_i)$ is close to zero with

$$\frac{P(D_i = 1|G_i, E_i)}{1 - P(D_i = 1|G_i, E_i)} \approx P(D_i = 1|G_i, E_i),$$

and hence the above model approximates a multiplicative model on the scale of the absolute risk of the disease.

TABLE 24.1
Odds ratio table for binary factors G and E.

	$E = 0$	$E = 1$
$G = 0$	$1 \;(= OR_{00})$	$\exp(\beta_E) \;(= OR_{01})$
$G = 1$	$\exp(\beta_G) \;(= OR_{10})$	$\exp(\beta_G + \beta_E + \beta_{GE}) \;(= OR_{11})$

24.2.1.2   Multiplicative Interaction

A departure from the multiplicative model in Eq. (24.1) is called a multiplicative interaction, which can be measured by testing whether an additional interaction term is zero or not, i.e.,

$$H_0 : \beta_{GE} = 0, \tag{24.2}$$

in the following model:

$$\mathrm{logit}\{P(D_i = 1 | G_i, E_i)\} = \beta_0 + \beta_G G_i + \beta_E E_i + \beta_{GE} G_i E_i. \tag{24.3}$$

Consider Table 24.1 that shows 2×2 odds ratios, OR_{ge}, ($g = 0, 1$ and $e = 0, 1$), assuming two levels for G and E for simplicity. The null hypothesis of a multiplicative interaction in Eq. (24.2) is equivalent to:

$$H_0 : OR_{11} = OR_{10} OR_{01}. \tag{24.4}$$

That is, the odds ratio when an individual is exposed to both environmental and genetic risk factors (OR_{11}) is equivalent to the product of the odds ratios when one is exposed to only one of the two factors, i.e., $OR_{10} OR_{01}$.

Without loss of generality, we assume in Table 24.1 that $G = 1$ and $E = 1$ corresponds to "at-risk" categories, so that $OR_{10} \geqslant 1$ and $OR_{01} \geqslant 1$. When the joint effect is larger than the product of two marginal odds ratios, i.e., $OR_{11} > OR_{10} OR_{01}$ ($\beta_{GE} > 0$), the interaction is called supra-multiplicative while it is called sub-multiplicative when the direction is opposite, i.e., $OR_{11} < OR_{10} OR_{01}$ ($\beta_{GE} < 0$).

24.2.2   Additive model

An additive model assumes G_i and E_i act additively on the risk of the disease itself, i.e.,

$$P(D_i = 1 | G_i, E_i) = b_0 + b_G G_i + b_E E_i \,.$$

A departure from this model is called an additive interaction, which can be tested by $H_0 : b_{GE} = 0$ in the following model:

$$P(D_i = 1 | G_i, E_i) = b_0 + b_G G_i + b_E E_i + b_{GE} G_i E_i. \tag{24.5}$$

Consider Table 24.2, which shows a disease risk, $R_{ge} = P(D = 1 | G = g, E = e)$ for $g, e = 0, 1$. The null hypothesis $H_0 : b_{GE} = 0$ implies that the risk difference (not the odds-ratio) associated with G_i is constant across levels of E_i, i.e.,

$$R_{11} - R_{01} = R_{10} - R_{00}. \tag{24.6}$$

24.2.2.1   Approximating an additive model using a logistic regression

It is challenging to estimate the parameters of the additive model because constraints are needed to guarantee that fitted probabilities are between 0 and 1 under the use of a non-standard link function. There have been numerous methods to fit this model through approximations. As one way to approximate the additive model, dividing Eq. (24.6) by R_{00}

TABLE 24.2

Disease risk table for binary factors G and E.

	$E = 0$	$E = 1$
$G = 0$	$b_0 \ (= R_{00})$	$b_E \ (= R_{01})$
$G = 1$	$b_G \ (= R_{10})$	$b_G + b_E + b_{GE} \ (= R_{11})$

gives $RR_{11} = RR_{10} + RR_{01} - 1$, where RR_{ge} is a relative risk for $G = g$ and $E = e$ (with a reference status of $G = 0$ and $E = 0$). Assuming a rare disease, a relative risk can be approximated by an odd ratio, and hence Eq. (24.6) is equivalent to $OR_{11} = OR_{10} + OR_{01} - 1$, which can be expressed as $\exp(\beta_G + \beta_E + \beta_{GE}) = \exp(\beta_G) + \exp(\beta_E) - 1$ (see Table 24.1). This implies that the additive interaction in Eq. (24.5) can be tested by:

$$H_0 : \exp(\beta_G + \beta_E + \beta_{GE}) = \exp(\beta_G) + \exp(\beta_E) - 1, \tag{24.7}$$

using a logistic regression model. While this relation only holds for binary G and E, analogous expressions can be derived for G and E with larger numbers of categories (Han *et al.*, 2012). Thus, for categorical G and E, the additive model can be re-written using a logistic model in the form of:

$$\text{logit}\{P(D_i = 1|G_i, E_i)\} = \beta_0 + \beta_G G_i + \beta_E E_i + \log\left\{\frac{\exp(\beta_G G_i) + \exp(\beta_E E_i) - 1}{\exp(\beta_G G_i + \beta_E E_i)}\right\}. \tag{24.8}$$

24.2.2.2 Testing and null hypotheses

There are several ways for testing for an additive interaction, including likelihood ratio tests using the null hypothesis in Eq. (24.7), as well as Wald tests based on various test statistics. To introduce a few well-known Wald-tests for additive interaction (Rothman *et al.*, 2008), Relative Excess Risk Due to Interaction ($RERI$) is defined as:

$$RERI = RR_{11} - RR_{01} - RR_{10} + 1 = \exp(\beta_G + \beta_E + \beta_{GE}) - \exp(\beta_G) - \exp(\beta_E) + 1$$

with H_0: $RERI = 0$.

Attributable Proportion due to interaction (AP) is defined as:

$$AP = \frac{RERI}{RR_{11}} = \frac{\exp(\beta_G + \beta_E + \beta_{GE}) - \exp(\beta_G) - \exp(\beta_E) + 1}{\exp(\beta_G + \beta_E + \beta_{GE})} \quad \text{with } H_0: AP = 0.$$

Synergy index (S) is defined as:

$$S = \frac{RR_{11} - 1}{(RR_{10} - 1) + (RR_{01} - 1)} = \frac{\exp(\beta_G + \beta_E + \beta_{GE}) - 1}{(\exp(\beta_G) - 1) + (\exp(\beta_E) - 1)} \quad \text{with } H_0: S = 1.$$

All of these tests could be performed by first obtaining parameter estimates from a logistic regression model that is saturated with respect to the effects of G and E and then using them to obtain estimates of the various quantities defined above. Variance estimates can be obtained by delta method, and Wald tests could be performed accordingly (Hosmer and Lemeshow, 1992).

24.2.3 Liability threshold model (probit model)

When the effects of G_i and E_i are assumed to be additive on the probit scale, a model can be presented as follows:

$$P(D_i = 1 | G_i, E_i) = \Phi(\gamma_0 + \gamma_G G_i + \gamma_E E_i)$$

(Falconer, 1967). This model is equivalent to having a latent trait Y_i modeled as:

$$Y_i = \gamma_0 + \gamma_G G_i + \gamma_E E_i + \varepsilon_i,$$

where $\varepsilon_i \sim N(0, 1)$ and $D_i = 1$ if $Y_i > C$; that is, one becomes affected by the disease if the value of a latent trait is above a certain clinical threshold C. This is also known as a liability threshold (LT) model. In statistical genetics, this model has been widely used for estimation of heritability partly because of computational convenience. The scale of a liability threshold model is similar to a logistic scale; hence, modeling gene-environment interaction using this model may not contribute additional insights compared to a logistic model (Han *et al.*, 2015). There are some other nonstandard models discussed in the literature (Clayton, 2012).

24.3 Various methods for inference

In this section, we will describe alternative methods for inference for gene-environment interactions under case-control designs. Here, we assume the goal is to analyze an interaction between a single genetic factor (G) and a single environmental exposure (E), adjusting for additional covariates. Typically, the genetic factor corresponds to a categorical variable, e.g., the genotype status associated with individual single nucleotide polymorphisms (SNPs) that are commonly studied in GWAS. Throughout we let n_1 denote the number of cases and n_0 the number of controls, so $n = n_0 + n_1$ is the number of individuals in the case-control sample.

24.3.1 Prospective likelihood

24.3.1.1 Logistic regression and a prospective likelihood

Standard analyses of case-control studies are typically based on a prospective likelihood for case-control data that does not take into account the retrospective nature of the sampling design. When no assumption is made about the joint distribution of covariates, including genetic and environmental factors and other confounders, such prospective treatment of case-control data is known to be efficient (Prentice and Pyke, 1979). In particular, if the disease risk is modeled by a logistic regression, retrospective and prospective maximum-likelihood analysis of the case-control data provide the same estimates of the association parameters. A prospective likelihood is given as follows:

$$L = \prod_{i=1}^{n} P(D_i = d_i | G_i, E_i) = \prod_{i=1}^{n} p_i^{d_i} (1 - p_i)^{1-d_i}, \tag{24.9}$$

where the specification of p_i can vary depending on the disease risk model being assumed. For example,

$$p_i = \frac{\exp(\beta_0 + \beta_G G_i + \beta_E E_i + \beta_{GE} G_i E_i)}{1 + \exp(\beta_0 + \beta_G G_i + \beta_E E_i + \beta_{GE} G_i E_i)}$$

when the saturated logistic regression model in Eq. (24.3) is assumed. In this model, additional covariates or confounding factors can be readily included as separate terms. The corresponding log likelihood is given as:

$$\ell = \sum_{i=1}^{n} \{d_i \log p_i + (1 - d_i) \log(1 - p_i)\}.$$

24.3.2 Data example using R

24.3.2.1 Multiplicative interaction using a prospective likelihood

A multiplicative interaction based on a prospective likelihood of the saturated logistic regression in Eq. (24.3) can be tested using a null hypothesis $H_0 : \beta_{GE} = 0$ using Wald tests, score tests, or likelihood-ratio tests. Any standard statistical package implements a logistic regression model based on a prospective likelihood. While the `glm()` function can be used to conduct this analysis in R, we will use the `snp.logistic()` function in the `CGEN` package that can perform a variety of other gene-environment interaction methods that we will demonstrate throughout this chapter. A SNP variable is typically coded as binary (0 or 1), ordinal (0, 1, or 2), or continuous variables. In the following codes, we will use an example of binary coding, but other coding is also available. "NAT2" is the variable for SNP rs1495741 in NAT2 (coded as 1 for carriers of the variant or 0 for noncarriers of the variant in rs1495741), and "CIGEVER" is a smoking status (0: never smokers versus 1: current and former smokers). The "covnames2" includes a list of covariates such as age and study. The "UML" ("Unconstrained Maximum Likelihood") option will provide a result based on a prospective likelihood:

```
> library(CGEN)

> out=snp.logistic(data=MYDAT, response.var="Case", snp.var="NAT2",
 main.vars=covnames2, int.vars=c("CIGEVER"))

> covnames2
 [1] "CIGEVER" "age_cat_base_50_54" "age_cat_base_55_59" "age_cat_base_60_64"
 [5] "age_cat_base_65_69" "age_cat_base_70_74" "age_cat_base_75p" "gender_MALE"

> getSummary(out$UML)
                   Estimate    Std.Error    Z.value       Pvalue
Intercept          0.20756883  0.12077634   1.7186216  8.568330e-02
CIGEVER            0.94606992  0.05626514  16.8144946  1.911156e-63
gender_MALE        0.38614751  0.04906386   7.8703048  3.537783e-15
age_cat_base_50_54 -0.23121909  0.08939330  -2.5865372  9.694569e-03
age_cat_base_55_59 -0.18076623  0.08271378  -2.1854427  2.885641e-02
age_cat_base_60_64 -0.20947928  0.08050718  -2.6019949  9.268322e-03
age_cat_base_65_69 -0.23263617  0.08269483  -2.8131887  4.905285e-03
age_cat_base_70_74 -0.19012601  0.08649859  -2.1980245  2.794736e-02
age_cat_base_75p   0.14157312  0.09399661   1.5061513  1.320283e-01
NAT2               0.01752099  0.05984870   0.2927548  7.697096e-01
NAT2:CIGEVER       0.15681855  0.06973414   2.2488059  2.452485e-02
```

The summary of the NAT2 × Smoking interaction results are shown in Table 24.3, with the multiplicative interaction P-value of 0.0245. Table 24.4 shows the sub-group analysis results for tests for associations between NAT2 and bladder cancer risk stratified by smoking status (never versus ever). These results suggest that among individuals who ever smoked,

TABLE 24.3
Evaluation of multiplicative interaction for NAT2 × Smoking on
bladder cancer risk. (*OR* and *SE* denote odds ratio and standard
error.)

Method	*OR*	P-value	Beta estimate	*SE*
Prospective likelihood	1.17	0.0245	0.157	0.0697
Retrospective likelihood	1.19	0.0021	0.172	0.0563
Case-only method	1.17	0.0147	0.155	0.0634
Empirical Bayes Estimator	1.19	0.0024	0.171	0.0567

the variant in NAT2 increases the risk of bladder cancer by 19% ($OR = 1.19$, $P = 1 \times 10^{-6}$),
while this variant does not affect the risk among never smokers (i.e., supra-multiplicative
interaction).

24.3.2.2 Additive interaction using a prospective likelihood

Tests for additive interactions can also be performed based on a prospective likelihood.
For example, we can perform a likelihood ratio test by comparing two models as follows:
First, we fit the full model in Eq. (24.3) based on a prospective likelihood using a maximum
likelihood method, and then fit the reduced model on which the null hypothesis in Eq. (24.7)
is imposed (Han *et al.*, 2012). The parameters in the reduced model can be estimated by
maximum likelihood using the `optim()` function in R. Then a likelihood ratio test, *LRT*, is
distributed as χ_1^2 under the null hypothesis for binary factors, G and E. Of course, this test
can be extended to more general cases, where G or E is a categorical variable with more
than two categories. This can lead to a test with larger degrees of freedom. This likelihood
ratio test for an additive interaction is implemented in the `additive.test()` function in
CGEN as well as the Wald tests for *RERI*, *S*, and *AP*.

```
out2=additive.test(data=MYDAT, response.var="Case", snp.var="NAT2",
    exposure.var=c("CIGEVER"), main.vars=covnames2,
    op=list(genetic.model=1,indep=F))
```

In the above code, `enetic.model=1` denotes using a dominant model (carrier versus non-
carrier), and `indep=F` specifies a prospective likelihood (versus retrospective likelihood for
`indep=T`). A more general genetic model can be also implemented using `genetic.model=3`,
which will lead to a larger degree of freedom test. The following output shows that the
P-value of the additive test is P = 0.00026. Table 24.5 shows that the difference of risks
between the mutation noncarriers versus carriers is 0.02 among never smokers while the
difference is larger among ever smokers (0.58), the significance of which is assessed in the
additive interaction test (LRT=13.30 and P-value = 0.000264).

```
> out2$pval.add
[1] 0.0002641841
```

TABLE 24.4
Odds ratios (*OR*) for bladder cancer associated with NAT2
genotype status stratified by smoking status: a prospective
likelihood is used.

Smoking	OR	95% CI	P-value
Never	1.02	0.90-1.14	0.77
Ever	1.19	1.11-1.28	1.10×10^{-6}

TABLE 24.5
Odds-ratios for bladder cancer risk associated with NAT2 genotype and smoking status.

	Never	Ever	Odds-ratio difference
NAT2 fast acetylation genotype	1	1.91 (1.27, 2.98)	0.91
NAT2 slow acetylation genotype	1.02 (0.90-1.15)	2.49 (1.70, 3.09)	1.47
Odds-ratio difference	0.02	0.58	

```
> out2$LRT.add
[1] 13.30865

> out2$or.tb
          [,1]      [,2]
[1,] 1.000000 1.914731
[2,] 1.021648 2.492126
```

24.3.3 Case-only design

In examining gene-environment interactions, investigators often may find that in some settings it is realistic to assume that genetic factors and environmental exposures are independent in the underlying population (Mukherjee and Chatterjee, 2008). This is a plausible assumption because the genetic variation an individual receives from their parent is determined during meiosis, and hence is randomly determined at birth rather than being affected by subsequent environmental exposures. Genetic susceptibility is unlikely to influence various exogenous exposures such as environmental pollutants or occupation exposures. On the other hand, this assumption can become questionable for endogenous exposures, such as biomarkers. The case-only design is one of the nontraditional methods that depend on an assumption of gene-environment independence in the underlying population, which can be used for testing for multiplicative interactions (Piegorsch *et al.*, 1994).

24.3.3.1 Methods

Consider the 2×4 table given in Table 24.6, where G and E are binary factors, with r_{dge} and p_{dge} denoting the observed cell count and the unknown true cell probability, respectively, for the configuration $D = d$, $G = g$, and $E = e$. As shown in Eq. (24.4), a multiplicative interaction parameter is given as

$$\psi = \frac{OR_{11}}{OR_{10}OR_{01}},$$

TABLE 24.6
Data for a case-control study with binary genetic (G) and environmental factors (E) on cases $(D = 1)$ and controls $(D = 0)$.

	$G = 0$		$G = 1$		Total
	$E = 0$	$E = 1$	$E = 0$	$E = 1$	
$D = 0$	r_{000}	r_{001}	r_{010}	r_{011}	n_0
$D = 1$	r_{100}	r_{101}	r_{110}	r_{111}	n_1

the ratio between the odds ratio when one is exposed both to environmental and genetic risks (OR_{11}) and the product of the odds ratios when exposed to only one of the two factors, i.e., $OR_{10}OR_{01}$. Note that

$$OR_{11} = \frac{p_{000}p_{111}}{p_{011}p_{100}}, \quad OR_{01} = \frac{p_{000}p_{110}}{p_{010}p_{100}}, \quad \text{and} \quad OR_{10} = \frac{p_{000}p_{101}}{p_{001}p_{100}}.$$

Therefore, the interaction parameter ψ can be written as:

$$\psi = \frac{OR_{11}}{OR_{10}OR_{01}} = \frac{p_{001}p_{010}p_{100}p_{111}}{p_{000}p_{011}p_{101}p_{110}}.$$

Equivalently,

$$\log(\psi) = \beta_{CC} = \log\left(\frac{p_{111}p_{100}}{p_{110}p_{101}}\right) - \log\left(\frac{p_{011}p_{000}}{p_{010}p_{001}}\right) \doteq \beta_{CO} - \theta_{GE}. \tag{24.10}$$

The first term in Eq. (24.10) is a measure of gene-environment association in the case population while the second term,

$$\theta_{GE} = \log\left(\frac{p_{011}p_{000}}{p_{010}p_{001}}\right),$$

is a measure of gene-environment association in the underlying control population. When the gene-environment independence assumption holds in the underlying population, i.e., $\theta_{GE} = 0$, the log of the multiplicative interaction parameter is reduced to β_{CC}, which is equivalent to simply testing for gene-environment association using case-only data. Therefore, we can perform a case-only based interaction test using the assumption that there is no correlation between G and E in a sample that is restricted to cases alone. It is easy to see that the case-only test will be much more powerful than its case-control counterpart because the latter is affected by the estimation uncertainty associated with θ_{GE}. This test can easily be conducted using a simple chi-square test of independence between two variables or using logistic or polytomous regressions using any statistical analysis package.

24.3.3.2 Limitations

One major limitation of the case-only design is that, while the case-only method has improved power over the traditional methods when G and E are independent in the underlying population, this method has a large type I error if the independence assumption is violated (Albert *et al.*, 2001). In addition, the case-only method is for testing for interaction only, and hence the regression parameters for main effects of G and E cannot be estimated.

24.3.3.3 Data illustration using NAT2 and smoking data

We applied this method to the NAT2 and smoking example for bladder cancer. First, testing for correlation between NAT2 and smoking among controls shows that G and E are independent (P-value = 0.69) using the following R code:

```
lm0=glm(CIGEVER ~ NAT2+., data=MYDAT2, subset=(Case==0), family=binomial)
```

Then we performed a logistic regression to test for an association between NAT2 and smoking among cases only, adjusting for a set of covariates using the following code:

```
lm1=glm(CIGEVER ~ NAT2+., data=MYDAT2, subset=(Case==1), family=binomial)
```

Table 24.3 summarizes the results for the case-only test for NAT2 × Smoking interaction, which show improved significance (P = 0.0147 versus 0.0245) and standard error (SE = 0.0634 versus 0.069) compared to the standard case-control based method shown in Table 24.3.

24.3.4 Log-linear model

To overcome the limitations of the case-only method that can only estimate the parameters for interactions, but not for main effects of G and E, Umbach and Weinberg (1997) considered a log-linear modeling technique on case-control data. While the connection between a logistic regression and log-linear modeling has been well known (Bishop *et al.*, 2007), Umbach and Weinberg (1997) showed the maximum-likelihood estimates of all parameters of a logistic regression model can be obtained more efficiently by dropping some terms from the log-linear model under the assumption of the gene-environment independence.

24.3.4.1 General log-linear model for a multiplicative interaction test using both cases and controls

Let r_{dge} and u_{dge} denote the observed cell count and expected cell count for the configuration $D = d$, $G = g$ and $E = e$ (see Table 24.6). The following saturated log-linear model of u_{dge} fully parameterizes the eight cells in Table 24.6:

$$\log u_{dge} = \beta_{00} + \beta_{0,G}G + \beta_{0,E}E + \beta_{0,GE}GE + \beta_0 D + \beta_G DG + \beta_E DE + \beta_{GE} DGE. \quad (24.11)$$

Here, the parameters β_{00}, $\beta_{0,G}$, $\beta_{0,E}$ and $\beta_{0,GE}$ parameterize the joint distribution of E and G among controls. The relation between Eq. (24.11) and the logistic regression in Eq. (24.3) is through $\text{logit}\{P(D|G, E)\} = \log u_{1ge} - \log u_{0ge}$. The models in Eq. (24.3) and in Eq. (24.11) have the same description for the disease with β_G, β_E and β_{GE} having exactly the same interpretation in both models. Hence the null hypothesis for a multiplicative interaction is $H_0 : \beta_{GE} = 0$. A maximum likelihood approach can be used to estimate the parameters in the log-linear model based on Poisson distributions. If the parameters that describe the joint distribution of G and E among controls ($D = 0$) are left completely saturated, then the maximum-likelihood estimates of the disease odds-ratio parameters from this model will be the same as those obtained from the standard prospective logistic regression analysis of case-control data.

24.3.4.2 Incorporating the gene-environment independence assumption

The assumption of gene-environment independence can be imposed by $\beta_{0,GE} = 0$, which implies no association between G and E among controls. Then the maximum likelihood estimator of β_{GE} under the following constrained model is equivalent to the estimator under the case-only design in the simple setting of the $2 \times 2 \times 2$ table described above. The log-linear model, however, can provide the estimates for the main effects of G and E, β_G and β_E:

$$\log u_{dge} = \beta_{00} + \beta_{0,G}G + \beta_{0,E}E + \beta_0 D + \beta_G DG + \beta_E DE + \beta_{GE} DGE.$$

24.3.5 Retrospective likelihood approach

Chatterjee and Carroll (2005) developed a general method using a retrospective likelihood that exploits the gene-environment independence assumption for testing for multiplicative interaction, but can use both cases and controls to estimate all of the parameters in a general logistic regression model. This method, by using a profile-likelihood approach, avoids dealing with potentially high-dimensional parameters associated with specification of joint distributions of genetic and environmental risk factors, including additional covariates, which is required in the log-linear modeling approach. This method has been extended to take into account gene-gene or gene-environment dependence due to population stratification by conditioning the likelihood on appropriate variables (S), such as self-reported ethnicity and/or principal components of population stratification markers (Price *et al.*, 2006).

24.3.5.1 Retrospective likelihood and gene-environment independence assumption

A retrospective likelihood is given as

$$L^R = \prod_{i=1}^{n} P(G_i, E_i, S_i | D_i), \tag{24.12}$$

where

$$P(G, E, S | D) = \frac{P(D|G, E, S)P(G|E, S)P(E, S)}{\sum_{G,E,S} P(D|G, E, S)P(G|E, S)P(E, S)},$$

and a logistic disease model is assumed for $P(D|G, E, S)$ as in Eq. (24.3) with additional variable S (population stratification) included as a covariate:

$$\text{logit}\{P(D = 1|G, E, S)\} = \beta_0 + \beta_G G + \beta_E E + \beta_{GE} GE + \beta_S S.$$

The joint distribution for E and S remains nonparametric. $P(G|E, S)$ could be modeled as:

$$P(G = 1|E, S) = H(\eta_0 + \eta_1 S + \theta E), \tag{24.13}$$

where $H(u) = (1 + \exp(-u))^{-1}$. The gene-environment independence assumption can be simply imposed by $\theta = 0$.

24.3.5.2 Profile likelihood

Chatterjee and Carroll (2005) showed that the parameter estimates that maximize the retrospective likelihood in Eq. (24.12) can be obtained alternatively by maximization of a "profile likelihood":

$$\begin{aligned} L^P &= \prod_{i=1}^{n} P(D_i = d_i, \ G_i = g_i | E_i = e_i, S_i = s_i, \ R = 1) \\ &= \prod_{i=1}^{n} \frac{\exp\{\phi(d_i, g_i, e_i, s_i)\}}{\sum_{d,g} \exp\{\phi(d, g, e_i, s_i)\}}. \end{aligned} \tag{24.14}$$

Here, R indicates the selection mechanism for the case-control design, and

$$\phi(d, g, e, s) = d\left(\beta_0 + \beta_G g + \beta_E e + \beta_{GE} ge\right) + I(g = 1)\log 2 + g\log\left(\frac{p_s}{1 - p_s}\right),$$

where p_s is the minor allele frequency of SNP G, and SNP genotype probabilities in stratum s are specified assuming Hardy-Weinberg equilibrium (HWE) as

$$P(G_i = 0|S_i = s) = (1 - p_s)^2, \quad P(G_i = 1|S_i = s) = 2p_s(1 - p_s), \quad P(G_i = 2|S_i = s) = p_s^2.$$

For continuous S, such as principal components, $P(G_i|S_i)$ can be modeled in terms of a polytomous regression model.

24.3.5.3 A multiplicative interaction based on a retrospective likelihood and NAT2 and smoking interaction

The null hypothesis for a multiplicative interaction is: $H_0 : \beta_{GE} = 0$ in Eq. (24.14). The method for testing for a multiplicative interaction based on the retrospective likelihood (profile likelihood) is implemented in snp.logistic() function in CGEN:

```
out=snp.logistic(data=MYDAT, response.var="Case", snp.var="NAT2",
main.vars=covnames2, int.vars=c("CIGEVER"), strata.var=studynames)
```

In the above code, S is specified in "strat.var," which is a list of variable names for study centers in this example:

```
studynames = c("study_group_ATBC","study_group_CPSII", "study_group_Europe",
"study_group_HPFS", "study_group_Italy", "study_group_LA", "study_group_NEBL",
"study_group_NHS", "study_group_PLCO", "study_group_SPBC")
```

The option $CML ("Constrained Maximum Likelihood") provides results under a retrospective approach while $UML ("Unconstrained Maximum Likelihood") is used for a standard prospective likelihood shown in Section 24.3.1. The summary of the results using the retrospective likelihood is shown in Table 24.3, which shows improved significance for testing a multiplicative interaction (P = 0.00219) compared to the standard case-control test (P = 0.024) or the case-only test (P = 0.0147) in Table 24.3. In addition, the full estimates of regression parameters such as the main effect of NAT2 (β_G= 0.0037) as well as smoking (β_E=0.952) are provided.

```
getSummary(out$CML)
                     Estimate   Std.Error      Z.value         Pvalue
Intercept          0.20116287  0.12028791   1.67234484   9.445634e-02
CIGEVER            0.95238968  0.05325942  17.88209051   1.626234e-71
gender_MALE        0.38755338  0.04902525   7.90517932   2.675482e-15
age_cat_base_50_54 -0.22909722 0.08930383  -2.56536846   1.030663e-02
age_cat_base_55_59 -0.17934219 0.08263852  -2.17020105   2.999162e-02
age_cat_base_60_64 -0.20710992 0.08043464  -2.57488454   1.002736e-02
age_cat_base_65_69 -0.23415267 0.08263204  -2.83367901   4.601553e-03
age_cat_base_70_74 -0.18592294 0.08640857  -2.15167247   3.142316e-02
age_cat_base_75p    0.14224878 0.09392764   1.51445064   1.299116e-01
NAT2               0.00371818  0.05365879   0.06929302   9.447564e-01
NAT2:CIGEVER       0.17259364  0.05634495   3.06316070   2.190124e-03
```

24.3.5.4 An additive interaction based on a retrospective likelihood and the NAT2 and smoking example

Recently Han *et al.* (2012) proposed a likelihood ratio test for an additive interaction that exploits the gene-environment independence assumption. Basically it is similar to the likelihood ratio test described in Section 24.3.1, where the likelihood is calculated using the profile-likelihood in Eq. (24.14) instead of the prospective likelihood. Similarly, other tests for additive interactions such as *RERI*, *S*, and *AP* can be also performed by estimating the regression parameters using the profile-likelihood that assumes the gene-environment independence assumption. These methods are implemented in the additive.test() function (indep=T option) in CGEN package. The following result shows that LRT is 13.8 with the corresponding P-value = 0.00020, with a similar level of significance compared to the one based on the prospective likelihood.

```
out2.add =additive.test(data=MYDAT, response.var="Case", snp.var="NAT2",
exposure.var=c("CIGEVER"),main.vars=covnames2,op=list(genetic.model=2,indep=T),
strata.var=studynames)

> out2.add$LRT.add
[1] 13.80


> out2.add$pval.add
[1] 0.00020
```

24.3.6   Empirical Bayes shrinkage estimation

A major limitation for the methods that rely on the gene-environment independence assumption, such as case-only, log-linear, and retrospective methods, is that they have the potential for large bias when the underlying assumption is violated (Albert *et al.*, 2001). Mukherjee and Chatterjee (2008) proposed an empirical Bayes type method that uses a weighted average of the case-control and case-only estimators of the multiplicative interaction, yielding an acceptable trade-off between bias and efficiency. A stochastic framework is used for allowing for uncertainty around the gene-environment independence assumption, which estimates the uncertainty parameter using data.

24.3.6.1   The method description for binary G and E

Consider the 2×4 table in Table 24.6 and the equation in Eq. (24.10). Then the relationship between the case-control (β_{CC}) and case-only (β_{CO}) based maximum likelihood estimators for the multiplicative interaction parameter is given as:

$$\hat{\beta}_{CC} = \log\left(\frac{r_{001}r_{010}r_{100}r_{111}}{r_{000}r_{011}r_{101}r_{110}}\right) = \log\left(\frac{r_{111}r_{100}}{r_{110}r_{101}}\right) - \log\left(\frac{r_{011}r_{000}}{r_{010}r_{001}}\right) = \hat{\beta}_{CO} - \hat{\theta}_{GE}.$$

Note that the first term represents the measure of gene-environment association in the case population (i.e., case-only test statistic) while the second term

$$\hat{\theta}_{GE} = \log\left(\frac{r_{011}r_{000}}{r_{010}r_{001}}\right)$$

is the measure of gene-environment association among controls. The Empirical Bayes type estimator is provided as following:

$$\hat{\beta}_{EB} = \frac{\hat{\sigma}_{CC}^2}{\hat{\theta}_{GE}^2 + \hat{\sigma}_{CC}^2}\,\hat{\beta}_{CO} + \frac{\hat{\theta}_{GE}^2}{\hat{\theta}_{GE}^2 + \hat{\sigma}_{CC}^2}\,\hat{\beta}_{CC},$$

where $\hat{\sigma}_{CC}^2$ is the estimated variance of case-control estimator, $\hat{\beta}_{CC}$. Here the intuition is that $\hat{\theta}_{GE}$ is a measure of bias of the case-only method, and the EB method provides more weight to the case-control method when this bias is large. How much weight will be given is calibrated by $\hat{\sigma}_{CC}^2$, which is the variance of the less efficient case-control estimator. If the gene-environment independence assumption is violated, i.e., true $\theta_{GE} \neq 0$, then the EB estimator asymptotically will behave the same as the case-control estimator. However, when gene-environment independence holds, the asymptotic weight for the EB estimator will be nonzero for both case-control and case-only estimators and thus will have efficiency in between.

24.3.6.2   General approach

A general approach for deriving EB-type shrinkage estimators for all of the parameters of a general logistic regression model was also proposed by Mukherjee and Chatterjee (2008), and Chen *et al.* (2009). Note that in Mukherjee and Chatterjee (2008), the EB estimator is proposed using a profile-likelihood that requires specifying a model for gene-environment correlation using some underlying parameters. On the other hand, Chen *et al.* (2009) proposed an EB type estimator, which is implemented in `CGEN`, that allows an arbitrary type of gene-environment correlation without need to specify any such model.

24.3.6.3   Data example

The method for testing for multiplicative interactions based on the EB type approach is implemented in `snp.logistic()` function in the `CGEN` package with an `$EB` output option. The option `$UML` produces outputs under the unconstrained MLE (i.e., equivalent to a standard method based on a prospective likelihood) while `$CML` produces outputs under the constrained ML (i.e., retrospective likelihood). The codes and results based on the EB method are shown below. The beta estimate and SE based on the EB method fall between the results based on the retrospective and prospective likelihoods (see Table 24.3), but closer to the ones under the retrospective likelihood because the data show almost no evidence of gene-environment association in the underlying population (see Section 24.3.3) with $P = 0.69$.

```
out2=snp.logistic(data=MYDAT, response.var="Case", snp.var="NAT2",
main.vars=covnames2, int.vars=c("CIGEVER"), strata.var=studynames)
```

```
names(out2)
[1] "UML"        "CML"        "EB"          "model.info"
```

```
getSummary(out2$EB)
```

	Estimate	Std.Error	Z.value	Pvalue
Intercept	0.201180840	0.12035613	1.6715463	9.461382e-02
CIGEVER	0.952310945	0.05330760	17.8644488	2.231254e-71
gender_MALE	0.387552223	0.04902966	7.9044440	2.691322e-15
age_cat_base_50_54	-0.229098415	0.08931619	-2.5650266	1.031679e-02
age_cat_base_55_59	-0.179342615	0.08264566	-2.1700184	3.000545e-02
age_cat_base_60_64	-0.207111969	0.08045427	-2.5742818	1.004484e-02
age_cat_base_65_69	-0.234152157	0.08264015	-2.8333945	4.605651e-03
age_cat_base_70_74	-0.185932836	0.08646835	-2.1502993	3.153155e-02
age_cat_base_75p	0.142248746	0.09392890	1.5144300	1.299168e-01
NAT2	0.004415267	0.05392923	0.0818715	9.347489e-01
NAT2:CIGEVER	0.171825660	0.05675563	3.0274644	2.466148e-03

24.4   Testing for genetic association in the presence of gene-environment interaction

24.4.1   Joint test of a main effect of G and an interaction effect of G and E

In testing for genetic associations to identify susceptibility loci for complex diseases, there have been interests in allowing for interaction with environmental risk factors. The underlying rationale is that allowing for interactions for testing for association could increase the power for detecting a gene when such interactions exist. Kraft *et al.* (2007) showed that a joint test of genetic association and interaction has robust performance over a wide range of underlying models although it could be less powerful than a marginal association test when there is no evidence of gene-environment interaction.

24.4.1.1   Null hypothesis for joint test

Revisiting the saturated model in Eq. (24.3),

$$\text{logit}\{P(D_i = 1|G_i, E_i)\} = \beta_0 + \beta_G G_i + \beta_E E_i + \beta_{GE} G_i E_i,$$

the null hypothesis of the joint test is given as: $H_0 : \beta_G = \beta_{GE} = 0$. Note that this test has increased degrees of freedom compared to a marginal association test, which can lead to a decrease in power when there is no interaction effect, i.e., $\beta_{GE} = 0$.

24.4.1.2   Different likelihoods and methods with examples

Joint tests can be performed under various likelihoods with or without the assumption of gene-environment independence. For example, a standard prospective likelihood can be used for conducting a joint test as follows:

```
out2=snp.logistic(data=MYDAT, response.var="Case", snp.var="NAT2",
main.vars=covnames2, int.vars=c("CIGEVER"), strata.var=studynames)

wt=getWaldTest(out2, c("NAT2", "NAT2:CIGEVER"))
```

Here, the function `getWaldTest()` in CGEN was used for testing the joint effects of association ("NAT2") and interaction("NAT2:CIGEVER"), which produces the results of the joint test under the prospective likelihood ("UML"), retrospective likelihood ("CML"), and the empirical Bayes type method ("EB"):

```
names(wt)
[1] "UML" "CML" "EB"

> wt$UML
$test
[1] 23.82947
$df
[1] 2
$pvalue
[1] 6.691092e-06
```

The summarized results for the joints tests under the three methods are shown in Table 24.7. Among the three methods in Table 24.7, the retrospective approach that uses the gene-environment independence assumption is the most powerful while the standard approach based on the prospective likelihood is the least powerful. The power of the EB method that uses this assumption in a data-adaptive way lies between these two methods.

24.4.2   Maximum score test

While a joint test can be powerful when the assumed interaction exists, the increased degrees of freedom of this test (versus a marginal association test) can lead to a reduced power when such interaction effects are relatively small or when these effects do not exist. Recently,

TABLE 24.7
Joint test: Test of association between NAT2 and BC risk in
the presence of NAT2 × Smoking interaction.

Method	Wald test	Degrees of freedom	P-value
Prospective likelihood	23.83	2	6.69×10^{-6}
Retrospective likelihood	31.06	2	1.80×10^{-7}
Empirical Bayes type	30.82	2	2.02×10^{-7}

Han *et al.* (2015) proposed a new score test for genetic association allowing for potential interactions under a wide range of disease risk models, incorporating multiplicative, additive, and liability threshold models as well as supra- and sub-multiplicative models. This method has shown to have improved power compared to joint tests or standard association tests over a range of risk models.

24.4.2.1 Methods

Focusing on the main effect of G, a score based on the multiplicative model in Eq. (24.1) can be derived by taking the first derivative in terms of β_G:

$$ S_{mult} = \left. \frac{\partial \log L}{\partial \beta_G} \right|_{\beta_G=0} = \sum_{i=1}^{n} G_i (D_i - \mu_i). \tag{24.15} $$

Under the null hypothesis of $H_0 : \beta_G = 0$, the log-likelihood based on the prospective likelihood is written as:

$$ \ell = \log L = \sum_{i=1}^{n} D_i \log \mu_i + (1 - D_i) \log(1 - \mu_i), $$

where

$$ \mu_i = \mu_i(E_i; \beta_E) = \text{logit}\{P(D_i = 1 | G_i, E_i)\} = \beta_0 + \beta_E E_i. $$

Han *et al.* (2015) showed that a score based on the additive model in Eq. (24.8) is given as:

$$ S_{add} = \left. \frac{\partial \log L}{\partial \beta_G} \right|_{\beta_G=0} = \sum_{i=1}^{n} \exp(\beta_E E_i)^{-1} G_i (D_i - \mu_i). \tag{24.16} $$

Here, the term $\exp(\beta_E E_i)^{-1}$, the inverse of the odds ratio for exposure E_i, acts as a weight. This implies that, for exposures that are positively associated with the disease risk (i.e., $\beta_E > 0$), subjects are down-weighted with increasing levels of exposure by a degree that depends on the strength of association (β_E) between disease and exposure. Thus, by using weighted score tests, it is possible to account for the heterogeneous genetic effects by exposure levels without incurring additional degrees of freedom. However, a particular form of weight will be optimal only under a certain model for gene-environment interactions. In an effort to build more robust score tests, Han *et al.* (2015) proposed a general score approach, which does not assume any specific disease risk model, but encompasses a wide range of alternative models:

$$ S(\theta) = \sum_{i=1}^{n} \omega_i^\theta G_i \{D_i - \mu_i\}, \tag{24.17} $$

where $\omega_i = \exp(\beta_E E_i)$ and the index parameter θ is allowed to vary over a range of values on the real line. For example, optimal weight can be obtained by setting $\theta = -1$, under the additive model and $\theta = 0$ under the multiplicative model in Eq. (24.15). The optimal weight function for the probit model (i.e., liability threshold model) is expected to lie between -1 and 0, where the genetic odds-ratio decreases by increasing level of exposure, but the rate of decrease is expected to be much more modest than that for the additive model. For any given θ, one can construct a score test of the form $T(\theta) = S(\theta)/\sqrt{V(\theta)}$, where $V(\theta) = \text{var}\{S(\theta)\}$. Thus, the final test statistic takes the form $T = \max_{\theta} |T(\theta)|$, where $\theta \in [L, \ U]$. This integrates a class of disease risk models where the model is chosen based on the evidence from data, without an arbitrary choice of models. The P-value of this maximum test is calculated using an extreme value theory (Davies, 1977). This method was also extended to incorporate the assumption of gene-environment independence (Han *et al.*, 2015).

24.5   Discussion

In this chapter, we reviewed various methods for detecting gene-environment interactions under a range of disease risk models that include multiplicative and additive models and different inferential procedures. While a prospective likelihood is commonly used for conducting traditional interaction tests in case-control studies, a retrospective likelihood can be useful to improve power by incorporating the gene-environment independence assumption. In addition, unlike the case-only design, the estimates of all regression parameters (such as the main effects of G and E) can readily be obtained by using the retrospective likelihood approach while still exploiting the gene-environment independence assumption.

A joint test of association allowing for gene-environment interaction can provide improved power for detecting genetic associations compared to a marginal association test when the assumed interactions exist. We have shown that a joint test can also be performed under various likelihoods including a retrospective likelihood that provides additional power when G and E are independent in the underlying population. A maximum score test was developed to overcome the potential loss of power of a joint test due to increased degrees of freedom. This method provides a unified approach that integrates a class of disease risk models by maximizing over a class of score tests, each of which involves modified standard tests of genetic association through a weight function. This weight function reflects the potential heterogeneity of the genetic effects by levels of environmental exposures. There are several other methods for testing for gene-environment interaction that were not discussed in this chapter. For example, tree-based methods (Breiman, 2001), multifactor dimensionality reduction (MDR, Ritchie *et al.*, 2001), and Bayesian network analysis (Baurley *et al.*, 2010) have been developed to explore higher-order gene-gene and gene-environment interactions (Hutter *et al.*, 2013; Cordell, 2002).

The challenges of gene-environment interaction analysis include replication issues. While various GWAS findings of the main effects of SNPs have been replicated by independent studies for many complex diseases (http://www.ebi.ac.uk/gwas/), relatively few interactions have been reproduced. It is likely that the sample sizes of GWAS that have required measurements on environmental exposures are not yet adequate to reliably identify gene-environment interactions of modest magnitude. Thus, while more powerful statistical methods for detecting interactions are helpful, ultimately studies with larger sample sizes are needed to identify interactions. While it will be always hard to rule out statistical interactions of very small magnitudes, a reasonable goal for the future will be to at least identify parsimonious models that adequately describe the risks of diseases associated with a combination of genetic and environmental risk factors. The lack of reporting of interaction in current studies so far indicates that linear logistic models, i.e., multiplicative models, in general are a good starting point for building models for evaluating the joint effects of genetic and environmental factors (Chatterjee *et al.*, 2016).

Bibliography

Albert, P. S., Ratnasinghe, D., Tangrea, J., and Wacholder, S. (2001). Limitations of the case-only design for identifying gene-environment interactions. *American Journal of Epidemiology*, **154**, 687–693.

Baurley, J. W., Conti, D. V., Gauderman, W. J., and Thomas, D. C. (2010). Discovery of complex pathways from observational data. *Statistics in Medicine*, **29**, 1998–2011.

Bishop, Y. M., Fienberg, S. E., and Holland, P. W. (2007). *Discrete Multivariate Analysis: Theory and Practice*. Springer, New York.

Breiman, L. (2001). Random forests. *Machine Learning*, **45**, 5–32.

Chatterjee, N. and Carroll, R. J. (2005). Semiparametric maximum likelihood estimation exploiting gene-environment independence in case-control studies. *Biometrika*, **92**, 399–418.

Chatterjee, N. and Mukherjee, B. (2008). Statistical approaches to studies of gene-gene and gene-environment interaction. In T. R. Rebbeck, C. B. Ambrosone, and P. G. Shields, editors, *Molecular Epidemiology: Applications in Cancer and Other Human Diseases*, pages 145–169. CRC Press, Boca Raton, FL.

Chatterjee, N., Shi, J., and Garcia-Closas, M. (2016). Developing and evaluating polygenic risk prediction models for stratified disease prevention. *Nature Reviews Genetics*, **17**, 392–406.

Chen, Y.-H., Chatterjee, N., and Carroll, R. J. (2009). Shrinkage estimators for robust and efficient inference in haplotype-based case-control studies. *Journal of the American Statistical Association*, **104**, 220–233.

Clayton, D. (2012). Link functions in multi-locus genetic models: Implications for testing, prediction, and interpretation. *Genetic Epidemiology*, **36**, 409–18.

Clayton, D. and McKeigue, P. M. (2001). Epidemiological methods for studying genes and environmental factors in complex diseases. *The Lancet*, **358**, 1356–1360.

Cordell, H. J. (2002). Epistasis: What it means, what it doesn't mean, and statistical methods to detect it in humans. *Human Molecular Genetics*, **11**, 2463–2468.

Davies, R. B. (1977). Hypothesis testing when a nuisance parameter is present only under the alternative. *Biometrika*, **64**, 247–254.

Eichler, E. E., Flint, J., Gibson, G., Kong, A., Leal, S. M., Moore, J. H., and Nadeau, J. H. (2010). Missing heritability and strategies for finding the underlying causes of complex disease. *Nature Reviews Genetics*, **11**, 446–450.

Falconer, D. (1967). The inheritance of liability to diseases with variable age of onset, with particular reference to diabetes mellitus. *Annals of Human Genetics*, **31**, 1–20.

Figueroa, J. D., Han, S. S., Garcia-Closas, M., Baris, D., Jacobs, E. J., Kogevinas, M., Schwenn, M., Malats, N., Johnson, A., Purdue, M. P., *et al.* (2014). Genome-wide interaction study of smoking and bladder cancer risk. *Carcinogenesis*, **35**, 1737–1744.

Garcia-Closas, M., Malats, N., Silverman, D., Dosemeci, M., Kogevinas, M., Hein, D. W., Tardon, A., Serra, C., Carrato, A., Garcia-Closas, R., *et al.* (2005). NAT2 slow acetylation, GSTM1 null genotype, and risk of bladder cancer: Results from the Spanish Bladder Cancer Study and meta-analyses. *The Lancet*, **366**, 649–659.

Han, S. S., Rosenberg, P. S., Garcia-Closas, M., Figueroa, J. D., Silverman, D., Chanock, S. J., Rothman, N., and Chatterjee, N. (2012). Likelihood ratio test for detecting gene (G)-environment (E) interactions under an additive risk model exploiting G-E independence for case-control data. *American Journal of Epidemiology*, **176**, 1060–1067.

Han, S. S., Rosenberg, P. S., Ghosh, A., Landi, M. T., Caporaso, N. E., and Chatterjee, N. (2015). An exposure-weighted score test for genetic associations integrating environmental risk factors. *Biometrics*, **71**, 596–605.

Hosmer, D. W. and Lemeshow, S. (1992). Confidence interval estimation of interaction. *Epidemiology*, **3**, 452–456.

Hutter, C. M., Mechanic, L. E., Chatterjee, N., Kraft, P., and Gillanders, E. M. (2013). Gene-environment interactions in cancer epidemiology: A National Cancer Institute Think Tank report. *Genetic Epidemiology*, **37**, 643–657.

Kraft, P., Yen, Y.-C., Stram, D. O., Morrison, J., and Gauderman, W. J. (2007). Exploiting gene-environment interaction to detect genetic associations. *Human Heredity*, **63**, 111–119.

Maas, P., Barrdahl, M., Joshi, A. D., Auer, P. L., Gaudet, M. M., Milne, R. L., Schumacher, F. R., Anderson, W. F., Check, D., Chattopadhyay, S., *et al.* (2016). Breast cancer risk from modifiable and nonmodifiable risk factors among white women in the United States. *JAMA Oncology*, **2**, 1295–1302.

Mandel, J. S., Silverman, D. T., McLaughlin, J. K., and Wacholder, S. (1992). Selection of controls in case-control studies: I. Principles. *American Journal of Epidemiology*, **135**, 1019–1028.

Mukherjee, B. and Chatterjee, N. (2008). Exploiting gene-environment independence for analysis of case–control studies: An empirical Bayes-type shrinkage estimator to trade-off between bias and efficiency. *Biometrics*, **64**, 685–694.

Ottman, R. (1996). Gene-environment interaction: Definitions and study designs. *Preventive Medicine*, **25**, 764–770.

Piegorsch, W. W., Weinberg, C. R., and Taylor, J. A. (1994). Non-hierarchical logistic models and case-only designs for assessing susceptibility in population-based case-control studies. *Statistics in Medicine*, **13**, 153–162.

Prentice, R. L. and Pyke, R. (1979). Logistic disease incidence models and case-control studies. *Biometrika*, **66**, 403–411.

Price, A. L., Patterson, N. J., Plenge, R. M., Weinblatt, M. E., Shadick, N. A., and Reich, D. (2006). Principal components analysis corrects for stratification in genome-wide association studies. *Nature Genetics*, **38**, 904–909.

Ritchie, M. D., Hahn, L. W., Roodi, N., Bailey, L. R., Dupont, W. D., Parl, F. F., and Moore, J. H. (2001). Multifactor-dimensionality reduction reveals high-order interactions among estrogen-metabolism genes in sporadic breast cancer. *The American Journal of Human Genetics*, **69**, 138–147.

Rothman, K. J., Greenland, S., and Walker, A. M. (1980). Concepts of interaction. *American Journal of Epidemiology*, **112**, 467–470.

Rothman, K. J., Greenland, S., and Lash, T. L. (2008). *Modern Epidemiology*. Lippincott Williams & Wilkins, Philadelphia.

Rothman, N., Garcia-Closas, M., Chatterjee, N., Malats, N., Wu, X., Figueroa, J. D., Real, F. X., Van Den Berg, D., Matullo, G., Baris, D., *et al.* (2010). A multi-stage genome-wide association study of bladder cancer identifies multiple susceptibility loci. *Nature Genetics*, **42**, 978–984.

Thomas, D. (2010). Gene-environment-wide association studies: Emerging approaches. *Nature Reviews Genetics*, **11**, 259–272.

Thompson, W. D. (1991). Effect modification and the limits of biological inference from epidemiologic data. *Journal of Clinical Epidemiology*, **44**, 221–232.

Umbach, D. M. and Weinberg, C. R. (1997). Designing and analysing case-control studies to exploit independence of genotype and exposure. *Statistics in Medicine*, **16**, 1731–1743.

Wacholder, S., Silverman, D. T., McLaughlin, J. K., and Mandel, J. S. (1992a). Selection of controls in case-control studies: II. Types of controls. *American Journal of Epidemiology*, **135**, 1029–1041.

Wacholder, S., Silverman, D. T., McLaughlin, J. K., and Mandel, J. S. (1992b). Selection of controls in case-control studies: III. Design options. *American Journal of Epidemiology*, **135**, 1042–1050.

Wacholder, S., Chatterjee, N., and Hartge, P. (2002). Joint effect of genes and environment distorted by selection biases implications for hospital-based case-control studies. *Cancer Epidemiology Biomarkers & Prevention*, **11**, 885–889.

Walter, S. and Holford, T. (1978). Additive, multiplicative, and other models for disease risks. *American Journal of Epidemiology*, **108**, 341–346.

25

Two-Stage Testing for Genome-Wide Gene-Environment Interactions

James Y. Dai, Li Hsu, and Charles Kooperberg

Fred Hutchinson Cancer Research Center

25.1 Introduction

In genome-wide association studies, agnostic searches for gene-environment interactions (G×E) are routinely conducted (Hunter, 2005; Hutter *et al.*, 2013; Thomas, 2010), though with limited success. The statistical interaction in a logistic regression model, defined as deviation from an additive contribution of two predictors on the logit-transformed risk scale, demands a much larger sample size to reach the same power than a genetic association with a similar effect size (Smith and Day, 1984). This inadequate power is exacerbated by the necessity of a multiple-testing correction for millions of genetic variants that are being interrogated one at a time, even though the vast majority of these genetic variants have no G×E. Progress has been made to improve efficiency of design and estimation for a single variant G×E test by incorporating the assumptions such as independence of G and E in the population and the Hardy-Weinberg equilibrium (Chatterjee and Carroll, 2005; Chen *et al.*, 2012; Mukherjee and Chatterjee, 2008), as covered in Chapter 24. In this chapter, efficient two-stage procedures are presented for genome-wide searches of G×E focusing on the "more promising" genetic variants for G×E interrogation.

Suppose Y is a dichotomized disease outcome, E is an environmental exposure of interest, and G_j is the jth genetic variant of m variants under investigation. For ease of notation, henceforth the subscript j is suppressed, except when the error rate for multiple tests is analyzed. Suppose a case-control sample has been drawn for testing G×E. A logistic regression model with a multiplicative gene-environment interaction is defined as

$$\text{logit}\{P(Y = 1|G, E)\} = \beta_0 + \beta_1 G + \beta_2 E + \beta_3 G \times E. \tag{25.1}$$

Other variables for confounding adjustment or improving estimation precision can be incorporated in model (25.1). The most common form of genetic variants is the single nucleotide polymorphism (SNP), typically with two alleles at each locus, denoted by A and a. There are three possible genotypes, AA, Aa, and aa. If the inheritance model is log-additive, $G = 0, 1$, and 2 indicating the number of variant alleles. Under the dominant model, $G = 1$ if the genotype is AA or Aa and 0 otherwise; under the recessive model, $G = 1$ if the genotype is AA and 0 otherwise; under the unrestricted model, G are two indicator variables for heterozygous and homozygous variant genotypes. Without loss of generality G is henceforth assumed to be binary. The interest is to test H_0: $\beta_3 = 0$ versus H_1: $\beta_3 \neq 0$.

When G and E are independent in the control population, for example, as approximated in the situation when the disease is rare and G and E are independent in the population, the case-only estimator of θ_1, defined in

$$\text{logit}\{P(G = 1|E, Y = 1)\} = \theta_0 + \theta_1 E, \tag{25.2}$$

is a more efficient estimator of β_3 (Piegorsch *et al.*, 1994); also see Chapter 24 for more details. If E is binary, the case-only estimator can be similarly obtained by fitting a logistic regression model with E as outcome and G as predictor; however, if E is continuous, which is common in epidemiological studies, there is no closed form for testing variants to relate the case-only association parameter in a linear model regressing E on G with the interaction parameter β_3 in (25.1). The test based on the case-only estimator is more powerful than the standard interaction test under model (25.1) (Piegorsch *et al.*, 1994); however, the type I error can be substantially inflated if the independence assumption of G and E is violated.

To protect the family-wise error rate at the level of 0.05 in genome-wide association studies, the p-value cut-off for individual SNPs is typically set at a staggering level: 5×10^{-8}, the convention used in practice for accounting for approximately one million independent SNPs. This is clearly an uninformed approach to allocating the type I error rate to each SNP, given the vast majority of SNPs are known to be neutral. If it is possible to sift the SNPs for the ones that are more likely involved in an interaction, then focusing G×E testing only on these SNPs would reduce the burden of multiple testing substantially. A two-stage testing procedure is thus defined as follows: the first-stage is to screen SNPs and the second stage is to test G×E only on SNPs selected in the first stage. Developing along this line of reasoning, two requirements arise for screening statistics: they must be uncorrelated with G×E test statistics (orthogonality), so that the step of screening for promising SNPs can be ignored in multiple-testing correction for G×E; they must be informative on G×E test statistics for variants that indeed have G×E, so that the screening step would enrich true G×E variants, thereby improving power.

In this chapter, two carefully constructed screening statistics are presented for case-control studies: marginal genetic association and gene-environment correlation, both of which are informative for selecting variants with G×E. However, because of the required orthogonality condition, the pair of a screening statistic and a testing statistic must be carefully chosen: whether to conduct G×E testing by the standard interaction estimator in (25.1) or by the case-only estimator in (25.2) depends on the screening statistic being used. Many efforts have been devoted to devise informative screening statistics and optimize the power performance under a wide range of G×E scenarios that may occur in a genome-wide study. Several two-stage procedures will be presented, each of which may perform better in some specific scenarios but not in others.

The presentation in this chapter focuses on conceptual developments of respective orthogonality (under the null) and informativeness (under the alternative) conditions for various pairs of screening and testing statistics in two-stage testing approaches. In Section 25.2, the orthogonality condition is examined for proper control of the family-wise error rate. The two main screening statistics are presented in Section 25.3. The asymptotic independence between the pairs of screening and testing statistics is proved and a pedagogical example is given. In Section 25.4, several procedures combining the two screening statistics are discussed, ending with an example for power comparison. An application to a study of post-menopausal hormone therapy and colorectal cancer risk is shown in Section 25.5. The chapter closes with a summary of the merits of two-stage procedures and further extensions.

25.2 Orthogonality, type I error control, and power

When a two-stage testing procedure for genome-wide G×E is used, the distributions of test statistics for those genetic variants that pass the first-stage filtering are conditional on the corresponding filtering statistics being greater than a pre-specified threshold. It is therefore different from their marginal distributions. Multiple-testing adjustment, for example a Bonferroni correction, has to account for the conditional distributions induced by such screening. However, if the screening statistic and the testing statistic are independent, the screening step can be ignored and the multiple-testing adjustment is only needed for genetic variants being tested in the second stage. This seemingly intuitive result is formally proved for the family-wise error rate in Theorem 1 in Dai *et al.* (2012).

Briefly, suppose a two-stage testing procedure is applied to data collected from n participants. In the first stage a screening statistic $\widehat{\zeta}_j$ is computed to filter m genetic variants at the significance level α_0, $0 < \alpha_0 < 1$, so that m_0 of the m variants pass the filtering. At the second stage, each of these m_0 SNPs is tested for G×E by a test statistic $\widehat{\vartheta}_j$ at level α/m_0. If the asymptotic distribution of $\widehat{\zeta}_j$ and $\widehat{\vartheta}_j$ has zero covariance, a simple probabilistic derivation shows that the two-stage procedure preserves the family-wise error rate at level α for large m and n. The proof applies to locally correlated SNPs as the linkage disequilibrium between SNPs decreases with the inter-SNP distance.

The independence of the screening and testing statistics protects the validity of the two-stage procedure. However, for such procedure to be useful, it should outperform the naïve one-stage testing procedure without screening. It is therefore of interest to investigate the power function of the two-stage procedure. Among the various two-stage procedures that will be presented in Section 25.3, $\widehat{\zeta}_j$ and $\widehat{\vartheta}_j$ are asymptotic independent both under the null hypothesis ($\beta_{3j} = 0$) and under the alternative hypothesis ($\beta_{3j} \neq 0$). This remarkable property simplifies the expression of the power function for a genetic variant with G×E as the product of the probability of passing the filtering and the power for the second-stage testing. Let $Z_{\widehat{\zeta}_j}$ and $Z_{\widehat{\vartheta}_j}$ denote the z-scores corresponding to $\widehat{\zeta}_j$ and $\widehat{\vartheta}_j$. The power function for the two-stage procedure is

$$\text{Power} = P(|Z_{\widehat{\zeta}_j}| > q_{\alpha_0/2}|\text{H}_1) \times P(|Z_{\widehat{\vartheta}_j}| > q_{\alpha/(2m\alpha_0)}|\text{H}_1), \qquad (25.3)$$

where H_1 is the alternative hypothesis, and $q_{\alpha_0/2}$ and $q_{\alpha/(2m\alpha_0)}$ are upper quantiles of a standard normal distribution. Strictly speaking, the power function above is approximate because the number of tests in the second stage is evaluated at the expectation $m\alpha_0$. Since the number of tests is typically large, this approximation is fairly accurate. Sensitivity analysis may be performed by varying the number of tests between, e.g., $m\alpha_0 - 1.96\text{sd}$ and $m\alpha_0 + 1.96\text{sd}$, where $\text{sd} = \{m\alpha_0(1 - \alpha_0)\}^{1/2}$. Inspection of the power function reveals that, when $\beta_{3j} \neq 0$, it is necessary to ensure that $\zeta_j \neq 0$ and the probability of passing screening is sufficiently high. Otherwise the first component of the power function will be α_0, resulting in abysmal power.

In summary, screening and testing statistics must be carefully paired to have valid type I error control and good power. Several pairs have been proposed: the marginal association statistic and the standard (multiplicative) interaction (Kooperberg and LeBlanc, 2008); the marginal association statistic and the case-only estimator (Dai *et al.*, 2012; Hsu *et al.*, 2012); and the G-E correlation statistic and the standard (multiplicative) interaction (Murcray *et al.*, 2009). Not every screening test statistic can be matched up with every test for G×E. For example, the G-E correlation statistic is not independent of the case-only estimator. The following section examines case-by-case the orthogonality condition in these paired statistics.

25.3 Pairs of screening and G×E testing statistics

25.3.1 Marginal genetic association with disease risk

Define a marginal genetic association model as follows,

$$\text{logit}\{P(Y = 1|G)\} = \gamma_0 + \gamma_1 G. \tag{25.4}$$

If the genetic variant G interacts with an environmental factor on the risk of Y, quite plausibly it would also exhibit some degree of marginal association with Y irrespective of the level of the environmental factor, unless genetic associations within environmental strata cancel out in marginalization. The latter scenario, sometimes called a qualitative interaction, does not occur frequently in epidemiological studies (Weiss, 2008). This argument forms the rationale for the marginal genetic association being used as a screening statistic for discovering G×E. It is a natural and sensitive filter: the set of SNPs with marginal association is of interest biologically, which is often the primary target of a genome-wide association study, and the power to detect a marginal genetic association is typically much higher than G×E testing. This idea was first proposed to test for genome-wide gene × gene interactions (Kooperberg and LeBlanc, 2008).

After screening by marginal genetic association, the second-stage G×E testing can be performed either by the standard case-control estimator in (25.1) or by the case-only estimator in (25.2), as orthogonality holds for both estimators. The asymptotic independence between maximum likelihood estimators $\widehat{\gamma}_1$ and $\widehat{\beta}_3$ in models (25.4) and (25.1) can be proved more generally for nested generalized linear models with a canonical link function (Dai *et al.*, 2012). Briefly, let $\mathbf{X}_1 = (1, G, E, G \times E)$ denote the design matrix for the bigger model (25.1), and let $\mathbf{X}_2 = (1, G)$ denote the design matrix for the smaller model (25.4). The asymptotic covariance matrix of the score functions for parameters in (25.4) and (25.1), denoted by $\mathbf{B}_{12}$, can be expressed as $\mathbb{E}\{(\mathbf{X}_1^T \mathbf{X}_2)\text{var}(Y \mid \mathbf{X}_1)\}$. It follows that the asymptotic covariance matrix of $(\widehat{\beta}_0, \widehat{\beta}_1, \widehat{\beta}_2, \widehat{\beta}_3)$ and $(\widehat{\gamma}_0, \widehat{\gamma}_1)$ is $\mathbf{\Sigma} = \mathbf{A}_1^{-1} \mathbf{B}_{12} \mathbf{A}_2^{-1}$, where $\mathbf{A}_1 = \mathbb{E}\{(\mathbf{X}_1^T \mathbf{X}_1)\text{var}(Y \mid \mathbf{X}_1)\}$ and $\mathbf{A}_2 = \mathbb{E}\{(\mathbf{X}_2^T \mathbf{X}_2)\text{var}(Y \mid \mathbf{X}_2)\}$, which are the negative expectation of the partial derivatives of the score functions for (25.1) and (25.4), respectively. Because $\mathbf{X}_2$ is a sub-matrix in $\mathbf{X}_1$, some algebra shows that the components corresponding to covariance between $(\widehat{\beta}_2, \widehat{\beta}_3)$ and $(\widehat{\gamma}_0, \widehat{\gamma}_1)$ in $\mathbf{\Sigma}$ are zero.

Similarly, the asymptotic covariance between the marginal association estimator $(\widehat{\gamma}_0, \widehat{\gamma}_1)$

in model (25.4) and the case-only estimator $(\widehat{\theta}_0, \widehat{\theta}_1)$ in (25.2) can be derived and the components of the covariance matrix corresponding to $\widehat{\theta}_1$ and $(\widehat{\gamma}_0, \widehat{\gamma}_1)$ can be shown to be 0. The asymptotic independence between the marginal association estimator $\widehat{\gamma}_1$ and the case-only estimator $\widehat{\theta}_1$ then follows.

25.3.2 Correlation of G and E

The correlation of G and E in a case-control sample is modeled by

$$\text{logit}\{P(G = 1|E)\} = \delta_0 + \delta_1 E. \tag{25.5}$$

If there is a G×E, the correlation between G and E is different for cases and controls. Thus, unless the overall correlation between G and E cancels out between cases and controls, there will be a nonzero G-E correlation over all subjects. In fact, when the disease is rare and G-E independence holds in the population, the observed G-E correlation in the combined case-control sample is essentially a tempered version of the case-only estimator of G×E, because G-E independence would roughly hold in controls. Therefore, genetic variants that show correlations with E can be screened for testing G×E (Murcray *et al.*, 2009).

The correlation screening statistic is orthogonal to the standard case-control estimator $\widehat{\beta}_3$ in (25.1). Let $\mathbf{X}_3 = (1, E)$. Following the law of iterated expectations, the asymptotic covariance matrix between the score functions for (25.5) and (25.1) can be expressed as

$$\mathbb{E}_{E,G}[\mathbf{X}_1^T \mathbf{X}_3 \{G - \mathbb{E}(G \mid E)\} \mathbb{E}_{Y|G,E}\{Y - \mathbb{E}(Y \mid G, E)\}] = 0.$$

However, the correlation screening statistic is not orthogonal to the case-only estimator $\widehat{\theta}_1$ in (25.2). The asymptotic covariance between the two estimators $(\widehat{\delta}_0, \widehat{\delta}_1)$ and case-only estimators $(\widehat{\alpha}_0, \widehat{\theta}_1)$ is $\{\mathbb{E}[\mathbf{X}_2^T \mathbf{X}_2 \mathbb{E}(E|G)]\}^{-1}$. The two estimators, $\widehat{\delta}_1$ and $\widehat{\theta}_1$, are indeed positively correlated, which violates the orthogonality assumption, and hence they cannot be used as a pair of screening and G×E testing statistics.

25.3.3 Illustration of why these two screening statistics are informative for G×E

As a pedagogical example, a data set of 500 cases and 500 controls was generated with one binary E with $P(E = 1) = 0.5$ and 400 binary genetic variants each with $P(G = 1) = 0.5$; the main effects of each of these SNPs are set to zero. Half of the variants were selected to have an interaction effect on disease risk with odds ratio 2.5 and the other half had null interaction effect. For each variant the following estimators were calculated: correlation between G and E, the marginal association of G with disease risk, the case-control G×E interaction by model (1), and the case-only G×E by model (2). Figure 25.1 shows the pairwise scatterplots of these associations of 400 SNPs with the "x" representing the variants that have G×E and the "o" representing the variants that have no G×E.

Several observations are made based on this figure. First, compared to variants without interaction, variants with interactions have larger values for the G-E correlation and the marginal association of G with disease risk, indicating that these two screening statistics can indeed help prioritize variants for G×E testing. Second, the case-control G×E estimator is independent of both the marginal association estimator screening and the G-E correlation estimator given any value of β_3, as the two clusters corresponding to no interaction and nonzero interaction show no correlation. Third, the case-only G×E estimator is independent of the marginal association estimator; however, there is a clear linear relationship between the case-only G×E estimator and the G-E correlation even for variants with no interaction, suggesting that if G-E correlation screening were paired with the case-only G×E testing without accounting for the screening, the type I error rate would be inflated.

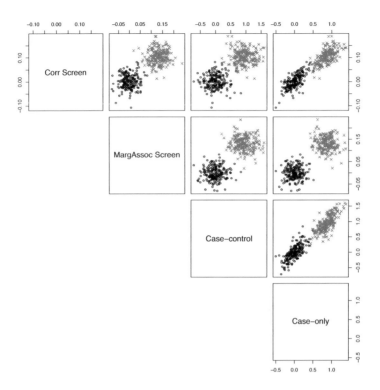

FIGURE 25.1

Pairwise scatterplots of estimates of interaction effect and screening for 400 genetic variants. The "x" and "o" represent SNPs with and without interaction effects, respectively. Corr Screen refers to the correlation between G and E; MargAssoc Screen refers to the association of G with disease risk; Case-control and Case-only refer to the interaction effects of G×E with disease risk by model (25.1) and (25.2), respectively.

25.4   Combinations of genetic association and G-E correlation screening statistics

The power performance of marginal association and G-E correlation as screening statistics for G×E testing depends on the type of interaction. A two-stage procedure using marginal association to screen genetic variants and testing interaction in a standard case-control model is more powerful when the interaction is quantitative, i.e., the magnitude of effect for G (but not the direction) differs for different levels of E or vice versa (Figure 25.2 (a)). On the other hand, when the interaction is qualitative (Figure 25.2 (b)), i.e., the direction of effect for G differs for different levels of E, the G-E correlation screening is more powerful (Dai *et al.*, 2012). The power of G-E correlation as the screening statistic is also affected by the G-E correlation in the population: it yields poor power when G and E have positive interaction but negative correlation in population, or vice versa (Mukherjee *et al.*, 2012).

To optimize power, a natural approach is to allocate the overall significance for genetic variants that pass the screening into two parts: a fraction ρ for the G-E correlation screening and the rest for the marginal association screening (Murcray *et al.*, 2011). However it is

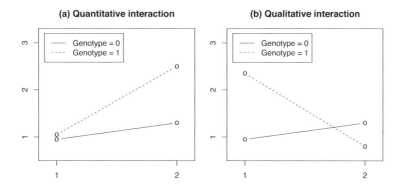

FIGURE 25.2
Two types of G×E interaction for a binary genotype and a binary environmental factor.

difficult to determine the optimal ρ when the types and the sizes of interactions are unknown. To improve the adaptiveness of the screening step, more sophisticated procedures to combine the strength of both screening test statistics have been developed.

25.4.1 Cocktail combination

Let p^{marg} denote the p-value for testing $\gamma_1 = 0$, and let p^{corr} denote the p-value for testing $\delta_1 = 0$. An adaptive screening based on both p-values can be formulated as

$$p^{screen(I)} = p^{marg}I(p^{marg} \leq c) + p^{corr}I(p^{marg} > c),$$

where $I(\cdot)$ denotes the indicator function, and c is a pre-specified constant. This is the first screening p-value constructed in the cocktail approach (Hsu *et al.*, 2012), using marginal genetic association as the primary screening and G-E correlation as the secondary.

The G×E testing statistic is then chosen according to the screening statistic being used. If $p^{screen(I)} = p^{marg}$, the testing statistic can be either the case-only estimator if the G-E independence is known to hold (e.g., E is a randomized treatment assignment in clinical trials), or the robust empirical Bayes (EB) estimator in case that the G-E independence assumption may be violated (Mukherjee and Chatterjee, 2008). This is because the marginal genetic association is orthogonal to both the standard case-control and the case-only G×E estimators. Now if $p^{screen(I)} = p^{corr}$, the testing statistic has to be based on the standard case-control G×E estimator, as the G-E correlation is correlated with the case-only estimator. Hsu *et al.* (2012) showed that $p^{screen(I)}$ is orthogonal to the G×E testing statistics, and the type I error is maintained. The powerful case-only estimator for G×E is thus cautiously incorporated in the testing procedure. This choice of the marginal association as the primary screening compares favorably in power performance to the alternative formulation using the G-E correlation as the primary component (Hsu *et al.*, 2012).

An alternative way of constructing an adaptive screening statistic, avoiding a pre-specified constant c as in $p^{screen(I)}$, is to choose the more significant one out of the two screening statistics, i.e.,

$$p^{screen(II)} = \min(p^{marg}, p^{corr}).$$

Similarly, if $p^{screen(II)} = p^{corr}$, G×E can be tested by the standard case-control estimator; if $p^{screen(II)} = p^{marg}$ the testing can be the powerful case-only or EB estimator. The preservation of the type I error control is more subtle than using $p^{screen(I)}$ for screening, because in the scenario where the marginal association and the case-only/EB estimator are chosen, $p^{screen(II)}$ uses the information in the G-E correlation ($p^{marg} < p^{corr}$) that is not orthogonal to the case-only estimator. Let p^{co} denote the p-value for the case-only estimator used in the G×E testing, and let p^{cc} denote the p-value for the standard case-control G×E testing. For every observed screening p-value cut-off, denoted as α_0, the joint probability of rejecting the G×E null hypothesis at level α can be written as

$$P(p^{co} < \alpha, p^{corr} \geq \alpha_0 \mid p^{marg} = \alpha_0)f(p^{marg} = \alpha_0)$$
$$+ P(p^{cc} < \alpha, p^{marg} \geq \alpha_0 \mid p^{corr} = \alpha_0)f(p^{corr} = \alpha_0).$$

Conditional on the marginal association test statistic, the p-values based on case-only and G-E correlation test statistics can be shown to be positively correlated. As a result the first term is bounded above by

$$P(p^{co} < \alpha \mid p^{marg} = \alpha_0)P(p^{corr} \geq \alpha_0 \mid p^{marg} = \alpha_0)f(p^{marg} = \alpha_0)$$
$$= \alpha P(p^{corr} \geq \alpha_0 \mid p^{marg} = \alpha_0)f(p^{marg} = \alpha_0),$$

where the equality follows from the orthogonality of the marginal association and the case-only estimators. Since the case-control estimator is independent of both screening statistics, the second term equals $\alpha P(p^{marg} \geq \alpha_0 \mid p^{corr} = \alpha_0)f(p^{corr} = \alpha_0)$. It follows that conditional on the cocktail screening $p^{screen(II)}$, the type I error of G×E testing is less than or equal to α.

25.4.2   EDG×E combination

Rather than choosing one of the two screening statistics, it is also appealing to use the marginal genetic association and the G-E correlation together in a combined statistic. Define an adjusted genetic association as follows,

$$\text{logit}\{P(Y = 1|G, E)\} = \beta_0 + \beta_{adj}G + \beta_2 E. \tag{25.6}$$

By the law of iterative expectations, the covariance of the score function for (25.6) and the score function for (25.5) is zero and hence $\text{Cov}(\widehat{\beta}_{adj}, \widehat{\delta}_1) = 0$. Furthermore, model (25.6) is nested in model (25.1), and following the same derivation as the independence between $\widehat{\theta}_1$ and $\widehat{\beta}_3$, $\text{Cov}(\widehat{\beta}_{adj}, \widehat{\beta}_3) = 0$. A χ_2^2 screening statistic can therefore be constructed, paired with testing by the standard case-control interaction: let S_{dg} be the χ_1^2 statistic corresponding to the hypothesis $\beta_{adj} = 0$ in (25.6), and let S_{ge} be the χ_1^2 statistic corresponding to the hypothesis $\delta_1 = 0$ in (25.5). One immediate way to combine the strength of both screening statistics is to use $S_{dg} + S_{ge}$, a χ_2^2 statistic due to independence of $\widehat{\beta}_{adj}$ and $\widehat{\delta}_1$.

A variation of this procedure is to combine the marginal association statistic in (25.4) and the G-E correlation in (25.5) directly, the so-called EDG×E approach (Gauderman *et al.*, 2013). A cautionary note is that, without adjusting for E, the marginal genetic association estimator $\widehat{\gamma}_1$ is not necessarily independent of the G-E correlation estimator $\widehat{\delta}_1$. Therefore a simple sum of the squared z-scores for $\widehat{\gamma}_1$ and $\widehat{\delta}_1$ without accounting for the correlation between the two test statistics is not distributed as χ_2^2. Nevertheless, the orthogonality between $(\widehat{\gamma}_1, \widehat{\delta}_1)$ and $\widehat{\beta}_3$ protects the validity of two-stage testing for G×E, even when the distribution of the combined screening statistic is not properly modeled in the first stage.

25.4.3   Power comparison

The power of two-stage testing procedures is compared with the standard case-control G×E estimator and the empirical Bayes (EB) estimator as introduced in Chapter 24. The

EB estimator combines the case-only and the case-control estimators using a weight, with greater weight given to the more efficient case-only estimator if the G-E independence is likely to hold and to the more robust case-control estimator otherwise. All derivations for the case-only estimator apply to the EB estimator.

Extensive simulations have been conducted to compare power performance of various screening statistics and the results can be found in Dai *et al.* (2012), Hsu *et al.* (2012) and Gauderman *et al.* (2013). Briefly, the marginal genetic association screening can increase power substantially particularly if variants have main genetic effects; however it can also lose power if the interaction model results in a null or small marginal association. A similar performance is observed for correlation screening. The hybrid screening statistics are like a double insurance and help guard potential power loss if a particular interaction model does not result in a marginal association or G-E correlation, but not both.

Here only two hybrid screening statistics, cocktail *screen(II)* followed by the EB estimator for G×E testing and EDG×E screening followed by the case-control estimator, are compared with the case-control and EB estimators. The power is computed algebraically using an R package for two-stage testing, `powerGWASinteraction`, which is available from CRAN (`http://cran.us.r-project.org/`). Specifically, consider a case-control study. Under model (25.1), both the Z-statistics for marginal genetic association and correlation of G and E, as well as their correlation, are derived and computed. This forms the basis for calculation of the probability of each hybrid screening statistic passing the pre-specified screening threshold. The power for a two-step procedure for G×E testing is then obtained by (25.3).

Briefly, consider a genome-wide case-control association study of $n = 20,000$ cases and $20,000$ controls with 1 million independent genetic variants. The disease prevalence is set to be 0.01 and the frequencies of G and E are 0.4 and 0.2, respectively. The family-wise type I error rate is controlled at 0.05, and the first stage significance level for screening, α_0, is taken as 0.001. Figure 25.3 shows that the two-stage testing with hybrid screening statistics, cocktail and EDG×E, deliver consistently good power compared to approaches without screening under all scenarios considered. Both the conventional case-control and EB estimators are very powerful under some scenarios, but can lose substantial power under other scenarios. The two-stage procedures that screen using only marginal association or G-E correlation, but not both, in general perform not as robustly as the hybrid procedures (results omitted). See also Hsu *et al.* (2012) and Gauderman *et al.* (2013).

25.4.4   Practical consideration

The power of two-stage testing can be sensitive to the choice of the threshold for the first stage screening. A stringent threshold may filter out variants with G×E, whereas a relaxed threshold may not reduce the burden of multiple comparisons enough to gain sufficient power for detecting G×E. Since the truth is unknown, it is difficult to determine *a priori* an appropriate threshold. To ease this difficulty, genetic variants may be grouped into multiple bins according to the strength of their screening statistics. Less stringent significance levels are then assigned to bins with stronger screening statistics and more stringency given to bins with weaker screening statistics, while maintaining an overall type I error at a pre-specified level for genome-wide G×E testing.

For example, one strategy is to rank genetic variants according to the significance of the screening statistics, and group these variants sequentially into bins of different sizes such as 5, 10, 20, 40, etc. (Ionita-Laza *et al.*, 2007). Variants in these bins are then assigned with varying levels of significance. For the aforementioned bin sizes, the corresponding levels are $\alpha/(2 \cdot 5)$, $\alpha/(4 \cdot 10)$, $\alpha/(8 \cdot 20)$, $\alpha/(16 \cdot 40)$, ..., to keep an overall type I error at α. An issue of grouping ranked variants into bins is that many variants are in linkage

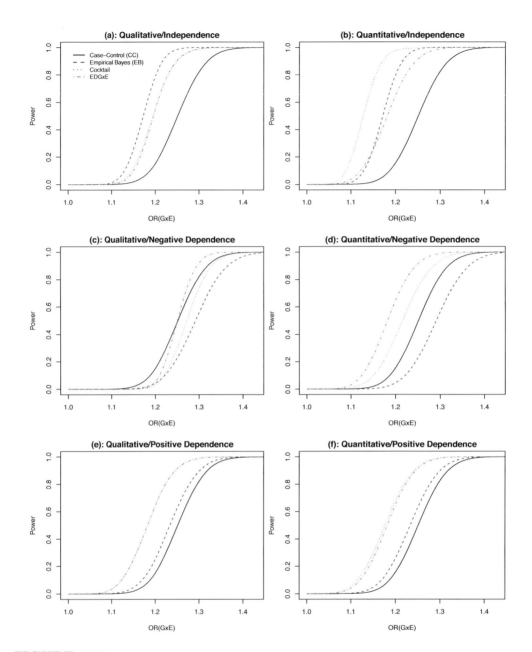

FIGURE 25.3
Power comparison of two hybrid two-stage testing, cocktail and EDG×E, and no-screening case-control (CC) and empirical Bayes (EB) G×E testing. Scenarios (a) and (b) are under qualitative and quantitative interaction, respectively, with independent G and E. The odds ratio (OR) of the main effect of E is 1.2, and the OR of the main effect of G is 1.05 under the quantitative interaction model and 0.95 under the qualitative model. Scenarios (c) and (d) are similar to (a) and (b) except that G and E are negatively correlated with OR 0.95. Scenarios (e) and (f) are similar to (a) and (b) except that G and E are positively correlated with OR 1.05.

disequilibrium. If a variant has a strong screening statistic, all correlated variants also have strong screening statistics and then a bin could have many correlated variants all tagging the same G×E causal variant. To avoid this problem, correlated variants may be first pruned by, for example, linkage disequilibrium or distance, before variants are grouped in bins.

25.5   Post-menopausal hormone therapy and colorectal cancer

Colorectal cancer is one of the most commonly diagnosed cancers and one of the leading causes of cancer death (Ferlay *et al.*, 2015). It has a sizable genetic component and well-established lifestyle and environmental risk factors (Peters *et al.*, 2015; Potter, 1999). The Genetics and Epidemiology Colorectal Cancer Consortium (GECCO) includes cohort and case-control studies conducted in North America, Australia, and Europe (Peters *et al.*, 2013). A key strength of this consortium is the large sample size with over 40,000 participants from well-characterized studies with detailed data on key environmental risk factors for colorectal cancer, and genome-wide genotyping data. For illustration, a genome-wide search of G×E with use of post-menopausal hormone therapy, here, specifically, estrogen plus progestin therapy (E+P), using two-stage testing procedures is shown here. The E+P use has been consistently shown to be associated with a reduced risk of developing colorectal cancer (Lin *et al.*, 2012). However, the underlying mechanisms of how such use influences colon carcinogenesis are largely unknown. It is therefore of interest to investigate genetic modifiers of colorectal cancer risk associated E+P use. The overall analysis results have been described previously (Garcia-Albeniz *et al.*, 2016).

There were a total of 10,835 post-menopausal women in GECCO: 5,419 cases and 5,416 controls, among whom 1,283 (11.8%) used estrogen plus progestin (E+P). Compared to nonusers of any HT, the OR (odds ratio) for colorectal cancer was 0.76 (95% CI 0.64 – 0.90, p = 0.0015) for women who used E+P. The conventional case-control analysis did not yield any variant that reached the genome-wide significance level of 5×10^{-8}. The EB test identified a significant interaction of variant rs964293 with OR = 0.62 (95% CI 0.53 – 0.73, p = 9.1×10^{-9}). The same variant was also identified by the CO test with OR = 0.63 (95% CI 0.55 – 0.74, p = 2.4×10^{-9}).

Both the cocktail and EDG×E screening approaches were performed. The multi-tiered testing described in Section 25.4.4 was used for two-stage testing. Correlated variants were pruned by distance. Specifically, SNPs were ranked according to the p-values of the screening statistics. Starting from the top ranked SNP and moving down the list, if a SNP was within 50Kb of any of the variants ranked higher, it was pruned. This results in about 40,000 roughly independent variants. They were then binned into groups of 5, 10, 20, 40, … SNPs and the corresponding significance levels for the groups were $\alpha/(2 \cdot 5)$, $\alpha/(4 \cdot 10)$, $\alpha/(8 \cdot 20)$, $\alpha/(16 \cdot 40)$, …, to give an overall type I error control of $\alpha = 0.05$.

The same variant, rs964293, showed a statistically significant interaction with E+P use on CRC risk for both the cocktail and EDG×E approaches (Table 25.1). For the cocktail screening, the correlation screening drove the screening signal. As a result, only the conventional case-control estimator can be used for testing G×E. The p-value for the case-control testing p^{cc} is 2.8×10^{-5}, exceeding the significance level for the bin, $\alpha = 3.1 \times 10^{-4}$, to which the SNP belongs. This p-value would not have reached the genome-wide significance level if screening were not performed. Similarly, the same SNP also passed the bin-level significance with the EDG×E screening. Both the cocktail and EDG×E screening assigned the variant in the same bin; however, the cocktail screening ranked this variant higher than EDG×E, 17 versus 35. This is because the screening signal only came from the correlation

TABLE 25.1
Results of the cocktail and EDG×E two-stage testing for SNP rs964293.

Method	p^{corr}	p^{marg}	p^{screen}	Rank	Bin	α_{bin}	p^{cc}
Cocktail	5.1×10^{-6}	0.99	5.1×10^{-6}	17	3	3.1×10^{-4}	2.8×10^{-5}
EDG×E	5.1×10^{-6}	0.99	3.0×10^{-6}	35	3	3.1×10^{-4}	2.8×10^{-5}

and EDG×E lost slight efficiency compared to the cocktail if the screening signal came from only one of the two screening statistics.

Since pruning could potentially filter out true G×E variants, as a comparison the genetic variants that were pruned out were brought back to the same bin as the variants with which they are tagged. A permutation test was conducted to calculate the effective number of independent tests in each bin and the significance level was adjusted accordingly. There was no additional G×E interaction that reached the genome-wide significance.

25.6 Summary

The interest in identifying G×E and G×G interactions has been recently revived because the availability of large-scale genome-wide association and next generation sequencing studies allows for a comprehensive interrogation of these interactions. As shown in simulations, the two-stage testing approach, in which variants are screened for their potential to be involved in interactions and only those that pass the screening are formally tested for interactions, can greatly enhance power for detecting interaction in a genome-wide search. In practice, however, the anticipated power improvement by two-stage procedures has not resulted in a proliferation of new G×E findings. This may be because the effect sizes for G×E are more modest than those evaluated in simulation, and the sample sizes for genome-wide G×E studies have not reached an adequate level. There are also other possible reasons, for example, simulations do not usually account for the complexity of environmental risk factors such as measurement error and heterogeneity across studies. Larger sample sizes and better measurements of environmental risk factors may hold promise to improve detection of G×E in such scenarios.

EDG×E, the sum of the chi-squared test statistics from marginal association and G-E correlation, is powerful when both screening statistics show evidence from the interaction. In contrast, the cocktail screening statistic is particularly powerful if marginal association screening is more informative when variants that have interaction effect also have main effect in the same direction. The power gain for the cocktail approach also comes from that the efficient case-only or EB estimator that exploits gene-environment independence can be used for testing G×E. It is worth noting that conditional on one of the marginal association estimators, the case-only estimator, and the correlation estimator, the other two of these three are correlated. This can be seen from a simple case of binary G, binary E, and binary disease status for which a 2×2×2 table can be formed, and given one of the estimators, the other two estimators are perfectly correlated. Various combinations of screening statistics followed by either the standard case-control or the more efficient case-only test, to some degree, are just different ways to use the same information in such a 2×2×2 table.

The two-stage testing procedures can be casted into the framework of "weighted hypothesis procedures" (Roeder and Wasserman, 2009). In this framework the threshold for each variant to be declared statistically significant is multiplied by a weight w (≥ 0), relaxing the threshold when $w > 1$ and decreasing it if $w < 1$. To control the overall type I error, the only

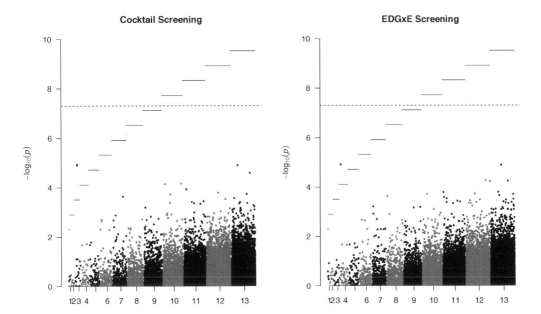

FIGURE 25.4

Manhattan plot of G×E with estrogen plus progestin use with colorectal cancer using both the cocktail (left) and EDG×E (right) methods. The variants are ordered along the X-axis by the size of the screening statistics. Gray and black bands correspond to groups of SNPs that are tested at the second stage with the same significance cut-off. The initial group size is 5 variants, and each successive group includes twice as many as variants as the preceding group. Along the Y-axis the $-\log 10$(p-value) for the second stage testing is displayed. The stepped horizontal line corresponds to the significance level for each group; the horizontal dashed-line would be the genome-wide significance for a one-stage procedure. Variant rs964293 is marked by an "x".

requirement is that the average weight is one. For example, the Bonferroni correction gives each test an equal weight. In contrast, the two-stage testing assigns a much larger weight to selected variants, but a zero weight to those that are not selected. Use of an informative weighting scheme leads to a significant improvement of power. The screening statistics that are introduced in this chapter provide a natural basis for selecting the weights. Another example of weight assignment may be to partition SNPs into bins such that variants belonging to the same bin receive the same weight and variants ranked higher by screening statistics are given greater weight (Hsu *et al.*, 2012; Ionita-Laza *et al.*, 2007), as we did for the colorectal cancer example. However, despite the informativeness of screening statistics, it remains to be difficult to select weights that are robust against a wide range of interaction scenarios, as would likely to be the case in a genome wide search of G×E.

The two-stage testing procedure can be applied to joint testing of main genetic effect and gene-environment interaction under model (25.1) (Kraft *et al.*, 2007), where G×E is exploited to improve power of detecting genetic association. The G-E correlation can be used as a screening statistic as it is easily shown to be independent of the joint test using the same technique as in Dai *et al.* (2012). A variation of this joint test can be obtained by combining the squared Z-statistics for the marginal test of genetic association and the test for G×E into a 2 degrees of freedom test. This way one can make use of the more efficient case-only or EB estimators for G×E. The marginal genetic association statistic here needs to adjust for E to ensure independence of the correlation statistic and the marginal association statistic.

The two-stage testing procedures can also be applied to genome-wide search of gene-gene (G×G) interaction. The computation required for calculating G-G correlation is on the order of the square of P variants. Algorithms that do not require iterative numerical methods are best; however, they are limited in fitting regression models, e.g., accounting for population structure. An approximation solution is to calculate the G-G correlation stratified by major groups of ancestry determined by principal components of genome-wide variants, though such approximation may fail to account for subtle population substructures. For marginal genetic association screening, the association signals for each pair of genetic variants can be combined in various ways. Using the minimum of the two Z-statistics works out to select a group of SNPs and test all pairwise interactions (Kooperberg and LeBlanc, 2008); using the maximum of the two Z-statistics is selecting a group of SNPs and testing them against all other SNPs. Another possibility would be to use a χ^2 combination of the two Z-statistics. Which combination or which screening statistic is more informative depends on the type of G-G interaction.

There are many open questions: decision rule and weight choice based on screening statistics in order to achieve robust power for detecting interaction; multiple testing adjustment for correlated SNPs (linkage disequilibrium); additive versus multiplicative interaction in relation to biological interaction. Future research along these lines may further improve the effectiveness and broad applicability of the two-stage approaches to genome-wide discovery of G×E and G×G interaction.

Acknowledgment

This work is supported by R01 HG006124, R01 HL114901, R01 CA189532, R01 CA195789, R21 CA214612, and P01 CA53996. The authors thank the Genetics and Epidemiology of Colorectal Cancer Consortium (GECCO; U01 CA137088; R01 CA059045) investigators and staff for their dedication, and the study participants for making the consortium possible. For a full description of the included studies (CCFR, DACHS, DALS, MEC, NHS, OFCCR, PLCO, PMH-CCFR, VITAL, WHI) and their funding sources, please see Peters *et al.* (2013).

Bibliography

Chatterjee, N. and Carroll, R. J. (2005). Semiparametric maximum likelihood estimation exploiting gene-environment independence in case-control studies. *Biometrika*, **92**, 399–418.

Chen, J., Kang, G., VanderWeele, T., Zhang, C., and Mukherjee, B. (2012). Efficient design of gene-environment interaction studies: Implications of Hardy-Weinberg equilibrium and gene-environment independence. *Statistics in Medicine*, **31**, 2516–2530.

Dai, J. Y., Kooperberg, C., LeBlanc, M., and Prentice, R. L. (2012). Two-stage testing procedures with independent filtering for genome-wide gene-environment interaction. *Biometrika*, **99**, 929–944.

Ferlay, J., Soerjomataram, I., Dikshit, R., Eser, S., Mathers, C., Rebelo, M., Parkin, D. M., Forman, D., and Bray, F. (2015). Cancer incidence and mortality worldwide: Sources, methods and major patterns in GLOBOCAN 2012. *International Journal of Cancer*, **136**, E359–E386.

Garcia-Albeniz, X., Rudolph, A., Hutter, C., White, E., Lin, Y., Rosse, S. A., Figueiredo, J. C., Harrison, T. A., Jiao, S., Brenner, H., *et al.* (2016). CYP24A1 variant modifies the association between use of oestrogen plus progestogen therapy and colorectal cancer risk. *British Journal of Cancer*, **114**, 221–229.

Gauderman, J., Zhang, P., Morrison, J. L., and Lewinger, J. P. (2013). Finding novel genes by testing G×E interactions in a genome-wide association study. *Genetic Epidemiology*, **37**, 603–613.

Hsu, L., Shuo, J., Dai, J. Y., Hutter, C., and Kooperberg, C. (2012). A powerful cocktail strategy for detecting genome-wide gene-environment interaction. *Genetic Epidemiology*, **36**, 183–94.

Hunter, D. J. (2005). Gene-environment interactions in human diseases. *Nature Reviews Genetics*, **6**, 287–298.

Hutter, C. M., Mechanic, L. E., Chatterjee, N., Kraft, P., and Gillanders, E. M. on behalf of the NCI Gene-Environment Think Tank (2013). Gene-environment interactions in cancer epidemiology: A National Cancer Institute Think Tank report. *Genetic Epidemiology*, **37**, 643–657.

Ionita-Laza, I., McQueen, M. B., Laird, N. M., and Lange, C. (2007). Genomewide weighted hypothesis testing in family-based association studies, with an application to a 100K scan. *The American Journal of Human Genetics*, **81**, 607–614.

Kooperberg, C. and LeBlanc, M. (2008). Increasing the power of identifying gene-gene interactions in genome-wide association studies. *Genetic Epidemiology*, **32**, 255–263.

Kraft, P., Yen, Y.-C., Stram, D. O., Morrison, J., and Gauderman, W. J. (2007). Exploiting gene-environment interaction to detect genetic associations. *Human Heredity*, **63**, 111–119.

Lin, K. J., Cheung, W. Y., Lai, J. Y., and Giovannucci, E. L. (2012). The effect of estrogen vs. combined estrogen-progestogen therapy on the risk of colorectal cancer. *International Journal of Cancer*, **130**, 419–430.

Mukherjee, B. and Chatterjee, N. (2008). Exploiting gene-environment independence for analysis of case-control studies: An empirical Bayes approach to trade off between bias and efficiency. *Biometrics*, **64**, 685–694.

Mukherjee, B., Ahn, J., Gruber, S. B., and Chatterjee, N. (2012). Testing gene-environment interaction in large-scale case-control association studies: Possible choices and comparisons. *American Journal of Epidemiology*, **175**, 177–190.

Murcray, C. E., Lewinger, J. P., and Gauderman, J. W. (2009). Gene-environment interaction in genome-wide association studies. *American Journal of Epidemiology*, **169**, 219–226.

Murcray, C. E., Lewinger, J. P., Conti, D. V., Thomas, D. C., and Gauderman, W. J. (2011). Sample size requirement to detect gene-environment interactions in genome-wide association studies. *Genetic Epidemiology*, **35**, 201–210.

Peters, U., Jiao, S., Schumacher, F. R., Hutter, C. M., Aragaki, A. K., Baron, J. A., Berndt, S. I., Bézieau, S., Brenner, H., Butterbach, K., *et al.* (2013). Identification of genetic susceptibility loci for colorectal tumors in a genome-wide meta-analysis. *Gastroenterology*, **144**, 799–807.

Peters, U., Bien, S., and Zubair, N. (2015). Genetic architecture of colorectal cancer. *Gut*, **64**, 1623–1636.

Piegorsch, W. W., Weinberg, C. R., and Taylor, J. A. (1994). Non-hierarchical logistic models and case-only designs for assessing susceptibility in population based case-control studies. *Statistics in Medicine*, **13**, 153–162.

Potter, J. D. (1999). Colorectal cancer: Molecules and populations. *Journal of the National Cancer Institute*, **91**, 916–932.

Roeder, K. and Wasserman, L. (2009). Genome-wide significance levels and weighted hypothesis testing. *Statistical Science*, **24**, 398.

Smith, P. G. and Day, N. E. (1984). The design of case-control studies: The influence of confounding and interaction effects. *International Journal of Epidemiology*, **13**, 356–365.

Thomas, D. (2010). Gene-environment-wide association studies: Emerging approaches. *Nature Reviews Genetics*, **11**, 259–272.

Weiss, N. S. (2008). Subgroup-specific associations in the face of overall null results: Should we rush in or fear to tread? *Cancer Epidemiology Biomarkers & Prevention*, **17**, 1297–1299.

26

Family-Based Case-Control Approaches to Study the Role of Genetics

Clarice R. Weinberg, Min Shi, and David M. Umbach

National Institute of Environmental Health Sciences, NIH

26.1 Introduction

Family-based study designs offer a useful alternative to population-based designs, particularly for studies of genetic contributions to conditions that develop early in life, such as birth defects, childhood cancers, or psychiatric disorders. This chapter will provide an introduction to methods based on genetic studies of nuclear families where at least one offspring has developed the condition of interest.

To delineate the scope of the chapter, we will consider designs that exploit apparent distortions in transmissions of relevant alleles to affected offspring. We focus on two simple designs: the case-parents design, where the affected child and available parents are genotyped, and the discordant sibling design, where at least one affected sibling and at least one unaffected sibling are genotyped. A principal use, but not the only use, for these designs is to study the relationship between heritable genetic factors and disease. For this purpose, they have a distinct advantage over population-based case-control designs, as they offer inherent robustness to bias arising from hidden genetic population structure (see Chapter 23 for a definition and discussion of this problem). They can have other advantages as well.

For consideration of methods that broaden the case-control setting to allow both cryptic and known relatedness among some of the participants, mixed models can be useful, as described in Chapter 27 by Golan and Rosset. The genotype data can be used to estimate a kinship correlation matrix for the random effects, as has been described (Euahsunthornwattana *et al.*, 2014). We caution the reader, however, that statistical dependencies can involve shared environments and not just kinship, so that additional measures to control nongenetic sources of dependency may be needed (Zhang and Pan, 2015). Hybrid designs will also not be considered here (Weinberg and Umbach, 2005).

This chapter is organized as follows. It begins with some genetic background and describes some general features of these family-based designs. It then provides an overview of analytic approaches that have been developed for the case-parents design. Next, specific topics such as missing data are considered, as are other aspects of genetic risk, such as maternal effects (effects on the child of the mother's genotype expressed prenatally) and parent-of-origin effects, that can be analytically probed with this design but not with a case-control design. The chapter then outlines features of discordant-sibling designs and provides some power comparisons across the designs. It closes by describing how to assess gene-by-environment interaction and multi-SNP effects with these designs.

26.2   Genetic background

Genetic variation among people is typically measured by genotyping diallelic single nucleotide polymorphisms (SNPs). These are loci on the genome where a single base pair is different for some individual chromosomes, so that there are exactly two versions (two distinct *alleles*) in the population. The more common of the two alleles is sometimes referred to as the "wild" type and the rarer of the two as the "variant" or the "mutant" allele. These alleles are transmitted from parents to child and, for the "autosomes" (the 22 chromosomes that are not the sex chromosomes X or Y), one allele was inherited from the mother and the other from the father via the gametes. Because each person has two copies of each autosomal chromosome, each carries 0, 1, or 2 copies of each autosomal variant. The human genome contains at least 38 million such SNPs (The 1000 Genomes Project Consortium, 2012). A genotyping assay typically reports how many copies of the variant are present at each SNP locus but does not report whether or not variants at two nearby loci are on the same parental chromosome. This missing information is referred to as "phase ambiguity" and it causes problems when one would like to assess risk associated with a particular haplotype (a set of neighboring SNPs on the same strand of DNA).

In the meiotic formation of gametes (sperm and oocyte), *recombinations* occur, often through crossover, which can break up a haplotype string of base pairs. SNP alleles that are located near each other on the same chromosome often tend to be inherited together, a phenomenon termed *linkage*, because their proximity reduces the probability of an intervening meiotic recombination event. The resulting proximity-related correlations in transmission, together with stochastic effects of genetic drift, selection for fitness over ancestral history, and the existence of incompletely assimilated ("admixed") subpopulations, have caused the counts of alleles at nearby SNPs to be correlated, especially if the ancestral mutation was relatively recent, creating *linkage disequilibrium* (LD). One practical implication of this biology is that the analyst needs to be aware that a statistical association between a SNP and a disease is often not causal: instead it often exists because the SNP that happened to be genotyped is in LD with some other SNP or haplotype that is causative.

26.3   Benefits and limitations of designs based on nuclear families

When genetic variants are of interest as risk factors for disease, population-based case-control studies can be subject to bias from what is known as *genetic population stratification*, a kind of confounding caused by nonrandom mating across subpopulations that vary in both their allele frequencies and in their baseline risk of the disease. Such subpopulations may be distinguished by ethnicity, geography (e.g., residence on a particular island), or some other factor that is related to susceptibility to the disease, prevalence of the allele and within-group mate selection. When such subpopulations are not readily distinguishable to the analyst, the usual remedy of stratified analysis is unavailable. Methods for indirectly adjusting for the resulting confounding in a population-based case-control study are provided in Chapter 23. Both case-parents and case-siblings study designs inherently resist bias due to genetic population stratification when testing for genetic effects. Case-parent approaches achieve this robustness by basing the inference on transmissions, a strategy that in effect enlists the parents of each case as perfectly matched genetic controls. Discordant sibling designs use full siblings as the perfectly matched genetic controls. Both designs can provide information that alleviates phase ambiguity for multi-SNP analyses.

Another problem that can influence population-based approaches is cryptic relatedness, where cases and controls that are treated as independent observations in a logistic analysis may actually have shared ancestry and not be fully independent. Methods for adjusting for that problem are provided in Chapter 27. Studies based on nuclear families are less subject to that problem (Bennett and Curnow, 2001).

Both the case-parent design and the discordant sibling design can be used to circumvent potential confounding of the offspring genome by the maternal genome. The mother's genome in part determines the offspring genome, but her genetic variants can also influence the prenatal environment in which the fetus develops. For example, a variant in a maternal gene that governs a detoxification pathway could make the embryo vulnerable to a teratogen (regardless of whether the causative variant allele was transmitted to the fetus) and that genetic variant would be (as a noncausal epiphenomenon) more commonly found in affected offspring than in population-based control offspring. This is one reason that genetic factors identified in a population-based case-control study may not always imply a causal role for the inherited genotype of the offspring. Unlike a case-control study or a discordant sibling study, the case-parents design can readily disentangle effects of the fetally inherited genotype from prenatal effects due to the maternal genotype. In fact, the case-parent design can be applied to the study of pregnancy complications, such as preeclampsia, where the 'case' can be thought of as the pregnancy itself, and both genomes could play a role in the etiology.

Finally, family-based designs can have important practical advantages. Parents of a newborn with a birth defect or of a child with cancer are often both nearby and motivated to contribute good quality data to research. The same would hold for parents of a young adult cancer patient and, presumably, for the siblings of adult patients. With the case-parents design, survival bias can also be avoided because parents can be included even if the affected offspring is unavailable due to elective termination of the pregnancy or death of the offspring.

Nevertheless, some caution is in order for family-based studies. If one enrolls affected individuals who are old enough that their parents or siblings will be selectively available, e.g., due to genotype effects on survival, then missingness can be informative and bias can result, both in testing and in estimation of the relative risks. In the U.S. population such attrition could become a serious concern for case ages above 50 (http://www.cdc.gov/

nchs/data/databriefs/db26.pdf). In populations with lower life expectancy, bias due to genotype-related attrition could be a problem even for younger diagnoses.

Another issue is that, even though missing data methods can be usefully employed when some individual genotype data are missing, the inclusion of ethnic minority families can result in estimation problems if missingness is related to ethnicity and thus to allele frequency. Stratification by ethnicity becomes necessary but produces problems related to low cell counts. This sparseness can be a problem even if the missingness is noninformative within each subpopulation.

Another major limitation is that, with studies based on cases and their parents, one cannot estimate main effects of nongenetic factors. The discordant sibling design does not face this limitation. A tetrad design that extends the case-parents design by including an unaffected sibling overcomes this limitation and enables inclusion of nongenetic factors but will not be further considered here (Shi *et al.*, 2013).

26.4   Methods of analysis for the case-parents design

Transmission-based approaches using nuclear families were originally described by Rubinstein *et al.* (1981) and Falk and Rubinstein (1987), and a conditional-logistic-regression-based method of analysis was first proposed by Self *et al.* (1991). The classical population-based case-control design allows one to test the null hypothesis that a given genetic variant is not marginally associated with the disease of interest, whereas a family-based design is best thought of as testing a null that the marker under study is not in linkage with any disease-causing variant. Rejection of this null yields a more direct causal inference that either the variant itself increases risk of the disease or it is linked to a nearby correlated variant or set of variants that increases risk.

The most basic unit of study considered is the case-parent triad, with one affected offspring and both parents genotyped (though a case-parent-grandparent study can be even more informative (Mitchell and Weinberg, 2005)). The key assumption underlying all methods of analysis is that SNP alleles are transmitted randomly; that is, via Mendelian inheritance. In short, we assume that each heterozygous parent from the source population is equally likely to have transmitted the minor allele and the wild-type allele to their offspring. The fundamental insight that forms the basis for inference with this design is that, if sampling into the study is not random but is based on the offspring having developed the disease of interest, a disease-related allele will appear to have been selectively over-transmitted to affected offspring from heterozygous parents. That apparent transmission distortion does not have its basis in the underlying biology, but in the disease-based sampling that generated the case-parent triads.

Mendelian transmission requires that certain assumptions hold for the source population: equal likelihood of transmission to viable gametes, equal likelihood of fertilization success, equal probability of survival to birth and equal probability of survival long enough to be at risk of the condition under study. While it is known that *transmission ratio distortion* does occur in certain mammals, e.g., due to *meiotic drive*, gamete competition or differential prenatal survival, thus far there is no compelling evidence that transmission ratio distortion happens in humans (Meyer *et al.*, 2012). We therefore assume that in the source population offspring of a heterozygous parent are equally likely to have inherited either allele, and thus control-parent triads are not needed for valid inference.

For the following sections, let us assume that the study has measured genotypes for a sample of unrelated case-parent triads, with no missing genotype data or missing family members. We initially consider a single, diallelic autosomal locus and denote the "wild-type" allele as "A" and the "variant" allele as "a."

26.4.1 Pseudo-sibling approaches

The first method proposed to usefully exploit these assumptions (Self *et al.*, 1991) was devised for studying associations between human leukocyte antigen (HLA) genetics and aplastic anemia. Under the null hypothesis that no particular allele is associated with risk, the two pairs of alleles carried by the parents of cases should be equally likely to produce any of 4 possible pairs of alleles in their offspring. With this fact in mind, Self et al. recognized that purely hypothetical children could usefully serve as controls in a conditional logistic model based on families with an affected offspring. Methods based on such "pseudo-siblings" offer flexible modeling through conditional logistic regression (Cordell *et al.*, 2004; Wise *et al.*, 2016).

26.4.2 Transmission-based approaches

An alternative and closely related approach to testing, which is also widely used, enumerates transmissions from informative, i.e., heterozygous, parents to affected offspring. Let b be the number of heterozygous parents who transmitted the a allele and c be the number who instead transmitted the A allele. The transmission disequilibrium test (TDT) (Spielman *et al.*, 1993) is a McNemar's test:

$$TDT = \frac{(b-c)^2}{b+c}.$$

(For each triad where transmission is ambiguous because both parents and the affected offspring are heterozygous, one adds 0.5 to b and 0.5 to c.) Under the null and with large numbers of informative families, the TDT statistic is distributed as chi-squared with 1 degree of freedom. Several extensions have been proposed to the TDT (Gordon *et al.*, 2004; Spielman and Ewens, 1998).

A related approach, called the family-based association test (FBAT) (Laird and Lange, 2006, 2008), calculates the mean product of the offspring trait (which could be binary or continuous) and the difference between the observed coded offspring genotype (e.g., number of copies of allele a) and its expected value conditional on a sufficient statistic for the parental genotypes. The statistic is

$$U = \sum_{ij} T_{ij} \left\{ X_{ij} - E(X_{ij}|S_i) \right\}.$$

Here, i indexes the family, j indexes nonfounders, e.g., offspring, in the family, X_{ij} is a coded genotype for person ij, T_{ij} is the trait value (which is 1 for everyone in a case-parent study), and S_i is a family-specific sufficient statistic that depends on which genotypes are missing and on the available genotypes (Laird and Lange, 2006; Rabinowitz and Laird, 2000). For a case-parent study with no missing genotypes, the FBAT statistic is equivalent to a test based on the mean paired difference between the total number of copies transmitted and the total number not transmitted, so that the TDT and FBAT are asymptotically equivalent. Both the TDT and FBAT are fully nonparametric, but neither provides relative risk estimates for the association between disease and one or two inherited copies of allele a compared to no copies.

26.4.3   Count-based approach

An alternative approach makes use of Poisson regression (Weinberg *et al.*, 1998). Let M, F, and C denote the number of copies of the variant allele carried by the mother, father and affected offspring, respectively. One fits the following log-linear model to the 15-nomial corresponding to all possible 3-tuples (M, F, C) of case-parent genotypes, where the unit of analysis is now the case-parent triad (and not transmissions):

$$\ln\{E(N_{M,F,C})\} = \mu_{\{M,F\}} + \beta_1 I_{(C=1)} + \beta_2 I_{(C=2)} + \ln(2) I_{(M=F=C=1)}. \qquad (26.1)$$

Here, the subscripted "I" is an indicator function that is 1 or 0 corresponding to whether the subscripted parenthetical expression is true or false, and the final term is an "offset" that doubles the count for the (1,1,1) cell, reflecting the fact that there are two ways to inherit a single copy when both parents are heterozygous. The intercept terms depend on the six possible pairs of (unordered) parental genotypes, i.e., the set $\{M, F\}$, and serve to impose conditioning on the set of parental genotypes without imposing any constraints on their relative numbers.

These "mating type" parameters have sometimes been misinterpreted as representing the log-relative frequencies of the six parental mating types in the source population. That interpretation is incorrect because even under the null hypothesis, population stratification will tend to distort the relative contributions of particular pairs of parental genotypes for parents of affected individuals due to variation in risk of disease across genetically diverse subpopulations. Thus the distribution of genotypes in parents of cases need not resemble the distribution of parental genotypes in the source population. A related point is that the design and analysis, by conditioning on parental genotypes, also inherently protects against bias due to self-selection of parents that may be jointly case- and genotype-related. Such self-selection can be related to factors such as access to medical care and therapeutic abortion, lifestyle differences, and even gene variants that might influence healthy people to altruistically volunteer for research studies. Self-selection is much less important for family-based studies where the controls are inherently matched to the cases than for population-based case-control studies where sampling of suitable controls remains an ongoing and possibly worsening challenge.

The expected cell counts reflect Mendelian transmission under the null. Under alternatives, they are distorted according to R_1 and R_2, which correspond to $\exp(\beta_1)$ and $\exp(\beta_2)$, the relative risks for offspring who inherit one or two copies, respectively, compared to no copies. Note that this structure is equivalent to that assumed by the TDT and FBAT under the null; and, therefore, all require the same assumptions for validity. The log-linear approach, however, specifies a risk-related particular distortion of the counts under alternatives. No rare disease assumption is required; and, unlike the population-based case-control study, the case-parent design with the log-linear model provides estimates of relative risks. Simplified coding of genotype effects can also be used: for example, for a genetic effects model that is log-additive in the number of copies C carried by the child, one replaces the "co-dominant" coding $\beta_1 I_{(C=1)} + \beta_2 I_{(C=2)}$ in (26.1) with βC.

Alternatively, one can maximize a likelihood, as proposed by Schaid and Sommer (1993), which explicitly conditions on parental genotypes. If the case-parent triad data are complete, relative risk estimation and testing will be completely equivalent to those of the log-linear model.

Sporadically missing individual SNP data and whole genomes that are missing for missing family members are commonplace in family-based studies. Naive exclusion of those families for which the missing data cannot be inferred from the observed data can produce bias (Curtis and Sham, 1995). Inclusion of families with missing genotype data is possible with FBAT (Horvath *et al.*, 2001) but is more straightforward under the log-linear framework. Under noninformative missingness, the expectation-maximization (EM) algorithm can be used to maximize the observed-data likelihood for the log-linear model and avoid bias, maintain the nominal Type I error rate and recover much of the lost efficiency (Weinberg, 1999a). Models have also been developed to avoid bias when it is feared that missingness is informative (Allen *et al.*, 2003).

26.4.4 Further uses for the case-parents design

26.4.4.1 Maternal effects

For young-onset conditions such as birth defects or psychiatric conditions like schizophrenia, the prenatal environment can be important. The maternal genome influences that environment directly, regardless of which variants are transmitted to the fetus. For example a genetic variant that influences the expression of an enzyme with a role in detoxifying a teratogen could cause a congenital malformation. Such an effect would incidentally result in a higher prevalence of the allele in cases compared to population-based (but not sibling) controls through confounding, because the maternal genome influences that of her offspring. The ability to disentangle maternally mediated, prenatally-acting genetic effects from long term effects of fetally inherited genotypes is a major advantage of case-parent studies over population-based case-control studies (Wilcox *et al.*, 1998) and discordant sibling case-control studies. The following extension of model (26.1) to incorporate maternal effects is easily fit using standard software if the triad genotype data are complete:

$$
\begin{aligned}
&\ln\{E(N_{M,F,C})\} \\
&= \ \mu_{\{M,F\}} + \beta_1 I_{(C=1)} + \beta_2 I_{(C=2)} + \alpha_1 I_{(M=1)} + \alpha_2 I_{(M=2)} + \ln(2) I_{(M=F=C=1)}.
\end{aligned}
\tag{26.2}
$$

The maternal and offspring effects in this model are orthogonal, meaning that the estimates for maternal relative risks, namely $\exp(\alpha_1)$ and $\exp(\alpha_2)$, do not depend on whether the offspring terms have been included in the model or not (and vice versa), when the genotype data are complete. This orthogonality cannot, however, be counted on if there are missing data, as there typically will be.

In model (26.2) for maternal effects, the father in effect serves as the genetic control for the mother. The assumption required for this inference to be valid is parental mating symmetry, that is, that exchanging the mother's and the father's genotypes provides two pairs of parental genotypes that are equally likely in the population. This assumption can be violated. For example, couples with an African-American husband and a European-American wife may be more common than the other way around. Mitchell proposed a remedy that would be robust to mating asymmetries: one can study distortion in transmissions of alleles from the maternal grandparents to the mothers of affected individuals (Mitchell, 1997), effectively treating the mother as the "case." Mating asymmetries in either the parental or the grandparental generations would not invalidate that approach.

Another approach is to carry out a hybrid study where one recruits couples who are parents of controls and genotypes those couples (Weinberg and Umbach, 2005). If the control parents are analyzed using a log-linear model with their own distinct set of mating type parameters and maternal parameters, then the assumption of mating symmetry can be tested, using the maternal parameters and a 2 degree-of-freedom likelihood ratio test. If the test of mating symmetry fails, and if one can assume there is no population stratification, then analysis of maternal effects can nonetheless be carried out by using the control parents in an extended log-linear model. If exposure data are also collected for the control offspring, main effects for the exposure and gene-by-environment interactions can also be assessed.

26.4.4.2   Parent-of-origin effects

The effect of a variant allele can sometimes depend on whether it was inherited from the mother or from the father, due to "epigenetic" mechanisms such as *imprinting*. The log-linear model is able to identify such second-order effects (Weinberg, 1999b). One can often unambiguously infer the parental origin of inherited alleles when the three genotypes are known. The exception is when $M = F = C = 1$. However, the EM algorithm can be used for those heterozygous offspring with indeterminate parental source. Inclusion of an indicator variable for the event that the offspring inherited a single copy that was derived from the father (as an arbitrary coding choice) will allow testing for imprinting effects based on that coefficient. One should not include an additional parameter for maternally derived alleles or the model will be over-parameterized and indeterminate.

26.5   Designs that include siblings

One family-based alternative to the case-parents design for genetic studies that use members of nuclear families is the discordant sibling design. This design enrolls a set of siblings who share both parents and where at least one sibling is affected and at least one is unaffected. The simplest design of this type is the discordant sibling-pair design, with one case and one control. As with case-parent triads, the matching on family counteracts potential bias induced by population structure on genetic associations. This robustness to bias accrues even if one does not directly utilize Mendelian transmission. Although they can be subject to survival bias, discordant case-sibling designs are more useful than the case-parent design for diseases with onset later in life when parents may be unavailable for genotyping.

A common approach to the analysis of discordant sibling designs is via conditional logistic regression. Genetic effects in the conditional logistic model can be coded using co-dominant, dominant, recessive or log-additive modes of inheritance. Because control siblings provide nongenetic information, this design allows the study of nongenetic main effects – a definite benefit compared to the case-parents design. Because the discordant sibling design is a matched case-control study, the conditional logistic analysis estimates odds ratio parameters, not the relative risk parameters estimated by log-linear models applied to case-parents data.

Hybrid approaches can also be used. Studies that include some families with case-parent triads and some with sibships can be jointly analyzed by treating the sibships as having parental genotypes missing by design (O'Brien *et al.*, 2016; Shi *et al.*, 2013).

Because the discordant sibling design does not collect parental genotypes, testing or estimating maternal effects or parent-of-origin effects is not possible with this design. Another issue that must be kept in mind is that siblings are correlated for unmeasured factors that tend to be shared within families, including genetic background and early life exposures. To the extent that those unmeasured factors interact with the measured factors under study, parameters related to both genetic and environmental effects can be subject to bias with a case-sibling approach.

Use of a discordant sibling design requires attention to the usual concerns for a finely matched epidemiologic study and some additional concerns related to genetic architecture. First, and speaking in terms of the sibling-pair design, care must be taken that the control sibling was unaffected by the disease under study at the age when the case sibling became affected. Similarly, for exposures, investigators should consider a 'reference age' for exposure assessment for both case and control siblings to ameliorate issues associated with opportunity for exposure (e.g., having experienced menopause or puberty) and secular trends in environmental factors. A reasonable choice for this referent age is the minimum of the age at diagnosis of the case and the ages at interview of the matched control siblings. A troubling implication of this choice of referent age is that many cases may need to recall their exposures farther back in time than would be required for controls, which argues for recruitment of cases very soon after diagnosis. In addition, investigators should be cognizant of the possibility of recall bias arising from differential exposure-interview intervals for siblings of different ages.

One additional complication for a design that includes multiple unaffected siblings is that the odds ratio parameter can be heterogeneous across families if, as is typical, the SNP under study is not the causative SNP but is associated with the outcome only because it is in linkage disequilibrium with a nearby causative SNP or set of SNPs. The true odds ratio will be 1 for siblings whose parents carry the marker allele but do not happen to carry the causative SNP. For other sibships, it could be less than 1 or more than 1, as determined by the true (unmeasured) genotype of the parents. If all sibships are simply case-control pairs, then testing based on these families will be valid, and the estimated odds ratio will be interpretable as a marginal, family-based parameter. On the other hand, if multiple controls are included for some families, the estimated standard error can be subject to error, due to this heterogeneity. A remedy for the problem involves repeatedly sampling a case and control sibling at random from each family to generate many data sets which each include only discordant pairs, and then combining the results (Rieger *et al.*, 2001).

The genotypes of siblings provide information about the genotypes of their parents. Consequently, another way to think about such a discordant sibling design would be to view it as related to a case-parents design with missing information: the parental genotypes are missing but the studied siblings provide genetic information that restricts the set of possible parental genotypes. From this viewpoint, FBAT's capabilities for the analysis of case-parent triads with partially missing genetic information can be used to test for genetic associations with disease. FBAT's approach conditions on a sufficient statistic for the complete set of missing parental alleles and thereby must allow for all the alleles the parents might have carried given the genotypes in the sibship. The necessary computations can be demanding, particularly for multi-SNP or haplotype analyses. Alternatively, one can use the EM algorithm in conjunction with a log-linear model analysis for the case-parents design, an approach which also must account for all the possible sets of missing parental alleles. Dudbridge *et al.* (2011) proposed a third alternative that conditions on only the set of alleles transmitted into the sibship, ignoring any possible untransmitted ones. Although less robust than accounting for all possible parental genotypes, this alternative approach is computationally efficient and has power comparable to FBAT's for both single SNP and haplotype analyses.

Shi *et al.* (2013) examined the log-linear EM approach to missing-parents analysis for a discordant sibling design where each family has exactly one case sibling and one or more control siblings. They found that for discordant sibling pairs the missing-parents approach offers no efficiency advantage over conditional logistic regression. However, as the number of control siblings increases, the efficiency of the missing-parents approach exceeds that of conditional logistic regression for both genetic effects and gene-environment interactions. An additional benefit of the missing-parents approach is that, under mild additional assumptions, the investigator could incorporate information from singleton cases (either without a control sibling or whose control sibling was unavailable) or from singleton controls (those who are known to have a case as a sibling but the case's genotype was unavailable). In this sense, the missing-parents approach overcomes in the genetic context what is a sticky problem for matched pair case-control designs in general – how to proceed when one of the pair is missing crucial data or simply unavailable.

26.6 G×E interaction in family-based studies

Although main effects of exposures (or other covariates) on risk cannot be studied using a case-parent approach, departures from multiplicative joint effects of environmental and genetic factors can be studied (Umbach and Weinberg, 2000; Kistner *et al.*, 2009). Case-sibling designs enable estimation of both main effects and G×E interaction and can be made more efficient by imposing an assumption that G and E are independent conditional on the parental genotypes (Chatterjee *et al.*, 2005). Here the environmental exposure can either be one experienced during pregnancy (for example, if the outcome is a pregnancy complication) or one experienced by the offspring after birth. Under a multiplicative joint effect (the null model for assessing multiplicative interactions), the transmission distortion for a causative allele is the same for exposed and unexposed individuals; the relative risk(s) are the same for both exposure groups. Under alternative scenarios, the relative risk(s) differ by exposure group and so one tests for whether the relative risk for the variant allele depends on exposure status.

A required assumption in this gene-by-environment analysis is that the inherited genotype does not influence the exposure, conditional on the genotypes of the parents. This assumption can sometimes be violated, e.g., by an allele that influences alcohol metabolism if the exposure of interest is alcohol. Note that, unlike the population-wide G×E independence required for valid case-only analysis (Piegorsch *et al.*, 1994), the required conditional-on-family G×E independence assumption is weak: it can only plausibly be violated if there is a causal effect of the variant (or another variant in LD with it) on E conditional on parents.

If family history of disease affects exposure, the assessment of exposure-disease association could be biased in a population-based case-control study. The problem is that family history can reflect effects of the proband case's allele in ancestors, and knowledge of that same family history might cause individuals to avoid exposures believed to be related to risk. For example, if one's mother died of lung cancer, one might both carry the genetic variant that caused her illness and be more motivated to quit smoking. However, as stated above, for studies based on nuclear families, all we need to assume is that, conditional on the parental genotypes, inheritance of the allele does not influence exposure. Inferences from case-parent studies are based on whether transmission of the allele is differential by exposure status among cases. This conditioning blocks any bias due to family history-exposure nonindependence. Because the siblings are perfectly matched on family history, a discordant sibling design is also protected against this bias, provided the allele itself does not influence exposure.

If the exposure is continuous, one can use a polytomous logistic model to assess G×E interaction (Kistner *et al.*, 2009) using the case-parents design. A case-pseudo-sibling analysis can also be used (Cordell, 2009b). These methods exploit the fact that the level of exposure will appear to influence the probability of transmission of an interacting allele.

One convenient feature of the case-parents design compared to a case-control approach for G×E interaction is that one does not need to ensure that the main effects model for the exposure has been correctly specified. The obvious corresponding limitation, however, is that the main effects for the exposure cannot be studied with a case-parent approach. One also must forego assessment of an additive model for G×E. However, if some families provide both an affected and an unaffected offspring, then both main effects and the interaction can be studied (Shi *et al.*, 2011). With such a quad design, one can also test an additive model for interaction, e.g., using the relative excess risk due to interaction approach (Hosmer and Lemeshow, 1992).

Although assessment of multiplicative G×E interactions using a family-based design is usually assumed to be robust to bias from population stratification, a phenomenon referred to as exposure-related population stratification can cause bias in estimation and testing of G×E interactions with population-based case-control studies, case-parents studies and case-sibling studies (Shi *et al.*, 2011). Exposure-related population stratification arises when there are unidentified subpopulations that differ in background risk of the disease and in prevalence of both the exposure and the allele of interest. Specifically, if the variant under study is in linkage with a causative SNP and is not causative itself, which is probably often the case for GWAS-based "hits," and if the strength of that linkage and the exposure prevalence both vary with subpopulation, then a case-parent study and a case-sibling study can be biased (Shi *et al.*, 2011).

G×E interactions are fundamentally about heterogeneity in genotype effects across exposure categories or heterogeneity in exposure effects across genotype categories. Another heterogeneity-related issue has to do with analysis of sub-phenotypes based on, e.g., tumor subtypes, age at onset, or categories of risk or severity of the condition. With case-parents data, assessment of heterogeneity in the association of a SNP with an outcome across such subtypes can be accomplished, similarly to G×E analysis. One extends the log-linear model to allow distinct mating type stratification parameters for the subtypes and tests a model that constrains the subtype-specific relative risks to be the same against one that allows those relative risk parameters to differ across subtypes. For a population-based case-control study, analysis of subtype heterogeneity can use polytomous logistic regression with subtypes as the response categories.

26.7 Power considerations

One might wonder how the efficiencies for the case-parent design or a discordant-sibling design for studying association with a single SNP compare with that for a population-based case-control design. To make the genotyping cost comparable, consider a case-parent study with N independent case-parent triads and a population-based case-control study with N cases and $2N$ controls. We also consider a population-based case-control study with N cases and N controls, and a case-sibling study with N cases and either 1 sibling or 2 siblings per case. Depending on the costs of recruiting, the expense for the case-parent design or a case-sibling design could fall between the two population-based case-control designs. The former is analyzed using model (26.1). The population-based and discordant-sibling case-control designs are analyzed using logistic regression and conditional logistic regression, respectively; each uses a similar model to (26.1) but without the mating type parameters or any adjustments for population stratification. Power calculations were based on noncentrality parameters calculated using the deviance associated with the expected cell counts (Agresti, 1990). Figure 26.1 shows the chi-squared noncentrality parameters for the five designs, with $N = 300$, as a function of the frequency of the minor allele at the SNP under study. We report power for the (somewhat idealized) two-control-sibling option to offer a design where the genotyping burden is equivalent to that of the case-parent approach; we caution that the reported power may be optimistic because the conditional logistic analysis employed cannot properly account for among-control-sibling correlations.

Based on Figure 26.1, the case-parents design offers power similar to that for a case-control design with the same number of cases and an equal number of controls under a log-additive risk model, and it slightly outperforms the case-control design under dominant or recessive scenarios. However, if one instead doubles the number of controls in the case-control study to equalize the genotyping effort with the case-parents study, the power is

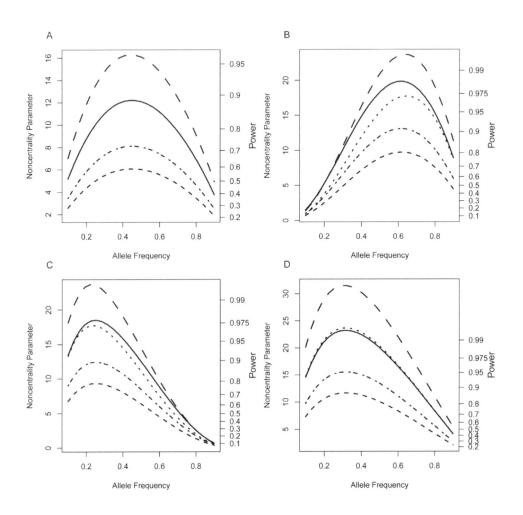

FIGURE 26.1

Chi-squared noncentrality parameter and power for a 2 degree-of-freedom test of genetic effects in relation to minor allele frequency for five designs: a population-based case-control study with 300 cases and 300 controls (dotted curve); a case-parent study with 300 cases (solid curve); a case-control study with 300 cases and 600 controls (long dashes); a discordant sibling study with one control sibling per case (medium long dashes); and a discordant sibling study with two control siblings per case (dash dot). Panels: A. $R_1 = 1.5$, $R_2 = 2.25$; B. $R_1 = 1$, $R_2 = 2$; C. $R_1 = 2$, $R_2 = 2$; and D. $R_1 = 2$, $R_2 = 3$. In panel A for the log-additive relative risk model, the dotted curve and the solid curve completely overlay.

better for a population-based case-control study. The case-sibling designs do less well. These calculations assume no population stratification and no bias due to differential participation of cases and controls. Thus, the added robustness gained by a case-parent study can come at a cost in power compared to a population-based study.

As would be expected, power for detecting multiplicative G×E is modest compared to power for finding main effects of the genotypes. Let I_1 (I_2) be the ratios of the R_1 (R_2) for exposed versus the R_1 (R_2) for unexposed. Figure 26.2 shows noncentrality parameters (for a 2 degree-of-freedom chi-squared) and corresponding power for a test of $I_1 = I_2 = 1$ using a likelihood ratio test for $N = 300$ families. The scenarios assumed are all $I_1 = 1$ and $I_2 = 2$ and the relative risks for the unexposed are the same as those in the scenarios depicted in Figure 26.1. Designs include case-parents and case-siblings with either one or two controls for each case.

The power for multiplicative interaction was slightly better for a case-parent design than for a case-control design with equal numbers of cases and controls. Power for a case-sibling study, even with only a single sibling, was considerably better than either a case-parent or a population-based case-control study. These calculations assumed, however, that exposures are independent among siblings; correlations among siblings' exposures would tend to reduce the power.

26.8 Multi-SNP methods

One might also want to study multi-SNP effects on risk, either for tightly linked SNPs and their associated haplotypes, or for more distant SNPs and possible epistatic effects. If there are multi-SNP effects on risk, the marginal effects of single SNPs can be badly attenuated so that corresponding single-SNP tests can have poor power (Shi and Weinberg, 2011).

A number of methods for detecting epistasis have been proposed (see Cordell (2009a), Steen (2012) and Wei *et al.* (2014) for reviews), but most of them are not intended for family-based studies. Trio "logic regression," available in the `trio` package in R, is an adaptation of the logic regression method (Ruczinski *et al.*, 2003) for analyzing case-parents data (Li *et al.*, 2010). It searches for the optimal combinations of binary risk factors or Boolean combinations of the original predictors that best differentiate transmitted from nontransmitted genotypes. Schwender *et al.* (2011) proposed a bagging version of the trio logic regression implemented by the `trioFS` function in the `trio` package. The multifactor dimensionality reduction (MDR) data mining approach, originally designed for case-control data, has also been adapted for detecting epistasis based on a modest numbers of SNPs in general nuclear families, as MDR-PDT (Martin *et al.*, 2006).

Several haplotype/multi-marker-based approaches have also been developed for family data. As distinct from the haplotype-based approaches, multi-marker-based approaches use genotypes directly without trying to estimate the unobservable haplotypes and assign phase. The TRIad MultiMarker (TRIMM) test, for example, is based on the genotypes of the cases and their complements (the hypothetical sibling who would have carried the parental alleles not transmitted to the case) (Shi *et al.*, 2007). One can use either the largest standardized statistic squared, max Z^2 (over the studied SNPs), or a composite statistic based on both the max Z^2 and Hotelling's T^2 as the test statistic. One then evaluates statistical significance via permutations. Zhang *et al.* (2007) extended the Pedigree Disequilibrium Test (PDT) (Martin *et al.*, 2000) to handle multiple SNPs for general nuclear families, and Wang *et al.* (2015) further extended it to the Optimal p-value Threshold Pedigree Disequilibrium Test (OPTPDT), which allows for selection of a subset of SNPs based on a p-value threshold

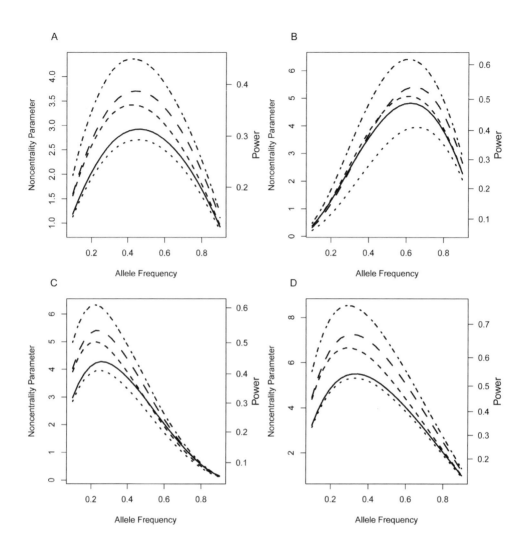

FIGURE 26.2

Chi-squared noncentrality parameter and power for a 2 degree-of-freedom test of G×E interaction in relation to minor allele frequency for five designs: a population-based case-control study with 300 cases and 300 controls (dotted curves), a case-parents study with 300 cases (solid curves), a population-based case-control study with 300 cases and 600 controls (long-dashed curves), a discordant sibling study with one control per case (medium dashes) and a discordant sibling study with two controls per case (dash dot). For sibships, the calculations assume within-family independence, as described by Chatterjee *et al.* (2005). Panels: A. $I_1 = 1.5$, $I_2 = 2.25$; B. $I_1 = 1$, $I_2 = 2$; C. $I_1 = 2$, $I_2 = 2$; and D. $I_1 = 2$, $I_2 = 3$ where I_1 and I_2 are interaction parameters (the ratios of genotype relative risks for exposed versus unexposed) among those carrying one or two copies of the variant allele, respectively. In all panels, the relative risk for the exposure is 1.2 and the relative risks for carrying one or two copies of the variant allele compared to zero copies are 1.2 and 1.44, respectively.

to calculate a test statistic. The optimal p-value threshold and the statistical significance are determined by a permutation procedure. Other multi-marker methods include methods based on comparing LD patterns between sets of transmitted and nontransmitted alleles (Yu and Wang, 2011), methods based on haplotype-similarity (Zhang *et al.*, 2003), and a multivariate extension of the Family-Based Association Test (FBAT) (Rakovski *et al.*, 2007).

Haplotype-based approaches have to handle the complication of haplotype phasing (with the exception of the X chromosome, where phase can be assigned unambiguously (Wise *et al.*, 2015) but they may be more powerful if the condition is indeed caused by a specific haplotype (which could influence the structure and function of the protein product) or set of haplotypes. Horvath *et al.* (2004) extended FBAT to haplotype FBAT by conceptualizing the haplotypes as a single multi-allelic marker. The missing phase information is handled by conditioning on the sufficient statistics in a way analogous to how FBAT handles missing genotypes. Other family-based methods for haplotypes include: Haplin (Gjessing and Lie, 2006), which extends log-linear case-parents analysis from single SNPs to haplotypes; an extension of the "association in the presence of linkage" (APL) test (Chung *et al.*, 2006); Unphased (Dudbridge, 2008); FamLBL (Wang and Lin, 2014); and methods based on haplotype sharing (Allen and Satten, 2007).

Multi-SNP and haplotype analyses are also possible with discordant sibling designs. Conditional logistic regression models can also include terms either for several SNPs simultaneously or for haplotypes (if phases are known) – offering ways to analyze multiple SNPS. The FBAT (Laird and Lange, 2008) and Dudbridge *et al.* (2011) approaches to missing information also allow inferences about haplotypes.

With the advances of genotyping and sequencing technology large amounts of data on rare variants are becoming available. Due to sparseness, rare variants are usually grouped together for analysis. Methods for analyzing rare variants for family-based studies include rare variant extensions of the TDT (He *et al.*, 2014), the family-based burden test (Choi *et al.*, 2014; De *et al.*, 2013) and variance-component-based tests (De *et al.*, 2013; Choi *et al.*, 2014; Wang and Lin, 2014).

For a smaller number of SNPs, e.g., based on sequencing of a particular gene, a family-based sequence kernel association test (FB-SKAT) can be used (Ionita-Laza *et al.*, 2013). One conditions on the parental genotypes and uses the fact that individuals with similar phenotypes should have similar genotypes if the region under study is related to risk. For FB-SKAT tests based on multiple SNPs, the power for N triads is similar to that based on a population-based study with N cases and N controls – similar to the results for single SNPs in Figure 26.1. How to include triads with a missing family member in FB-SKAT remains unclear.

26.9 Summary

Family-based approaches can be considered viable alternatives to case-control approaches when the disease shows strong evidence for heritability. Such studies use parents when the onset is young and unaffected sibling(s) when the onset is older. Their advantages include robustness against genetic population stratification, protection from self-selection biases, easy access to family members, improved motivation of participants, ability to assess maternally mediated prenatal genetic effects and parent-of-origin effects (for case-parents), ability to identify regions with *de novo* mutations (case-parents), and improved power for assessing gene-by-environment interaction (discordant siblings). However, the costs can include loss of ability to assess exposure main effects (case-parents), loss of ability to assess additive interactions (case-parents), and limits on generalizability (discordant siblings).

Acknowledgment

The authors thank Drs. Dmitri Zaykin, Katie O'Brien and Heather Cordell for helpful comments and discussions on the chapter.

Bibliography

Agresti, A. (1990). *Categorical Data Analysis*. John Wiley & Sons, New York.

Allen, A. S. and Satten, G. A. (2007). Statistical models for haplotype sharing in case-parent trio data. *Human Heredity*, **64**, 35–44.

Allen, A. S., Rathouz, P. J., and Satten, G. A. (2003). Informative missingness in genetic association studies: Case-parent designs. *The American Journal of Human Genetics*, **72**, 671–680.

Bennett, S. and Curnow, R. N. (2001). Consanguinity and the transmission/disequilibrium test for allelic association. *Genetic Epidemiology*, **21**, 68–77.

Chatterjee, N., Kalaylioglu, Z., and Carroll, R. (2005). Exploiting gene-environment independence in family-based case-control studies: Increased power for detecting associations, interactions and joint effects. *Genetic Epidemiology*, **28**, 138–156.

Choi, S., Lee, S., Cichon, S., Nöthen, M. M., Lange, C., Park, T., and Won, S. (2014). FARVAT: A family-based rare variant association test. *Bioinformatics*, **30**, 3197–3205.

Chung, R. H., Hauser, E. R., and Martin, E. R. (2006). The APL test: Extension to general nuclear families and haplotypes and examination of its robustness. *Human Heredity*, **61**, 189–199.

Cordell, H., Barratt, B., and Clayton, D. (2004). Case/pseudo-control analysis in genetic association studies: A unified framework for detection of genotype and haplotype associations, gene-gene and gene-environment interactions, and parent-of-origin effects. *Genetic Epidemiology*, **26**, 167–185.

Cordell, H. J. (2009a). Detecting gene-gene interactions that underlie human diseases. *Nature Reviews Genetics*, **10**, 392–404.

Cordell, H. J. (2009b). Estimation and testing of gene-environment interactions in family-based association studies. *Genomics*, **93**, 5–9.

Curtis, D. and Sham, P. C. (1995). A note on the application of the transmission disequilibrium test when a parent is missing. *The American Journal of Human Genetics*, **56**, 811–812.

De, G., Yip, W. K., Ionita-Laza, I., and Laird, N. (2013). Rare variant analysis for family-based design. *PLoS One*, **8**, e48495.

Dudbridge, F. (2008). Likelihood-based association analysis for nuclear families and unrelated subjects with missing genotype data. *Human Heredity*, **66**, 87–98.

Dudbridge, F., Holmans, P. A., and Wilson, S. G. (2011). A flexible model for association analysis in sibships with missing genotype data. *Annals of Human Genetics*, **75**, 428–438.

Eu-ahsunthornwattana, J., Miller, E. N., Fakiola, M., Wellcome Trust Case Control Consortium, Jeronimo, S. M. B., Blackwell, J. M., and Cordell, H. J. (2014). Comparison of methods to account for relatedness in genome-wide association studies with family-based data. *PLoS Genetics*, **10**, e1004445.

Falk, C. and Rubinstein, P. (1987). Haplotype relative risks: An easy, reliable way to construct a proper control sample for risk calculations. *Annals of Human Genetics*, **51**, 227–233.

Gjessing, H. K. and Lie, R. T. (2006). Estimating single- and double-dose effects of fetal and maternal disease gene haplotypes. *Annals of Human Genetics*, **70**, 382–396.

Gordon, D., Haynes, C., Johnnidis, C., Patel, S. B., Bowcock, A. M., and Ott, J. (2004). A transmission disequilibrium test for general pedigrees that is robust to the presence of random genotyping errors and any number of untyped parents. *European Journal of Human Genetics*, **12**, 752–761.

He, Z., O'Roak, B. J., Smith, J. D., Wang, G., Hooker, S., Santos-Cortez, R. L., Li, B., Kan, M., Krumm, N., Nickerson, D. A., Shendure, J., Eichler, E. E., and Leal, S. M. (2014). Rare-variant extensions of the transmission disequilibrium test: Application to autism exome sequence data. *The American Journal of Human Genetics*, **94**, 33–46.

Horvath, S., Xu, X., and Laird, N. M. (2001). The family based association test method: Strategies for studying general genotype–phenotype associations. *European Journal of Human Genetics*, **9**, 301–306.

Horvath, S., Xu, X., Lake, S. L., Silverman, E. K., Weiss, S. T., and Laird, N. M. (2004). Family-based tests for associating haplotypes with general phenotype data: Application to asthma genetics. *Genetic Epidemiology*, **26**, 61–69.

Hosmer, D. W. and Lemeshow, S. (1992). Confidence interval estimation of interaction. *Epidemiology*, **3**, 452–456.

Ionita-Laza, I., Lee, S., Makarov, V., Buxbaum, J. D., and Lin, X. (2013). Family-based association tests for sequence data, and comparisons with population-based association tests. *European Journal of Human Genetics*, **21**, 1158–1162.

Kistner, E. O., Shi, M., , and Weinberg, C. R. (2009). Using cases and parents to study multiplicative gene-by-environment interaction. *American Journal of Epidemiology*, **170**, 393–400.

Laird, N. M. and Lange, C. (2006). Family-based designs in the age of large-scale gene-association studies. *Nature Reviews Genetics*, **7**, 385–394.

Laird, N. M. and Lange, C. (2008). Family-based methods for linkage and association analysis. *Advances in Genetics*, **60**, 219–252.

Li, Q., Fallin, M. D., Louis, T. A., Lasseter, V. K., McGrath, J. A., Avramopoulos, D., Wolyniec, P. S., Valle, D., Liang, K. Y., Pulver, A. E., and Ruczinski, I. (2010). Detection of SNP-SNP interactions in trios of parents with schizophrenic children. *Genetic Epidemiology*, **34**, 396–406.

Martin, E. R., Monks, S. A., Warren, L. L., and Kaplan, N. L. (2000). A test for linkage and association in general pedigrees: The pedigree disequilibrium test. *The American Journal of Human Genetics*, **67**, 146–154.

Martin, E. R., Ritchie, M. D., Hahn, L., Kang, S., and Moore, J. H. (2006). A novel method to identify gene-gene effects in nuclear families: The MDR-PDT. *Genetic Epidemiology*, **30**, 111–123.

Meyer, W. K., Arbeithuber, B., Ober, C., Ebner, T., Tiemann-Boege, I., Hudson, R. R., and Przeworski, M. (2012). Evaluating the evidence for transmission distortion in human pedigrees. *Genetics*, **191**, 215–232.

Mitchell, L. (1997). Differentiating between fetal and maternal genotypic effects, using the transmission test for linkage disequilibrium (letter). *The American Journal of Human Genetics*, **60**, 1006–1007.

Mitchell, L. E. and Weinberg, C. R. (2005). Evaluation of offspring and maternal genetic effects on disease risk using a family-based approach: The "pent" design. *American Journal of Epidemiology*, **162**, 676–685.

O'Brien, K. M., Shi, M., Sandler, D. P., Taylor, J. A., Zaykin, D. V., Keller, J., Wise, A. S., and Weinberg, C. R. (2016). A family-based, genome-wide association study of young-onset breast cancer: Inherited variants and maternally mediated effects. *European Journal of Human Genetics*, **24**, 1316–1323.

Piegorsch, W., Weinberg, C., and Taylor, J. (1994). Non-hierarchical logistic models and case-only designs for assessing susceptibility in population-based case-control studies. *Statistics in Medicine*, **13**, 153–162.

Rabinowitz, D. and Laird, N. (2000). A unified approach to adjusting association tests for population admixture with arbitrary pedigree structure and arbitrary missing marker information. *Human Heredity*, **50**, 211–223.

Rakovski, C. S., Xu, X., Lazarus, R., Blacker, D., and Laird, N. M. (2007). A new multi-marker test for family-based association studies. *Genetic Epidemiology*, **31**, 9–17.

Rieger, R. H., Kaplan, N. L., and Weinberg, C. R. (2001). Efficient use of siblings in testing for linkage and association. *Genetic Epidemiology*, **20**, 175–191.

Rubinstein, P., Walker, M., Carpenter, C., Carrier, C., Kressner, J., Falk, C., and Ginsberg, F. (1981). Genetics of HLA disease associations: The use of the haplotype relative risk (HRR) and the "haplo-delta" (Dh) estimates in juvenile diabetes from three racial groups (abstract). *Human Immunology*, **3**, 384.

Ruczinski, I., Kooperberg, C., and LeBlanc, M. (2003). Logic regression. *Journal of Computational and Graphical Statistics*, **12**, 475–511.

Schaid, D. and Sommer, S. (1993). Genotype relative risks: Methods for design and analysis of candidate-gene association studies. *The American Journal of Human Genetics*, **53**, 1114–1126.

Schwender, H., Bowers, K., Fallin, M. D., and Ruczinski, I. (2011). Importance measures for epistatic interactions in case-parent trios. *Annals of Human Genetics*, **75**, 122–132.

Self, S., Longton, G., Kopecky, K., and Liang, K. (1991). On estimating HLA-disease association with application to a study of aplastic anemia. *Biometrics*, **47**, 53–61.

Shi, M. and Weinberg, C. R. (2011). How much are we missing in SNP-by-SNP analyses of genome-wide association studies? *Epidemiology*, **22**, 845–847.

Shi, M., Umbach, D. M., and Weinberg, C. R. (2007). Identification of risk-related haplotypes with the use of multiple SNPs from nuclear families. *The American Journal of Human Genetics*, **81**, 53–66.

Shi, M., Umbach, D. M., and Weinberg, C. R. (2011). Family-based gene-by-environment interaction studies: Revelations and remedies. *Epidemiology*, **22**, 400–407.

Shi, M., Umbach, D. M., and Weinberg, C. R. (2013). Case-sibling studies that acknowledge unstudied parents and permit the inclusion of unmatched individuals. *International Journal of Epidemiology*, **42**, 298–307.

Spielman, R. S. and Ewens, W. J. (1998). A sibship test for linkage in the presence of association: The sib transmission/disequilibrium test. *The American Journal of Human Genetics*, **62**, 450–458.

Spielman, R. S., McGinnis, R. E., and Ewens, W. J. (1993). Transmission test for linkage disequilibrium: The insulin gene region and insulin-dependent diabetes mellitus (IDDM). *The American Journal of Human Genetics*, **52**, 506–516.

Steen, K. V. (2012). Travelling the world of gene-gene interactions. *Briefings in Bioinformatics*, **13**, 1–19.

The 1000 Genomes Project Consortium (2012). An integrated map of genetic variation from 1,092 human genomes. *Nature*, **491**, 56–65.

Umbach, D. and Weinberg, C. (2000). The use of case-parent triads to study joint effects of genotype and exposure. *American Journal of Human Genetics*, **66**, 251–261.

Wang, M. and Lin, S. (2014). FamLBL: detecting rare haplotype disease association based on common SNPs using case-parent triads. *Bioinformatics*, **30**, 2611–2618.

Wang, Y. T., Sung, P. Y., Lin, P. L., Yu, Y. W., and Chung, R. H. (2015). A multi-SNP association test for complex diseases incorporating an optimal P-value threshold algorithm in nuclear families. *BMC Genomics*, **16**, 381.

Wei, W. H., Hemani, G., and Haley, C. S. (2014). Detecting epistasis in human complex traits. *Nature Reviews Genetics*, **15**, 722–733.

Weinberg, C. (1999a). Allowing for missing parents in genetic studies of case-parent triads. *American Journal of Human Genetics*, **64**, 1186–1193.

Weinberg, C. (1999b). Methods for detection of parent-of-origin effects in genetic studies of case-parent triads. *American Journal of Human Genetics*, **65**, 229–235.

Weinberg, C. R. and Umbach, D. M. (2005). A hybrid design for studying genetic influences on risk of diseases with onset early in life. *The American Journal of Human Genetics*, **77**, 627–636.

Weinberg, C. R., Wilcox, A. J., and Lie, R. T. (1998). A log-linear approach to case-parent-triad data: Assessing effects of disease genes that act either directly or through maternal effects and that may be subject to parental imprinting. *The American Journal of Human Genetics*, **62**, 969–978.

Wilcox, A. J., Weinberg, C. R., and Lie, R. T. (1998). Distinguishing the effects of maternal and offspring genes through studies of "case-parent triads". *American Journal of Epidemiology*, **148**, 893–901.

Wise, A. S., Shi, M., and Weinberg, C. R. (2015). Learning about the X from our parents. *Frontiers in Genetics*, **6**, 15.

Wise, A. S., Shi, M., and Weinberg, C. R. (2016). Family-based multi-SNP X chromosome analysis using parent information. *Frontiers in Genetics*, **7**, 20.

Yu, Z. and Wang, S. (2011). Contrasting linkage disequilibrium as a multilocus family-based association test. *Genetic Epidemiology*, **35**, 487–498.

Zhang, S., Sha, Q., Chen, H. S., Dong, J., and Jiang, R. (2003). Transmission/disequilibrium test based on haplotype sharing for tightly linked markers. *The American Journal of Human Genetics*, **73**, 566–579.

Zhang, Y. and Pan, W. (2015). Principal component regression and linear mixed model in association analysis of structured samples: Competitors or complements? *Genetic Epidemiology*, **39**, 149–155.

Zhang, Z., Zhang, S., and Sha, Q. (2007). A multi-marker test based on family data in genome-wide association study. *BMC Genetics*, **8**, 65.

27

Mixed Models for Case-Control Genome-Wide Association Studies: Major Challenges and Partial Solutions

David Golan

Technion - Israel Institute of Technology

Saharon Rosset

Tel Aviv University

27.1 Introduction

Case-control studies have been used in genetics from its early days. The intuitive idea that when a condition is rare, it is worthwhile to make an effort to collect a large sample of cases was obvious to the fathers of the field even before concepts such as statistical power were introduced. It is therefore no wonder that as the technical capability to genotype genetic markers emerged, it was often applied in the context of a case-control study of a disease such as diabetes, schizophrenia or hypertension.

In parallel to the progress in human genetics, animal breeders were developing a set of tools to optimize selection in pedigrees of livestock. Since the 1970s, the major workhorse of that field was the linear mixed model (LMM), used to model polygenic phenotypes – phenotypes driven by a plethora of genetic variants – and leverage the genetic information embedded in the pedigree.

In recent years, as it became apparent that many common human diseases are highly polygenic, a need to bring the two concepts – case-control studies and LMMs – onto a single framework emerged. We describe some of the recent efforts done in this direction in this chapter. For ease of exposition, we begin by describing the concept of a linear mixed model in the context of animal breeding and human genetics. We then describe the problems caused when trying to apply such methods to case-control studies, and discuss ways to solve them.

27.2   LMM overview

27.2.1   Background and intuition

A linear mixed model (LMM) is an extension of the standard linear regression model, wherein the variables are divided into two groups: fixed effects and random effects. Fixed effects are modelled as parameters, i.e., fixed, but unknown, quantities, while random effects are modelled as being drawn from a random distribution – typically a Gaussian distribution with mean zero and an unknown variance. Intuitively, this formulation allows accounting for the random effects, while not specifically estimating the value of each random effect. This is done by integrating the random effects out, resulting in a linear regression model with a nonidentity covariance matrix (where samples which have similar random-effects values have stronger correlations and vice versa).

To illustrate this idea, consider the following toy example: A researcher is interested in modelling some biometric measure as a function of time (e.g., weight of children). For that purpose she measures the weight of several toddlers once a month over a year, starting at the age of two. However, it is obvious that each subject has a different starting point at time $t = 0$. When using basic linear regression, accounting for this heterogeneity requires adding an indicator variable per individual, dramatically inflating the number of parameters in the model and increasing the standard errors of each estimate. The idea behind LMMs is to realize that the between-individuals differences are not the focus of interest of this specific study, and so it is counter-productive to "waste" information on estimating the per-individual effect. Instead, each individual's intercept term is treated as being drawn from some distribution. Treating the intercept as random captures the between-individual differences without requiring per-individual parameters, thus reducing the overall number of parameters while increasing accuracy and power for the parameters of interest. Instead of adding one parameter for each individual, we add only a single parameter – the variance of the intercept. This variance captures the extent of the heterogeneity. The key is that the observations of each individual share the value of the random effect, and so, after integrating it out, they become highly correlated: If a child is seen as high weight at the first time point, we expect her to continue being relatively high weight at following time points.

27.2.2   Formulation and estimation

To put these ideas in a more rigorous form, we write down the linear mixed effect model:

$$Y = X\beta + Zu + e,$$

where $Y_{n\times 1}$, $X_{n\times p}$, $\beta_{p\times 1}$ and $e_{n\times 1}$ take their usual roles as in a standard linear regression model (outcome, covariates, regression coefficients and i.i.d noise drawn from a $N(0, \sigma_e^2)$, respectively). The important addition is Zu where $Z_{n\times m}$ is another set of covariates, similar to X but for which we are not interested in specific estimates of the coefficients, and $u_{m\times 1}$

which are the associated random effects drawn from $N(0, \sigma_u^2)$. This model can be expressed through the multivariate normal distribution of $\boldsymbol{Y}$:

$$\boldsymbol{Y} \mid \boldsymbol{u} \sim N(\boldsymbol{X}\boldsymbol{\beta} + \boldsymbol{Z}\boldsymbol{u}, \boldsymbol{I}_{n \times n}\sigma_e^2).$$

Note how we condition on $\boldsymbol{u}$ but not on $\boldsymbol{\beta}$, because only the former is a random variable. Assuming the covariates in $\boldsymbol{Z}$ were standardized to have mean 0 and variance 1, and integrating $\boldsymbol{u}$ out, we get the unconditional distribution of $\boldsymbol{Y}$:

$$\boldsymbol{Y} \sim N(\boldsymbol{X}\boldsymbol{\beta}, \boldsymbol{Z}\boldsymbol{Z}^T\sigma_u^2 + \boldsymbol{I}_{n \times n}\sigma_e^2).$$

Notice how $\boldsymbol{Z}$ no longer affects the mean of the distribution. Instead, it appears as a component of the covariance matrix. This is the reason why this component of the model is also often referred to as a "variance component." Another useful representation of this model is to define $\sigma_g^2 = m\sigma_u^2$, and $\boldsymbol{G} = \frac{1}{m}\boldsymbol{Z}\boldsymbol{Z}^T$, and replace the $\boldsymbol{Z}\boldsymbol{u}$ term by $\boldsymbol{g} \sim N(\boldsymbol{0}, \boldsymbol{G}\sigma_g^2)$ so that the model can be written as:

$$\boldsymbol{Y} = \boldsymbol{X}\boldsymbol{\beta} + \boldsymbol{g} + \boldsymbol{e}.$$

This representation can be useful when the specific values of $\boldsymbol{Z}$ are unknown, but $\boldsymbol{G}$ can somehow be calculated or estimated using external data, as will be the focus of this chapter. LMMs can be naturally extended to accommodate several variance components, each with a different variance parameter.

The primary uses of LMMs are:

Estimation and testing of fixed and random effects. Once the distribution of $\boldsymbol{Y}$ is specified, one can proceed to estimate the fixed effects ($\boldsymbol{\beta}$) and the variance of each group of random effects using maximum likelihood approaches. Specifically, the common approach for estimating variance components is known as restricted maximum likelihood (REML). This is then often used to test hypotheses about either the fixed or random effects, most commonly of the form $H_0 : \boldsymbol{\beta} = 0$.

Prediction. Given $\boldsymbol{x}$ and $\boldsymbol{z}$, the covariates associated with a newly observed individual for whom the outcome y is unknown, we would like to predict y with the greatest possible accuracy. For a simple linear regression model, the answer is simply taking the covariate vector $\boldsymbol{x}$ and multiplying it by the estimated coefficients $\hat{\boldsymbol{\beta}}$: $\hat{y} = \boldsymbol{x}^T\hat{\boldsymbol{\beta}}$. This practice yields unbiased estimates. However, when attempting prediction in the LMM case, things are not so simple. One could adopt the same approach, but since the effects of the random components are not directly estimated, the vector of covariates $\boldsymbol{z}$ will not contribute directly to the predicted value of y, and will only affect the variance of the prediction, resulting in an unbiased but inefficient estimate. Instead, one can use the correlation between the realized values of $\boldsymbol{Z}\boldsymbol{u}$, to attempt a better guess at the realization of $\boldsymbol{z}\boldsymbol{u}$ for the new sample. This is achieved by computing the conditional distribution of the outcome of the new sample conditional on the full data set, by using the following property of the multivariate normal distribution. Assume we sampled n individuals, but the outcome for the ith individual is unknown. The conditional distribution of y_i given the rest of the outcomes ($\boldsymbol{y}_{-i}$) is given by:

$$y_i|\boldsymbol{y}_{-i} \sim N\big(\boldsymbol{x}_i^T\boldsymbol{\beta} + \boldsymbol{\Sigma}_{i,-i}\boldsymbol{\Sigma}_{-i,-i}^{-1}(\boldsymbol{y}_{-i} - (\boldsymbol{X}\boldsymbol{\beta})_{-i}), \boldsymbol{\Sigma}_{i,-i}\boldsymbol{\Sigma}_{-i,-i}^{-1}\boldsymbol{\Sigma}_{-i,i}\big), \quad (27.1)$$

where $\boldsymbol{\Sigma} = \boldsymbol{Z}\boldsymbol{Z}^T\sigma_u^2 + \boldsymbol{I}\sigma_e^2$, and positive/negative indices indicate the extraction/removal of rows or columns, respectively. Intuitively, we use information from different samples that have a high correlation with the new sample, to improve its prediction accuracy. The practice of using the conditional distribution is known as BLUP (Best Linear Unbiased Predictor).

27.3   LMMs in genetics

Linear mixed models have been extensively used in genetics, and in particular have been popular in the animal-breeding literature and practice for many years (Mrode, 2014). Historically, the major focus of interest was breeding selection – choosing which sires and dames to mate in order to improve a specific trait, or phenotype, in the next generation (e.g., dairy yield). The phenotype is the outcome y, the covariates X are measured and observed quantities (e.g., nutrition type, the farm where the animal was raised, etc.) and the Z matrix is the matrix of genetic variants. In many cases, the phenotype is influenced by many such variants, a situation which is typically referred to as a highly-polygenic phenotype or a complex phenotype. In such situations there are simply too many genetic variants to be included in the model, as they dramatically outnumber the samples. Moreover, even if there were enough samples to allow including all the genetic variants, up until roughly 20 years ago, actually measuring – or genotyping – these variants was either impossible or prohibitively expensive. So the problem posed by such genetic studies is double: the variables are both too many and unobserved. The solution put forward by LMMs is to skip the representation of the model that includes Z, directly to the variance components representation, and use pedigree information to estimate G, and plug the estimate into the equations.

The existence of pedigree information that allows to estimate the correlation accurately is quite unique to this domain, and explains the unique success of LMMs in the context of animal breeding long before genotyping became possible and affordable. In short, the DNA of an offspring is a mix of DNA segments from both parents. On average, each parent contributes 50% of the DNA (note that this is true in expectation only). Hence, when we look at the realizations of the random vector g for parent-offspring pairs, they have a correlation of 0.5 (under additivity assumptions on the genetic architecture, which we will not delve into here). Similarly, for any known relationship, one can compute the expected correlation: grandparent-grandchild pairs would have a correlation of 0.25, as would avuncular pairs, while second cousins would have a correlation of $\frac{1}{8}$, and unrelated individuals would have a zero correlation. For these reasons g is typically referred to as the "genetic" effect, while G is referred to as the "kinship," or "genetic relationship" matrix. Similarly, e is referred to as the "environmental" effect (which combines unmeasured effects and random noise). Thus animal breeders could utilize their pedigree information to compute an (approximate) genetic correlation matrix $\hat{G}$, and use it for prediction with BLUP, thus predicting which breeding choices would result in the best (predicted) yield.

Applications extend beyond prediction. One could be interested in estimating fixed effects (e.g., nutrition type, local weather) while controlling for genetic effects. For example one could ask whether an observed difference in yield is due to controllable living conditions or accumulated genetic differences. To answer such questions one needs to control the genetic differences in different farms. Again, this is achieved by using LMM with $\hat{G}$, thus controlling for the genetic effect, and estimating or testing the fixed effects.

Lastly, it is often of interest to estimate $h^2 = \sigma_g^2/\mathrm{var}(y)$, which is referred to as the (narrow-sense) heritability, the fraction of phenotypic variance which is explained by genetics. This magnitude is specifically important in the context of animal breeding, as it signifies how effective would the breeding actually be: high heritability implies a considerable genetic basis of the trait, so selective breeding would be very effective. Zero heritability means no genetic basis, so random breeding would be just as effective. This is captured by the famous *breeder's equation*: $R = h^2 S$ where R is the expected difference in phenotype between the previous and current generations, h^2 is the heritability, and S is the difference between the average phenotype in the population and the average phenotype of the selected parents (Plomin *et al.*, 1990). As the selection progresses and the phenotype improves, the relevant variants become more and more frequent in the population, until they are fixated, thus reducing the role of genetic diversity and reducing the heritability.

27.3.1   Moving to GWAS

As genotyping technologies emerged and prices plummeted, genome-wide association studies (GWAS) became more and more affordable and a major dogma for human genetics research. When performing GWAS, one genotypes thousands of individuals at hundreds of thousands of genomic loci and scans the genome for loci which are significantly associated with the measured phenotype. Several major differences exist between the human-centric GWAS and the animal breeding practice. First, the typical goal of the GWAS is not improved breeding, but rather identifying loci which harbor causative variants (hoping to implicate genes near these loci, thus leading to better understanding of a disease and novel therapeutics). Second, when dealing with humans, one has less control over the design of the study compared to cattle. The vast genetic heterogeneity in humans is mostly undocumented, and pedigrees are not as carefully maintained for human populations as they are in the animal breeding business. Lastly, unlike carefully bred animals, human populations are structured, where geographic, ethnic and other factors are correlated with genetic differences. Many of these issues can be addressed by applying LMMs to GWAS.

The use of LMMs in GWAS was pioneered by Kang *et al.* (2008, 2010). They consider the problem of association tests of a polygenic phenotype, in a highly structured population (wild-type and domesticated mice). They note that testing the association of a single SNP (say, x_1) involves assuming a univariate model:

$$y_i = \beta_1 x_{i1} + e_i,$$

to estimate β_1 and test its significance, while in fact the true model is polygenic, and so the fitted model should be:

$$y_i = \beta_1 x_{i1} + \sum_{k>1} u_k x_{ik} + \eta_i,$$

where we use the notation u_k to emphasize the connection (which we will soon establish) to the random effects in the mixed model definition above. Due to the population structure, many of the SNPs have different frequencies in each population, resulting in a considerable dependence between them. Running a univariate scheme ignores the effect of the other SNPs, effectively modelling them as part of the error, so we have $e_i = \sum_{k>1} u_k x_{ik} + \eta_i$. Since the SNPs are correlated, due to the major genome-wide differences in allele frequencies between the populations, this results in a correlation between the tested SNP and the noise term. In other words, both the value of x_{i1} and the value of $\sum_{k>1} u_k x_{ik}$ depend on which population the sample is drawn from, and so the covariate, x_{i1}, and the noise term, e_i, are dependent. In addition, the same dependencies lead to correlations between the noise terms of same-population samples. Both the dependency between the covariate and the noise, and the correlation between different noise terms, violate the basic assumptions required for inference in the regression setting, thus resulting in inflated type-1 error rates. To solve this problem, they adopt the LMM framework and treat the SNPs which are not directly tested as random effects. The effects u_k are treated as identically and independently distributed random variables drawn from a distribution with mean 0 and variance σ_u^2. Higher values of σ_u^2 imply larger effects. Hence, there is an additional "genetic effect," $g_i = \sum_{k>1} u_k x_{ik}$, with variance σ_g^2, and the model becomes:

$$y_i = \beta_1 x_{i1} + g_i + e_i,$$

where the genetic effects are positively correlated between genetically similar individuals and vice versa. This is exactly the same LMM formulation used before, with the major difference being the way that G is obtained. Instead of using pedigree data, the correlation between any two individuals is estimated using the observed genotypes (after centering and scaling):

$$G_{ij} = \text{cor}(g_i, g_j) = \frac{1}{m} \sum_{k=1}^{m} \frac{(x_{ik} - 2f_k)(x_{jk} - 2f_k)}{2f_k(1 - f_k)},$$

where f_k is the allele frequency of the kth SNP. Note that this is only an estimate of the true correlation for several reasons. First, the true causal SNPs affecting the phenotype are not necessarily genotyped. Second, the correlation is estimated using all genotyped SNPs, thus including many noncausal SNPs (adding noise to the estimate). However, the estimated correlation is an unbiased estimate of the true kinship (Zuk *et al.*, 2012). Several works focus on improving the estimation of G, either by modelling LD (Speed *et al.*, 2012), accounting for cryptic relatedness (Crossett *et al.*, 2013) or trying to pick out only the causal SNPs (or the SNPs which best tag those SNPs) (Golan and Rosset, 2011). However, for our discussion, we treat the estimated G as the true G, and note that this is an interesting area for future research.

While this approach was first applied to mouse GWAS, the methodology as described is well suited to human GWAS as well, and indeed the LMM approach to GWAS gained popularity as it was repeatedly shown that accounting for the subtle genetic similarities between individuals in a GWAS increases power and reduces type-1 error rates (Yu *et al.*, 2006; Yang *et al.*, 2014). In addition, it was shown that accounting for the genetic correlation by using LMMs is appropriate for controlling for population structure (which is a common problem in human GWAS), as well as for cryptic relatedness, and that LMMs outperform the previously preferred principal component analysis (PCA) approach in addressing these issues (Yang *et al.*, 2014). At the same time, methods for efficient estimation emerged and enabled applying these methods to progressively larger GWAS (e.g. Kang *et al.*, 2010; Lippert *et al.*, 2011; Zhou and Stephens, 2012).

The state of the art methods in terms of speed and memory requirements are BOLT-LMM (Loh *et al.*, 2015b) and BOLT-REML (Loh *et al.*, 2015a), which are the first to provide a method to estimate an LMM that is not cubic in the number of individuals, allowing their application to GWAS as large as $50,000$ individuals.

At the same time, LMMs were used to address a different burning question in human genetics: the problem of the missing heritability (Maher, 2008). Despite the clear evidence from twin and family studies that many traits and diseases are highly genetic (e.g., height, type-1 and type-2 diabetes, multiple sclerosis, schizophrenia and more), GWAS were only able to identify a handful of variants associated with these traits and diseases, and these variants accounted for only a fraction of the heritability expected from twin studies. Specifically for height, commonly cited numbers are 80% heritability from twin studies, and $< 20\%$ heritability explained by discovered genetic variants. One leading theory explaining this gap was that these phenotypes are driven by a large number of variants with small effects, and that GWAS are under-powered to detect most of the causal variants. Yang *et al.* (2010) used the LMM framework to address this question: assuming that the effect of each variant is drawn from a Gaussian distribution, the model of the phenotype is an LMM, and the estimates of the variance components can be used to estimate the heritability: $h^2 = \sigma_g^2/(\sigma_g^2 + \sigma_e^2)$. Their seminal paper showed that the fraction of heritability of height explained by a set of $500K$ genotyped SNPs is considerably larger than the heritability explained by the genome-wide significant hits alone, suggesting that height is indeed driven, to the large part, by a plethora of common variants with small effects.

Their work sparked a wave of follow-up work adopting and adapting the LMM framework for various heritability-related goals. One popular approach is to partition the SNPs to l groups, and compute a correlation matrix $\boldsymbol{G}_i$ for each group. The variances $\sigma_{g1}^2, ..., \sigma_{gl}^2$ are estimated simultaneously, capturing the heritability explained by each group. This practice was used, for example, to partition the heritability by chromosomes (Yang *et al.*, 2013), by *cis/trans* effects (Price *et al.*, 2011) or by functional annotations (Gusev *et al.*, 2014).

27.4 The mixed modelling challenge for case-control GWAS

So far, we discussed LMMs in the context of studies where sampling is random and the phenotype in question is quantitative. However, in many scenarios one or both of these assumptions does not hold. In particular, the most important use of GWAS is for studying human diseases, where the phenotype is usually binary (affected/healthy), and (relative) rarity of the disease requires the adoption of case-control sampling schemes. In this setting, the problems addressed by using LMMs are still present, but application of LMMs is much less straightforward. In this section we describe how LMMs are extended in these situations and what problems arise.

27.4.1 Modelling discrete phenotypes

Quite often, the phenotype in question is discrete rather than quantitative, specifically binary like disease phenotypes. In traditional regression settings (fixed-effects modelling), this is often addressed by moving from linear models to the generalized linear models (GLM; McCullagh and Nelder, 1989) framework, where instead of assuming $Y = \boldsymbol{x}^T\boldsymbol{\beta} + e$, we move to assuming $g(P(Y = 1|\boldsymbol{x})) = \boldsymbol{x}^T\boldsymbol{\beta}$, for an appropriate link function g. The most common approaches are the probit and logit link functions:

$$\text{Probit}: \quad g(p) = \Phi^{-1}(1 - p)$$

$$\text{Logit}: \quad g(p) = \log\left(\frac{p}{1 - p}\right),$$

where Φ is the standard normal cumulative distribution function. The well-known logistic regression approach is simply a GLM with the logit link.

In the generalized linear mixed models (GLMM) literature in statistics, the binary situation is often addressed by the same approach that generalizes the linear mixed model through use of a link function (Breslow and Clayton, 1993):

$$g(P(\boldsymbol{Y} = 1|\boldsymbol{X}, \boldsymbol{Z}, \boldsymbol{u})) = \boldsymbol{X}\boldsymbol{\beta} + \boldsymbol{Z}\boldsymbol{u},$$

where the probability operation and the link function are applied to the vector $\boldsymbol{Y}$ element-wise, and we still assume that $u_i \sim N(0, \sigma_u^2)$. While this model is well defined, estimation and inference in this model is a much more complex task than in the standard LMM setting, since the normally distributed vector is now unobserved. If the link function used is probit, the setting falls under the more general category of Gaussian process regression and classification, which has been widely studied in the machine learning literature (Rasmussen and Williams, 2005). The state of the art solutions developed in this area, including expectation-propagation (EP) (Rasmussen and Williams, 2005) and Markov-Chain Monte Carlo approaches (MCMC) (Frigola *et al.*, 2013), can offer practical solutions to GWAS-sized problems. Such solutions can address all aspects of the GWAS problem discussed above: fixed effects estimation/testing, variance components (heritability) estimation, and prediction.

In the context of genetics, Wright (1934) put forward the liability threshold model (LTM) to address the issue of binary phenotypes. In the mixed model version of LTM, one assumes the existence of a latent phenotype vector $\boldsymbol{L} = \boldsymbol{X\beta} + \boldsymbol{Zu} + \boldsymbol{e}$, which follows the same normal assumptions of the standard LMM:

$$\boldsymbol{L} \mid \boldsymbol{u} \sim N(\boldsymbol{X\beta}, \boldsymbol{ZZ}^T \sigma_u^2 + \boldsymbol{I}\sigma_e^2), \tag{27.2}$$

$$\boldsymbol{Y} = \mathbb{I}(\boldsymbol{L} > T), \tag{27.3}$$

where again the indicator function $\mathbb{I}$ is applied to its argument element-wise. The observed phenotype is determined by the latent phenotype crossing or not crossing a threshold T, set such that the probability of crossing T is exactly the prevalence of the disease in the population. In the GLMM context, LTM is simply a GLMM with a probit link function, since it gives (again, interpreted element-wise):

$$P(\boldsymbol{Y} = 1 | \boldsymbol{X}, \boldsymbol{Z}, \boldsymbol{u}) = P(\boldsymbol{L} > T | \boldsymbol{X}, \boldsymbol{Z}, \boldsymbol{u}) = 1 - \Phi\left(\frac{T - (\boldsymbol{X\beta} + \boldsymbol{Zu})}{\sigma_e}\right).$$

An important development in the analysis of genetic data under LTM was the presentation by Dempster and Lerner (1950) of a mathematical connection between the heritability on the observed (Y) scale, i.e., $h_o^2 = \text{cov}(Y, g)/\text{var}(Y)$, and the heritability on the liability scale, i.e., $h_l^2 = \text{cov}(L, g)/\text{var}(L) = \sigma_g^2/(\sigma_g^2 + \sigma_e^2)$:

$$h_l^2 = \frac{K(1-K)}{\varphi(T)^2} h_o^2,$$

where K is the prevalence of the phenotype, T is the liability threshold, and φ is the density of the standard Gaussian distribution. Note that although under the assumed liability threshold model, the genetic and environmental components do not combine additively on the observed scale (and hence $\text{var}(Y) \neq \text{var}(g) + \sigma_e^2$), the formal definition of h_o^2 is still well defined, and complies with the result. Importantly, this is a relationship between the parameters of the model, and so it suggests that estimates of the heritability on the observed scale can be transformed to an estimate of the "true" heritability. One such estimate can be obtained using a method known as Haseman-Elston regression (Haseman and Elston, 1972), whereby the $O(n^2)$ products of binary phenotypes $Y_i \times Y_j$ are regressed on the kinship values G_{ij}. Thus within the LTM we have two competing approaches for estimating heritability: (i) via maximum likelihood GLMM or (ii) by estimating heritability in the observed scale, while ignoring the binary nature of the phenotype altogether (e.g., by using the "moment-based" regression estimator), followed by the correction of Dempster and Lerner to transform the observed-scale estimate to the liability scale, which is the scale of interest.

A different approach which is often practiced in the genetics community is to ignore the binary nature of the phenotype and apply regular LMM's to the data, as if Y were a quantitative, normally distributed phenotype. While this practice is clearly unsubstantiated from a probabilistic perspective, it leads in practice to useful methods, especially for prediction. It can be thought of as using Y as a surrogate of the unobserved L.

27.4.2   Case-control sampling

So far we have assumed that samples are randomly drawn from the population. However, quite often this is not the case, with the prime example being case-control studies. In case-control studies, one is interested in studying a (relatively) rare outcome, e.g., a disease which affects $< 1\%$ of the population. In such scenarios, a random sample from the population would include a very small fraction of affected individuals (cases), and so the efficiency of the statistical analysis would be compromised. The common strategy to address this problem is to make an effort to sample more cases than their random share in the population, e.g., by recruiting cases using ads or at clinics and hospitals directly, and separately sampling healthy controls from a "similar" population (to mitigate the effects of population structure and other confounders). The resulting sample is then subjected to GWAS.

This seemingly innocent sampling approach has the potential to create major implications in the statistical analysis of the resulting data, which has been the subject of a long and storied line of work in the statistics literature (Anderson, 1972; Prentice and Pyke, 1979; Scott and Wild, 1997, 2001; Chatterjee and Carroll, 2005; Clayton, 2012). Here we concentrate on some of the aspects of this area which are most relevant to mixed models analysis of case-control GWAS.

It is first important to note one situation where case-control sampling can be mostly ignored. The famous result by Prentice and Pyke (1979), building on earlier work by Anderson (1972), shows that if we are assuming that $P(Y|\boldsymbol{x})$ follows a fixed-effects GLM with a logit link function in the population, with an intercept:

$$P(Y = 1|\boldsymbol{x}) = \frac{\exp(\alpha + \boldsymbol{x}^T\boldsymbol{\beta})}{1 + \exp(\alpha + \boldsymbol{x}^T\boldsymbol{\beta})},$$

then the parameters $\boldsymbol{\beta}$ can be estimated from a case-control sample from the population, and inference carried out on them, while ignoring the fact that such sampling has taken place. This result is extremely useful and widely used, but it represents the exception rather than the norm in analyzing case-control data. Even if no random effects are assumed, but we move away from the logit link (say, to probit), important aspects of this result no longer hold. Once we also include random effects and move to a mixed model (say, using LTM), we can no longer ignore the case-control sampling and hope to obtain meaningful results.

More concretely, the typical probabilistic mixed model in case-control GWAS still assumes that the GLMM (specifically, probit GLMM through the LTM) holds at the population level without the case-control sampling. This is often justified by a Central Limit Theorem (CLT) type of argument, for example, that the genetic effect is the sum of many small effects drawn from the same distribution and therefore follows a normal distribution by virtue of the CLT. Thus, in the population we still assume the model (27.2) and (27.3). Once we move to case-control sampling, then in the sampled population the probabilistic setting is significantly changed. Formally, we add sampling variables S which encode the sampling process, i.e., in case-control sampling the liability is sampled not from $P(L)$, but from $P(L \mid S = 1)$, and similarly for all other quantities. In this setting, it is easy to see that (Golan *et al.*, 2014):

1. The distributions of the liability L, the genetic effect g, and the environmental effect e are no longer normal.

2. The genetic effect g and the environmental effect e are no longer independent, because cases are oversampled, and these tend to have both a high value of g and a high value of e, so that L passes the threshold T (this is apparent in the right panel of Figure 27.2).

These effects are demonstrated in Figures 27.1 and 27.2.

Maximum-likelihood based statistical modelling and estimation of GLMMs with case-control sampling in this setting is to our knowledge an unsolved problem. The Gaussian-process literature discussed previously does not offer EP or MCMC solutions to this problem,

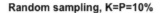

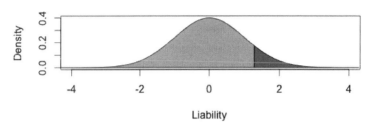

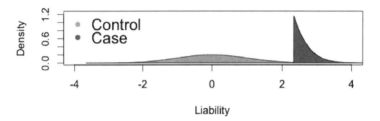

FIGURE 27.1

Comparison of the distribution of the liability in a random sample and a case-control sample of a discrete phenotype. We simulated two studies using the liability threshold model: a random sampling study of a relatively common disease phenotype ($K = 10\%$, top panel), where the liability follows a normal distribution as expected; and a balanced ($P = 50\%$) case-control study where the phenotype is relatively rare ($K = 1\%$, bottom panel). In the latter case, the oversampling of cases results in an oversampling of the right tail of the distribution, and the distribution is obviously no longer normal.

and we are not aware of other work offering practical computational solutions to this problem (which can be thought of as a high-dimensional integration problem).

However, as discussed before, using LMMs to analyze GWAS offers a unique combination of major benefits, including their ability to control for population structure and model cumulative effect of many small genetic effects, and the efficient computational tools that exist for computing LMMs. Because of this, many researchers have sought to analyze case-control studies by applying standard (normal) LMMs to the data, and using the results in association testing (Lippert *et al.*, 2011), heritabililty estimation (Lee *et al.*, 2011), and genetic risk prediction (Speed and Balding, 2014). In some of these cases, the results of LMM were "corrected" to account for case-control sampling (Lee *et al.*, 2011).

The fundamental difficulty in all these efforts is that the probabilistic model assumed by the LMM does not hold at all: As just demonstrated, the distributions of the elements of the LTM (liability, genetic effect and environmental effect) and their correlation structure are fundamentally influenced by the sampling. Not surprisingly, we are not aware of any theory that can describe the distribution of estimates derived by applying standard LMMs to case-control GWAS, and developing such a theory seems like a worthy goal for future research. Consequently, we do not believe that tasks concentrated on statistical estimation, inference and testing in case-control GWAS (like association testing and heritability estimation) should be based on LMMs. A slightly different case is presented by genetic risk

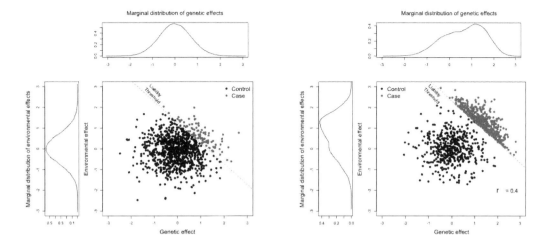

FIGURE 27.2
The effects of case-control sampling on the marginal and joint distribution of the genetic and environmental effects. We simulated genetic and environmental effects for unrelated individuals with $\sigma_g^2 = \sigma_e^2$ (so $h^2 = 0.5$). Phenotypes were determined using a liability threshold model without fixed effects using for either a common phenotype ($K = 10\%$, left panel) or a rare phenotype ($K = 1\%$, right panel). In the former scenario, random sampling was applied, while in the latter scenario, cases were oversampled to achieve a balanced study ($P = 50\%$). The joint distributions are illustrated in the middle panels while the marginal distributions of the random effects are illustrated in the side panels.

prediction, where the goal is to predict the phenotype of new individuals, based on their genotypes. Since this task carries with it an objective measure of performance that does not need to be tied to probabilistic inference, methods based on LMMs can be justified. However, they should be thought of as algorithmic predictive modelling approaches, rather than a well-founded probabilistic model of case-control GWAS.

27.5 Methods for mixed modelling of case-control GWAS

After reviewing the general challenge, in this section we review some of the recent methods for addressing the major tasks in case-control GWAS under the mixed-models paradigm. We try to emphasize methods that take into account the complex probabilistic model in this setting and offer valid solutions (if partial and suboptimal, compared to the currently impractical alternative of solving the full case-control GLMM problem).

27.5.1 Association testing and estimation of fixed effects

Association testing is the main original intended use of GWAS (as expressed in the term itself), and naturally it has been extensively applied to case-control GWAS. Ultimately, association testing seeks to test a null hypothesis for the association between each variant genotyped in a GWAS (typically counting the number of minor alleles $0, 1, 2$) and the phenotype in question. The simplest approach treats this through standard univariate tests: Armitage's test for trend, chi-square tests on contingency tables, likelihood-based tests (G test, score test) on logistic regression, etc. All of these tests are statistically valid for case-control GWAS (since under the null, the sampling does not affect the distribution of the statistic) and have been extensively used in GWAS (e.g. Burton *et al.*, 2007).

Already in the early days of GWAS, the statistical genetics community came to the realization that population structure and linkage disequilibrium (LD) are critical aspects of the problem. Univariate tests which ignore them give results that are statistically valid, but may yield many uninteresting findings, as the truly causative findings are often heavily masked by noise resulting from population structure and/or LD. This is because the presence of the above factors, especially population structure, imply that many noncausative genetic variants will be significantly associated with the phenotype through their correlation with causative variants, and these can be spread throughout the genome. Early efforts to correct this problem (beyond traditional genomic control approaches; Devlin and Roeder, 1999) concentrated on explicitly modelling structure through the use of principal components (PCs). These were then added as additional fixed effects to a regression model, or regressed out of both the genetic variants and the phenotype, before testing (Price *et al.*, 2006). Under the assumption that a few PCs successfully capture population structure, this approach is reasonable. However, as previously described, the use of mixed models for controlling population and genetic structure has been demonstrated to be the most effective and general approach in many settings both in terms of power and controlling for type-1 errors (Yang *et al.*, 2014).

Thus there is an obvious interest in taking advantage of the mixed models conceptual framework in case-control GWAS as well. The first option is to apply LMMs to this problem "out of the box," ignoring both the discrete phenotype and the sampling (see, e.g., Lippert *et al.*, 2011; Speed and Balding, 2014), assuming that the 0/1 phenotype follows the LMM normal distribution. This is difficult to justify as has been discussed, and indeed leads empirically to low power (Yang *et al.*, 2014).

We are aware of two recent papers that made an effort to adapt the mixed model framework to association testing in case-control GWAS (Weissbrod *et al.*, 2015; Hayeck *et al.*, 2015). The common idea to these two methods is to start from replacing the 0/1 case-control status by an estimate of the liability L, and doing so while taking into account the probabilistic structure (i.e., considering the distribution $P(L|S = 1)$).

Weissbrod *et al.* (2015) take advantage of the similarity between BLUP and ridge regression prediction (which are equivalent when no fixed effects are present), to formulate the liability estimation problem as a penalized probit regression problem:

$$\hat{L} = Z\hat{u} + \epsilon$$

$$\hat{u} = \arg\min_{u} \sum_{i=1, y_i=1}^{n} \log\left(\Phi(\frac{T - z_i^T u}{\sigma_e})\right) + \sum_{i=1, y_i=0}^{n} \log\left(1 - \Phi(\frac{T - z_i^T u}{\sigma_e})\right) + \frac{1}{2\sigma_u^2}\|u\|^2.$$

This calculation assumes that the variances $\sigma_g^2 = m\sigma_u^2, \sigma_e^2$ are known in advance, and the resulting $\hat{L}$ is the maximum aposteriori (MAP) estimate of $L|S = 1$. The authors then plug this $\hat{L}$ into a regular LMM to perform the association testing, and demonstrate that the resulting power is superior to that of standard LMMs or PC-based correction for structure. However, as demonstrated in Figures 27.1 and 27.2 there is no reason to assume that $\hat{L}$ (or indeed the true unobserved liability L) has a normal distribution under case-control sampling; hence the second part of their solution still fails to fully take the case-control sampling into account.

The paper by Hayeck *et al.* (2015) takes a different approach to estimating the liability.

They use the fact that given the phenotype vector $\boldsymbol{Y}$, and all liabilities but one $\boldsymbol{L}_{-i}$, the distribution of the missing liability is a truncated normal:

$$L_i \mid \boldsymbol{L}_{-i}, Y_i = 1 \ \sim \ TN(\mu_i, \sigma_i^2, T, \infty),$$
$$L_i \mid \boldsymbol{L}_{-i}, Y_i = 0 \ \sim \ TN(\mu_i, \sigma_i^2, -\infty, T),$$

where μ_i, σ_i^2 are the conditional mean and variance, calculated as in Eq. (27.1). This allows them to design a simple Gibbs sampling algorithm for generating random samples of "representative" liability vectors $\boldsymbol{L}$ for the case-control probabilistic model. These are averaged to calculate a "posterior mean" liability vector $\hat{\boldsymbol{L}}$. This vector is then used as if it were a normally distributed LMM response in a score test of the null of no association for each genetic variant. Hence for this approach too, the second part fails to take the probabilistic structure into account. The superiority of the approach over standard LMMs and trend test in terms of power is demonstrated in both simulations and real data.

Beyond testing, actual estimation of the association parameters (fixed effects) is usually considered a by-product of the process. We are not aware of specific efforts to estimate fixed effects within mixed-model analysis of case-control GWAS. This is in contrast to the problem of estimating variance components and heritability, discussed next.

27.5.2   Estimating variance components (heritability)

The first attempt to estimate the variance of the genetic random effect (i.e., the heritability) in the context of case-control GWAS was by Lee *et al.* (2011). They describe a procedure in the spirit of Dempster and Lerner (1950): First code the phenotype as a 0/1 variable, treat it as quantitative and apply a standard LMM method (in their case, REML as implemented in GCTA; Yang *et al.*, 2011). Then, apply a post hoc correction to correct the errors and biases introduced by the fact that, in fact, the method applied was inappropriate. Specifically, Lee *et al.* (2011) obtain an "observed scale" heritability estimate $\hat{h}_o^2$, which is the heritability of the synthetic 0/1 phenotype, and transform it to the desired "liability scale" heritability using the following relationship:

$$\hat{h}_l^2 = \frac{K^2(1-K)^2}{P(1-P)\varphi(T)^2}\hat{h}_o^2,$$

where K is the prevalence of the disease in the population, and P the percentage of cases in the study (typically $P \gg K$ in case-control studies).

While the method of Lee *et al.* (2011) has become extremely popular, evidence from both simulation studies and actual studies show that it, in fact, produces downwards-biased estimates (Yang *et al.*, 2014; Golan *et al.*, 2014). Strikingly, this bias appears to increase with sample size, as demonstrated by simulations in Golan *et al.* (2014) and using real data in Loh *et al.* (2015a), who used downsampling of a huge GWAS to demonstrate how the estimates decrease as the size of the sample increases.

Recently, Golan *et al.* (2014) developed an alternative method that does not suffer from the same problems as the method of Lee *et al.* (2011). They adopt the moments-method approach of Haseman and Elston (1972) to obtain estimates that are unbiased despite the complicated underlying probabilistic model. The basic idea is to look at the relationship between two correlations: the correlation between the phenotypes of pairs of individuals (phenotypic correlation) and the correlation between the genotypes of pairs of individuals (the genetic correlation). Higher heritability implies that high genetic correlation should yield high phenotypic correlation, and low heritability implies no such relationship. More formally, Golan et al. express the product of the phenotypes of any two individuals, as a function f of the true underlying heritability, the genetic correlation, and the fixed effects, where f itself depends on the actual design of the study (specifically P) and the properties of the disease (specifically K):

$$\mathbb{E}(y_i y_j \mid S = 1; G_{ij}, h^2) = f(h^2, G_{ij}),$$

where the conditioning on $S = 1$ indicates the fact that both individuals were selected for the study. Note that we assume that the phenotypes are centered and scaled so $\mathbb{E}(y_i y_j) = \mathrm{cor}(y_i, y_j)$. Next, f is approximated using its Taylor series approximation:

$$f(h^2, G_{ij}) = a_0 + a_1 G_{ij} h^2 + \mathcal{O}(G_{ij}^2).$$

Recall that G_{ij} is the correlation between the genotypes of individuals i and j (over the set of causal SNPs). Since individuals in the GWAS study are typically unrelated, and assuming a highly polygenic disease (so the number of causal variants is high), the values of G_{ij} are relatively small, so is the error term $\mathcal{O}(G_{ij}^2)$. Hence the first order approximation is satisfactory, resulting in an (approximated) linear relationship between the phenotypic correlation and the genetic correlation.

In this situation, one can use linear regression to estimate the slope $a_1 h^2$ (by regressing the products $y_i y_j$ onto G_{ij} for all pairs $i \neq j$). To obtain an estimate of the heritability, all that is left is to compute the constant a_1, which is the value of the first derivative of f at $G_{ij} = 0$. While f itself is generally intractable, it is tractable for the special case of $G_{ij} = 0$. The key to obtaining a_1 is to write down the joint density of the liability of individuals i and j, and integrate this density over the region that corresponds to their phenotypes (e.g., $l_i > t$ and $l_j > t$ if both are cases). While generally this double integral has no closed form, for the special case of $\mathrm{cor}(l_i, l_j) = 0$ the double integral can be written as a product of two single (and tractable) integrals, as the individuals are now independent.

Golan et al. show how this can be done for various study designs (e.g., case-control and extreme phenotype sampling). Importantly, the computation explicitly involves the conditioning on the selection variable $S = 1$, so it accounts for the effects of the nonrandom selection. The resulting estimates are unbiased (by virtue of being first moments estimators) and fast to compute ($O(n^2)$ instead of the usual $O(n^3)$ of most REML based methods). The method is named PCGC (for regressing phenotype correlations on genetic correlations) and a fast and memory-efficient implementation of PCGC regression can be found in the software reference list at the end of the chapter.

The application of PCGC regression to a wide range of GWAS in Golan *et al.* (2014) demonstrated that the fraction of heritability explained by common variants is larger than estimated by the method of Lee et al. (for example, the estimated heritability of multiple sclerosis explained by common variants increased from 30% (Lee *et al.*, 2013) to 45% (Golan *et al.*, 2014) using the same data), and recent applications of PCGC regression for other phenotypes show similar results (Loh *et al.*, 2015a; Jiang *et al.*, 2015). Importantly, a recent paper used a huge GWAS of schizophrenia (involving 50,000 individuals) to show that estimates using the method of Lee et al. indeed decrease as the sample size increases, and that PCGC regression yields the correct estimate (i.e., a similar estimate to the estimates obtained when applying Lee et al.'s method to very small subsets of the data which have a very small bias due to their size).

27.5.3 Prediction

The prediction problem is essentially different from the problems of estimating fixed or random effects. For these statistical inference problems, one is interested in unraveling some ground truth (the true heritability of a disease or the true effect size of a SNP), or making a scientific discovery (identifying a novel causal locus). In contrast, the prediction problem comes with its objective and measurable metric of success – predictive accuracy. In this case, applying methods which are not theoretically justified, but yield good performance, is legitimate, as evidenced by the popularity of the application of out-of-the-box machine-learning methods such as support vector machines or elastic-nets for phenotype prediction (e.g., Abraham *et al.*, 2013). However, machine learning methods typically make no assumptions regarding the data, and take as input only a feature matrix (the genotyped SNPs) and an outcome vector (the phenotype). In contrast, GWAS in general, and case-control GWAS in particular, does have several unique characteristics: a highly polygenic nature of many phenotypes; a unique structure of correlations between the SNPs (linkage disequilibrium); the existence of population structure, which is captured by the correlation matrix G; and, of course, the artifacts introduced by the nonrandom sampling scheme in case-control studies. As discussed earlier, LMMs are particularly suited to take advantage of these features in the case of randomly sampled phenotypes, and often outperform other methods, including "simple" classifiers which are based only on genome-wide significant SNPs (e.g., Purcell *et al.*, 2009). Given these results, it is only natural to apply LMMs to the problem of prediction using a case-control GWAS as reference panel.

One popular approach is to code the binary phenotype as 0/1, and use standard LMM methods for prediction (e.g., using BLUP, or its recent extension multiBLUP (Speed and Balding, 2014) on the coded phenotype). The application of LMM-based methods aims to utilize their advantages for improved prediction. However, the same logic implies that a BLUP-like method that accounts for the quirks introduced by case-control sampling should out-perform naive BLUP methods as it takes full advantages of the unique features of the case-control GWAS problem, namely, assumes a highly additive model, captures population structure, *and* accounts for the nonrandom sampling.

This intuition is captured by GeRSI – a method for genetic risk score inference which accounts for case-control sampling (Golan and Rosset, 2014). Here the authors find the conditional distributions of the genetic and environmental effects $e_i \mid g, e_{-i}, Y_i$ and $g_i \mid g_{-i}, e, Y_i$, which turn out to be truncated normal distributions, similarly to the conditional distribution of the liabilities in Hayeck *et al.* (2015) described earlier. Once the conditional distributions are specified, Gibbs sampling is used to sample the posterior distribution of the genetic effect of an individual with an unknown phenotype, and these samples can be used to compute the posterior risk prediction (intuitively, higher posterior value of the genetic effect translates to higher risk). Simulations and application to real data show that GeRSI outperforms its BLUP equivalent.

27.6   Conclusion

The problem of mixed-modelling analysis of case-control studies in general, and case-control GWAS in particular, is unique in its combination of high importance and popularity, extreme difficulty, and paucity of computationally effective and statistically valid approaches. Indeed, while several of the approaches we presented here offer statistically valid solutions to specific aspects, we are aware of no fully valid approaches based on maximum-likelihood principles or Bayesian principles for estimation or testing in case-control GWAS. An intriguing question is whether this is because this problem is simply too difficult from a computational and statistical perspective, or whether it is a matter of getting the right communities and capabilities involved. In particular, the Gaussian processes literature does offer efficient solutions to GWAS-sized problems with binary phenotypes and natural sampling (Rasmussen and Williams, 2005; Frigola *et al.*, 2013). If these EP and MCMC approaches can be adapted to dealing with case-control sampling, they may present an important opportunity. We note that recent research efforts in our group have been focused on this direction, and we are hopeful that a solution may be found.

One common critique of the mixed effects approach is that while many phenotypes are considered to be highly polygenic, it is not reasonable that all of the SNPs have identically distributed nonzero effects. Several methods try to address this issue by introducing an indicator variable for every SNP, indicating whether the SNP has a nonzero effect, and another parameter p which is the proportion of causal SNPs. Then, p can be jointly estimated with the other parameters of the model using MCMC-based methods (Golan and Rosset, 2011; Guan and Stephens, 2011). These models were recently extended to allow for a richer distribution of the effect sizes of SNPs, jointly modelling several scales of effect sizes (Moser *et al.*, 2015). These models are promising as they allow for a more realistic modelling of the genetic architecture and yield posterior probabilities of causality per SNP, as well as an overall estimate of the proportion of causal SNPs. While some efforts were made to modify these models to address some of the issues discussed here (Zhou *et al.*, 2013), we still view the problem of extending these approaches to account for case-control sampling in a way which is scalable for large GWAS as an open problem of great interest and potential importance.

27.7   Software reference list

GCTA A software package (Yang *et al.*, 2011) containing an implementation of BLUP for standard LMM and an implementation of the biased heritability estimation method of (Lee *et al.*, 2011), as well as many other useful functions for data handling (e.g., computing GRMs).
http://cnsgenomics.com/software/gcta/

PCGC Regression A memory-efficient implementation of the PCGC method (Golan *et al.*, 2014) implemented by Bhatia *et al.* (2015).
https://github.com/gauravbhatia1/PCGCRegression/

LTSOFT A software package implementing various liability-threshold related functions, including the computation of posterior liabilities of Hayeck *et al.* (2015).
http://www.hsph.harvard.edu/alkes-price/software/

LEAP Implementation of the MAP liability for case-control GWAS of Weissbrod *et al.* (2015).
https://github.com/omerwe/LEAP

GeRSI Prediction of case-control status using LMMs which takes the case-control sampling scheme into account (Golan and Rosset, 2014).
https://sites.google.com/site/davidgolanshomepage/software/gersi

GEMMA A software package which includes the Sparse Bayesian regression (BSLMM) models of Zhou *et al.* (2013).
http://www.xzlab.org/software.html

Bibliography

Abraham, G., Kowalczyk, A., Zobel, J., and Inouye, M. (2013). Performance and robustness of penalized and unpenalized methods for genetic prediction of complex human disease. *Genetic Epidemiology*, **37**, 184–195.

Anderson, J. A. (1972). Separate sample logistic discrimination. *Biometrika*, **59**, 19–35.

Bhatia, G., Gusev, A., Loh, P.-R., Vilhjálmsson, B. J., Ripke, S., Purcell, S., Stahl, E., Daly, M., de Candia, T. R., Kendler, K. S., *et al.* (2015). Haplotypes of common SNPs can explain missing heritability of complex diseases. *bioRxiv*, page doi: https://doi.org/10.1101/022418.

Breslow, N. E. and Clayton, D. G. (1993). Approximate inference in generalized linear mixed models. *Journal of the American Statistical Association*, **88**, 9–25.

Burton, P. R., Clayton, D. G., Cardon, L. R., Craddock, N., Deloukas, P., Duncanson, A., Kwiatkowski, D. P., McCarthy, M. I., Ouwehand, W. H., Samani, N. J., *et al.* (2007). Genome-wide association study of 14,000 cases of seven common diseases and 3,000 shared controls. *Nature*, **447**, 661–678.

Chatterjee, N. and Carroll, R. J. (2005). Semiparametric maximum likelihood estimation exploiting gene-environment independence in case-control studies. *Biometrika*, **92**, 399–418.

Clayton, D. (2012). Link functions in multi-locus genetic models: Implications for testing, prediction, and interpretation. *Genetic Epidemiology*, **36**, 409–418.

Crossett, A., Lee, A. B., Klei, L., Devlin, B., and Roeder, K. (2013). Refining genetically inferred relationships using treelet covariance smoothing. *The Annals of Applied Statistics*, **7**, 669–690.

Dempster, E. R. and Lerner, I. M. (1950). Heritability of threshold characters. *Genetics*, **35**, 212–236.

Devlin, B. and Roeder, K. (1999). Genomic control for association studies. *Biometrics*, **55**, 997–1004.

Frigola, R., Lindsten, F., Schön, T. B., and Rasmussen, C. (2013). Bayesian inference and learning in Gaussian process state-space models with particle MCMC. In C. Burges, L. Bottou, M. Welling, Z. Ghahramani, and K. Weinberger, editors, *Advances in Neural Information Processing Systems 26*, pages 3156–3164. Curran Associates, Inc.

Golan, D. and Rosset, S. (2011). Accurate estimation of heritability in genome wide studies using random effects models. *Bioinformatics*, **27**, i317–i323.

Golan, D. and Rosset, S. (2014). Effective genetic-risk prediction using mixed models. *The American Journal of Human Genetics*, **95**, 383–393.

Golan, D., Lander, E. S., and Rosset, S. (2014). Measuring missing heritability: Inferring the contribution of common variants. *Proceedings of the National Academy of Sciences*, **111**, E5272–E5281.

Guan, Y. and Stephens, M. (2011). Bayesian variable selection regression for genome-wide association studies and other large-scale problems. *The Annals of Applied Statistics*, **5**, 1780–1815.

Gusev, A., Lee, S. H., Trynka, G., Finucane, H., Vilhjálmsson, B. J., Xu, H., Zang, C., Ripke, S., Bulik-Sullivan, B., Stahl, E., *et al.* (2014). Partitioning heritability of regulatory and cell-type-specific variants across 11 common diseases. *The American Journal of Human Genetics*, **95**, 535–552.

Haseman, J. K. and Elston, R. C. (1972). The investigation of linkage between a quantitative trait and a marker locus. *Behavioral Genetics*, **2**, 3–19.

Hayeck, T. J., Zaitlen, N. A., Loh, P.-R., Vilhjalmsson, B., Pollack, S., Gusev, A., Yang, J., Che, G.-B., Goddard, M. E., Visscher, P. M., Patterson, N., and Price, A. L. (2015). Mixed model with correction for case-control ascertainment increases association power. *American Journal of Human Genetics*, **96**, 720–730.

Jiang, L., Liu, L., Cheng, Y., Lin, Y., Shen, C., Zhu, C., Yang, S., Yin, X., and Zhang, X. (2015). More heritability probably captured by psoriasis genome-wide association study in Han Chinese. *Gene*, **573**, 46–49.

Kang, H. M., Zaitlen, N. A., Wade, C. M., Kirby, A., Heckerman, D., Daly, M. J., and Eskin, E. (2008). Efficient control of population structure in model organism association mapping. *Genetics*, **178**, 1709–1723.

Kang, H. M., Sul, J. H., Service, S. K., Zaitlen, N. A., Kong, S.-y., Freimer, N. B., Sabatti, C., Eskin, E., *et al.* (2010). Variance component model to account for sample structure in genome-wide association studies. *Nature Genetics*, **42**, 348–354.

Lee, S. H., Wray, N. R., Goddard, M. E., and Visscher, P. M. (2011). Estimating missing heritability for disease from genome-wide association studies. *The American Journal of Human Genetics*, **88**, 294–305.

Lee, S. H., Harold, D., Nyholt, D. R., Goddard, M. E., Zondervan, K. T., Williams, J., Montgomery, G. W., Wray, N. R., and Visscher, P. M. (2013). Estimation and partitioning of polygenic variation captured by common SNPs for Alzheimer's disease, multiple sclerosis and endometriosis. *Human Molecular Genetics*, **22**, 832–841.

Lippert, C., Listgarten, J., Liu, Y., Kadie, C. M., Davidson, R. I., and Heckerman, D. (2011). Fast linear mixed models for genome-wide association studies. *Nature Methods*, **8**, 833–835.

Loh, P.-R., Bhatia, G., Gusev, A., Finucane, H. K., Bulik-Sullivan, B. K., Pollack, S. J., de Candia, T. R., Lee, S. H., Wray, N. R., Kendler, K. S., *et al.* (2015a). Contrasting genetic architectures of schizophrenia and other complex diseases using fast variance-components analysis. *Nature Genetics*, **47**, 1385–1392.

Loh, P.-R., Tucker, G., Bulik-Sullivan, B. K., Vilhjalmsson, B. J., Finucane, H. K., Salem, R. M., Chasman, D. I., Ridker, P. M., Neale, B. M., Berger, B., *et al.* (2015b). Efficient Bayesian mixed-model analysis increases association power in large cohorts. *Nature Genetics*, **47**, 284–290.

Maher, B. (2008). The case of the missing heritability. *Nature*, **456**, 18–21.

McCullagh, P. and Nelder, J. (1989). *Generalized Linear Models*. Chapman & Hall, London, 2nd edition.

Moser, G., Lee, S. H., Hayes, B. J., Goddard, M. E., Wray, N. R., and Visscher, P. M. (2015). Simultaneous discovery, estimation and prediction analysis of complex traits using a Bayesian mixture model. *PloS Genetics*, **11**, e1004969.

Mrode, R. A. (2014). *Linear Models for the Prediction of Animal Breeding Values*. Cabi, Wallingford, UK, 3rd edition.

Plomin, R., DeFries, J., and McClearn, G. (1990). *Behavior Genetics: A Primer*. WH Freeman and Company, New York.

Prentice, R. L. and Pyke, R. (1979). Logistic disease incidence models and case-control studies. *Biometrika*, **66**, 403–411.

Price, A. L., Patterson, N. J., Plenge, R. M., Weinblatt, M. E., Shadick, N. A., and Reich, D. (2006). Principal components analysis corrects for stratification in genome-wide association studies. *Nature Genetics*, **38**, 904–909.

Price, A. L., Helgason, A., Thorleifsson, G., McCarroll, S. A., Kong, A., and Stefansson, K. (2011). Single-tissue and cross-tissue heritability of gene expression via identity-by-descent in related or unrelated individuals. *PLoS Genetics*, **7**, e1001317.

Purcell, S. M., Wray, N. R., Stone, J. L., Visscher, P. M., O'Donovan, M. C., Sullivan, P. F., Sklar, P., Ruderfer, D. M., McQuillin, A., Morris, D. W., *et al.* (2009). Common polygenic variation contributes to risk of schizophrenia and bipolar disorder. *Nature*, **460**, 748–752.

Rasmussen, C. E. and Williams, C. K. I. (2005). *Gaussian Processes for Machine Learning*. The MIT Press, Cambridge, MA.

Scott, A. J. and Wild, C. J. (1997). Fitting regression models to case-control data by maximum likelihood. *Biometrika*, **84**, 57–71.

Scott, A. J. and Wild, C. J. (2001). Maximum likelihood for generalised case-control studies. *Journal of Statistical Planning and Inference*, **96**, 3–27.

Speed, D. and Balding, D. J. (2014). MultiBLUP: improved SNP-based prediction for complex traits. *Genome Research*, **24**, 1550–1557.

Speed, D., Hemani, G., Johnson, M. R., and Balding, D. J. (2012). Improved heritability estimation from genome-wide SNPs. *The American Journal of Human Genetics*, **91**, 1011–1021.

Weissbrod, O., Lippert, C., Geiger, D., and Heckerman, D. (2015). Accurate liability estimation improves power in ascertained case-control studies. *Nature Methods*, **12**, 332–334.

Wright, S. (1934). An analysis of variability in number of digits in an inbred strain of guinea pigs. *Genetics*, **19**, 506.

Yang, J., Benyamin, B., McEvoy, B. P., Gordon, S., Henders, A. K., Nyholt, D. R., Madden, P. A., Heath, A. C., Martin, N. G., Montgomery, G. W., *et al.* (2010). Common SNPs explain a large proportion of the heritability for human height. *Nature Genetics*, **42**, 565–569.

Yang, J., Lee, S. H., Goddard, M. E., and Visscher, P. M. (2011). GCTA: a tool for genome-wide complex trait analysis. *The American Journal of Human Genetics*, **88**, 76–82.

Yang, J., Lee, T., Kim, J., Cho, M.-C., Han, B.-G., Lee, J.-Y., Lee, H.-J., Cho, S., and Kim, H. (2013). Ubiquitous polygenicity of human complex traits: Genome-wide analysis of 49 traits in Koreans. *PLoS Genet*, **9**, e1003355.

Yang, J., Zaitlen, N. A., Goddard, M. E., Visscher, P. M., and Price, A. L. (2014). Advantages and pitfalls in the application of mixed-model association methods. *Nature Genetics*, **46**, 100–106.

Yu, J., Pressoir, G., Briggs, W., Bi, I., Yamasaki, M., Doebley, J., McMullen, M., Gaut, B., Nielsen, D., Holland, J., Kresovich, S., and Buckler, E. (2006). A unified mixed-model method for association mapping that accounts for multiple levels of relatedness. *Nature Genetics*, **38**, 203–208.

Zhou, X. and Stephens, M. (2012). Genome-wide efficient mixed-model analysis for association studies. *Nature Genetics*, **44**, 821–824.

Zhou, X., Carbonetto, P., and Stephens, M. (2013). Polygenic modeling with Bayesian sparse linear mixed models. *PLoS Genetics*, **9**, e1003264.

Zuk, O., Hechter, E., Sunyaev, S. R., and Lander, E. S. (2012). The mystery of missing heritability: Genetic interactions create phantom heritability. *Proceedings of the National Academy of Sciences*, **109**, 1193–1198.

28

Analysis of Secondary Phenotype Data under Case-Control Designs

Guoqing Diao

George Mason University

Donglin Zeng and Dan-Yu Lin

University of North Carolina at Chapel Hill

28.1 Introduction

Although the primary objective of case-control studies is to assess the effects of genetic variants between cases and controls, secondary phenotypes are often collected in such studies without much extra cost. For example, in the Diabetes Genetics Initiative (DGI) study, there were 1,464 patients with type 2 diabetes and 1,467 controls from Finland and Sweden, while at the same time, a variety of secondary phenotype traits were available for these patients, including anthropometric measures, glucose tolerance and insulin secretion, lips and apoliporoteins and blood pressure. These secondary phenotypes are typically the exposures/risk-factors of interest for the main outcome. In the Wellcome Trust Case Control Consortium (WTCCC), a case-control study consisting of 1,924 U.K. type-2 diabetes patients and 2,938 U.K. population controls, body mass index (BMI) and adult height were also measured as secondary traits in the study. With the availability of second phenotype information, it is cost-effective to study the association between genetic variants and these additional traits without need to conduct new studies. Indeed, the DGI study identified association of a particular single nucleotide polymorphism (SNP) in an intron of glucokinase regulatory protein with serum triglycerides in both case and control groups.

However, due to the biased sampling nature of a case-control design, analysis of secondary phenotype data can no longer proceed as standard regression without accounting for this design. Otherwise, spurious association may be detected. A simple example is that a SNP is not associated with the secondary trait but associated with case-control status; thus, when the secondary trait is correlated with case-control status, a naive regression without accounting for the biased sampling design may lead to a false association between the SNP and this trait (for instance, see Figure 2 in Lin and Zeng (2009)).

There have been a number of methods developed to analyze secondary phenotype data, under different models and assumptions. In this chapter, we will provide a selective review of these methods and discuss the pro and con of each method. We will provide a numerical example to illustrate these methods. Finally, we will discuss other future problems arising from this secondary phenotype analysis.

28.2　Methods for secondary phenotype analysis

We first introduce some necessary notation, which will be used throughout the chapter. Let D denote the primary trait, i.e., the disease status, which takes value 1 for cases and 0 for controls. Also, let Y denote the secondary phenotype, G the genotype at a SNP, and $\mathbf{Z}$ a vector of covariates. Under an additive genetic model, the genotype G is defined as the number of minor alleles at the locus, whereas under dominant or recessive models G takes value 0 or 1. Unless otherwise specified, we use $\mathbf{Y}$ to denote multivariate secondary phenotypes and Z a scalar covariate. Additionally, we define $\mathbf{X} \equiv (G, \mathbf{Z})$.

Suppose that there are n subjects in a case-control study. The data consist of $\{(D_i, Y_i, G_i, \mathbf{Z}_i), i = 1, ..., n\}$. The number of cases (controls) are

$$n_d = \sum_{i=1}^{n} I(D_i = d), \qquad d = 0, 1,$$

where $I(\cdot)$ is an indicator function.

The joint distribution of a randomly sampled observation $(D, Y, \mathbf{X})$ from the target population is

$$P(D, Y, \mathbf{X}) = P(D, Y|\mathbf{X})P(\mathbf{X}) = P(D|\mathbf{X}, Y)P(Y|\mathbf{X})P(\mathbf{X}).$$

In the secondary data analysis, our main interest concerns the effects of $\mathbf{X}$ on the secondary phenotype Y, that is, we focus on modelling $P(Y|\mathbf{X})$. Because the sampling is conditional on the case-control status, the retrospective likelihood for an observation $(D, Y, \mathbf{X})$ from a case-control sampled data is

$$P(Y, \mathbf{X}|D) = \frac{P(D, Y, \mathbf{X})}{P(D)} = \frac{P(D|\mathbf{X}, Y)P(Y|\mathbf{X})P(\mathbf{X})}{P(D)}.$$

Therefore, proper analysis of the secondary data involves model specifications of

a) disease prevalence in the population, i.e., $P(D = 1)$;

b) conditional disease rate given $(Y, \mathbf{X})$, i.e., $P(D = 1|Y, \mathbf{X})$;

c) distribution of $\mathbf{X}$ in the target population;

d) distribution of Y given $\mathbf{X}$, i.e., $P(Y|\mathbf{X})$.

Different methods in literature impose different conditions on the above model leading to different properties.

28.2.1 Case-only or control-only methods

Case-only and control-only methods are based on the prospective likelihood

$$\prod_{i=1}^{n} I(D_i = d)P(Y_i|\mathbf{X}_i),$$

for $d = 1$ and 0, respectively.

Lin and Zeng (2009) discussed the scenarios under which the cases-only or control-only methods are valid. In particular, when the secondary phenotype is independent of the disease status conditional on $\mathbf{X}$, i.e., $P(D|\mathbf{X}, Y) = P(D|\mathbf{X})$, these two methods including the methods based on the combined samples of cases and controls are valid because $P(D|\mathbf{X}), P(\mathbf{X})$ and $P(D)$ do not involve parameters in $P(Y|\mathbf{X})$ and therefore can be factored out of the retrospective likelihood. Under the rare disease assumption, Li *et al.* (2010) showed that the control-only method is still valid; however, standard methods that also use cases result in biased estimates and highly inflated type I error if there is an interaction between Y and $\mathbf{X}$ on the risk of the primary disease.

When the disease is rare, say less than 1%, methods based on cases only or controls only can be appropriate under a logistic regression model for the disease probability with only main effects of Y and $\mathbf{X}$,

$$P(D = 1|Y, \mathbf{X}) = \frac{\exp(\gamma_0 + \boldsymbol{\gamma}_1^T \mathbf{X} + \gamma_2 Y)}{1 + \exp(\gamma_0 + \boldsymbol{\gamma}_1^T \mathbf{X} + \gamma_2 Y)}.$$

Under the rare disease assumption, $P(D = 1|Y, \mathbf{X}) \approx \exp(\gamma_0 + \boldsymbol{\gamma}_1^T \mathbf{X} + \gamma_2 Y)$. In this scenario, standard methods based on cases only, controls only, and the combination of cases and controls are still valid. However, as pointed out by Li *et al.* (2010), it is not true when there is an interaction effect between secondary phenotype and covariates on the disease status. Additionally, even when they are valid, the case-only or control-only methods may have reduced power since only part of the data is used in the analysis.

28.2.2 Weighting methods

A number of authors, see, for instance, Richardson *et al.* (2007) and Monsees *et al.* (2009), proposed the weighted approach to account for the case-control sampling. In a typical case-control study, we oversample the cases. The rationale of the weighted approach is to give more weights to the controls and less weights to cases. Specifically, one can solve the following weighted estimating equations

$$\sum_{i=1}^{n} w_i \mathbf{S}_{Y|\mathbf{X}}(Y_i, \mathbf{X}_i; \boldsymbol{\beta}) = \mathbf{0},$$

where $\mathbf{S}_{Y|\mathbf{X}}(\cdot)$ is a set of functions satisfying

$$E\{\mathbf{S}_{Y|\mathbf{X}}(Y, \mathbf{X}; \boldsymbol{\beta})\} = \mathbf{0},$$

and w_i is the sampling weight for the ith observation to be described later. Note that the above expectation is evaluated at the true model of Y given $\mathbf{X}$ in the target population. In a likelihood approach, $\mathbf{S}_{Y|\mathbf{X}}(Y, \mathbf{X}; \boldsymbol{\beta})$ can be the score functions, i.e., the first derivatives of $\log P(Y|\mathbf{X}; \boldsymbol{\beta})$ with respect to the unknown parameters $\boldsymbol{\beta}$. For example, for a binary secondary outcome, we may consider a logistic regression model

$$P(Y = 1|\mathbf{X}) = \frac{\exp(\boldsymbol{\beta}^T \mathbf{X})}{1 + \exp(\boldsymbol{\beta}^T \mathbf{X})}.$$

In this case, the score function takes the form

$$\mathbf{S}_{Y|\mathbf{X}} = \left\{ Y - \frac{\exp(\boldsymbol{\beta}^T \mathbf{X})}{1 + \exp(\boldsymbol{\beta}^T \mathbf{X})} \right\} \mathbf{X}.$$

For a continuous secondary phenotype, we may derive the score function from ordinary least squares

$$\mathbf{S}_{Y|\mathbf{X}} = (Y - \boldsymbol{\beta}^T \mathbf{X})\mathbf{X}.$$

For multivariate secondary phenotypes, Schifano *et al.* (2013) considered

$$\mathbf{S}_{\mathbf{Y}|\mathbf{X}} = \mathbf{X}^T \mathbf{R}^{-1}(\mathbf{Y} - \boldsymbol{\beta}^T \mathbf{X}),$$

where $\mathbf{R}$ is a working correlation matrix accounting for the correlations among multiple phenotypes and is allowed to be misspecified.

We now turn our attention to the weights w_i, which are defined as

$$w_i = \begin{cases} n_1^{-1} P(D = 1), & \text{if } D_i = 1, \\ n_0^{-1} P(D = 0), & \text{if } D_i = 0. \end{cases}$$

That is, the weights are the inverse of the sampling probabilities in the case-control study. Such approaches are called the inverse probability weighting (IPW) approaches. The IPW approach requires that the disease prevalence is known. When disease is rare, w_i is close to 0 for cases and hence the IPW method reduces to the control-only method.

28.2.3   Likelihood-based methods

Lin and Zeng (2009), He *et al.* (2012), Ghosh *et al.* (2013), and Tchetgen Tchetgen (2014) proposed likelihood-based estimation and inference based on the retrospective likelihood conditional on the disease status. Specifically, the retrospective likelihood based on a total of n subjects $\{(D_i, Y_i, \mathbf{X}_i), i = 1, ..., n\}$ takes the form

$$\prod_{i=1}^{n} \left\{ \frac{P(D_i = 1|Y_i, \mathbf{X}_i)P(Y_i|\mathbf{X}_i)P(\mathbf{X}_i)}{P(D_i = 1)} \right\}^{D_i} \left\{ \frac{P(D_i = 0|Y_i, \mathbf{X}_i)P(Y_i|\mathbf{X}_i)P(\mathbf{X}_i)}{P(D_i = 0)} \right\}^{1-D_i},$$

(28.1)

where

$$P(D_i = 1) = \int_{y,\mathbf{x}} P(D_i = 1|y, \mathbf{x})P(y|\mathbf{x})P(\mathbf{x})dyd\mathbf{x},$$

$$P(D_i = 0) = 1 - P(D_i = 1),$$

and

$$P(D_i = 0|Y_i, \mathbf{X}_i) = 1 - P(D_i = 1|Y_i, \mathbf{X}_i).$$

Lin and Zeng (2009) assume 1) that

$$P(Y = 1|\mathbf{X}) = \frac{\exp(\beta_0 + \boldsymbol{\beta}_1^T \mathbf{X})}{1 + \exp(\beta_0 + \boldsymbol{\beta}_1^T \mathbf{X})}$$

for a binary secondary phenotype and

$$Y|\mathbf{X} \sim N(\beta_0 + \boldsymbol{\beta}_1^T \mathbf{X}, \sigma^2)$$

for a continuous binary secondary phenotype, and 2) that

$$P(D = 1|Y, \mathbf{X}) = \frac{\exp(\gamma_0 + \boldsymbol{\gamma}_1^T \mathbf{X} + \gamma_2 Y)}{1 + \exp(\gamma_0 + \boldsymbol{\gamma}_1^T \mathbf{X} + \gamma_2 Y)}.$$

The marginal distribution of $\mathbf{X}$, $P(\mathbf{X})$ is left unspecified. Let $\boldsymbol{\beta}$ denote the parameters in the model $P(Y|\mathbf{X})$. The unknown parameters are then $(\gamma_0, \boldsymbol{\gamma}_1, \gamma_2, \boldsymbol{\beta}, P(\mathbf{x}))$. Assume that the data matrix for $(1, \mathbf{X}, Y)$ is of full rank. Lin and Zeng (2009) showed that these unknown parameters are identifiable when the disease is rare or the disease prevalence is known. However, when the disease prevalence is unknown and disease is not rare, the unknown parameters are weakly identifiable. Particularly, the estimation of γ_0 may not be numerically stable. When disease is rare,

$$P(D = 1 \,|\, Y, \mathbf{X}) \approx \exp(\gamma_0 + \boldsymbol{\gamma}_1^T \mathbf{X} + \gamma_2 Y)$$

and

$$P(D = 0 \,|\, Y, \mathbf{X}) \approx 1.$$

Then the retrospective likelihood function (28.1) becomes

$$\prod_{i=1}^{n} \left\{ \frac{P(Y_i|\mathbf{X}_i) P(\mathbf{X}_i) \exp(\boldsymbol{\gamma}_1^T \mathbf{X}_i + \gamma_2 Y_i)}{\int_{y, \mathbf{x}} P(y|\mathbf{x}) P(\mathbf{x}) \exp(\boldsymbol{\gamma}_1^T \mathbf{x} + \gamma_2 y)} \right\}^{D_i} \{P(Y_i|\mathbf{X}_i) P(\mathbf{X}_i)\}^{1 - D_i}. \qquad (28.2)$$

The maximization of the above likelihood (28.2) is involved. Lin and Zeng (2009) proposed to estimate $P(\mathbf{x})$ nonparametrically. Specifically, one treats the point masses $p_i = P(\mathbf{X}_i)$ as the unknown parameters and maximize the above likelihood function subject to the constraint $\sum_{i=1}^{n} p_i = 1$. A profile likelihood approach was then proposed to profile out $p_i, i = 1, .., n$, to obtain the maximum likelihood estimators. When the disease prevalence is known, one maximizes

$$\prod_{i=1}^{n} P(Y_i|\mathbf{X}_i) p_i \frac{e^{D_i(\gamma_0 + \boldsymbol{\gamma}_1^T \mathbf{X}_i + \gamma_2 Y_i)}}{1 + e^{\gamma_0 + \boldsymbol{\gamma}_1^T \mathbf{X}_i + \gamma_2 Y_i}}$$

subject to the constraint $\sum_{i=1}^{n} p_i = 1$ and

$$\sum_{i=1}^{n} p_i \int_y P(y|\mathbf{X}_i) \frac{e^{\gamma_0 + \boldsymbol{\gamma}_1^T \mathbf{X}_i + \gamma_2 y}}{1 + e^{\gamma_0 + \boldsymbol{\gamma}_1^T \mathbf{X}_i + \gamma_2 y}} dy = \pi_0,$$

where π_0 is the known value of $P(D = 1)$. By using the Lagrange multipliers and the profile likelihood approach, one can estimate the unknown parameters. Similar techniques were also used in empirical likelihood literature; for instance, see Qin and Lawless (1994) and Owen (2001). The resulting maximum likelihood estimators can be shown to be consistent and asymptotically normal. Furthermore, the limiting covariance matrix of the MLEs of the finite dimensional parameters attain the semiparametric efficiency bound and can be consistently estimated by the inverse of the negative Hessian matrix of the profile log-likelihood function. A user-friendly software implementing this efficient semiparametric likelihood-based method is available at `http://dlin.web.unc.edu/software/spreg-2/`.

By specifying the models for $P(D|\mathbf{X})$ and $P(Y|\mathbf{X})$, a particular conditional joint distribution of (D, Y) given $\mathbf{X}$ is induced. To allow more general form of joint distribution of (D, Y) given $\mathbf{X}$, Ghosh *et al.* (2013) propose to model the conditional distributions of D and Y given $\mathbf{X}$ and then introduce a certain association or correlation between D and

Y given $\mathbf{X}$. For example, when Y is also binary, Ghosh *et al.* (2013) consider the following models

$$P(D = 1|\mathbf{X}) = \frac{e^{\alpha_1 + \boldsymbol{\beta}_1^T \mathbf{X}}}{1 + e^{\alpha_1 + \boldsymbol{\beta}_1^T \mathbf{X}}}$$

and

$$P(Y = 1|\mathbf{X}) = \frac{e^{\alpha_2 + \boldsymbol{\beta}_2^T \mathbf{X}}}{1 + e^{\alpha_2 + \boldsymbol{\beta}_2^T \mathbf{X}}} :$$

Then an additional model is introduced to account for the association by modeling the conditional odds ratio between D and Y.

$$\log OR(D, Y|\mathbf{X}) = \log \left\{ \frac{P(D = 1, Y = 1|\mathbf{X})P(D = 0, Y = 0|\mathbf{X})}{P(D = 1, Y = 0|\mathbf{X})P(D = 0, Y = 1|\mathbf{X})} \right\} = \alpha_3 + \boldsymbol{\beta}_3^T \mathbf{X}.$$

When the secondary outcome is continuous, a latent variable V is introduced such that (V, Y) follows a bivariate normal distribution conditional on $\mathbf{X}$. Another latent variable U is then introduced to produce the logistic marginal for the disease model. Since the genotype at a SNP of interest is discrete, Ghosh *et al.* (2013) further propose to model the distribution $P(G)$ and $P(\mathbf{Z})$ separately and assume that

$$P(G_i, \mathbf{Z}_i) = P(G_i)P(\mathbf{Z}_i),$$

that is, the genotype at the SNP is independent of the covariates. The distribution of $\mathbf{Z}_i$ is modelled nonparametrically as in Lin and Zeng (2009) such that $P(\mathbf{Z}_i) = p_i$. The same technique was used to derive the profile likelihood function of other finite dimensional parameters.

Finally, Li *et al.* (2010) considered the case of a binary secondary phenotype Y. A logistic regression model is assumed for $P(Y = 1|G)$:

$$P(Y = 1|G) = \frac{e^{\beta_0 + \beta_1 G}}{1 + e^{\beta_0 + \beta_1 G}}.$$

Another logistic regression model is assumed for $P(D = 1|Y, G)$ including both main effects of Y and G and their interaction effect

$$P(D = 1|Y, G) = \frac{e^{\gamma_0 + \gamma_1 G + \gamma_2 Y + \gamma_{12} GY}}{1 + e^{\gamma_0 + \gamma_1 G + \gamma_2 Y + \gamma_{12} GY}}. \tag{28.3}$$

Assuming rare disease,

$$P(D = 1|Y, G) \approx e^{\gamma_0 + \gamma_1 G + \gamma_2 Y + \gamma_{12} GY}.$$

The main interest focuses on the parameter β_1. Li *et al.* (2010) showed that under the saturated disease model (28.3) and the rare disease assumption, the MLE of β_1 from Lin and Zeng (2009) is in fact the control-only estimator $(\widehat{\beta}_{1CO})$ and does not use any information from cases. To improve efficiency, Li *et al.* (2010) propose to combine the case and control estimators by inverse variance weighting that leads to

$$\widehat{\beta}_{1W} = w_{cc}\widehat{\beta}_{1CO} + (1 - w_{cc})\widehat{\beta}_{1CA},$$

where $\widehat{\beta}_{1CA}$ is the case-only estimator, $w_{cc} = \widehat{\sigma}_{CA}^2/(\widehat{\sigma}_{CA}^2 + \widehat{\sigma}_{CO}^2)$, and $\widehat{\sigma}_{CA}^2$ and $\widehat{\sigma}_{CO}^2$ are the variance estimators of $\widehat{\beta}_{1CA}$ and $\widehat{\beta}_{1CO}$, respectively. The estimator $\widehat{\beta}_{1W}$, however, is consistent only when $\gamma_{12} = 0$. To retain the efficiency gain of $\widehat{\beta}_{1W}$ when there is no interaction effect between Y and G on the disease status while maintaining the robustness of the control-only estimator, Li *et al.* (2010) proposed an adaptively weighted estimator which combines $\widehat{\beta}_{1W}$ and $\widehat{\beta}_{1CO}$ based on the interaction estimate $\widehat{\gamma}_{12}$. The weight is based on the bias of the model-based estimator (i.e., under the assumption of $\gamma_{12} = 0$) and variance of the model-free estimator. This allows a bias-variance trade-off between a less efficient but more robust estimator (i.e., $\widehat{\beta}_{1CO}$) and potentially a more efficient but biased estimator (i.e., $\widehat{\beta}_{1W}$). Note that this approach can be easily extended to accommodate multinomial and continuous outcome variables. In a related work, Li and Gail (2012) extended the above method to the setting where the disease rate is known by adaptively combining the estimators under the saturated model (28.3) and a reduced model without the interaction term.

28.2.4 Copula modelling

Copulas are commonly used in statistical literature to formulate multivariate distribution (Nelsen, 2006). The basic idea is that one first specifies the marginal distribution for each variable. After certain transformation on each marginal variable, the transformed variable follows a uniform distribution in $[0, 1]$. A copula, which is a multivariate distribution on marginally uniform random variables, is then used to introduce dependence structure among the multivariate variables. One popular copula is the Gaussian copula, which is constructed from multivariate normal distributions. Gaussian copulas are particularly useful for handling mixed types of outcomes such as continuous, discrete, and count data, etc. (Song *et al.*, 2009).

Recall that the retrospective likelihood methods described in Section 28.2.3 involve modelling the conditional joint distribution of (D, Y) given covariates $\mathbf{X}$. He *et al.* (2012) proposed to use Gaussian copula in the analysis of secondary outcome data in case-control studies. In particular, the authors derived the conditional joint distribution of D and possibly correlated multivariate continuous secondary outcomes given the genotype G at a SNP by using a Gaussian copula model. The marginal distribution of each secondary outcome is assumed to be from the exponential family. Assuming a standard logistic regression model for $P(D = 1|G)$, one can then maximize the retrospective likelihood to obtain the MLEs of the unknown parameters. Numerical studies suggested that the Gaussian copula method performs well compared to the method of Lin and Zeng (2009) especially when the correlation between disease status and the secondary outcome is high. On the other hand, it is worth to note that no other covariates except the discretely coded genotype are included in the Gaussian copula model of He *et al.* (2012). Hence, the computation does not involve the estimation of an infinite dimensional parameter, that is, the marginal distribution of the covariates.

In a related work, Zhang *et al.* (2013) proposed a copula model for testing the interaction effect between two risk factors on the disease rate under the case-control design. The two risk factors are allowed to be continuous or discrete. Furthermore, unlike the copula model in He *et al.* (2012), the marginal distributions of the two variables are completely unspecified and are estimated nonparametrically. This flexible and robust approach can be useful in detecting gene by environment interaction in genetic case-control studies.

28.2.5 Semiparametric regression models for secondary phenotype

The likelihood-based methods described in Section 28.2.3 typically assume a parametric model for $P(Y|\mathbf{X})$. For example, for a continuous secondary phenotype, it is common to assume that Y (possibly after a known transformation) given $\mathbf{X}$ follows a normal distribution. The maximum likelihood estimators under the correctly specified models are most efficient among all estimators under the same model. However, such parametric model assumptions can be violated in practice and hence lead to biased results.

Wei *et al.* (2013) proposed a robust regression estimation of Y given $\mathbf{X}$. Specifically, the authors consider a homoscedastic regression model

$$Y = \alpha_{true} + \mu(\mathbf{X}, \boldsymbol{\beta}_{true}) + \epsilon,$$

where α_{true} is an intercept, $\mu(\cdot)$ is a known function, and the residual error ϵ has mean 0 and is independent of $\mathbf{X}$, but the distribution of ϵ is unspecified. To estimate the parameter of interest $\boldsymbol{\beta}_{true}$, the authors derive the score function by differentiating $\{Y - \alpha - \mu(\mathbf{X}, \boldsymbol{\beta})\}^2$ with respect to $\boldsymbol{\beta}$ yielding

$$S\{R(\boldsymbol{\beta}), \mathbf{X}, \alpha, \boldsymbol{\beta}\} = \mu_\beta(\mathbf{X}, \boldsymbol{\beta})\{R(\boldsymbol{\beta}) - \alpha\}, \tag{28.4}$$

where $R(\boldsymbol{\beta}) = Y - \mu(\mathbf{X}, \boldsymbol{\beta})$ and μ_β is the first derivative of $\mu(\mathbf{X}, \boldsymbol{\beta})$ with respect to $\boldsymbol{\beta}$. In a case-control sampling scheme, the above score does not have mean 0. The authors cleverly proposed an adjustment of the score function such that it has mean 0 in general. The basic idea is to first estimate the distribution of $R(\boldsymbol{\beta})$ at fixed values of $\boldsymbol{\beta}$ and other parameters $\boldsymbol{\Omega}$ involved in the disease status model $P(D|Y, \mathbf{X})$. Denote the estimated distribution of $R(\boldsymbol{\beta})$ by $p_{est}\{R(\boldsymbol{\beta}), \boldsymbol{\Omega}\}$. Then α_{true} can be estimated by

$$\widetilde{\alpha}(\boldsymbol{\beta}, \boldsymbol{\Omega}) = \frac{n^{-1} \sum_{i=1}^{n} R_i(\boldsymbol{\beta}) p_{est}\{R_i(\boldsymbol{\beta}), \boldsymbol{\Omega}\}}{n^{-1} \sum_{i=1}^{n} p_{est}\{R_i(\boldsymbol{\beta}), \boldsymbol{\Omega}\}}.$$

Replacing α with $\widetilde{\alpha}$ in the score function (28.4), one obtains the adjusted score function. Provided $\widehat{\boldsymbol{\Omega}}$, a consistent estimator of $\boldsymbol{\Omega}$, one can then solve the adjusted score equation to estimate $\boldsymbol{\beta}_{true}$ and hence α_{true}. Assuming a rare disease or that the disease rate is known, one can estimate $\boldsymbol{\Omega}$ by fitting a standard logistic regression model on $P(D|Y, \mathbf{X})$. The estimator of $\boldsymbol{\beta}_{true}$ was shown to be consistent and asymptotically normal. The analytic expression of the limiting covariance matrix of the estimator, however, is difficult to implement. The authors then propose to use a bootstrapping method to estimate the covariance matrix, which can considerably increase the computation burden.

In a related work, Gazioglu *et al.* (2013) consider the nonparametric regression model

$$Y = g(Z) + \epsilon,$$

where Z is a continuous scalar covariate, $g(\cdot)$ is a completely unspecified function, and ϵ has mean 0 and is independent of Z, but its distribution is otherwise unspecified. The authors proposed to use penalized regression splines (Ruppert *et al.*, 2003) and approximate $g(z)$ by $\alpha + \mathbf{B}^T(x)\boldsymbol{\beta}$, where $\mathbf{B}(x) = \{b_1(x), ..., b_P(x)\}^T$ is a series of basis functions. One then estimates $\boldsymbol{\beta}$ by minimizing

$$\sum_{i=1}^{n} \{Y_i - \alpha - \mathbf{B}^T(Z_i)\boldsymbol{\beta}\}^2 + \lambda \boldsymbol{\beta}^T \Delta \boldsymbol{\beta},$$

where Δ is a penalty matrix and λ is a penalty or smoothing parameter. Under the case-control sampling scheme, ideas similar to those in Wei *et al.* (2013) were used to estimate α for fixed values of $\boldsymbol{\beta}$ and $\boldsymbol{\Omega}$. The estimator of $\boldsymbol{\beta}$ and α can then be calculated by solving the adjusted score equations. This approach also requires that the disease is rare or the disease rate is known. More recently, Rahman (2015) considered the same setting as in Gazioglu *et al.* (2013) and proposed a titled kernel estimator for $g(\cdot)$.

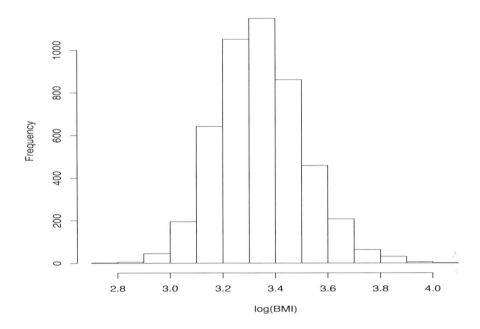

FIGURE 28.1
Histogram of log(BMI) for the FUSION study.

28.3   Numerical illustration

For illustration, we apply the likelihood-based method by Lin and Zeng (2009) and the IPW method to the Finland-United States Investigation of NIDDM Genetics (FUSION) study (Zeggini *et al.*, 2008). The goal of the FUSION study is to map and identify genetic variants that influence the risk of type 2 diabetes mellitus (T2D) or impact diabetes-related quantitative traits. For comparison, we also performed the case-only and control-only analyses and a simple analysis including both cases and controls and adjust for disease status in the model.

The data set consist of 4,792 subjects, among which 2,365 are cases and the other 2,427 are controls. The secondary phenotype of interest we consider here is body mass index (BMI). To approximate normality, we apply the log-transformation on the raw data (see Figure 28.1 for the histogram of log-transformed BMI data). In the case group, log(BMI) was observed in 2,290 subjects (mean = 3.406, sd = 0.162); and in the control group, 2,425 subjects had observed log(BMI) values (mean = 3.286, sd = 0.140). We include two environmental covariates in the model, age and gender. For each subject, genotypes at 224 SNPs on chromosome 6 were available. For the analysis, we consider the following additive genetic model for the secondary phenotype

$$\log(BMI) = \beta_{0j} + \beta_{1j} \times Age + \beta_{2j} \times Gender + \beta_{3j}SNP_j + \epsilon_j, \quad j = 1, ..., 224,$$

where ϵ_j is assumed to be normal. Per American Diabetes Association, the disease prevalence

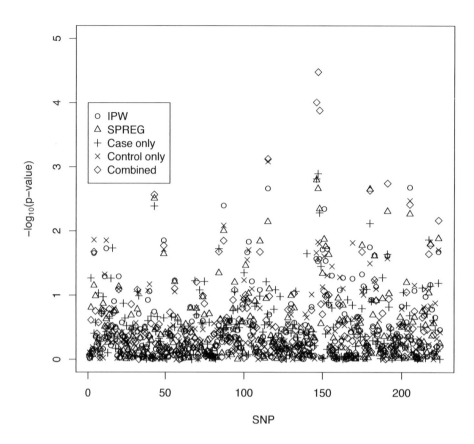

FIGURE 28.2
Results of testing the additive genetic effects on log(BMI) for the FUSION study.

was approximately 0.096 in 2005 and similar rates were observed in Finland. Therefore, we set the disease prevalence as 0.096 in the analysis. To apply the likelihood-based method of Lin and Zeng (2009), we use the software SPREG (http://dlin.web.unc.edu/software/spreg-2/). The command to run SPREG on a Linux platform is ./spreg fusion.dat fusion.out 0.096 2, where fusion.dat is the data file, fusion.out is the output file, 0.096 is the disease rate, and 2 is the number of environmental variables.

We use the Wald test statistics for all five methods to test the additive genetic effect on log(BMI) at each of the 224 SNPs. Figure 28.2 displays the plot of $-\log_{10}(p\text{-value})$ for both methods. As discussed in previous sections, the IPW method may not be efficient when disease rate is small. Therefore as expected, the likelihood-based method detected more SNPs with significant effects on log(BMI) at $\alpha = 0.005$. The likelihood-based method also detected more SNPs with significant effects than the case-only and control-only methods. These results are consistent with the simulation results presented in Lin and Zeng (2009). It is interesting that the combined method detected more SNPs with significant effects; however, as shown in Lin and Zeng (2009), the combined method tends to have inflated type I errors. Therefore, caution needs to be taken when interpreting results from the combined method. Table 28.1 presents the estimates of the genetic effects at the SNPs detected by the likelihood-based method at $\alpha = 0.005$. The standard error estimates using the IPW method, case-only and control-only methods are consistently larger than those using the likelihood-based method.

TABLE 28.1
Estimates of additive genetic effects at selected SNPs for the FUSION study. (Estimates and standard errors are multiplied by 100.)

SNP	IPW			SPREG			Case only			Control only			Combined		
	Est	SE	p-value	Est	SE	p-value	Est	SE	p-value	Est	SE	p-value	Est	SE	p-value
43	-0.739	0.551	0.180	-1.381	0.467	0.003	-2.008	0.699	0.004	-0.572	0.591	0.334	-1.377	0.459	0.003
146	-1.011	0.456	0.027	-1.197	0.379	0.002	-1.726	0.544	0.002	-1.155	0.503	0.022	-1.455	0.373	9.8e-5
147	-1.056	0.484	0.029	-1.212	0.395	0.002	-1.798	0.557	0.001	-1.307	0.535	0.015	-1.618	0.389	3.3e-5
148	-1.097	0.496	0.027	-1.170	0.412	0.004	-1.626	0.581	0.005	-1.350	0.558	0.016	-1.553	0.406	1.3e-4
180	-0.893	0.376	0.018	-0.978	0.320	0.002	-1.265	0.473	0.008	-0.880	0.409	0.032	-0.958	0.314	0.002
191	-0.989	0.439	0.024	-1.040	0.370	0.005	-1.259	0.553	0.023	-1.043	0.469	0.026	-1.136	0.364	0.002

28.4 Discussion

In this chapter, we provide a selective review of recent development on the analysis of secondary phenotype data under case-control studies. Due to limit of space, we are unable to provide detailed review of many other important works in the field,; to name a few, for example, Wang and Shete (2011), Wang and Shete (2012), Liu and Leal (2012), Tchetgen Tchetgen (2014), Chen *et al.* (2013), Wei *et al.* (2013), Song *et al.* (2016), and Ma and Carroll (2016).

Although there is a rich literature on the analysis of univariate secondary phenotype data under case-control designs, methods for multivariate secondary phenotype data are limited. Schifano *et al.* (2013) proposed to use the IPW method based on generalized estimating equations. However, IPW methods may not be efficient especially when disease is rare. He *et al.* (2012) proposed to use Gaussian copulas which can handle a mixed type of secondary outcome data. The performance may rely on the parametric assumption on the marginal distribution of each variable. Additionally, it is not clear how well the method will perform when covariates other than the genotype at a SNP are present. A future research would be along the direction of developing flexible and efficient methods for the analysis of multivariate secondary outcome data in case-control studies.

Acknowledgment

The authors thank Dr. Nilanjan Chatterjee for his helpful comments that have greatly improved this chapter.

Bibliography

Chen, H. Y., Kittles, R., and Zhang, W. (2013). Bias correction to secondary trait analysis with case-control design. *Statistics in Medicine*, **32**, 1494–1508.

Gazioglu, S., Wei, J., Jennings, E. M., and Carroll, R. J. (2013). A note on penalized regression spline estimation in the secondary analysis of case-control data. *Statistics in Biosciences*, **5**, 250–260.

Ghosh, A., Wright, F. A., and Zou, F. (2013). Unified analysis of secondary traits in case-control association studies. *Journal of the American Statistical Association*, **108**, 566–576.

He, J., Li, H., Edmondson, A. C., Rader, D. J., and Li, M. (2012). A Gaussian copula approach for the analysis of secondary phenotypes in case-control genetic association studies. *Biostatistics*, **13**, 497–508.

Li, H. and Gail, M. H. (2012). Efficient adaptively weighted analysis of secondary phenotypes in case-control genome-wide association studies. *Human Heredity*, **73**, 159–173.

Li, H., Gail, M. H., Berndt, S., and Chatterjee, N. (2010). Using cases to strengthen inference on the association between single nucleotide polymorphisms and a secondary phenotype in genome-wide association studies. *Genetic Epidemiology*, **34**, 427–433.

Lin, D. and Zeng, D. (2009). Proper analysis of secondary phenotype data in case-control association studies. *Genetic Epidemiology*, **33**, 256–265.

Liu, D. J. and Leal, S. M. (2012). A flexible likelihood framework for detecting associations with secondary phenotypes in genetic studies using selected samples: Application to sequence data. *European Journal of Human Genetics*, **20**, 449–456.

Ma, Y. and Carroll, R. J. (2016). Semiparametric estimation in the secondary analysis of case-control studies. *Journal of the Royal Statistical Society: Series B (Statistical Methodology)*, **78**, 127–151.

Monsees, G. M., Tamimi, R. M., and Kraft, P. (2009). Genome-wide association scans for secondary traits using case-control samples. *Genetic Epidemiology*, **33**, 717–728.

Nelsen, R. B. (2006). *An Introduction to Copulas*. Springer, New York, 2nd edition.

Owen, A. B. (2001). *Empirical Likelihood*. Chapman & Hall/CRC, Boca Raton.

Qin, J. and Lawless, J. (1994). Empirical likelihood and general estimating equations. *The Annals of Statistics*, **22**, 300–325.

Rahman, S. (2015). A tilted kernel estimator for nonparametric regression in the secondary analysis of case-control studies. *Statistics in Biosciences*, **7**, 322–347.

Richardson, D. B., Rzehak, P., Klenk, J., and Weiland, S. K. (2007). Analyses of case-control data for additional outcomes. *Epidemiology*, **18**, 441–445.

Ruppert, D., Wand, M. P., and Carroll, R. J. (2003). *Semiparametric Regression*. Cambridge University Press, Cambridge.

Schifano, E. D., Li, L., Christiani, D. C., and Lin, X. (2013). Genome-wide association analysis for multiple continuous secondary phenotypes. *The American Journal of Human Genetics*, **92**, 744–759.

Song, P. X.-K., Li, M., and Yuan, Y. (2009). Joint regression analysis of correlated data using Gaussian copulas. *Biometrics*, **65**, 60–68.

Song, X., Ionita-Laza, I., Liu, M., Reibman, J., and We, Y. (2016). A general and robust framework for secondary traits analysis. *Genetics*, **202**, 1329–1343.

Tchetgen Tchetgen, E. J. (2014). A general regression framework for a secondary outcome in case-control studies. *Biostatistics*, **15**, 117–128.

Wang, J. and Shete, S. (2011). Estimation of odds ratios of genetic variants for the secondary phenotypes associated with primary diseases. *Genetic Epidemiology*, **35**, 190–200.

Wang, J. and Shete, S. (2012). Analysis of secondary phenotype involving the interactive effect of the secondary phenotype and genetic variants on the primary disease. *Annals of Human Genetics*, **76**, 484–499.

Wei, J., Carroll, R. J., Müller, U. U., Keilegom, I. V., and Chatterjee, N. (2013). Robust estimation for homoscedastic regression in the secondary analysis of case-control data. *Journal of the Royal Statistical Society: Series B (Statistical Methodology)*, **75**, 185–206.

Zeggini, E., Scott, L. J., Saxena, R., Voight, B. F., Marchini, J. L., Hu, T., de Bakker, P. I., Abecasis, G. R., Almgren, P., Andersen, G., *et al.* (2008). Meta-analysis of genome-wide association data and large-scale replication identifies additional susceptibility loci for type 2 diabetes. *Nature Genetics*, **40**, 638–645.

Zhang, H., Qin, J., Landi, M., Caporaso, N., and Yu, K. (2013). A copula-model based on semiparametric interaction test under the case-control design. *Statistica Sinica*, **23**, 1505–1521.

Index